Neurophysiology: Brain-Stem Function and Control

Neurophysiology: Brain-Stem Function and Control

Editor: Rosalyn Pryor

AMERICAN
MEDICAL PUBLISHERS
www.americanmedicalpublishers.com

AMERICAN
MEDICAL PUBLISHERS
www.americanmedicalpublishers.com

Cataloging-in-Publication Data

Neurophysiology : brain-stem function and control / edited by Rosalyn Pryor.
p. cm.
Includes bibliographical references and index.
ISBN 979-8-88740-317-5
1. Neurophysiology. 2. Brain stem--Anatomy. 3. Brain stem--Diseases--Prevention.
4. Neurobiology. 5. Neuroanatomy. I. Pryor, Rosalyn.
QP355.2 .N483 2023
612.8--dc23

American Medical Publishers,
41 Flatbush Avenue,
1st Floor, New York,
NY 11217, USA

ISBN 979-8-88740-317-5 (Hardback)

Contents

Preface VII

Chapter 1 **TASK1 and TASK3 are Coexpressed with ASIC1 in the Ventrolateral Medulla and Contribute to Central Chemoreception in Rats** 1
Xia Wang, Ruijuan Guan, Xiaomei Zhao, Danian Zhu, Nana Song and Linlin Shen

Chapter 2 **Activation of Brainstem Neurons During Mesencephalic Locomotor Region-Evoked Locomotion in the Cat** 11
Ioan Opris, Xiaohong Dai, Dawn M. G. Johnson, Francisco J. Sanchez, Luz M. Villamil, Songtao Xie, Cecelia R. Lee-Hauser, Stephano Chang, Larry M. Jordan and Brian R. Noga

Chapter 3 **Effect of Different Movement Speed Modes on Human Action Observation: An EEG Study** 36
Tian-jian Luo, Jitu Lv, Fei Chao and Changle Zhou

Chapter 4 **The Role of Long Noncoding RNAs in Central Nervous System and Neurodegenerative Diseases** 51
Chang-Wei Wei, Ting Luo, Shan-Shan Zou and An-Shi Wu

Chapter 5 **Non-Invasive High Frequency Median Nerve Stimulation Effectively Suppresses Olfactory Intensity Perception in Healthy Males** 62
Ashim Maharjan, Mei Peng and Yusuf O. Cakmak

Chapter 6 **Post-Stroke Hemiplegic Gait: New Perspective and Insights** 76
Sheng Li, Gerard E. Francisco and Ping Zhou

Chapter 7 **Altered Neuromodulatory Drive may Contribute to Exaggerated Tonic Vibration Reflexes in Chronic Hemiparetic Stroke** 84
Jacob G. McPherson, Laura M. McPherson, Christopher K. Thompson, Michael D. Ellis, Charles J. Heckman and Julius P. A. Dewald

Chapter 8 **Differential Dopamine D1 and D3 Receptor Modulation and Expression in the Spinal Cord of Two Mouse Models of Restless Legs Syndrome** 99
Samantha Meneely, Mai-Lynne Dinkins, Miki Kassai, Shangru Lyu, Yuning Liu, Chien-Te Lin, Kori Brewer, Yuqing Li and Stefan Clemens

Chapter 9 **Electroacupuncture Inhibits Visceral Nociception via Somatovisceral Interaction at Subnucleus Reticularis Dorsalis Neurons in the Rat Medulla** 113
Lingling Yu, Liang Li, Qingguang Qin, Yutian Yu, Xiang Cui, Peijing Rong and Bing Zhu

Chapter 10 **Adjustment of Synchronization Stability of Dynamic Brain-Networks Based on Feature Fusion** 122
Haifang Li, Rong Yao, Xiaoluan Xia, Guimei Yin, Hongxia Deng and Pengfei Yang

Chapter 11 **Age-Related Changes in Neuromodulatory Control of Bladder Micturition Contractions Originating in the Skin** 137
Harumi Hotta, Harue Suzuki, Kaori Iimura and Nobuhiro Watanabe

Chapter 12 **Upregulation of AT_1 Receptor Mediates a Pressor Effect Through ROS-SAPK/JNK Signaling in Glutamatergic Neurons of Rostral Ventrolateral Medulla in Rats with Stress-Induced Hypertension** 148
Liping Jiang, Xuan Zhou, Hongyu Yang, Ruijuan Guan, Yanlei Xin, Jijiang Wang, Linlin Shen, Danian Zhu, Shulan Ma and Jin Wang

Chapter 13 **Parameters of Surface Electromyogram Suggest that Dry Immersion Relieves Motor Symptoms in Patients with Parkinsonism** 159
German G. Miroshnichenko, Alexander Yu Meigal, Irina V. Saenko, Liudmila I. Gerasimova-Meigal, Liudmila A. Chernikova, Natalia S. Subbotina, Saara M. Rissanen and Pasi A. Karjalainen

Chapter 14 **Reticulospinal Systems for Tuning Motor Commands** 176
Robert M. Brownstone and Jeremy W. Chopek

Chapter 15 **Optogenetic Activation of A11 Region Increases Motor Activity** 186
Kathrin Koblinger, Céline Jean-Xavier, Sandeep Sharma, Tamás Füzesi, Leanne Young, Shane E. A. Eaton, Charlie Hong Ting Kwok, Jaideep Singh Bains and Patrick J. Whelan

Chapter 16 **Monoaminergic Neuromodulation of Sensory Processing** 201
Simon N. Jacob and Hendrikje Nienborg

Chapter 17 **Effective Stimulation Type and Waveform for Force Control of the Motor Unit System: Implications for Intraspinal Microstimulation** 218
Hojeong Kim and Youngchang Ju

Permissions

List of Contributors

Index

Preface

The area of medicine which focuses on the diagnosis and monitoring of neurological diseases through the measurement and evaluation of nervous system function is known as neurophysiology. Brainstem is an important part of the nervous system which connects the brain to the spinal cord. There are majorly three parts of the brainstem, which includes the medulla oblongata, the midbrain and the pons, and sometimes the diencephalon. The brainstem plays a crucial role in conduction. This involves relaying the information from the body to the cerebellum and cerebrum, which pass through the brainstem. It also has integrative functions which plays an integral role in respiratory control, alertness, pain sensitivity control, cardiovascular system control, consciousness and awareness. This book is a compilation of chapters that discuss the most vital concepts and emerging trends in the field of neurophysiology. It provides comprehensive insights into brain-stem function and control. This book will prove to be immensely beneficial to students and researchers in this field.

The information contained in this book is the result of intensive hard work done by researchers in this field. All due efforts have been made to make this book serve as a complete guiding source for students and researchers. The topics in this book have been comprehensively explained to help readers understand the growing trends in the field.

I would like to thank the entire group of writers who made sincere efforts in this book and my family who supported me in my efforts of working on this book. I take this opportunity to thank all those who have been a guiding force throughout my life.

Editor

1

TASK1 and TASK3 are Coexpressed with ASIC1 in the Ventrolateral Medulla and Contribute to Central Chemoreception in Rats

Xia Wang[1†], Ruijuan Guan[1†], Xiaomei Zhao[1], Danian Zhu[1], Nana Song[2] and Linlin Shen[1,3*]*

[1]Department of Physiology and Pathophysiology, School of Basic Medical Sciences, Fudan University, Shanghai, China, [2]Division of Nephrology, Zhongshan Hospital, Fudan University, Shanghai, China, [3]Shanghai Key Laboratory of Medical Imaging Computing and Computer-Assisted Intervention, Fudan University, Shanghai, China

***Correspondence:**
Nana Song
song.nana@zs-hospital.sh.cn
Linlin Shen
llshen@shmu.edu.cn

†These authors have contributed equally to this work

The ventrolateral medulla (VLM), including the lateral paragigantocellular nucleus (LPGi) and rostral VLM (RVLM), is commonly considered to be a chemosensitive region. However, the specific mechanism of chemoreception in the VLM remains elusive. Acid-sensing ion channels (ASICs), a family of voltage-independent proton-gated cation channels, can be activated by an external pH decrease to cause Na^+ entry and induce neuronal excitability. TWIK-related acid-sensitive potassium channels (TASKs) are members of another group of pH-sensitive channels; in contrast to AISICs, they can be stimulated by pH increases and are inhibited by pH decreases in the physiological range. Our previous study demonstrated that ASICs take part in chemoreception. The aims of this study are to explore whether TASKs participate in the acid sensitivity of neurons in the VLM, thereby cooperating with ASICs. Our research demonstrated that TASKs, including TASK1 and TASK3, are colocalized with ASIC1 in VLM neurons. Blocking TASKs by microinjection of the non-selective TASK antagonist bupivacaine (BUP), specific TASK1 antagonist anandamide (AEA) or specific TASK3 antagonist ruthenium red (RR) into the VLM increased the integrated phrenic nerve discharge (iPND), shortened the inspiratory time (Ti) and enhanced the respiratory drive (iPND/Ti). In addition, microinjection of artificial cerebrospinal fluid (ACSF) at a pH of 7.0 or 6.5 prolonged Ti, increased iPND and enhanced respiratory drive, which were inhibited by the ASIC antagonist amiloride (AMI). By contrast, microinjection of alkaline ACSF decreased iPND and respiratory drive, which were inhibited by AEA. Taken together, our data suggest that TASK1 and TASK3 are coexpressed with ASIC1 in the VLM. Moreover, TASK1 and TASK3 contribute to the central regulation of breathing by coordinating with each other to perceive local pH changes; these results indicate a novel chemosensitive mechanism of the VLM.

Keywords: TASK1, TASK3, ventrolateral medulla, pH-sensitive, chemoreception

INTRODUCTION

Central chemoreceptors sense changes of H^+ concentration ($[H^+]$) in cerebrospinal fluid (CSF), play an important role in respiratory regulation and contribute to acid-base homeostasis. It is generally considered that chemoreceptors in the central nervous system (CNS) mainly detect CO_2, while carotid bodies (peripheral chemoreceptors) detect PCO_2 in the blood (Goridis and Brunet, 2010). CO_2 can be dissolved in CSF and penetrates membranes readily to generate H_2CO_3, which decomposes to H^+ and HCO_3^-. Therefore, the physiological stimulation of the central chemoreceptor is H^+ in the CSF and local extracellular fluid. It has been reported that chemoreceptors exist in many brain areas including raphe, retrotrapezoid nucleus (RTN), ventrolateral medulla (VLM), locus coeruleus (LC) and the nucleus of tractus solitaries (NTS). Among these chemosensitive areas, VLM is considered to specialize in central chemoreception (Millhorn and Eldridge, 1986). However, the mechanism of chemoreception by VLM neurons remains elusive. pH-sensitive ion channels, including acid-sensing ion channels (ASICs) and TWIK-related acid-sensitive potassium channels (TASKs), establish a new paradigm to study the chemosensory mechanism of the CNS. Molecular analysis has shown that ASICs contribute to the capacity of afferent neurons to monitor acidosis (Holzer, 2009). Our previous study also found that ASIC1 in the VLM contributes to chemoreception and the regulation of respiration (Song et al., 2016). However, it is unclear whether TASKs participate in central chemoreception.

TASKs are characterized by "leak" K^+ currents and play key roles in maintaining the rest membrane potential by adjusting the action potential duration and modulating the response to synaptic inputs (Honoré, 2007). TASKs are also pH-sensitive, which can be by inhibited by acidification and activated by alkalization. Among the three TASK subunits, TASK1 and TASK3 are widely expressed throughout the brain, including in the VLM and raphe nuclei (Washburn et al., 2002, 2003). These subunits are sensitive to extracellular protons with different sensitivities and contribute to the regulation of neuronal excitability (Bayliss et al., 2015). The pK value of TASK1 ranges from pH 7.3 to 7.5, and that of TASK3 ranges from pH 6.5 to 6.7 (Duprat et al., 2007). Their pH sensitivities are used to differentiate TASK1 from TASK3 (Hartness et al., 2001; Czirják and Enyedi, 2002; Washburn et al., 2003). TASKs in serotonergic raphe neurons exert pH and anesthetic sensitivity *in vitro* (Washburn et al., 2002). Inhibition of the TASKs by extracellular acidosis leads to an increased excitability of brainstem respiratory neurons (Duprat et al., 2007). Extracellular alkalization decreases the excitability of neurons expressing TASKs (Berg et al., 2004). In addition, they play a major functional role in the respiratory rhythm generation of the pre-Bötzinger complex (Koizumi et al., 2010). TASK1 and TASK3 appear to serve specific and distinct roles in chemoreception and respiratory control (Buehler et al., 2017).

It seems that both TASKs and ASICs are involved in the pH sensitivity of chemosensitive neurons in the CNS. However, the colocalization of TASKs and ASICs in chemosensitive neurons has not been addressed, and little is known about the cooperation of these two types of channels in respiratory regulation. In the current study, we hypothesized that TASKs and ASIC1 are coexpressed in the VLM and cooperate in the central control of respiration. In our present study, we found both ASIC1 and TASKs (1 and 3) expressed in the VLM of rats. We then investigated the role of ASIC1 and TASKs (1 and 3) in chemoreception. Our data showed that ASIC1 and TASKs (1 and 3) were colocalized in VLM neurons. The microinjection of different TASKs blockers, including a non-selective antagonist bupivacaine (BUP), a specific TASK1 antagonist anandamide (AEA) and a specific TASK3 antagonist ruthenium red (RR), into the VLM facilitated phrenic nerve discharge (PND). In addition, the microinjection of artificial CSF (ACSF) at a pH of 7.0 or 6.5 increased integrated PND (iPND), Inspiratory time (Ti) and respiratory drive, which were inhibited by the ASIC antagonist, amiloride (AMI). Contrarily, the microinjection of alkaline ACSF decreased iPND and respiratory drive, and this effect was attenuated by AEA. Our research indicated that TASKs and ASICs contribute to the central regulation of breathing by coordinating with each other to cause the perception of local pH changes. This investigation will help to establish a new understanding of the pH-sensing mechanism of chemosensitive neurons in the VLM.

MATERIALS AND METHODS

Animals

Male Sprague–Dawley rats (250–350 g, aged 3–4 months) were obtained from Shanghai Jiesijie Experimental Animal Co. Ltd. (Shanghai, China). All animals were kept in a room under a 12-h light-dark cycle, an ambient temperature of 22 ± 0.5°C and a relative humidity of 60 ± 2%. Food and water were given freely. The animal experiments were conducted in strict accordance with the US National Institutes of Health Guidelines for the Care and Use of Laboratory Animals and were approved by the Ethics Committee of Experimental Research, Shanghai Medical College, Fudan University. A total of 58 adult rats were used in this study. Maximal efforts were undertaken to minimize the number of animals and their suffering.

Drug Application

A nonselective ASIC inhibitor, AMI (Sigma Aldrich, St. Louis, MO, USA); a non-selective TASK antagonist, BUP (Sigma Aldrich, St. Louis, MO, USA); and a specific TASK3 antagonist, RR (Sigma Aldrich, St. Louis, MO, USA) were freshly prepared in ACSF immediately before administration. A specific TASK1 antagonist, AEA (Sigma Aldrich, St. Louis, MO, USA), was prepared in ethanol. The ACSF solutions were prepared at different pHs (8.0, 7.4, 7.0, 6.5, and 6.0). ACSF containing (mM) NaCl 130, $NaHCO_3$ 26, KCl 5, $CaCl_2$ 2.6, $MgSO_4$ 1.2, NaH_2PO_4 1.6, glucose 11 and sucrose 10 at pH 7.4 and ethanol served as the vehicle and volume controls.

Immunohistochemistry

Adult Sprague-Dawley rats were anesthetized with urethane (1 $g.kg^{-1}$) and perfused through the left ventricle with normal saline followed by 4% paraformaldehyde. After perfusion, the medullary was dissected, transferred to graded sucrose solutions (20% and 30%) until sinking and were cut into coronal sections at 25-μm thickness using a Leica freezing microtome. The slides were washed with 0.01 M PBS and blocked in 1% BSA for 1 h at room temperature. After blocking, the slides were incubated with a primary antibody against TASK1 or TASK3 (Alomone Laboratory, Israel, 1:100) diluted in 0.01 M PBS, and the controls were incubated with 0.01 M PBS without primary antibody overnight. The reaction was then detected using a Boshide avidin-biotin-HRP complex (ABC) immunohistochemical kit (Wuhan, China). Slices were dried in the drying oven and mounted with coverslips after dehydration and rendering transparent and were then observed and photographed under a microscope.

Immunofluorescence Technique

Slides were washed with 0.01 M PBS and then blocked with a 5% mixture of donkey and goat serum for 1 h at room temperature. After blocking, the slides were incubated with primary antibodies against TASK1 (Alomone Laboratory, Israel, 1:100), TASK3 (Alomone Laboratory, Israel, 1:100) and ASIC1 (Santa Cruz Biotechnology, Dallas, TX, USA, 1:100), Neurofilament-H (Abcam, Cambridge, MA, USA) which were diluted in 0.01 M PBS, overnight. After washing, the slides were incubated with goat anti rabbit IgG conjugated with cy3, donkey anti goat IgG conjugated with FITC, rabbit anti mouse IgG conjugated with DY light 405 (1:100, Beyotime Institute of Biotechnology, Haimen, China) for 1 h in the dark. The slides were then mounted in antifading medium (Beyotime Institute of Biotechnology), and fluorescence was detected using a Zeiss LSM confocal laser system.

Phrenic Nerve Discharge Recording

PND was recorded with platinum bipolar electrodes, which were amplified (filters set at 5.0 kHz) using a Polygraph System (NIHON KOHDEN) and digitized using a SMUP system (SMUP-E, Shanghai Medical College, Fudan University). The experiments were started after the phrenic activity was stabilized (approximately 30 min). The iPND was obtained as a moving average of the phrenic signal. Ti was averaged over 30 s. The value of each iPND and the period of Ti reflected the respiratory drive.

Microinjection

Rats were held in stereotaxic frames with their heads inclined forward at 45 degrees to the level of the dorsal surface of the brain stem after anesthetization. A stainless steel needle was used to unilaterally microinject 0.1 μL into the VLM (12.3 mm posterior, 2.2 mm lateral, and 10 mm dorsal from the bregma). At the end of the experiment, 2% pontamine sky blue was microinjected into the same injection point. The brains were then removed and fixed in 10% formalin solution. After 48 h, the brain stem was coronally sectioned (30 μm) and stained with neutral red to determine the injection site. Data was discarded, if injection site was out of VLM.

Statistical Analysis

Data are expressed as the means ± SD. The significance of differences among the groups was evaluated using the Student *t*-test or a one-way ANOVA test. A value of $p < 0.05$ was considered statistically significant.

RESULTS

Distribution of TASK1 and TASK3 in Rat VLM

The localization of TASK1 and TASK3 immunopositive cells was determined in the VLM of rats (**Figure 1**). According to rat brain atlases, TASK1-ir and TASK3-ir cells are mainly localized in the VLM, including the rostroventrolateral reticular nucleus (RVL) and the lateral paragigantocellular nucleus (LPGi).

Colocalization of TASK1 and TASK3 in VLM Neurons

To detect whether TASK1 and TASK3 are localized in VLM neurons, TASK1-ir and TASK3-ir cells were measured in rat VLM by double immunofluorescence. TASK1 and TASK3 were colocalized with neurofilaments, the biomarker for neurons. Furthermore, TASK1 and TASK3 were colocalized in VLM (**Figure 2**).

Coexpression of ASIC1 and TASK1 or TASK3 in VLM Neurons

We have previously shown that ASIC1 is expressed in VLM neurons and contribute to respiratory regulation (Song et al., 2016). Thus, we wondered whether ASIC1 is coexpressed with TASK1 or TASK3 in VLM neurons. Immunofluorescence was applied to observe the coexpression of ASIC1 and TASK1 or TASK3. Our data showed that ASIC1 was coexpressed with TASK1 and with TASK3 in VLM neurons (**Figure 3**).

The Effects of Non-selective TASK Antagonists on Respiration

To test whether TASKs in the VLM are involved in respiration that is controlled by the respiratory center, the non-selective TASK antagonist BUP was applied. BUP was known to block TASK1 and TASK3 channels (Kindler et al., 1999).We microinjected BUP (200 μM) into the VLM to observe the consequent changes of PND and iPND (**Figure 4A**). Microinjection of BUP triggered significant changes in iPND, Ti and respiratory drive (integrating the value of iPND/Ti). The iPND value was increased by approximately 35% from 1.08 ± 0.11 to 1.45 ± 0.15 arbitrary units ($p < 0.01$, $n = 6$, **Figure 4C**). The respiratory drive was also increased from 1.05 ± 0.07 to 1.56 ± 0.12 ($p < 0.01$, $n = 6$, **Figure 4D**). However, Ti was shortened from 0.36 ± 0.02 to 0.31 ± 0.02 s ($p < 0.05$, $n = 6$, **Figure 4B**). Additionally, the injection spot was confirmed by histological staining (**Figure 4E**). These results indicate that the inhibition of TASKs in VLM neurons leads to cell depolarization by decreasing K^+ efflux, thus stimulating respiration.

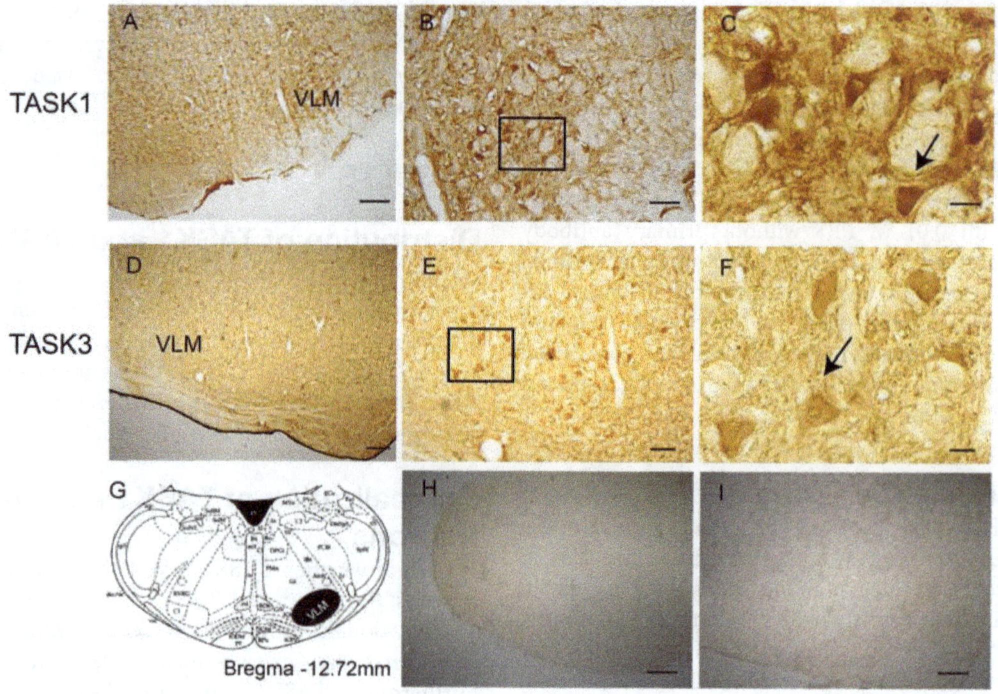

FIGURE 1 | The location of TWIK-related acid-sensitive potassium channel 1 and 3 (TASK1 and 3)-positive cells in the ventrolateral medulla (VLM) of SD rats. **(A)** TASK1-positive cells were located in the VLM of rats. **(B,C)** represent high-power visual fields of the area shown in **(A)**, showing a detailed view of TASK1-positive cells in the VLM. **(D)** TASK3-positive cells in the VLM of rats. **(E,F)** represent high-power visual fields of the area shown in **(D)**, showing a detailed view of TASK3-positive cells in the VLM. **(G)** Coronal diagram of the rat medulla; the area shown in black represents the distribution of TASK1 and TASK3. Cell morphology is indicated by the arrows shown in **(C,F)**. **(H–I)** Negative control. Scale bar: 200 μm **(A,D,H,I)**; 80 μm **(B,E)** and 20 μm **(C,F)**.

The Effects of TASK1 and TASK3 Selective Antagonists on Respiration

To determine the effects of TASK1 and TASK3 on respiration, we blocked TASK1 using AEA and blocked TASK3 using RR. It was reported that AEA was widely applied as TASK1 inhibitor (Maingret et al., 2001). RR was recently found to selectively inhibit TASK3 with little or no effect on TASK-1 (Berg et al., 2004). Microinjection of AEA (100 μM) increased iPND and respiratory drive from 0.97 ± 0.04 to 1.61 ± 0.15 ($p < 0.01$, $n = 5$, **Figures 5A,D**) and from 0.97 ± 0.04 to 1.69 ± 0.16 ($p < 0.001$, $n = 5$, **Figure 5E**), respectively. Ti was shortened from 0.31 ± 0.03 to 0.27 ± 0.03 s ($p < 0.05$, $n = 5$, **Figures 5C**). RR (10 μM) increased iPND from 1.07 ± 0.06 to 1.29 ± 0.07 ($p < 0.001$, $n = 5$, **Figures 5B,G**), enhanced respiratory drive from 1.07 ± 0.09 to 1.48 ± 0.12 ($p < 0.05$, $n = 5$, **Figure 5H**), and shortened Ti from 0.36 ± 0.02 to 0.31 ± 0.02 s ($p < 0.05$, $n = 5$, **Figure 5F**). Together, these results suggest that both TASK1 and TASK3 in the VLM are involved in the central regulation of respiration. Furthermore, inhibition of TASK1 and TASK3 in rat VLM stimulated breathing that is controlled by the respiratory center.

The Effect of ACSF With Different pH Values on Respiration

It has been reported that TASKs are sensitive to changes in extracellular proton chemoreception and that the inhibition of TASKs by extracellular acidosis leads to increased excitability of brainstem respiratory neurons (Duprat et al., 1997; Bayliss and Barrett, 2008). Conversely, activation by alkalization exerts an inhibitory effect. ASICs have been reported to be involved in the pH sensitivity in the CNS and are voltage-insensitive, proton-gated cation channels that are activated by extracellular acidification (Waldmann et al., 1997). AMI is widely used as a non-selective ASIC inhibitor (Waldmann et al., 1997; Baron and Lingueglia, 2015). We first microinjected ACSF at acidic pH (7.4, 7.0 and 6.5) into the VLM of rats and observed the resulting changes of respiratory activation (**Figures 6A–C**). Microinjection at pH 7.0 and 6.5 caused significant increases in iPND, Ti and respiratory drive, which were inhibited by AMI (**Figures 6D–F**). To explore the effect of TASK activation on respiration, we microinjected alkaline ACSF (pH 8.0) and found that alkaline ACSF triggers decreases of iPND and respiratory drive, which were inhibited by AEA (**Figures 7A,B,C,E,F**). However, microinjection of alkaline ACSF had no significant effect on Ti (**Figure 7D**).

DISCUSSION

The central chemoreflex is essential to the maintenance of circulatory acid-base homeostasis by adjusting the activity of breathing. However, the mechanism of chemoreflex has

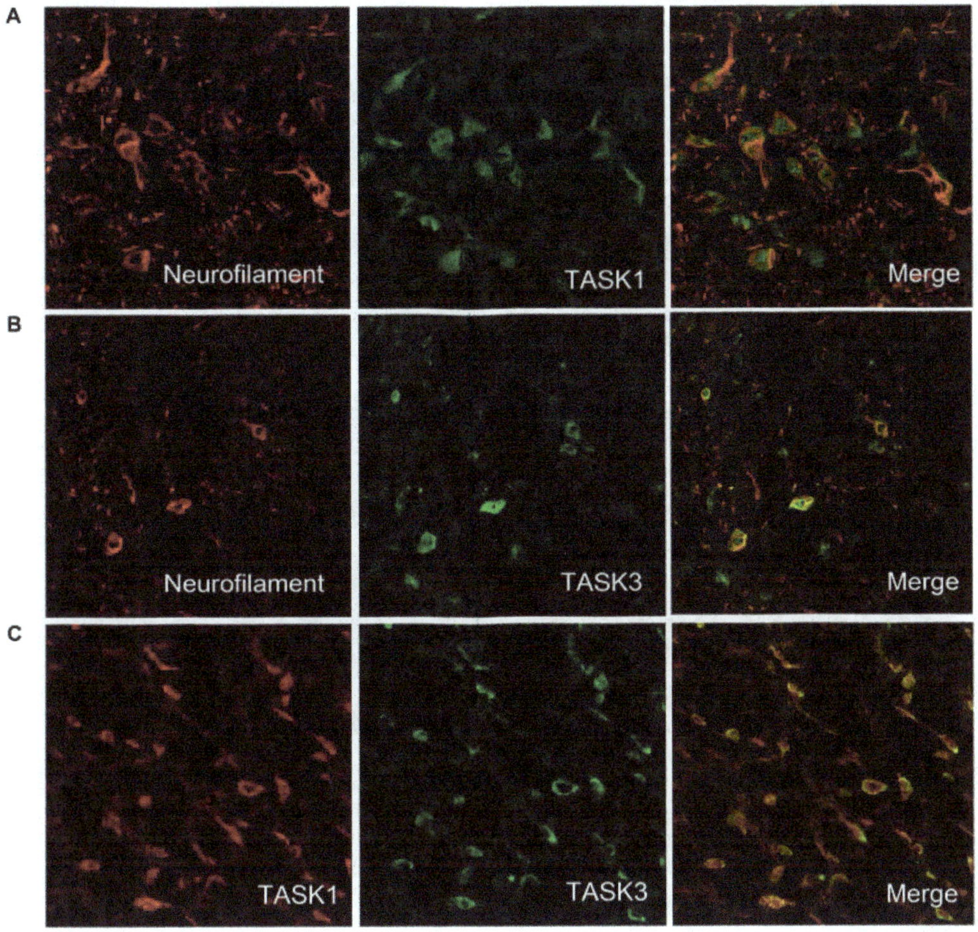

FIGURE 2 | TASK1 and TASK3 are expressed and colocalized in VLM neurons. **(A,B)** Representative confocal photomicrograph showing the colocalization of TASK1-ir and TASK3-ir (green) with neurofilament-ir (red) in the VLM. **(C)** Representative confocal photomicrograph showing the colocalization of TASK1 (red) and TASK3 (green) in the VLM. Original magnification, 200×.

remained unclear until now. Our previous study demonstrated that ASICs are expressed on the neurons of chemosensitive areas such as the lateral hypothalamus and VLM and contribute to respiratory regulation. In the present study, we focused on the role of another class of pH-sensitive ion channels, TASKs, in breathing regulation and their cooperation with ASICs in the central chemosensory system. We found that TASK1 and TASK3 are expressed in the VLM of rats. TASK1 and TASK3 cooperate with ASIC1 to participate in the central regulation of respiration. This might be the chemosensitive mechanism of the VLM.

The expression of TASKs in brain stem has been reported previously (Talley et al., 2001; Berg et al., 2004). TASK1 is expressed in the facial nucleus, ambiguous nucleus, hypoglossal nucleus and LC (Sirois et al., 2000; Bayliss et al., 2001), and TASK3 is expressed in the nucleus of the solitary tract, raphes and LC (Talley et al., 2001). ASICs, especially ASIC1 and ASIC2a, are widely expressed in the CNS (García-Añoveros et al., 1997; Waldmann et al., 1997; Alvarez de la Rosa et al., 2003). It has been reported that ASIC1 in NTS mediates chemosensitivity and is involved in the control of breathing (Huda et al., 2012). Acidification of the LH can stimulate breathing via the activation of ASIC1a on orexin neurons (Song et al., 2012). However, little is known about the coexpression of ASIC1 and TASKs (1 and 3) in the CNS. In the present study, we first examined the expression of TASK1 and TASK3 by localizing TASK1- and TASK3-positive cells in the VLM by immunohistochemistry. TASK1 and TASK3 subunits are colocalized with most serotonergic dorsal and caudal raphe neurons and with noradrenergic cells of the LC (Talley et al., 2001; Washburn et al., 2002). According to the immunofluorescence results, TASK1 and TASK3 coexpression were detected in the VLM, which indicates that heteromeric TASKs may also be involved in central chemoreception. Furthermore, ASIC1, which can be activated by extracellular acidification, was found to be coexpressed with TASK1 and TASK3, suggesting that TASKs may cooperate with ASIC1 and thereby participate in central respiratory regulation. The VLM neurons serve as central chemoreceptors mediating respiratory responses to hypoxia and/or hypercapnia (Wakai et al., 2015) Therefore, these morphological results lay the foundation for

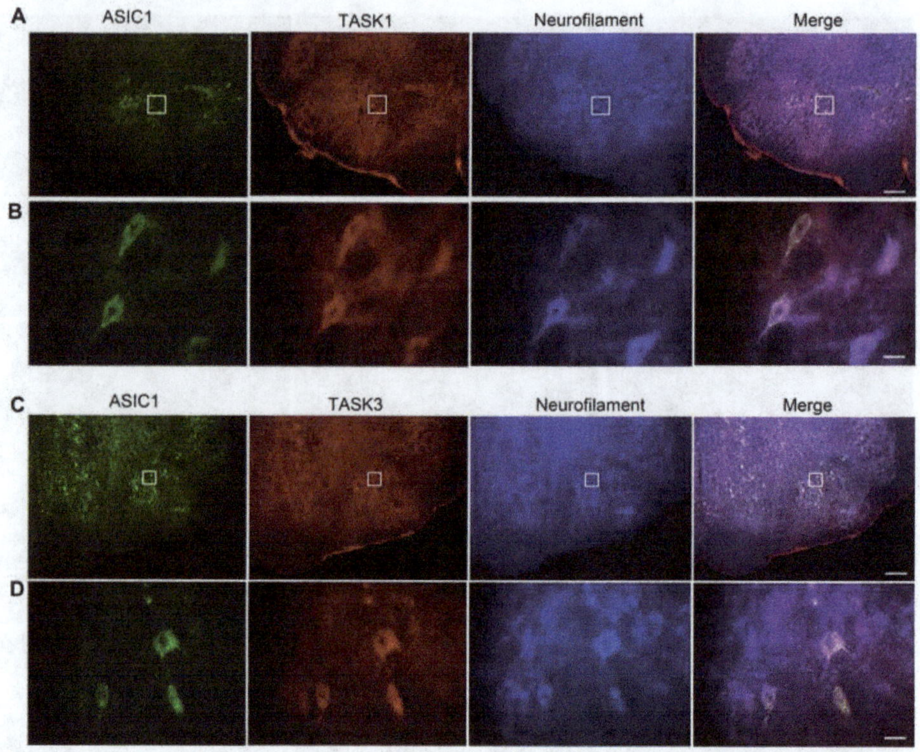

FIGURE 3 | Acid-sensing ion channel 1 (ASIC1), TASK1 and TASK3 are expressed and colocalized in the VLM neurons of adult rats. **(A)** Representative confocal photomicrographs showing the colocalization of ASIC1-ir (green), TASK1-ir (red) and neurofilament-H (blue) in the VLM. **(B)** Representative high power visual field of the area shown in **(A)**. **(C)** Representative confocal photomicrographs showing the colocalization of ASIC1-ir (green), TASK3-ir (red) and neurofilament-H (blue) in the VLM. **(D)** Representative high power visual field of the area shown in **(C)**. **(A–C)** Scale bar = 200 μm; **(B,D)** scale bar = 20 μm.

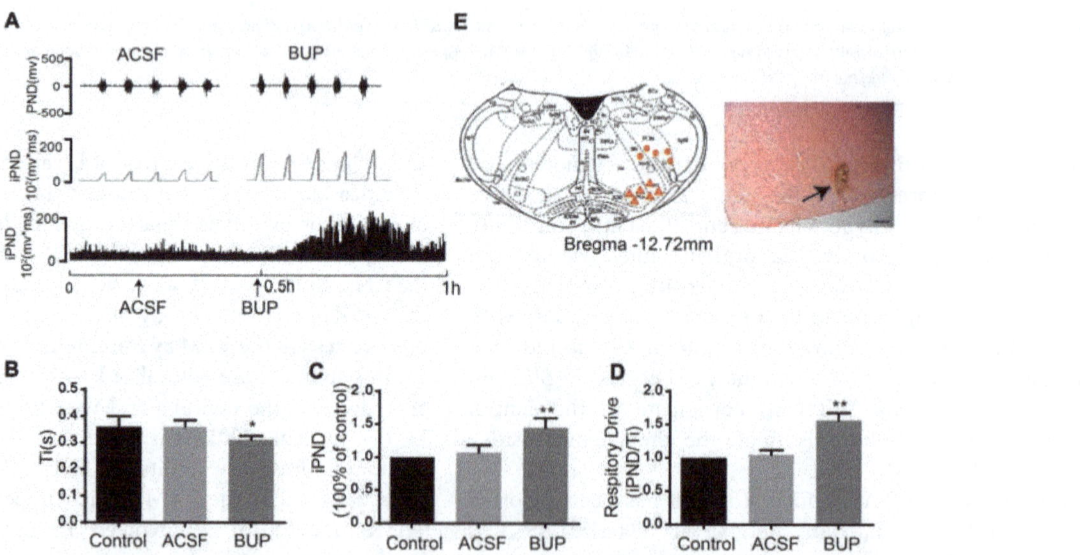

FIGURE 4 | The non-selective TASKs antagonist, bupivacaine (BUP) stimulated respiration of rats. **(A)** The phrenic nerve discharge (PND) was recorded from the same animal. The unilateral microinjection of 200 μM BUP into the VLM increased PND and integrated PND (iPND). The microinjection of artificial cerebrospinal fluid (ACSF; pH 7.4) served as a control. **(B)** Inspiratory time (Ti) was decreased by BUP injection. **(C)** Group data showing the effects of BUP on iPND. **(D)** Responses of the respiratory drive. Note that BUP stimulated respiration (*$p < 0.05$, **$p < 0.01$ relative to control; $n = 6$). **(E)** Histological staining with neutral red: the sky blue spot indicates the injection site in the VLM, and the injection plot was confirmed by comparison with the Bregma −12.72 mm coronal diagram in the Paxinos and Watson stereotaxic atlas of the rat brain. In the diagram, red arrowheads represent the injection points and dots signify injection points out of VLM.

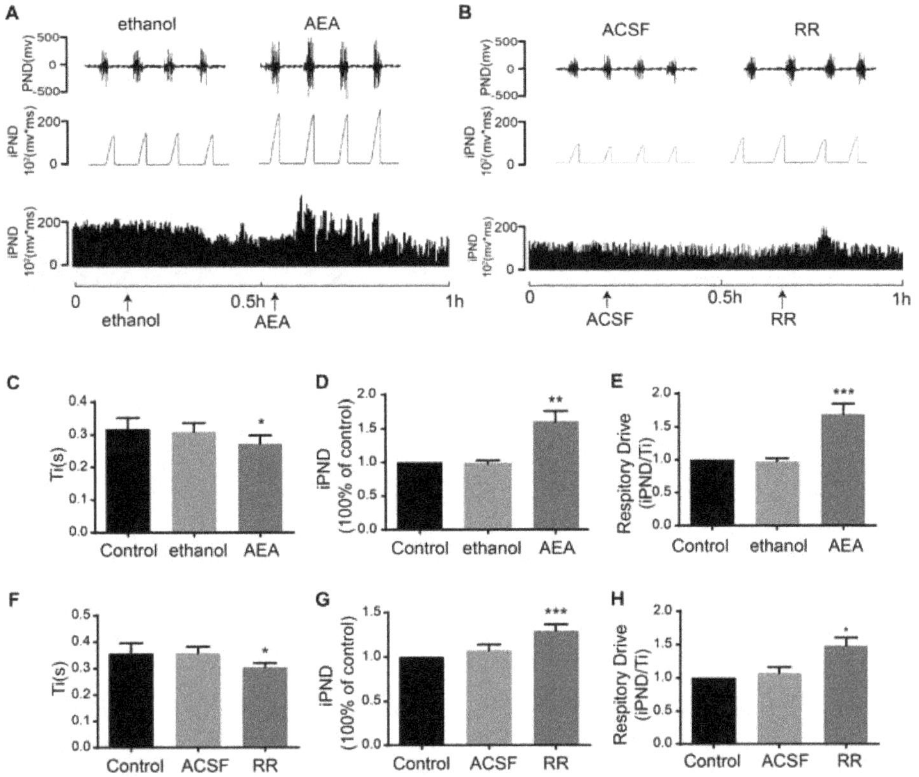

FIGURE 5 | TASK1 antagonist, anandamide (AEA) and TASK3 antagonist, ruthenium red (RR) stimulated the respiration of rats. **(A,B)** The PND was recorded from the same animal. The unilateral microinjection of 100 μM AEA and 10 μM RR into the VLM increased PND and iPND. The microinjection of ethanol and ACSF (pH 7.4) served as a control. **(C–F)** Ti was decreased by AEA and RR injection. **(D–G)** Group data showing the effects of AEA and RR on iPND. **(E–H)** Responses of the respiratory drive. Note that AEA and RR stimulated respiration, $^{*}p < 0.05$, $^{**}p < 0.01$, $^{***}p < 0.001$ relative to control; $n = 5$.

exploring the function of ASIC1 and TASKs (1 and 3) in the brainstem.

Recent studies have shown that TASK1 and TASK3 subunits generate a pH-sensitive and weakly rectifying K^+ current, which is critical for regulating the resting membrane potential and the excitability of respiration-related neurons (Duprat et al., 1997; Buckler et al., 2000; Kim et al., 2000; Bayliss et al., 2015). TASK1 and TASK3 are responsible for the pH sensitivity of serotonergic neurons in the dorsal and caudal raphe of mice (Washburn et al., 2002). *In vivo*, hypoxic and acidic responses are partially blunted in TASK1 and TASK3 knockout mice (Trapp et al., 2008). In the carotid body, TASK1 plays a key role in the control of ventilation peripherally in mice (Trapp et al., 2008). Despite these findings, the role of TASKs in the VLM in central respiratory regulation has not been reported yet. We determined the role of TASK1 and TASK3 in the central regulation of breathing by PND recording. TASK1 and TASK3 are both inhibited by local anesthetics, including BUP (Kindler et al., 1999; Kim et al., 2000). It has been demonstrated that TASK1 is directly inhibited by the AEA (Maingret et al., 2001), and TASK3 is selectively blocked by RR (Czirják and Enyedi, 2002). Therefore, a non-selective antagonist, BUP, a specific TASK1 antagonist, AEA, and a specific TASK3 antagonist, RR, were applied in an animal experiment. We found that the microinjection of BUP, AEA and RR stimulated breathing by increasing PND and iPND, shortened Ti, and enhanced respiratory drive, suggesting that the inhibition of TASK1 and TASK3 in VLM neurons blocked the background K^+ current, which contributes to producing the action potential and increases the excitability of inspiratory neurons. However, neither RR nor AEA are specific for TASKs channels. This is a shortcoming of the study. RR is a non-selective inhibitor of transient receptor potential (TRP) channels and AEA is agonist of both cannabinoid (CB) receptors and TRP channels (Watanabe et al., 2003; Kopczyńska, 2007). Indeed, it has been reported that CB receptors and TRP channels cooperate with each other in breathing regulation. Intravenous injection of AEA induced depression of breathing can be prevented by the CB1 antagonist AM281 (Kopczyńska, 2007; Iring et al., 2017). TRPV2 channel was found to be expressed in VLM (Nedungadi et al., 2012). However, TRPV2 channel is mainly stretch and thermo sensitive. TRPV1 is acidic sensitive, which can be activated by low pH. Our current study found that microinjection of either agonist (AEA) or antagonist (RR) of TRP channels into VLM stimulates breathing. Thus, we speculate that it is unlikely TRP take part in regulation of breathing by neurons of the VLM. Ordinarily, activation of CB receptors reduces neuronal excitability (den Boon et al., 2012). But, we found that microinjection of the agonist of CB receptors, AEA into the

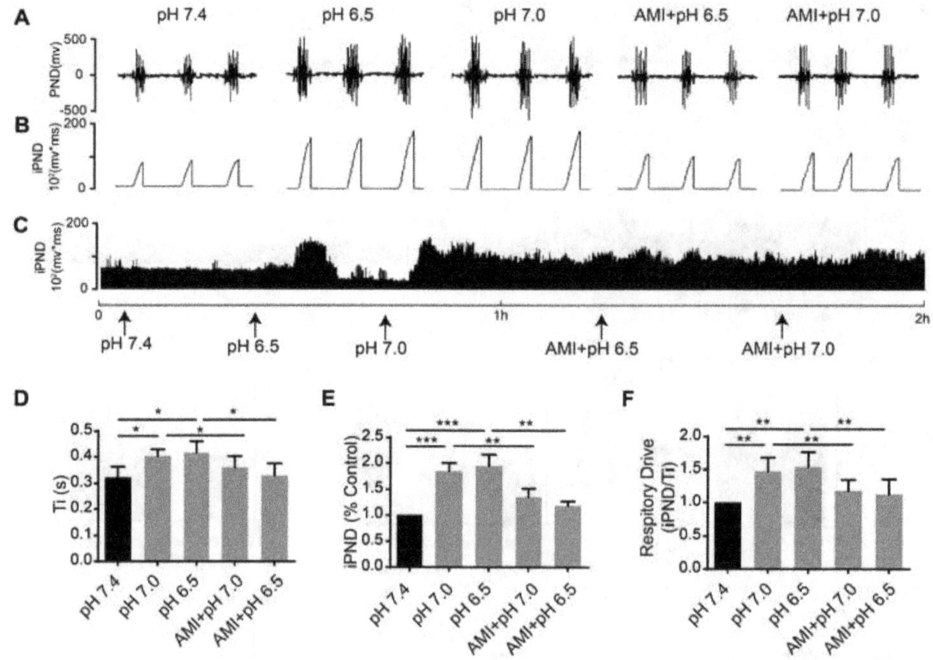

FIGURE 6 | ASIC antagonists attenuated the stimulatory effect of acidification on respiration in rat VLM. **(A–C)** The unilateral microinjection of 0.1 μL ACSF (pH 7.4, 7.0 and 6.5) into the VLM increased raw PND **(A)** and iPND **(B,C)**. AMI pre-treatment (100 μM) blocked this effect. The microinjection of ACSF (pH 7.4) served as a control. **(D–F)** Statistical data showing the effects of alkalization and AMI on Ti **(D)**, iPND **(E)** and respiratory drive **(F)**. *$p < 0.05$, **$p < 0.01$, ***$p < 0.001$, $n = 6$.

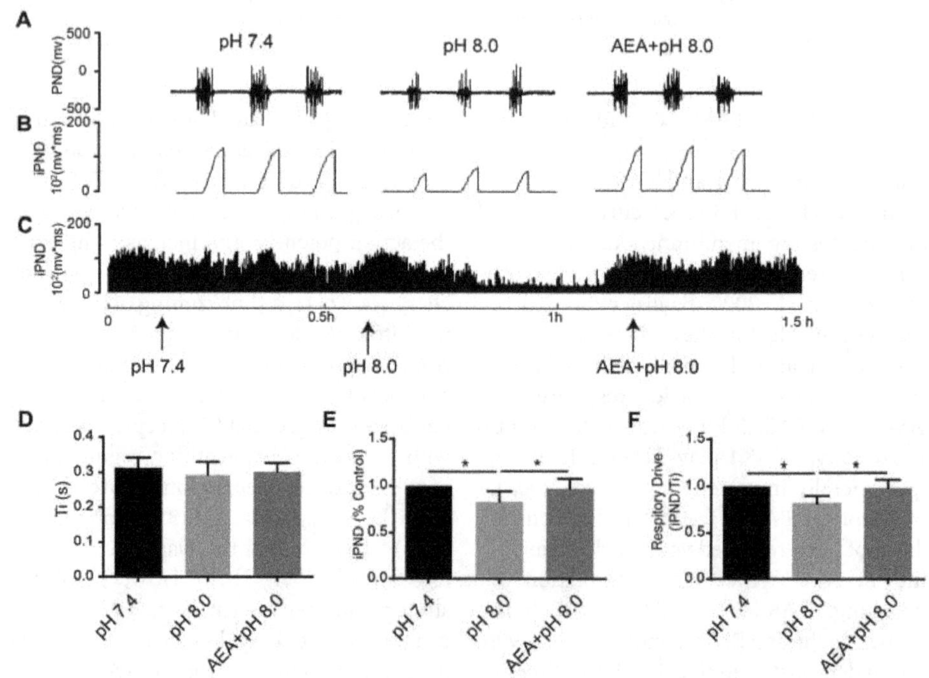

FIGURE 7 | TASK1 antagonists attenuated the subdued effect of alkalization on respiration in the rat VLM. **(A–C)** The unilateral microinjection of 0.1 μL ACSF (pH 8.0) into the VLM decreased raw PND **(A)** and iPND **(B,C)**. TASK1 antagonist AEA pre-treatment (100 μM) blocked this effect. The microinjection of ACSF (pH 7.4) served as a control. **(D–F)** Statistical data showing the effects of different levels of alkalization and AEA on Ti **(D)**, iPND **(E)** and respiratory drive **(F)**. *$p < 0.05$, $n = 6$.

VLM activated breathing. Thus, we consumed that it is unlikely the activation of CB receptor medicated respiratory regulation. However, there is no direct evidence to rule out the role of CB receptors and TRP channels in VLM mediated respiratory regulation. Further investigations are needed to explore the roles of TASKs channels in the central regulation of breathing.

It has been well documented that central respiratory chemoreceptors are located in the medullary raphe, nucleus tractus solitarius, VLM and hypothalamus (Funk, 2010). VLM, including RVL and LPGi, is a putative site for central chemoreception, (Corcoran et al., 2009). However, the specific pH sensing mechanism remains controversial. Therefore, we focused on the effect of ASIC1 and TASKs in the VLM on chemoreception.

TASKs are inhibited by extracellular acidification (Bayliss et al., 2003; Bayliss and Barrett, 2008; Enyedi and Czirják, 2010). The pH sensitivities of heterodimeric TASKs (1 and 3) and TASK1 (pK ~7.4) are closer to the physiological range than that of TASK-3 (pK ~6.8; Berg et al., 2004; Duprat et al., 2007). Thus, the acid-induced inhibition of TASK channel activity enhances nerve excitability. In addition to TASKs, ASICs have been reported to be involved in the pH sensitivity in the CNS; ASICs are voltage-insensitive, proton-gated cation channels that are activated by extracellular acidification (Waldmann et al., 1997). ASIC1 activation causes the entry of Na^+ and a little Ca^{2+}, which leads to the polarization and excitability of neurons. Because of the similar pKa values of TASK3 and ASIC1a and their coexpression in the VLM, we think that these proteins may work together to participate in respiratory regulation by central chemosensitive neurons. AMI is widely used to block ASICs and can reversibly inhibit ASICs (Champigny et al., 1998; Baron and Linguеglia, 2015). To investigate whether TASKs (1 and 3) and ASIC1 contribute to chemoreception in rats, we microinjected ACSF at pH values from 7.4 to lower pH levels dose-dependently in the absence and presence of AMI into VLM to observe the change of PND. Our results showed that the microinjection of ACSF at pH 7.0 and 6.5 obviously prolonged Ti, increased iPND, and enhanced respiratory drive. AMI inhibited this effect. On the contrary, the microinjection of ACSF at pH 8.0 decreased iPND and respiratory drive, which were inhibited by AEA. However, alkaline ACSF had no significant effect on Ti. One possible reason is that TASK1 and TASK3 exhibit different pH sensitivity. TASK-1 is activated strongly by alkalization pH over 7.3 (Duprat et al., 1997; Bayliss et al., 2001, 2015), whereas, TASK3 is nearly fully activated at pH 7.3, and additional alkalization has little effect on TASK-3 currents (Rajan et al., 2000; Bayliss et al., 2015). The results indicated that activation of TASK-1 may have minor effect on Ti. However, further studies are needed to explore the roles of TASKs in regulation of breathing.

Based on the data presented above, the inhibition of TASK1 and TASK3 in the VLM under physiological conditions stimulates respiration. The acidification of the VLM led to PND enhancement, which was caused by ASIC1 activation. The alkalization of the VLM reduced PND, which was mainly caused by TASK1 activation. This result indicates that ASIC1 and TASKs (1 and 3) coexist in the chemosensitive neurons of VLM and coordinate with each other to sense local pH fluctuations; this may be one of the mechanisms by which central chemosensitive neurons respond to pH changes.

In summary, extracellular pH is a critical signal in the central regulation of breathing. In the present study, we have shown that TASKs including TASK1 and TASK3 are expressed in the VLM of rats and are coexpressed with ASIC1 in VLM neurons. Furthermore, we have shown that local acidification of the VLM can stimulate respiration, mainly via ASIC1. Local alkalization weakens respiration, mainly via TASK1. Our findings support the notion that ASIC1, TASK1 and TASK3 are expressed on neurons in the VLM and participate in the chemical regulation of respiration in response to extracellular pH change under physiological conditions.

AUTHOR CONTRIBUTIONS

XW performed the *in vivo* and some of the *in vitro* experiments and prepared the manuscript. RG conducted some of the *in vitro* experiments. XZ and DZ analyzed some of the data. NS and LS designed the experiments and revised the manuscript.

FUNDING

This work was funded by a grant from the National Natural Science Foundation of China (Nos. 81470203 and 81500048).

REFERENCES

Alvarez de la Rosa, D., Krueger, S. R., Kolar, A., Shao, D., Fitzsimonds, R. M., and Canessa, C. M. (2003). Distribution, subcellular localization and ontogeny of ASIC1 in the mammalian central nervous system. *J. Physiol.* 546, 77–87. doi: 10.1113/jphysiol.2002.030692

Baron, A., and Lingueglia, E. (2015). Pharmacology of acid-sensing ion channels–Physiological and therapeutical perspectives. *Neuropharmacology* 94, 19–35. doi: 10.1016/j.neuropharm.2015.01.005

Bayliss, D. A., and Barrett, P. Q. (2008). Emerging roles for two-pore-domain potassium channels and their potential therapeutic impact. *Trends Pharmacol. Sci.* 29, 566–575. doi: 10.1016/j.tips.2008.07.013

Bayliss, D. A., Barhanin, J., Gestreau, C., and Guyenet, P. G. (2015). The role of pH-sensitive TASK channels in central respiratory chemoreception. *Pflugers Arch.* 467, 917–929. doi: 10.1007/s00424-014-1633-9

Bayliss, D. A., Sirois, J. E., and Talley, E. M. (2003). The TASK family: two-pore domain background K^+ channels. *Mol. Interv.* 3, 205–219. doi: 10.1124/mi.3.4.205

Bayliss, D. A., Talley, E. M., Sirois, J. E., and Lei, Q. (2001). TASK-1 is a highly modulated pH-sensitive 'leak' K^+ channel expressed in brainstem respiratory neurons. *Respir. Physiol.* 129, 159–174. doi: 10.1016/s0034-5687(01)00288-2

Berg, A. P., Talley, E. M., Manger, J. P., and Bayliss, D. A. (2004). Motoneurons express heteromeric TWIK-related acid-sensitive K^+ (TASK) channels containing TASK-1 (KCNK3) and TASK-3 (KCNK9) subunits. *J. Neurosci.* 24, 6693–6702. doi: 10.1523/JNEUROSCI.1408-04.2004

Buckler, K. J., Williams, B. A., and Honore, E. (2000). An oxygen-, acid- and anaesthetic-sensitive TASK-like background potassium channel in rat arterial chemoreceptor cells. *J. Physiol.* 525, 135–142. doi: 10.1111/j.1469-7793.2000.00135.x

Buehler, P. K., Bleiler, D., Tegtmeier, I., Heitzmann, D., Both, C., Georgieff, M., et al. (2017). Abnormal respiration under hyperoxia in TASK-1/3 potassium channel double knockout mice. *Respir. Physiol. Neurobiol.* 244, 17–25. doi: 10.1016/j.resp.2017.06.009

Champigny, G., Voilley, N., Waldmann, R., and Lazdunski, M. (1998). Mutations causing neurodegeneration in *Caenorhabditis elegans* drastically alter the pH sensitivity and inactivation of the mammalian H^+-gated Na^+ channel MDEG1. *J. Biol. Chem.* 273, 15418–15422. doi: 10.1074/jbc.273.25.15418

Corcoran, A. E., Hodges, M. R., Wu, Y., Wang, W., Wylie, C. J., Deneris, E. S., et al. (2009). Medullary serotonin neurons and central CO_2 chemoreception. *Respir. Physiol. Neurobiol.* 168, 49–58. doi: 10.1016/j.resp.2009.04.014

Czirják, G., and Enyedi, P. (2002). TASK-3 dominates the background potassium conductance in rat adrenal glomerulosa cells. *Mol. Endocrinol.* 16, 621–629. doi: 10.1210/mend.16.3.0788

den Boon, F. S., Chameau, P., Schaafsma-Zhao, Q., van Aken, W., Bari, M., Oddi, S., et al. (2012). Excitability of prefrontal cortical pyramidal neurons is modulated by activation of intracellular type-2 cannabinoid receptors. *Proc. Natl. Acad. Sci. U S A* 109, 3534–3539. doi: 10.1073/pnas.1118167109

Duprat, F., Lauritzen, I., Patel, A., and Honore, E. (2007). The TASK background K_2P channels: chemo- and nutrient sensors. *Trends Neurosci.* 30, 573–580. doi: 10.1016/j.tins.2007.08.003

Duprat, F., Lesage, F., Fink, M., Reyes, R., Heurteaux, C., and Lazdunski, M. (1997). TASK, a human background K^+ channel to sense external pH variations near physiological pH. *EMBO J.* 16, 5464–5471. doi: 10.1093/emboj/16.17.5464

Enyedi, P., and Czirják, G. (2010). Molecular background of leak K^+ currents: two-pore domain potassium channels. *Physiol. Rev.* 90, 559–605. doi: 10.1152/physrev.00029.2009

Funk, G. D. (2010). The 'connexin' between astrocytes, ATP and central respiratory chemoreception. *J. Physiol.* 588, 4335–4337. doi: 10.1113/jphysiol.2010.200196

García-Añoveros, J., Derfler, B., Neville-Golden, J., Hyman, B. T., and Corey, D. P. (1997). BNaC1 and BNaC2 constitute a new family of human neuronal sodium channels related to degenerins and epithelial sodium channels. *Proc. Natl. Acad. Sci. U S A* 94, 1459–1464. doi: 10.1073/pnas.94.4.1459

Goridis, C., and Brunet, J. F. (2010). Central chemoreception: lessons from mouse and human genetics. *Respir. Physiol. Neurobiol.* 173, 312–321. doi: 10.1016/j.resp.2010.03.014

Hartness, M. E., Lewis, A., Searle, G. J., O'Kelly, I., Peers, C., and Kemp, P. J. (2001). Combined antisense and pharmacological approaches implicate hTASK as an airway O_2 sensing K^+ channel. *J. Biol. Chem.* 276, 26499–26508. doi: 10.1074/jbc.M010357200

Holzer, P. (2009). Acid-sensitive ion channels and receptors. *Handb. Exp. Pharmacol.* 194, 283–332. doi: 10.1007/978-3-540-79090-7_9

Honoré, E. (2007). The neuronal background K2P channels: focus on TREK1. *Nat. Rev. Neurosci.* 8, 251–261. doi: 10.1038/nrn2117

Huda, R., Pollema-Mays, S. L., Chang, Z., Alheid, G. F., McCrimmon, D. R., and Martina, M. (2012). Acid-sensing ion channels contribute to chemosensitivity of breathing-related neurons of the nucleus of the solitary tract. *J. Physiol.* 590, 4761–4775. doi: 10.1113/jphysiol.2012.232470

Iring, A., Hricisák, L., and Benyó, Z. (2017). CB1 receptor-mediated respiratory depression by endocannabinoids. *Respir. Physiol. Neurobiol.* 240, 48–52. doi: 10.1016/j.resp.2017.02.011

Kim, Y., Bang, H., and Kim, D. (2000). TASK-3, a new member of the tandem pore K^+ channel family. *J. Biol. Chem.* 275, 9340–9347. doi: 10.1074/jbc.275.13.9340

Kindler, C. H., Yost, C. S., and Gray, A. T. (1999). Local anesthetic inhibition of baseline potassium channels with two pore domains in tandem. *Anesthesiology* 90, 1092–1102. doi: 10.1097/00000542-199904000-00024

Koizumi, H., Smerin, S. E., Yamanishi, T., Moorjani, B. R., Zhang, R., and Smith, J. C. (2010). TASK channels contribute to the K^+-dominated leak current regulating respiratory rhythm generation *in vitro*. *J. Neurosci.* 30, 4273–4284. doi: 10.1523/JNEUROSCI.4017-09.2010

Kopczyńska, B. (2007). The contribution of VR1 and CB1 receptors and the role of the afferent vagal pathway in modelling of cardio-respiratory effects of anandamide in rats. *Life Sci.* 80, 1738–1745. doi: 10.1016/j.lfs.2007.01.062

Maingret, F., Patel, A. J., Lazdunski, M., and Honore, E. (2001). The endocannabinoid anandamide is a direct and selective blocker of the background K^+ channel TASK-1. *EMBO J.* 20, 47–54. doi: 10.1093/emboj/20.1.47

Millhorn, D. E., and Eldridge, F. L. (1986). Role of ventrolateral medulla in regulation of respiratory and cardiovascular systems. *J. Appl. Physiol.* 61, 1249–1263. doi: 10.1152/jappl.1986.61.4.1249

Nedungadi, T. P., Dutta, M., Bathina, C. S., Caterina, M. J., and Cunningham, J. T. (2012). Expression and distribution of TRPV2 in rat brain. *Exp. Neurol.* 237, 223–237. doi: 10.1016/j.expneurol.2012.06.017

Rajan, S., Wischmeyer, E., Xin, L. G., Preisig-Muller, R., Daut, J., Karschin, A., et al. (2000). TASK-3, a novel tandem pore domain acid-sensitive K^+ channel. An extracellular histiding as pH sensor. *J. Biol. Chem.* 275, 16650–16657. doi: 10.1074/jbc.M000030200

Sirois, J. E., Lei, Q., Talley, E. M., Lynch, C. R., and Bayliss, D. A. (2000). The TASK-1 two-pore domain K^+ channel is a molecular substrate for neuronal effects of inhalation anesthetics. *J. Neurosci.* 20, 6347–6354. doi: 10.1523/jneurosci.20-17-06347.2000

Song, N., Guan, R., Jiang, Q., Hassanzadeh, C. J., Chu, Y., Zhao, X., et al. (2016). Acid-sensing ion channels are expressed in the ventrolateral medulla and contribute to central chemoreception. *Sci. Rep.* 6:38777. doi: 10.1038/srep38777

Song, N., Zhang, G., Geng, W., Liu, Z., Jin, W., Li, L., et al. (2012). Acid sensing ion channel 1 in lateral hypothalamus contributes to breathing control. *PLoS One* 7:e39982. doi: 10.1371/journal.pone.0039982

Talley, E. M., Solorzano, G., Lei, Q., Kim, D., and Bayliss, D. A. (2001). Cns distribution of members of the two-pore-domain (KCNK) potassium channel family. *J. Neurosci.* 21, 7491–7505. doi: 10.1523/JNEUROSCI.21-19-07491.2001

Trapp, S., Aller, M. I., Wisden, W., and Gourine, A. V. (2008). A role for TASK-1 (KCNK3) channels in the chemosensory control of breathing. *J. Neurosci.* 28, 8844–8850. doi: 10.1523/JNEUROSCI.1810-08.2008

Wakai, J., Takamura, D., Morinaga, R., Nakamuta, N., and Yamamoto, Y. (2015). Differences in respiratory changes and Fos expression in the ventrolateral medulla of rats exposed to hypoxia, hypercapnia and hypercapnic hypoxia. *Respir. Physiol. Neurobiol.* 215, 64–72. doi: 10.1016/j.resp.2015.05.008

Waldmann, R., Champigny, G., Bassilana, F., Heurteaux, C., and Lazdunski, M. (1997). A proton-gated cation channel involved in acid-sensing. *Nature* 386, 173–177. doi: 10.1038/386173a0

Washburn, C. P., Bayliss, D. A., and Guyenet, P. G. (2003). Cardiorespiratory neurons of the rat ventrolateral medulla contain TASK-1 and TASK-3 channel mRNA. *Respir. Physiol. Neurobiol.* 138, 19–35. doi: 10.1016/s1569-9048(03)00185-x

Washburn, C. P., Sirois, J. E., Talley, E. M., Guyenet, P. G., and Bayliss, D. A. (2002). Serotonergic raphe neurons express TASK channel transcripts and a TASK-like pH- and halothane-sensitive K^+ conductance. *J. Neurosci.* 22, 1256–1265. doi: 10.1523/jneurosci.22-04-01256.2002

Watanabe, H., Vriens, J., Prenen, J., Droogmans, G., Voets, T., and Nilius, B. (2003). Anandamide and arachidonic acid use epoxyeicosatrienoic acids to activate TRPV4 channels. *Nature* 424, 434–438. doi: 10.1038/nature01807

2

Activation of Brainstem Neurons During Mesencephalic Locomotor Region-Evoked Locomotion in the Cat

Ioan Opris[1], Xiaohong Dai[2], Dawn M. G. Johnson[1†], Francisco J. Sanchez[1], Luz M. Villamil[1], Songtao Xie[1†], Cecelia R. Lee-Hauser[1], Stephano Chang[1], Larry M. Jordan[2] and Brian R. Noga[1]*

[1] *The Miami Project to Cure Paralysis, Department of Neurological Surgery, University of Miami Miller School of Medicine, Miami, FL, United States,* [2] *Department of Physiology, Spinal Cord Research Centre, University of Manitoba, Winnipeg, MB, Canada*

***Correspondence:**
Brian R. Noga
bnoga@miami.edu

†Present address:
Dawn M. G. Johnson, National Institute of Mental Health, Bethesda, MD, United States
Songtao Xie, Department of Chemical and Natural Gas Engineering, Texas A&M University – Kingsville, Kingsville, TX, United States

The distribution of locomotor-activated neurons in the brainstem of the cat was studied by c-*Fos* immunohistochemistry in combination with antibody-based cellular phenotyping following electrical stimulation of the mesencephalic locomotor region (MLR) – the anatomical constituents of which remain debated today, primarily between the cuneiform (CnF) and the pedunculopontine tegmental nuclei (PPT). Effective MLR sites were co-extensive with the CnF nucleus. Animals subject to the locomotor task showed abundant *Fos* labeling in the CnF, parabrachial nuclei of the subcuneiform region, periaqueductal gray, locus ceruleus (LC)/subceruleus (SubC), Kölliker–Fuse, magnocellular and lateral tegmental fields, raphe, and the parapyramidal region. Labeled neurons were more abundant on the side of stimulation. In some animals, *Fos*-labeled cells were also observed in the ventral tegmental area, medial and intermediate vestibular nuclei, dorsal motor nucleus of the vagus, n. tractus solitarii, and retrofacial nucleus in the ventrolateral medulla. Many neurons in the reticular formation were innervated by serotonergic fibers. Numerous locomotor-activated neurons in the parabrachial nuclei and LC/SubC/Kölliker–Fuse were noradrenergic. Few cholinergic neurons within the PPT stained for *Fos*. In the medulla, serotonergic neurons within the parapyramidal region and the nucleus raphe magnus were positive for *Fos*. Control animals, not subject to locomotion, showed few *Fos*-labeled neurons in these areas. The current study provides positive evidence for a role for the CnF in the initiation of locomotion while providing little evidence for the participation of the PPT. The results also show that MLR-evoked locomotion involves the parallel activation of reticular and monoaminergic neurons in the pons/medulla, and provides the anatomical and functional basis for spinal monoamine release during evoked locomotion. Lastly, the results indicate that vestibular, cardiovascular, and respiratory centers are centrally activated during MLR-evoked locomotion. Altogether, the results show a complex pattern of neuromodulatory influences of brainstem neurons by electrical activation of the MLR.

Keywords: mesencephalic locomotor region, cuneiform nucleus, pedunculopontine nucleus, fictive locomotion, reticulospinal, monoamine, choline acetyltransferase, activity-dependent labeling

INTRODUCTION

Of the various higher brain centers that elicit locomotion when stimulated, the MLR, a key, phylogenetically preserved, regulatory node within the supraspinal locomotor circuit controlling spinal locomotor neurons (Shik et al., 1966, 1967; Grillner et al., 2008; Jordan et al., 2008), is increasingly looked at as a target for improving locomotion (freezing-of-gait) in Parkinson's disease (PD) and after spinal cord injury (SCI). The anatomical equivalent of this physiologically defined region was originally thought to be the CnF (Shik et al., 1966) and subsequent work confirmed this conclusion (Mori et al., 1989, 1992; Grillner et al., 1997; Jordan, 1998; Jordan and Sławińska, 2014; Takakusaki et al., 2016). The nearby cholinergic PPT has also been suggested to be the primary component of the MLR (Garcia-Rill et al., 1986, 1987, 2011). Recent optogenetic and chemogenetic experiments, however, have cast doubt on the role of the cholinergic PPT neurons in the initiation of locomotion (Lee et al., 2014; Roseberry et al., 2016; Capelli et al., 2017; Kroeger et al., 2017; Caggiano et al., 2018; Josset et al., 2018). Rather, these studies emphasize the key role for glutamatergic neurons, especially in CnF and SubCnF regions, for initiating locomotion and suggest that cholinergic neurons may only have a role in the modulation of ongoing locomotor activity or play a role in non-locomotor functions of the MLR.

The MLR does not directly project to the spinal cord but rather activates spinal neurons controlling locomotion (Noga et al., 1995, 2003; Dai et al., 2005) by activation of reticulospinal (RS) neurons in the brainstem (Shik et al., 1967; Orlovskii, 1970; Shefchyk et al., 1984; Garcia-Rill and Skinner, 1987; Noga et al., 1988, 1991, 2003). These in turn descend through the ventral funiculus (Steeves and Jordan, 1984; Noga et al., 1991, 2003). This pathway, considered to be the "command pathway" for the initiation of locomotion (Shik et al., 1967; Jordan, 1998), activates spinal locomotor neurons, in part, by the release of glutamate (Douglas et al., 1993; Hägglund et al., 2010). Such results are supported by optogenetic studies in the mouse, which were used to stimulate glutamatergic RS neurons within the lateral paragigantocellular (LPGi) nucleus (Capelli et al., 2017). Photo-stimulation of these neurons evokes short-latency high-speed locomotion, while ablation of this population significantly reduces the speed of glutamatergic MLR-evoked locomotion. LPGi neurons receive a predominant glutamatergic input from the CnF (Capelli et al., 2017). Glutamatergic RS neurons expressing the transcription factors Lhx3 and/or Chx10 within the MedRF that are activated during locomotion and receive anatomical inputs from the MLR have also been described (Bretzner and Brownstone, 2013), supporting this concept.

In addition to RS command neurons, there is evidence that monoaminergic neurons may play a key role in the activation of spinal locomotor networks. For example, intravenous administration of noradrenergic and serotonergic precursors produces reflex discharges that resemble locomotion (Jankowska et al., 1967; Viala and Buser, 1969). Since then, many studies have shown that monoaminergic drugs may evoke or modulate locomotion in spinally injured cats (Barbeau and Rossignol, 1991; Kiehn et al., 1992; Marcoux and Rossignol, 2000), rats (Cazalets et al., 1992; Kiehn and Kjærulff, 1996; Feraboli-Lohnherr et al., 1999; Sqalli-Houssaini and Cazalets, 2000; Antri et al., 2002), and mice (Christie and Whelan, 2005). Since MLR stimulation produces a similar effect as seen with L-DOPA administration to the spinal cord, it was suggested that the MLR activates a noradrenergic descending system which controls the spinal locomotor generating network (Grillner and Shik, 1973). This idea is supported by the presence of catecholamine-containing neurons in the vicinity of the MLR (Steeves et al., 1976), the demonstration of direct projections from the MLR to the monoaminergic nuclei (Edwards, 1975; Steeves and Jordan, 1984; Sotnichenko, 1985) and the observation that both noradrenergic (Rasmussen et al., 1986) and serotonergic neurons are rhythmically active during overground or treadmill locomotion (Veasey et al., 1995). Recent work in our laboratory has now shown that during MLR-evoked locomotion, spinal monoamine release is widespread and modulated on a timescale of seconds, in tandem with centrally generated locomotion (Noga et al., 2017). While this release is observed during MLR-evoked locomotion, it is not obligatory since depletion of spinal NE or 5-HT does not abolish the MLR's ability to evoke locomotion (Steeves et al., 1980).

To enable MLR-evoked locomotion the activity within brainstem microcircuits must be modulated. In this study we aimed to identify the brainstem neurons activated by electrical stimulation of the MLR as this method is the current clinical standard for targeted stimulation of deep brain structures. MLR sites were identified by their low electrical thresholds and best locomotor responses to stimulation. In the first series of experiments, we documented the distribution of locomotor-activated neurons within the mesencephalon, pons, and medulla using c-*Fos* immunohistochemistry (IHC) (Herdegen and Leah, 1998) as an activity-dependent marker of induced locomotion (Huang et al., 2000; Dai et al., 2005; Noga et al., 2009, 2011). To gain perspective on cells potentially generating locomotor movements, i.e., those that are centrally activated in the absence of peripheral afferent feedback, we used the fictive locomotion preparation in which animals are paralyzed by neuromuscular blockade and locomotor activity is monitored

---

Abbreviations: 4, trochlear nucleus; 5M, motor trigeminal nucleus; 5SL, laminar spinal trigeminal nucleus; 5SP, spinal trigeminal nucleus; 5ST, spinal trigeminal tract; 7, facial nucleus; 7G, genu of the facial nerve; 7N, facial nerve; AMB, nucleus ambiguus; BC, brachium conjunctivum; bcm, marginal nucleus of the brachium conjunctivum; CI, inferior central nucleus; CnF, cuneiform nucleus; CU, cuneate nucleus; dmnV, dorsal motor nucleus of the vagus; DRG, dorsal root ganglion; FF, fields of Forel; FTC, central tegmental field; FTG, gigantocellular tegmental field; FTL, lateral tegmental field; FTM, magnocellular tegmental field; FTP, paralemniscal tegmental field; GR, gracile nucleus; IC, inferior colliculus; IO, inferior olive nucleus; KF, Kölliker–Fuse nucleus; LC, locus ceruleus; LDT, laterodorsal tegmental nucleus; LLD, dorsal nucleus of the lateral lemniscus; LRI, lateral reticular nucleus internal division; LRN, lateral reticular nucleus; MedRF, medial reticular formation; MLR, mesencephalic locomotor region; NRM, nucleus raphe magnus; NRO, nucleus raphe obscurus; NRP, nucleus raphe pallidus; NTS, nucleus tractus solitarii; P, pyramidal tract; PAG, periaqueductal gray; PPR, post-pyramidal nucleus of the raphe; PPT, pedunculopontine tegmental nucleus; RFN, retrofacial nucleus; RVLM, rostral ventrolateral medulla; SC, superior colliculus; SO, superior olivary nucleus; SubC, subceruleus; SubCnF, subcuneiform region; TB, trapezoid body; VIN, inferior vestibular nucleus; VLN, lateral vestibular nucleus; VMN, medial vestibular nucleus; VRG, ventral respiratory group; VTA, ventral tegmental area.

by electroneurogram (ENG) recordings from peripheral nerves. Animals subject to treadmill locomotion, with consequent phasic, sensory feedback were also examined for comparative purposes. In a second series of experiments, *Fos*+ cells were inspected for co-localization with either dopamine-beta-hydroxylase (DβH), 5-hydroxytryptamine (5-HT), or choline acetyltransferase (ChAT) to determine whether noradrenergic, serotonergic, or cholinergic neurons are activated during MLR-evoked fictive locomotion. The results reveal the anatomical correlate of the MLR, the target descending locomotor pathway neurons and provide evidence for a central coupling of locomotor, vestibular, respiratory, and cardiovascular networks during locomotion. Preliminary results have been reported (Noga et al., 2008).

MATERIALS AND METHODS

Animal Preparation

Experimental procedures were approved by the local University IACUC committees in accordance with the National Institute of Health guidelines (NIH Publications No. 80-23; revised 1996). The number of animals used, and their pain and distress, were minimized. Experiments were performed on 10 adult female cats weighing between 1.9 and 4.3 kg subject to precollicular–postmammillary decerebration. Experimental procedures for treadmill and fictive locomotion experiments were as described previously (Dai et al., 2005; Noga et al., 2009). For fictive locomotion experiments, nerves to one flexor and extensor muscle supplying each of the hindlimbs and forelimbs were dissected, bilaterally, and mounted in tunnel electrodes. The head of each animal was fixed in a Transvertex headframe. In treadmill-locomotion (TL-1) and treadmill-control (TC-1 and TC-2) experiments, all four limbs were free to step on a treadmill belt, and the hindquarters were suspended by a sling under the abdomen. In fictive-locomotion (FL-1,2,3) and fictive-control (FC-1,2,3,4) experiments, the animals were suspended with all four limbs pendant. **Table 1** summarizes the procedural details of animals included in the present study.

Stimulation and Recording

The experimental setup is illustrated in **Figure 1**. Following a recovery period from the decerebration of 1.5–3 h, 4-limbed locomotion was evoked by electrical stimulation of the MLR (1.0 ms square wave pulses, 15–20 Hz) using monopolar stimulating electrodes (SNE-300; David Kopf Instruments, Tujunga, CA, United States) as previously described (Noga et al., 2009, 2011). Electrodes were stereotaxically inserted into the mesopontine tegmentum at an area bounded by posterior (P) 1–3 and lateral (L) 3.0–5.0 mm and included the CnF, bcm within the SubCnF region, and the PPT. Electrodes were typically advanced slowly while stimulating, thus limiting the stimulation of unrelated sites, until the optimal locomotor response was obtained. Thresholds were then tested. If no response was noted or if stimulation strength was high, the electrode was repositioned, and the procedure repeated. Final position was determined by the best locomotor response (greatest ENG amplitudes presenting in locomotor-like rhythms) provided by the lowest threshold at the specified frequency and pulse width. Tract coordinates and electrode depth were noted. In some experiments, electrodes were repositioned in small incremental steps and responses to electrical stimulation at the same strength (slightly above predetermined thresholds) were examined (**Figure 2**) as a further validation of the threshold test results. During the experiment, the strength of stimulation was adjusted to a level which was suitable to maintain locomotion for prolonged periods. Locomotion was monitored by visual confirmation of weight support and walking on the treadmill (treadmill experiments: belt speed: ~0.46 m/s) or from ENG recordings (fictive locomotion experiments). Representative ENG activity was obtained from the bouts of locomotion throughout the stimulation period (**Figures 1B, 2**). The ENG signals were amplified with AC-coupled amplifiers (bandwidth 300 Hz to 10 kHz), rectified and low-pass filtered (10 or 20 ms

TABLE 1 | Animals and experimental procedures.

ID	Study	Total time locomotion (min)	Time end of stim to perfusion (h)	Time decerebration to perfusion (h)	IHC procedures	Previous study designation
FL-1	1	157	1	9	DAB (Fos)	FL-1†
FL-2	1	210	1	9	DAB (Fos)	FL-2†
FL-3	2	262	1	10	Fluorescence (Fos, DβH, ChAT, 5-HT)	LC-1††
FC-1	1	<1	6	8.5	DAB (Fos)	FC-1†
FC-2	1	<1	6	8.5	DAB (Fos)	FC-2†
FC-3	1	No stim	–	9	DAB (Fos)	FC-4†
FC-4	2	<1	8	10	Fluorescence (Fos, DβH, ChAT, 5-HT)	C††
TL-1	1	322	1	9	DAB (Fos)	TL-1†
TC-1	1	<1	7	8.5	DAB (Fos)	TC-1†
TC-2	1	No stim	–	9	DAB (Fos)	TC-2†

Animals are assigned into different groups: fictive locomotion (FL); treadmill locomotion (TL); fictive control (FC); and treadmill control (TL). †Dai et al. (2005) and ††Noga et al. (2009, 2011).

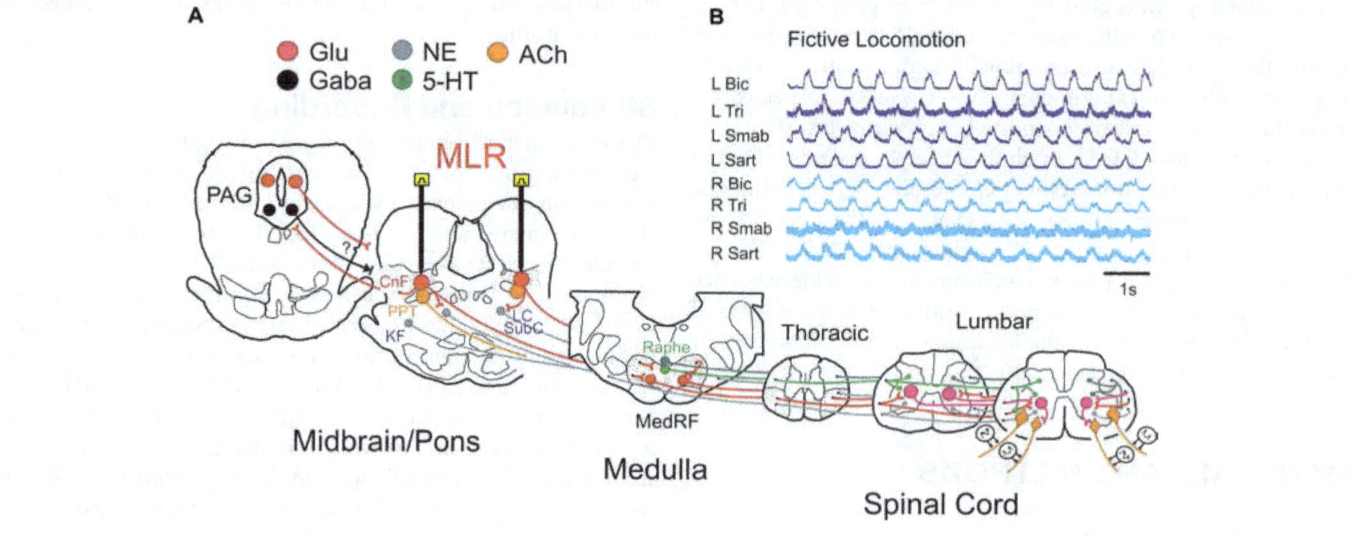

FIGURE 1 | Experimental schema illustrating the brainstem network involved in neuromodulation of locomotor command with stimulation of the MLR. **(A)** Schematic diagram of the brainstem showing the putative anatomical correlates of the MLR, the cuneiform (CnF), and pedunculopontine tegmental (PPT) nuclei, and their putative target neurons within the midbrain/pons and medulla: the periaqueductal gray (PAG), the glutamatergic reticulospinal (RS) neurons within the medial reticular formation (MedRF), the noradrenergic nuclei locus ceruleus (LC), subceruleus (SubC) and Kölliker–Fuse (KF), and the serotonergic nuclei (Edwards, 1975; Steeves and Jordan, 1984; Sotnichenko, 1985). Axons of RS, noradrenergic and serotonergic neurons innervate locomotor central pattern generator neurons (Steeves and Jordan, 1980; Noga et al., 2003, 2009, 2011, 2017). The projections of neurons releasing the neurotransmitters glutamate (Glu), acetylcholine (ACh), noradrenaline (NE), serotonin (5-HT), and gamma-aminobutyric acid (GABA) are depicted across the major relays in locomotion control. **(B)** Example of fictive locomotor activity as monitored by electroneurogram (ENG) recordings from peripheral nerves from all limbs. R, right; L, left; Bic, biceps brachii; Tri, triceps brachii; Smab, semimembranosus/anterior biceps, Sart, sartorius.

time constant), and subsequently digitized through a 1 MHz, 16 channel analog-to-digital converter (12 bit) at 2–4 kHz using customized software (Spinal Cord Research Centre, University of Manitoba, Canada).

Tissue Perfusion

In all of the experiments reported here, there was an 8.5–10 h interval between decerebration and perfusion to reduce *Fos* expression resulting from surgical procedures (**Table 1**). At the end of each locomotor experiment, after a 1 h interval with no-stimulation and immediately prior to perfusion, a small electrolytic lesion was made to mark the MLR stimulation site(s). Animals were re-anesthetized with either halothane or sodium pentobarbital (30 mg/kg) and perfused transcardially with normal saline (0.3 ml/g of animal weight) containing 0.1% $NaNO_2$ and 100 units/ml heparin, followed by 4% paraformaldehyde, 0.2% picric acid, in 0.1 M phosphate-buffered saline (PBS, 4°C), pH 7.4 (1 ml/g of animal weight). The brainstems were removed, post-fixed in the fixative solution for 5 h, and cryoprotected by washing in a solution containing 25% sucrose, 10% glycerol, and 0.001% sodium azide in 0.1 M phosphate buffer for several days.

Immunohistochemistry

The immunohistochemical analysis was carried out on brainstem tissue obtained from animals described in our previous publications on MLR-evoked spinal cord *Fos* expression (Dai et al., 2005; Noga et al., 2009, 2011). **Table 1** summarizes the designations (animal ID) for the present study and from previous studies. Frozen tissue sections of 20 (Dai et al., 2005) or 30 μm (Noga et al., 2009, 2011) thickness were sectioned in a sagittal or coronal plane with a sliding microtome and collected in 0.1 M PBS. To optimize immunohistochemical procedures, a small group of sections were randomly collected from the brainstem segments and a primary antibody dilution series performed. In addition, for the pre-adsorption control, cat tissue sections were incubated only with pre-immuno serum without the primary antibodies. Immunoreactivity was totally absent after omission of all primary antibodies. Controls conducted for double labeling demonstrated no cross-reactivity between primary antibodies and inappropriate secondary antibodies. Selected serial sections of the brainstem were processed to label c-*Fos* nuclear protein alone or co-localized with either DβH, 5-HT, or ChAT to identify activated noradrenergic, serotonergic, or cholinergic brainstem neurons. Two experimental protocols were followed. In Study 1, examining the distribution of activated neurons, *Fos* was stained using diaminobenzidine (DAB) IHC (Dai et al., 2005). Sections were incubated for 72 h in sheep polyclonal anti-*Fos* IgG (Cambridge Research Biochemical) 1:2,000. In Study 2, we examined the distribution of *Fos*-activated noradrenergic, serotonergic, or cholinergic neurons. Cells were stained for *Fos*, and either DβH, 5-HT, or ChAT using fluorescent immunohistochemical techniques (Noga et al., 2009, 2011). Sections were incubated 48 h in rabbit polyclonal anti-*Fos* IgG (PC38-100U: Oncogene Research Products/Calbiochem, San Diego, CA, United States) 1:2,500. Sections were then incubated for 48 h in either mouse monoclonal anti-DβH IgG (MAB308: Chemicon International, Temecula, CA, United States) 1:500, rat

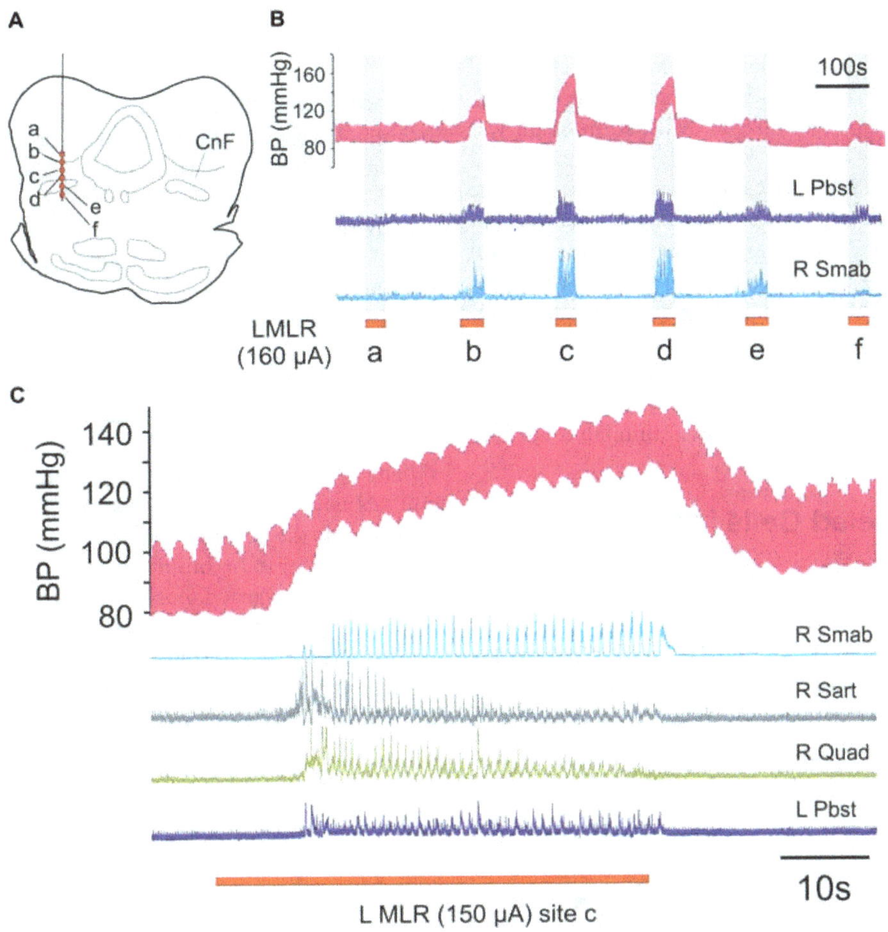

FIGURE 2 | Mapping of locomotor responses to electrical stimulation of the MLR and surrounding region of the midbrain. Stimulation of CnF and SubCnF sites **(A)** produces largest locomotor and pressor responses **(B)** in neuromuscular paralyzed and artificially ventilated decerebrate cats. Note reduced ENG responses in ventral stimulation locations. Locomotion monitored by electroneurogram recordings from hindlimb peripheral nerves. Blood pressure responses measured from indwelling catheter (carotid artery). **(C)** Locomotor and pressure responses to stimulation of site *c*. Low amplitude pressor responses (~0.4 Hz) result from artificial respiration of the animal. R, right; L, left; Pbst: posterior biceps/semitendinosus; Smab, semimembranosus/anterior biceps; Sart, sartorius; Quad, quadriceps.

monoclonal anti-5-HT IgG (MAB352: Chemicon International, Temecula, CA, United States) 1:100, or goat polyclonal anti-ChAT IgG (AB144P: Millipore) 1:100. Each secondary antibody was conjugated to a different fluorophore (Molecular Probes-Invitrogen, Carlsbad, CA, United States): Alexa 488 (green) for *Fos* (1:500; goat anti-rabbit, A-11008), Alexa 594 (red) for DβH (1:500; goat anti-mouse, A-11005), Alexa 594 for 5-HT (1:200; goat anti-rat; A-11007), and Alexa 594 for ChAT (1:200; donkey anti-goat).

Data Analysis and Interpretation

Anatomical landmarks from sagittal or coronal brainstem sections were identified using an atlas of the cat brainstem (Berman, 1968). The location of the stimulation sites were determined from depth measurements taken from the surface of the IC of the electrode along the reconstructed electrode tracks and also from a small electrolytic lesions made in the MLR prior to perfusion. For DAB experiments, sections were examined under a light microscope, and cellular architecture, as well as locations of labeled cells, were drawn using a camera lucida. For co-localization experiments, sections were examined with Zeiss Axioline microscopes using fluorescence microscopy. Cells were mapped using Neurolucida software. Cell counts were done using stereologic cell counting methods (Stereo Investigator 5.0, Microbrightfield Bioscience, Inc., Williston, VT, United States) giving estimates of cell number per sections and or nuclei. Cell positions of labeled neurons were determined by reconstruction of individual images of each section at 10× power. Confocal microscopy (Zeiss LSM510, with Ar multiline and HeN1 564) was used for high power examination of the three-dimensional structure of selected cells. Noradrenergic, cholinergic, and serotonergic cells were scanned in a series of optical sections and three-dimensional reconstructions were digitized. Serotonergic innervation of *Fos*-labeled reticular neurons (Di Prisco et al., 1994; Antri et al., 2008) was assessed using criteria previously established for spinal locomotor activated neurons (Noga et al., 2009).

RESULTS

Locomotion was evoked by stimulation of the MLR for a period of 2.5–5.5 h in four animals (FL-1, FL-2, FL-3, and TL-1; **Table 1**). In three animals (FL-1, FL-2, and TL-1), MLR stimulation was confined to one side (Study 1). In FL-3, both sides were stimulated during the testing period (Study 2). Control animals received the same surgical procedures as the locomotor test animals, except that they were not subject to the full locomotor task. Most control animals (FC-1, FC-2, FC-4, and TC-1) could produce locomotion with MLR stimulation but were only briefly stimulated. Sub-optimal sites were stimulated only briefly during the search for low threshold sites (see the section "Materials and Methods"), limiting their possible contribution to overall *Fos* expression. Two animals (FC-3 and TC-2) were neither stimulated nor had stimulating electrodes inserted.

Study 1: *Fos*-Labeled Cells in the Brainstem

Sagittal sections of the brainstems from two fictive locomotion animals (FL-1 and FL-2), one treadmill locomotion (TL-1), and five control animals (FC-1–3, TC-1, and TC-2) were stained for *Fos* using the DAB method and examined under the microscope. Representative photomicrographs illustrating the appearance of *Fos*-labeled neurons in the CnF and the SubCnF region (bcm) from FL-2 cat are shown in **Figure 3A**.

Locomotor Experiments

In animals subject to the locomotion protocol, the best locomotor responses were observed with stimulation within the CnF and SubCnF region (bcm), dorsal to the BC (**Figure 2**). At the frequencies used (15–20 Hz), the response produced by stimulation in more ventral sites including the BC and/or PPT was either of lower amplitude or consisted of erratic or tonic nerve activity. Stimulation of the MLR invariably increased blood pressure during the stimulation period, the amplitude of which was highest during stimulation of the best locomotor points (**Figure 2**). Stimulation strengths adjusted to maintain locomotor bouts over long periods of time ranged between 50 and 160 μA.

The distribution of *Fos*-labeled neurons from three locomotor animals is presented in **Figures 3** (FL-2) and 4 (FL-1 and TL-1). Overall, the distribution of labeled cells within fictive and treadmill locomotor animals was similar, indicating that *Fos* expression is governed more by the central drive than by afferent feedback. Labeled neurons were observed in several brainstem nuclei and were typically greater in number on the side of stimulation. (1) CnF: large numbers of cells were labeled in the CnF on the side of stimulation (*insets*, **Figures 3, 4**). Fewer cells

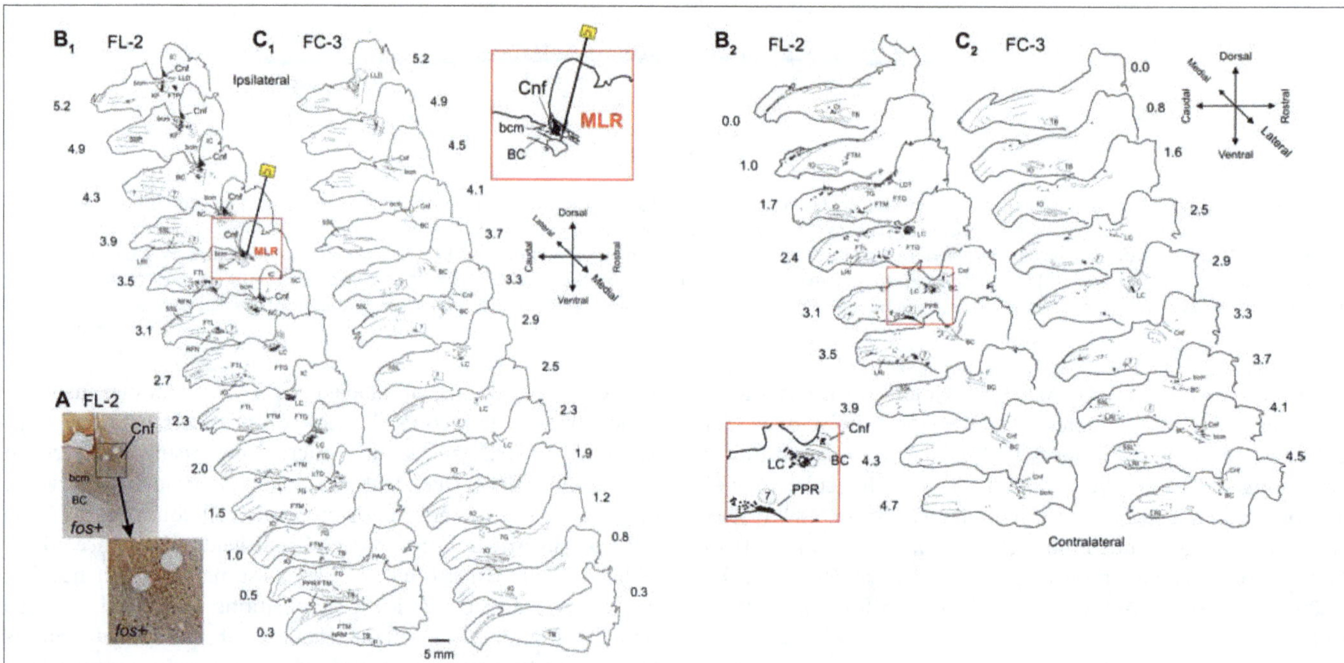

FIGURE 3 | Distribution of *Fos* labeled neurons in the brainstem of a MLR-evoked fictive locomotor cat compared to non-locomotor control cat. **(A)** Photomicrographs illustrating the appearance of *Fos* labeled neurons near the stimulation electrode in the CnF and SubCnF region. Inset: higher magnification image of indicated area. **($B_{1,2}$,$C_{1,2}$)** Camera lucida drawings showing distribution of *Fos* immunoreactive neurons in brainstem of fictive locomotor cat FL-2 and non-locomotor control cat FC-3, respectively. Images in **(B_1)** and **(B_2)** show distribution on side ipsilateral and contralateral to the stimulating electrode (indicated in sagittal section at 3.5 mm from midline), respectively. Images in **(C_1)** and **(C_2)** show distribution on right and left sides of the brainstem, respectively. Note dense labeling within the CnF, the bcm of the SubCnF region, the locus ceruleus (LC), the lateral tegmental field (FTL), the magnocellular tegmental field (FTM), and the parapyramidal region (PPR). Labeling was more robust on side of stimulation. Control animals show relatively low numbers of labeled cells. Each diagram includes all labeled cells from single sections at the indicated levels. Each dot represents one labeled cell in this and other figures. Insets: higher magnification of MLR stimulation site in **(B_1)** (lateral 3.5 mm) and LC/FTL/PPR region in **(B_2)** (contralateral 3.1 mm). Anatomical structures labeled in this and other figures are listed under Abbreviations.

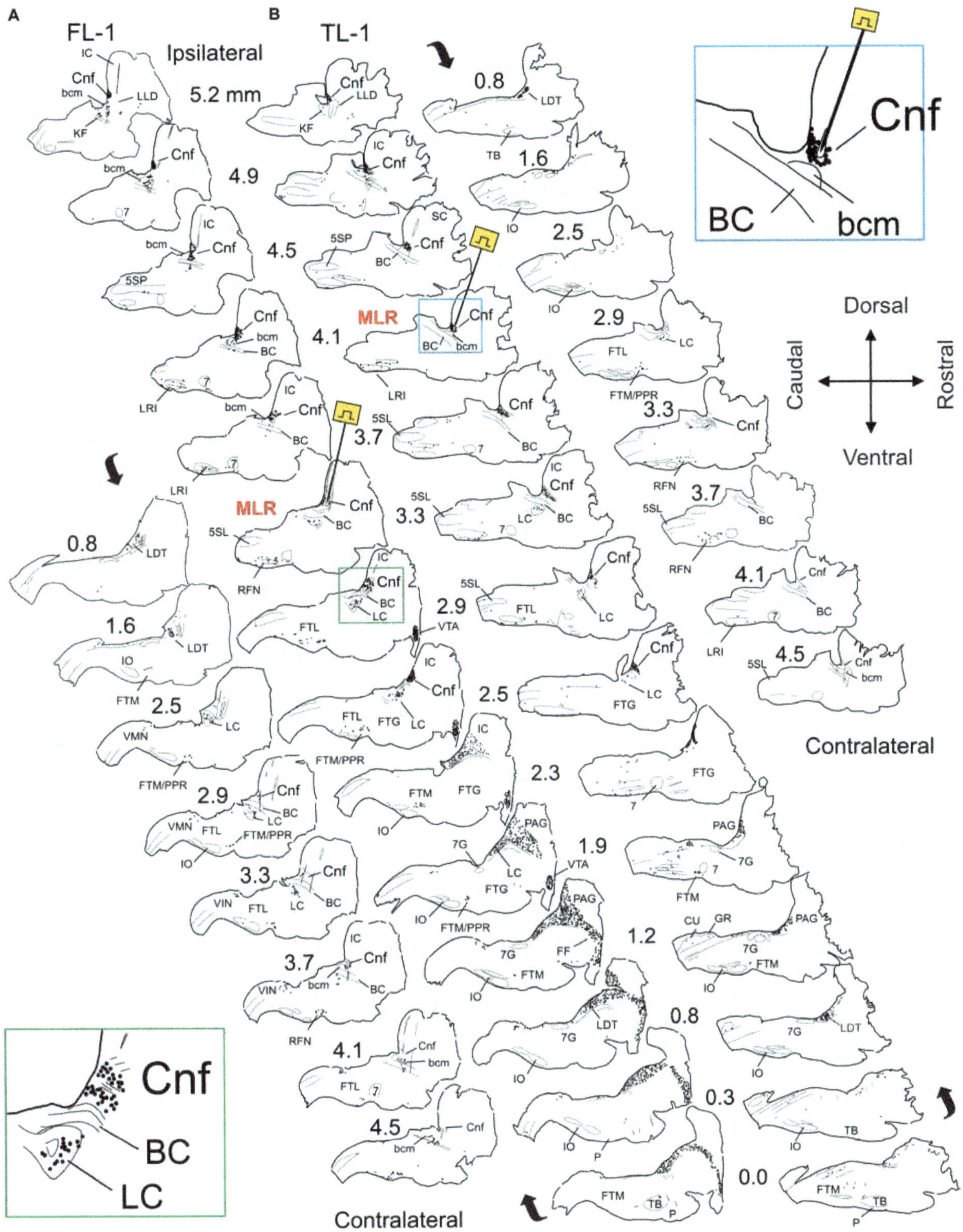

FIGURE 4 | Distribution of *Fos* labeled neurons in the brainstem of MLR-evoked fictive locomotor cat 1 (FL-1) and treadmill locomotor cat 1 (TL-1). **(A,B)** Camera lucida drawings showing distribution of *Fos* immunoreactive neurons in brainstem. Site of MLR stimulation electrodes indicated in sagittal sections at 3.3 and 4.1 mm lateral to midline for FL-1 **(A)** and TL-1 **(B)**, respectively. Note dense labeling within the CnF, bcm, the laterodorsal tegmental nucleus (LDT), the LC, the FTL, the FTM, and the PPR in both animals. Strong labeling was also observed in the periaqueductal gray (PAG) and ventral tegmental area (VTA) of FL-1 and less so in the PAG of TL-1. Labeling was more robust on side of stimulation. Insets: higher magnification of CnF/LC region in FL-1 (**A:** ipsilateral 2.9 mm) and MLR stimulation site in TL-1 (**B:** lateral 3.5 mm).

were observed in the contralateral CnF (e.g., FL-1; **Figure 4**). (2) bcm: cells in the bcm of the SubCnF region were labeled in all animals. (3) LC: cells in the LC were labeled bilaterally in all locomotor cats (**Figure 4**, *inset*). (4) KF: labeled cells were found bilaterally in the area of the KF. (5) PPT: a small group of labeled cells located rostral to the bcm and KF, in lateral sections on the side of stimulation (lateral L4.3–5.2) was seen in cat FL-2 (**Figure 3B**$_1$) but not cats FL-1 and TL-1 (**Figure 4**). *Fos*+ neurons were also observed more caudally in an area medial and ventral to the BC. The phenotype(s) of these neurons is not clear without ChAT immunostaining (Garcia-Rill et al., 1987) and cells in this area overlap with cells of the LC. (6) Laterodorsal tegmental nucleus (LDT): *Fos*+ cells were observed in the LDT on the ventromedial border of the caudal ventrolateral PAG in all locomotor animals (**Figure 3B**$_1$ – L0.5–1.5 and **Figures 4A,B** – L0.8–1.2). (7) PAG: many *Fos*-labeled neurons of the ipsilateral PAG were labeled at-level and rostral to the site of stimulation in FL-Cat1 (**Figures 3B1,2, 4A,B**). A small number of cells within the PAG of TL-1 was also labeled. (8) FF: a column of *Fos*+ cells extended rostrally and ventrally from the PAG (**Figure 4A** – L0–1.2) through the central gray and the FF toward the VTA of FL-1. (9) The VTA of Tsai was labeled on the side of stimulation of cat FL-1 (**Figures 3B1,2, 4A,B** – L1.9–2.9). It was not possible to evaluate the contralateral VTA since tissue along the cut edge of the brain (decerebration) was contaminated with blood cells. (10) FTL: numerous cells were labeled bilaterally in the FTL (L4.0–2.0) in all locomotor animals (**Figures 3B, 4A,B**). Most cells were located in an area bounded rostrally by the facial nucleus (7N), caudally by the LRI, and ventrally by the inferior olivary nucleus (IO) (**Figure 3B**$_2$, *inset*). Few, if any, cells were found in the LRI or the trigeminal nuclei (5SL and 5SP). Around L3, the length of this cell column shortened and was concentrated in the medulla near the ponto-medullary junction. The labeled cells in this area overlapped the areas occupied by the AMB and the RFN. (11) FTM: *Fos*-labeled cells were found bilaterally in an area immediately caudal to the TB and rostral to the IO from about L0.5 to 2.0 at the ponto-medullary junction in all locomotor animals. Some labeled cells also appeared in an area just dorsal to the TB. Cells toward the midline were in the region of the NRM and obscurus (NRO). (12) Dorsal medulla: a small group of cells located bilaterally in the dorsal medulla was labeled in locomotor cats (**Figures 3B, 4A,B**). Most of the cells were located in the area of the NTS, the dmnV, and the vestibular nuclei (VLN) (VIN, VMN) (L1–3.5). (13) CU and GR: a few labeled neurons were observed in the CU and GR of TL-1 (**Figure 4B**, L1.2) but not in FL-1 and FL-2. (14) Central canal: a strip of labeled neurons were observed surrounding the central canal in caudal brainstem sections of FL-2 (**Figure 3B**$_1$) but was not observed in FL-1 and TL-1.

Non-locomotor Control Experiments

Limited labeling in the various brainstem nuclei was seen in control animals, including those that were stimulated only briefly to ensure that the brainstem health was comparable to locomotor animals. Many hours elapsed between this brief locomotor bout and perfusion (**Table 1**) to minimize *Fos* expression in the Control animals. Labeling was not observed in the CnF nucleus of FC-3 (**Figures 3C1,2**), the non-stimulated control, although sparse labeling was seen in the bcm. This animal was representative of the other fictive locomotion cats and showed higher numbers of labeled cells in comparison to treadmill control animals (**Figure 5A**). The increased numbers of cells in the fictive-control animals as compared with the treadmill-control animals is most likely due to the additional sensory input produced by the nerve dissection surgery and placement of the animals in the spinal frame.

Comparisons of the Number of Labeled Cells in Locomotor and Control Animals

Fos labeling in the brainstem, MedRF, and LC of locomotor animals was much higher than that seen in their respective controls (**Figure 5**). In locomotor animals, the total number of labeled cells was highest in FL-1. This was primarily due to the large number of labeled cells within the PAG, although there was a scattering of labeled cells in the PAG of TL-1 (**Figure 4**: 1.9 and 1.2 lateral to midline). Inspection of panels from **Figures 3, 4** show that the number of labeled cells was also greater on the side of stimulation than on the opposite, unstimulated side. This is shown for the LC of locomotor animals in **Figure 5C**.

Study 2: Phenotyping of *Fos*-Labeled Cells in the Brainstem

A second set of experiments were done combining *Fos* IHC with staining for either DβH, ChAT, or 5-HT to identify noradrenergic, cholinergic, and serotonergic neurons, respectively. As in Study 1 animals, the best locomotor responses were obtained with stimulation within the CnF and SubCnF region (bcm), dorsal to the BC. Four-limbed locomotion was evoked by stimulation of both sides of the brainstem, either separately or together to maintain locomotor bouts lasting upward of 100 min at a time for a total of 262 min. Stimulation in more ventral sites failed to induce coordinated locomotion and instead evoked erratic or tonic nerve activity. The brainstem viability was comparable in control (FC-4) and locomotor (FL-3) cats since the control animal was also capable of four-limbed locomotion, but was stimulated only briefly (~1 min), 8 h before perfusion.

DβH/*Fos* Immunohistochemistry

Dopamine-beta-hydroxylase IHC was used to quantify the number of noradrenergic neurons in midbrain and pons activated during MLR-evoked lcocomotion. Numerous noradrenergic neurons were observed in the LC, SubC, and KF of both locomotor and control animals. Noradrenergic neurons were medium-sized oval, fusiform, or round (**Figures 6A–D**). Maps of *Fos*- and/or DBH-stained neurons within the brainstems of locomotor and control cats are illustrated in **Figures 6E,F**.

Locomotor experiment

As observed in Study 1 animals, abundant *Fos*-labeled neurons were observed in the CnF (sites of stimulation), the bcm or SubCnF region, FTC, PAG, LDT, LC, SubC, and KF of cat FL-3. *Fos*+ cells were generally symmetrically distributed in this bilaterally stimulated animal. Fewer neurons were labeled in the

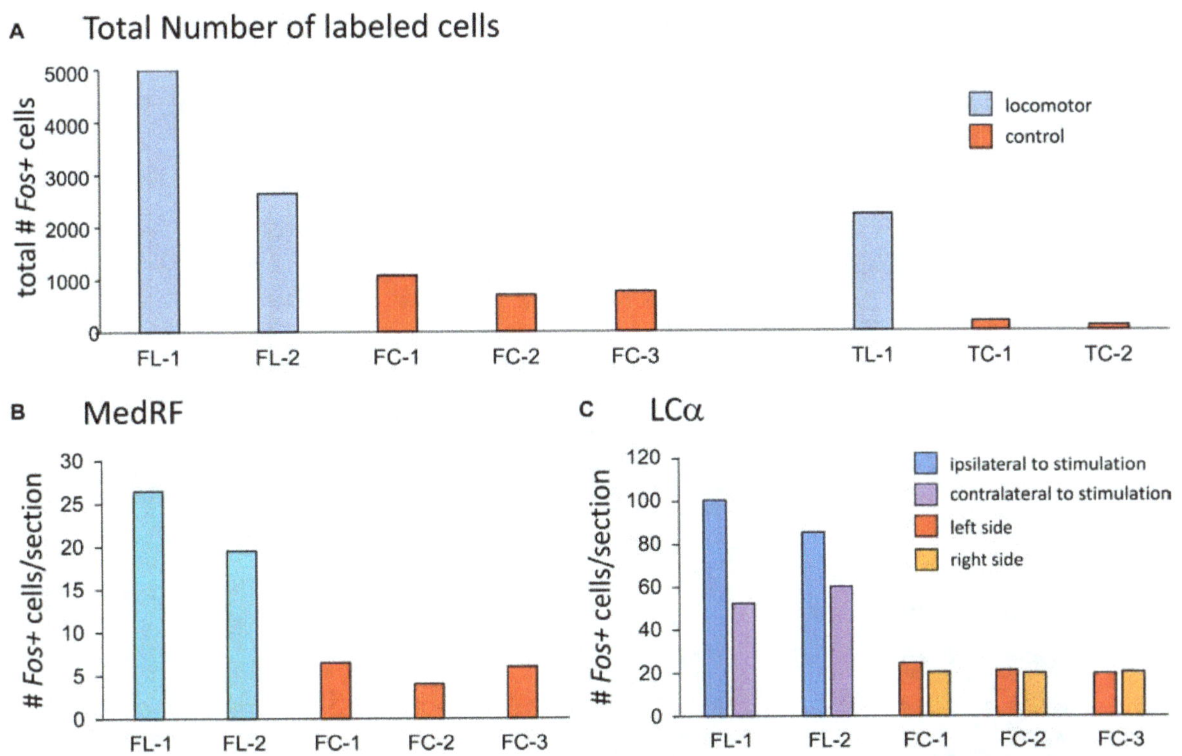

FIGURE 5 | Comparisons of numbers of *Fos*-labeled cells within the brainstem, MedRF, and locus ceruleus alpha (LCα) of MLR-evoked locomotor and control cats. The total number of labeled cells in both fictive and treadmill locomotor animals exceeds that observed in respective control animals **(A)**. Likewise, the number of *Fos*+ cells/section within the MedRF **(B)** and LCα **(C)** was consistently much higher that observed in control animals. The number of *Fos*-labeled cells/section in the LCα was higher on the side of stimulation.

superior (SC) and IC pontine FTL and FTG (**Figure 6E** - P4 and P5). Large numbers of *Fos*+ neurons in the LC/SubC and KF stained positive for DβH (**Figures 6A–D**), indicating that many of the Fos+ labeled cells in the LC region in Study 1 were likely noradrenergic (**Figure 5C**). While the majority of *Fos*+ noradrenergic neurons were located 1–2 mm away from the sites of stimulation, a scattering of *Fos*+ noradrenergic neurons were also observed in the parabrachial region nearer to the electrode stimulation site, as reported previously (Steeves et al., 1976).

Non-locomotor control

Like Study 1, few *Fos*-labeled cells were observed in the control animal (**Figure 6F**) than in the locomotor animal (**Figure 6E**). Furthermore, relatively few noradrenergic neurons in the control animal showed *Fos* expression. Interestingly, *Fos* co-expression in some sections was slightly higher on the side of the stimulation used to demonstrate that the control animal was capable of MLR-evoked locomotion.

Distribution of Fos-labeled DβH neurons

The rostro-caudal distribution of *Fos*+ cells observed in the brainstem of locomotor (FL-3) and control (FC-4) cats is illustrated in **Figure 7A**. In FL-3, the greatest number of *Fos*+ cells was found between P0.5 and P3.3, with a peak at P1.6 near the MLR stimulation site located at P1.8 (note that the electrolytic lesion used to mark the stimulation sites likely resulted in an underestimate of the number of *Fos*+ cells at that level). This represented a 6–144-fold increase in the number of *Fos*+ cells compared to the control animal. At more caudal levels (P3.7–5.0), the number of *Fos*-labeled neurons in the locomotor animal was 3–10 times greater than the control. The number of *Fos* immunoreactive noradrenergic neurons was also dramatically increased in the locomotor animal compared to the control (**Figure 7B**). The largest number of *Fos*+/DβH cells in FL-3 was found between P2.25 and P4.0 and peaked at P3.3 where all three noradrenergic nuclei (LC, SubC, and KF) were present. Between P2 and P4, ~75–100% of noradrenergic cells showed *Fos* co-expression. In contrast, relatively few noradrenergic neurons between P2-4 showed *Fos* labeling in the control animal (0–37%).

ChAT/*Fos* Immunohistochemistry

Choline acetyltransferase IHC was used to quantify the number of cholinergic neurons in midbrain and pons activated during MLR-evoked locomotion. Numerous cholinergic neurons were observed in the PPT, LDT, trochlear (4), and motor trigeminal (5M) nuclei of both locomotor and control animals. The neurons were medium-sized, irregular multipolar shaped. Photomicrographs taken from single sections through the LDT and PPT of cat FL-3 are illustrated in **Figures 8A–D**. Maps of *Fos*- and/or ChAT-stained neurons within the brainstems of locomotor and control cats are

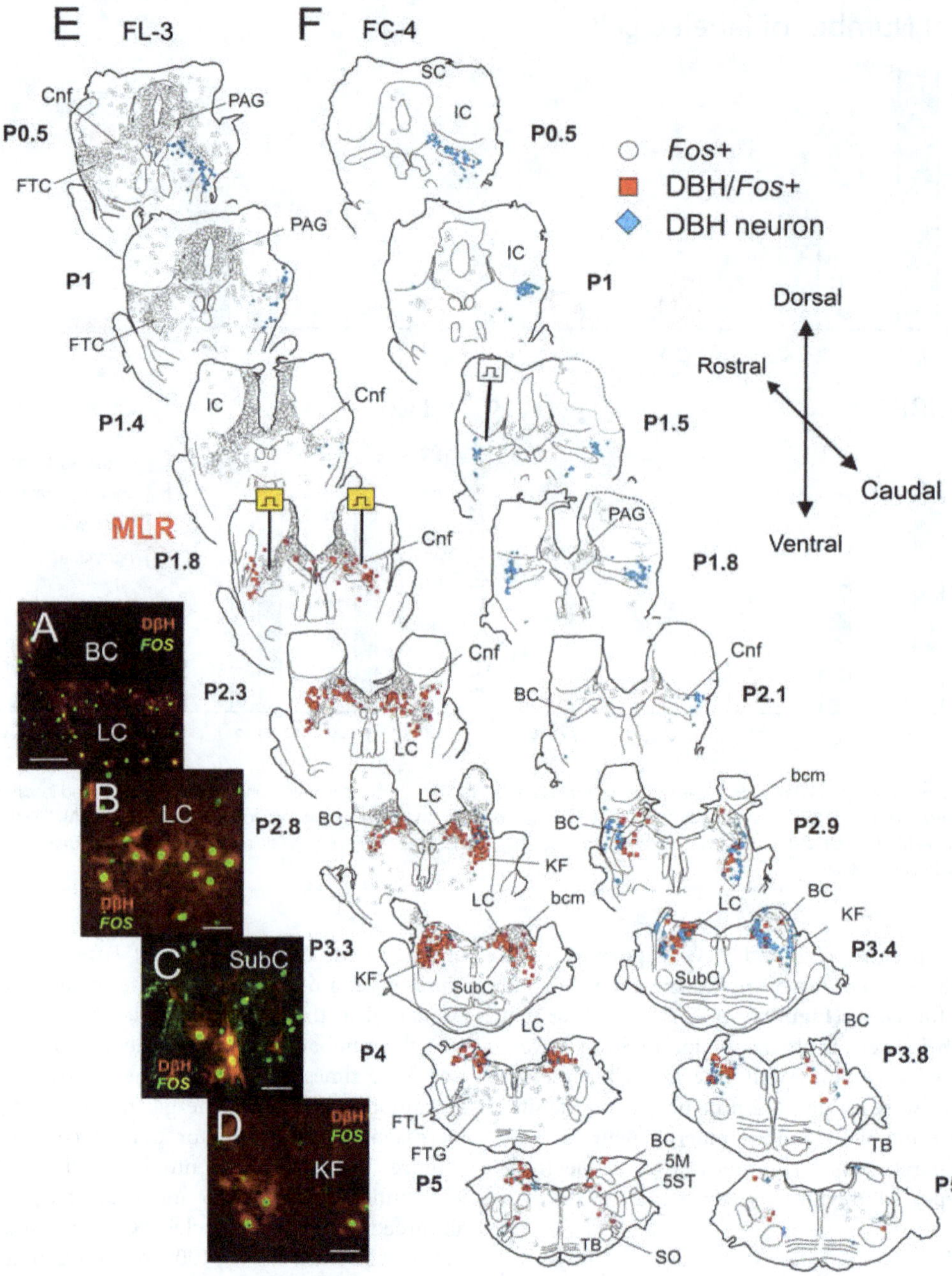

FIGURE 6 | Noradrenergic neurons within the locus ceruleus (LC), subceruleus (SubC), and Kölliker–Fuse (KF) nuclei show activity-dependent *Fos* labeling following MLR-evoked fictive locomotion in the decerebrate cat. **(A–D)** Immunocytochemical identification of noradrenergic locomotor-activated neurons co-stained with *Fos* (*green*) and dopamine-β-hydroxylase or DβH (red). Confocal photomicrographs of cells located in LC **(A,B)**, SubC **(C)**, and KF **(D)** of fictive locomotor cat 3 (FL-3). Note that some cells showed only *Fos* labeling. **(E,F)** Camera lucida drawings showing distribution of *Fos*, DβH/*Fos*, and DβH immunoreactive neurons in locomotor and control cats, respectively. MLR stimulation electrodes were located at posterior 1.8 (P1.8; Berman, 1968). Testing electrode in control cat FC-4 was found at P1.5. In the MLR locomotor cat, abundant *Fos*-labeled neurons were observed in the CnF (site of stimulation), the bcm or SubCnF region, the PAG, LDT, LC, and the FTL. Large numbers of *Fos*+ neurons in the LC/SubC and KF stained positive for DβH. A few scattered *Fos*+ cells were observed in the inferior colliculus (IC) and superior colliculus (SC). The control animal was only briefly stimulated (50 s of locomotor activity total), indicating comparable health of the brain stem and spinal cord. Fewer *Fos*-labeled neurons were observed in FC-4, although there were slightly more *Fos*-labeled cells on the side of the MLR stimulation test. Scale bar: 100 μm **(A)** and 40 μm **(B–D)**.

illustrated in **Figures 8E,F**. At their most rostral location, PPT neurons were observed more ventrolaterally within the tegmentum. Caudally, PPT neurons were observed loosely scattered around or ventral to the BC in areas occupied by noradrenergic neurons stained in other adjacent sections (**Figures 6E,F**).

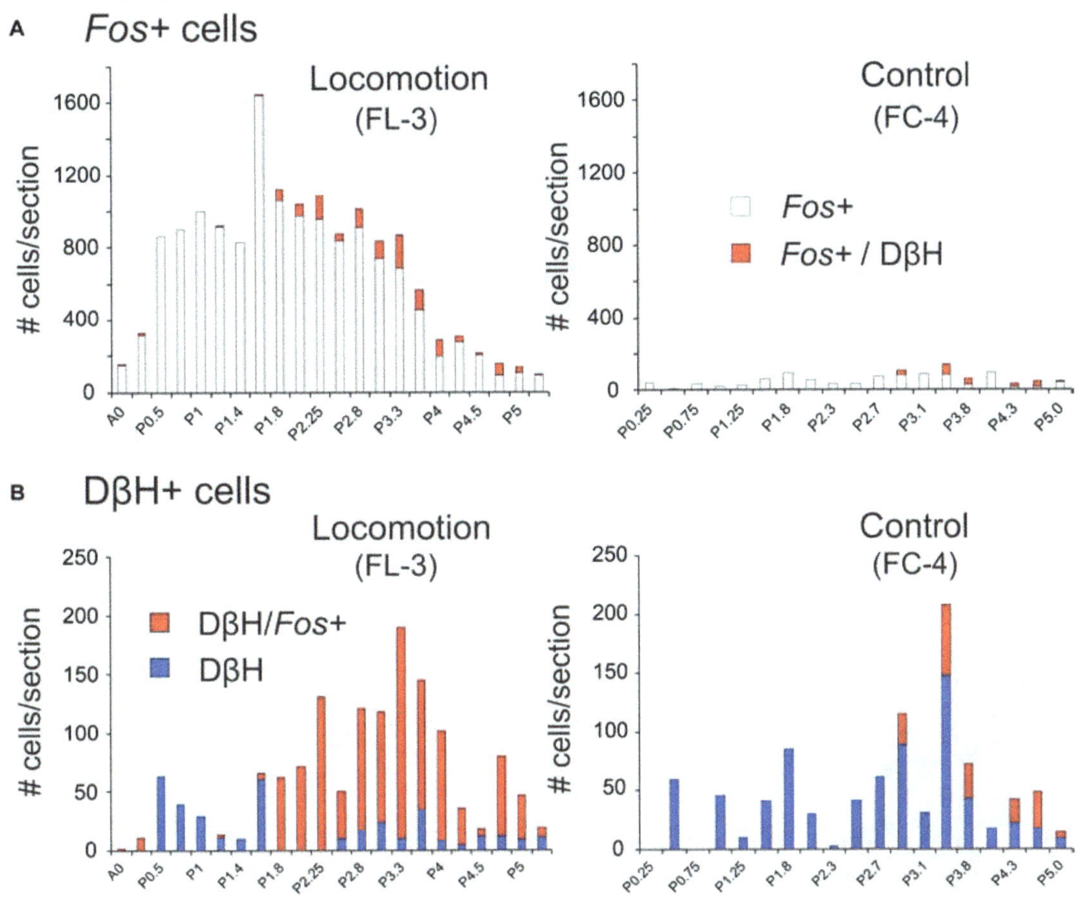

FIGURE 7 | Distribution of *Fos*+ neurons with or without co-labeling with DβH in the midbrain and pons following bilateral stimulation of the MLR. **(A)** The number of *Fos*-labeled cells increased tremendously in FL-3 compared to the non-locomotor control animal (FC-4). **(B)** Noradrenergic neurons showed dramatic increases in *Fos* expression in the locomotor animal. Numeration includes all labeled cells from single sections at the indicated levels.

Locomotor experiment

As observed in sections stained for *Fos* and DβH (**Figures 6E,F**), a large number of *Fos*-labeled neurons were observed in the CnF (sites of stimulation), bcm, PPT, FTC, PAG, LDT, LC, SubC, and KF. Caudally, a few neurons were labeled in the FTL and FTG (**Figure 8E** – P5.5 and P6). Relatively few cholinergic PPT neurons, however, stained positive for *Fos* (**Figure 8E**). Cholinergic PPT neurons were located ventral to sites producing the best locomotor response to electrical stimulation. In the LDT, a number of cholinergic neurons also stained positive for *Fos*. This group of cells accounted for about 50% of the double-labeled cholinergic neurons in the locomotor animal. Cholinergic motoneurons in cranial nerve nuclei [trochlear nucleus (4) and motor trigeminal nucleus (5M)] did not stain for *Fos*.

Non-locomotor control

As before, fewer *Fos*-labeled cells were observed in the control animal (**Figure 8F**) than in the fictive locomotor animal (**Figure 8E**). Likewise, few PPT cholinergic neurons showed *Fos* co-expression although there were a number of double labeled cells in the LDT. As in locomotor animals, no motor nuclei (4 and 5M) were double labeled.

Distribution of Fos-labeled ChAT neurons

The rostro-caudal distribution of ChAT and/or *Fos*+ cells in control and locomotor animals is shown in **Figure 9**. In FL-3, *Fos*+ cells peaked at P1.7 near the MLR stimulation sites (lesion visible at this level). This represented an approximately eightfold increase compared to the control. At more caudal levels (~P2.4–4.2), the number of *Fos*-labeled neurons showed a two to sevenfold increase in the locomotor cat. The number of *Fos*-immunoreactive cholinergic neurons was slightly increased in the locomotor animal (**Figure 9B**), the increase split between cholinergic neurons in the PPT and LDT. This increase was much less than that observed for noradrenergic neurons within the same area (**Figure 7B**).

5-HT/*Fos* Immunohistochemistry

Numerous serotonergic neurons were observed in the NRM, pallidus (NRP), obscurus (NRO), and PPR of locomotor and control animals. Photomicrographs of serotonergic and non-serotonergic reticular (FTM) neurons taken from single sections of the brainstem of cat FL-3 are illustrated in **Figures 10A–D**. Serotonergic neurons were medium-sized, oval, or fusiform and in the PPR, were intermingled with

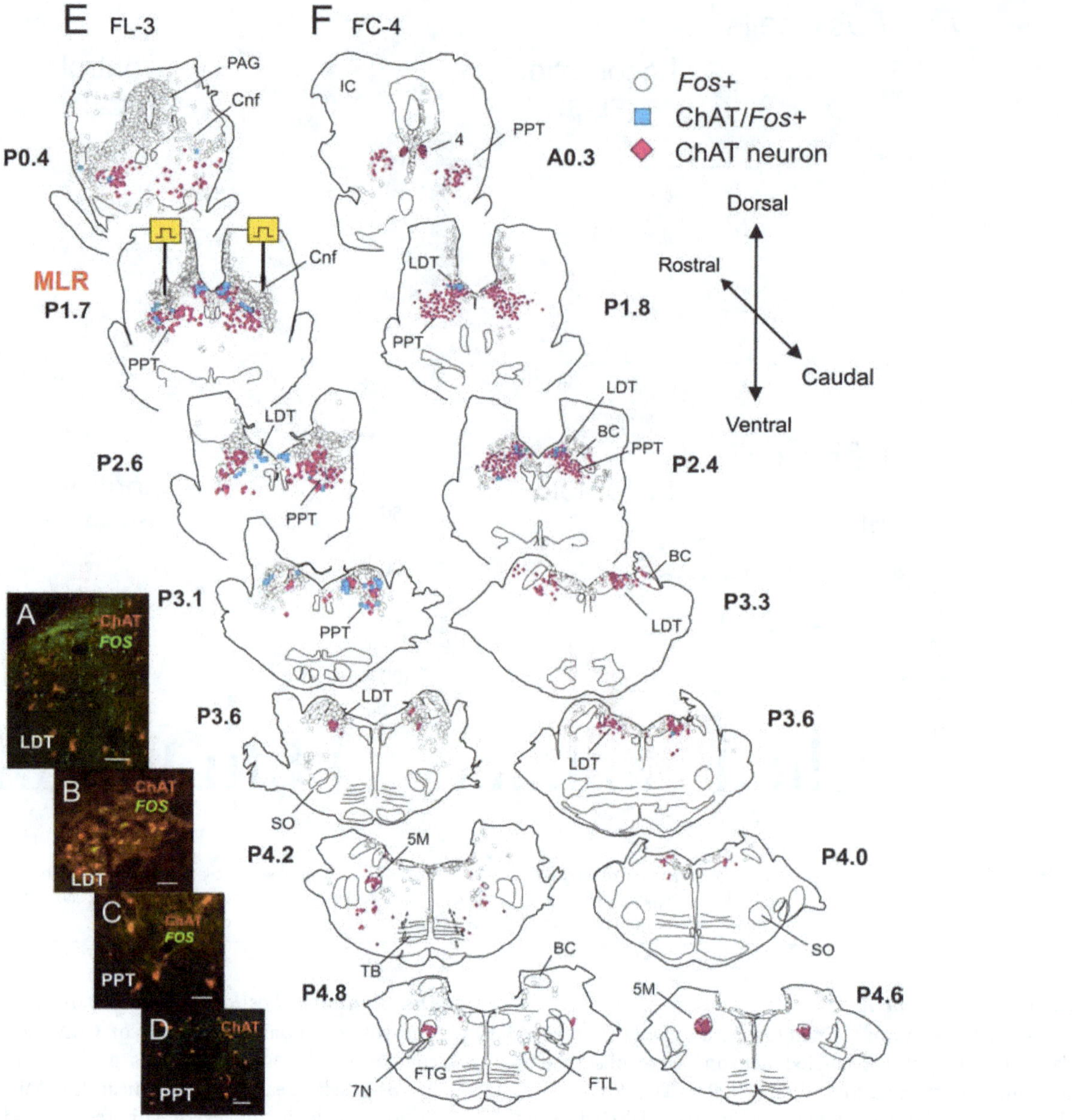

FIGURE 8 | Few cholinergic cells in midbrain and pons show activity dependent *Fos* labeling following MLR-evoked fictive locomotion in the decerebrate cat. **(A–D)** Confocal photomicrographs demonstrating *Fos* (*green*) and/or choline acetyltransferase (ChAT, *red*) immunoreactive cells in the brainstem between levels P0-5. Micrographs taken of cells located in the LDT **(A,B)** or PPT **(C,D)** of fictive locomotor cat FL-3. Few ChAT neurons in the PPT showed *Fos* labeling. **(E,F)** Camera lucida drawings showing distribution of *Fos*, ChAT/*Fos*, and ChAT immunoreactive neurons in locomotor FL-3 and control FC-4 cats, respectively. MLR stimulation sites, marked electrolytically, were located at approximately P1.7 (Berman, 1968) in FL-3. As in **Figure 4**, the MLR locomotor cat show abundant *Fos*-labeled neurons were observed in the CnF, bcm, PAG, LDT, LC, SubC, and the FTL. Some cholinergic neurons in the PPT and LDT (about equal numbers) showed *Fos* labeling although many non-cholinergic neurons in these areas also showed *Fos* expression. Relatively few *Fos*+ neurons were observed in the control animal. Scale bar: 100 μm **(A,D)** and 50 μm **(B,C)**.

other non-serotonergic neurons. In all areas of the medulla, serotonergic fibers formed a dense network surrounding many *Fos*-stained neurons (**Figure 10D**) and many cells in reticular and other areas appeared to be innervated by them (Noga et al., 2009). Maps of *Fos* and/or 5-HT stained neurons within the brainstems of locomotor and control cats are illustrated in **Figures 10E,F**.

Locomotor experiment

Many *Fos*-labeled cells were observed in the pons and medulla (P5.5–P14) following the locomotor task (**Figure 10E**). The distribution of these neurons was mostly symmetrical in this bilaterally stimulated animal. Abundant *Fos*-labeled neurons were found in the FTM, dorsal to the TB, and pyramids in a region laterally bounded by the superior olive (SO) and

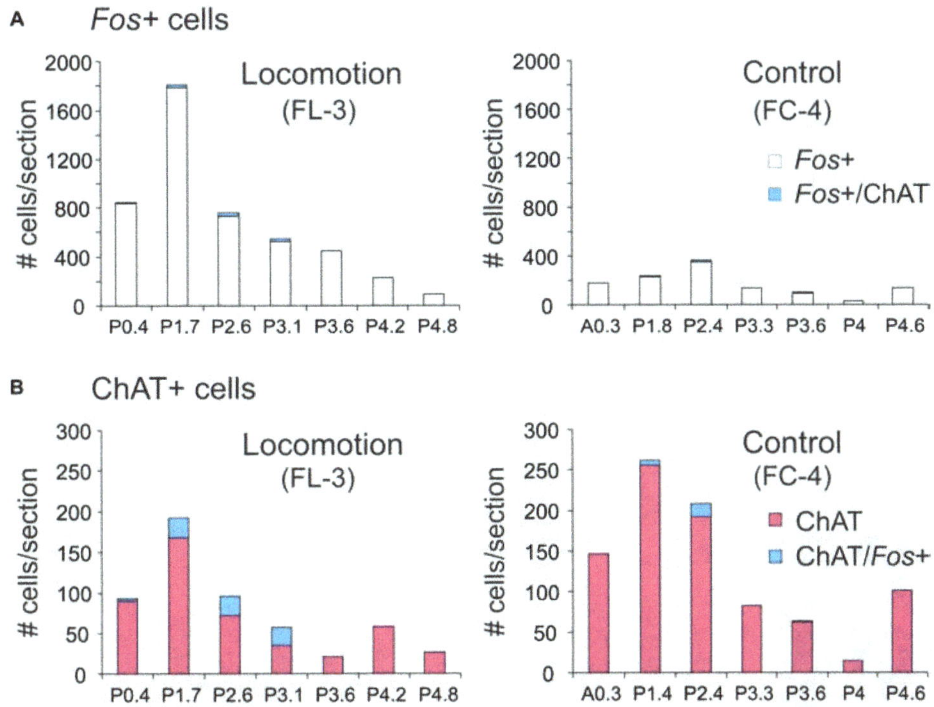

FIGURE 9 | Distribution of *Fos*+ neurons with or without co-labeling with ChAT in the midbrain and pons following bilateral stimulation of the MLR. **(A)** The number of *Fos*-labeled cells increased tremendously compared to the non-locomotor control animal. Relatively few *Fos*+ neurons were cholinergic. **(B)** Comparison of cholinergic neurons with or without *Fos* expression in the locomotor and control animals. Numeration includes all labeled cells from single sections at the indicated levels.

facial motor nucleus (7M). Relatively fewer cells were labeled in the FTG and more dorsally located FTL in this rostral area. This pattern of activated neurons corresponded with the MLR termination pattern described by Steeves and Jordan (1984). At the P8.5 level and caudally, ventrally located *Fos*+ neurons were found extending more laterally in the FTL. Numerous *Fos*+ neurons were also observed in the VMN and the VIN in rostral and caudal medulla. Relatively few labeled cells were observed within the lateral VLN. In caudal areas of the medulla, at the level of the inferior olivary nuclei (IO), large numbers of *Fos*+ cells were observed in the NTS of the dorsal respiratory group (DRG), the RFN of the VRG, the LRN, the RVLM, and the dmnV. Moderate labeling was observed in the FTM in caudal areas and scattered labeling of neurons were seen in the FTG. A small number of *Fos*+ cells was found within or bordering the AMB. Several serotonergic neurons in NRM were double labeled with *Fos*. Laterally, a large number of the serotonergic neurons within the PPR were also positive for *Fos* (P8.5).

Non-locomotor control

Like that observed in Study 1, maps constructed from brainstem segments in the control (FC-4) animal showed relatively few *Fos*-labeled neurons (**Figure 10F**). The difference between the control (**Figure 10F**) and fictive locomotor animals (**Figure 10E**) was striking. No serotonergic neurons in the control animal showed *Fos* labeling.

Distribution of Fos-labeled 5-HT neurons

The rostro-caudal distribution of 5-HT and/or *Fos*+ cells for control and locomotion experiments is shown in **Figure 11**. In the locomotor animal, the number of *Fos*+ cells/section found between P5.5 and P14 ranged from 250 to 684 and peaked at the P11 level in the caudal medulla (**Figure 11A**). In contrast, the number of *Fos*+ neurons/section in the control animal ranged between 7 and 64 neurons. At the peak level, this represented an approximately 34-fold increase in the number of *Fos*+ neurons in the locomotor animal compared to control. At other levels this increase ranged from 8- to 43-fold. Serotonergic immunoreactive boutons were found in close contact with many of these *Fos*+ neurons (**Figure 11A**). Overall, the percentage of *Fos*+ cells contacted by serotonergic fibers was ~60% (**Figure 7B**) with a range between 25 and 83%. The number of *Fos*-immunoreactive serotonergic neurons was increased in the locomotor animal compared to control (**Figure 11B**). The largest number of *Fos*+/5-HT cells was found at P8.5 at the level of the NRM and PPR. At this level, 38.5% of serotonergic neurons expressed *Fos* protein. In contrast, no serotonergic neurons between P5.5 and P14 in the control animal expressed *Fos*.

Overview of labeled cells in locomotor and control animals – Study 2

The distribution of brainstem *Fos*+ neurons in control and animals subject to MLR-evoked fictive locomotion is plotted in **Figure 12**.

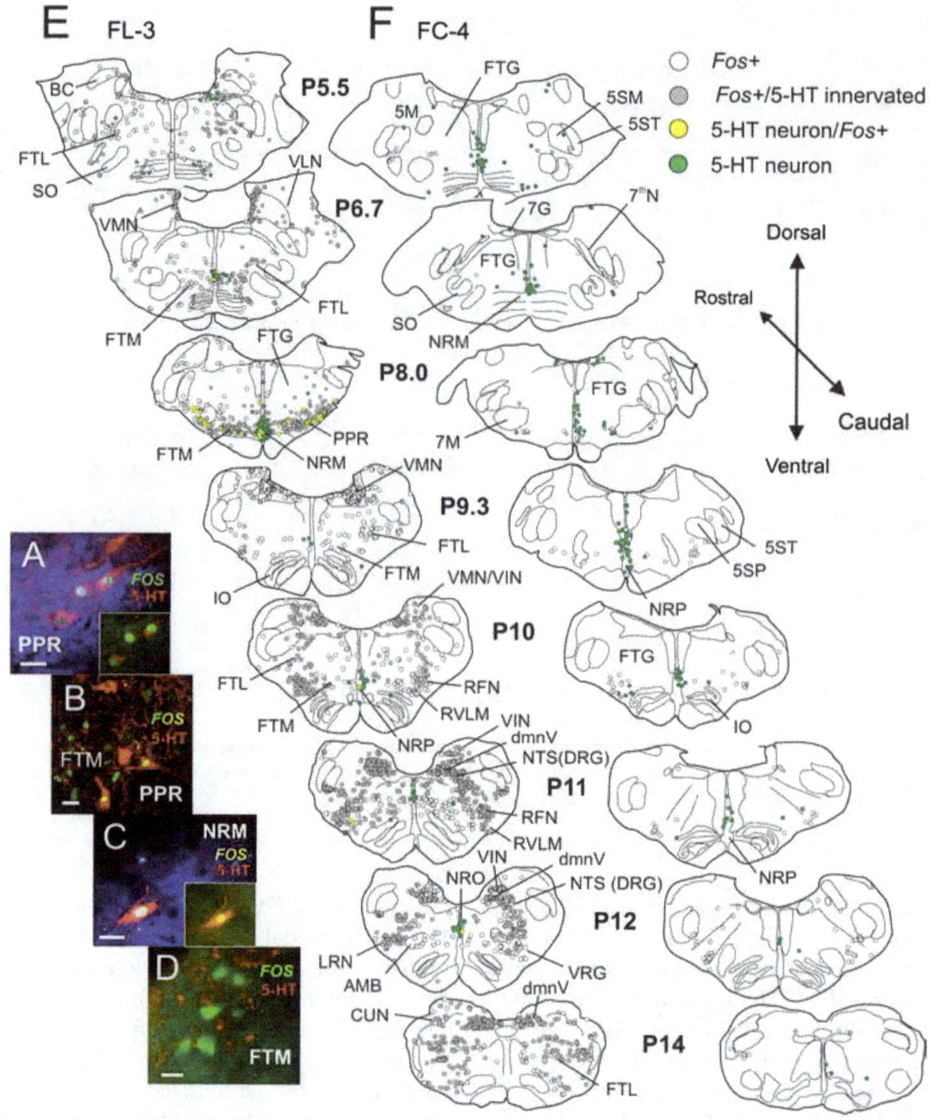

FIGURE 10 | Locomotor activated pontomedullary neurons: serotonergic cells within the raphe and parapyramidal region show activity-dependent *Fos* labeling following MLR-evoked fictive locomotion in the decerebrate cat. **(A–D)** Confocal photomicrographs of locomotor-activated neurons from FL-3 showing *Fos* nuclear labeling (*green*) with and without cytoplasmic co-localization of 5-HT (*red*). Photomicrographs taken from FTM, PPR, and nucleus raphe magnus (NRM). Micrographs enhanced (blue background) in **(A)** and **(C)** to better illustrate fine serotonergic fibers and varicosities in surrounding neuropil (insets show original micrographs). Note that *Fos*+ cells in the FTM (and other regions of the reticular formation) are surrounded by a dense network of serotonergic fibers, likely making close contacts with the neurons. **(E,F)** Camera lucida drawings of single sections between posterior levels P5.5–14 showing distribution of *Fos*, 5-HT/*Fos*+, and 5-HT immunoreactive neurons in locomotor FL-3 and control FC-4 cats, respectively. *Fos* neurons with serotonergic contacts (gray) are indicated. In the MLR locomotor cat, abundant *Fos*-labeled neurons were observed in the FTM, FTL, PPR, NRM, medial vestibular nucleus (VMN), inferior vestibular nucleus (VIN), dorsal motor nucleus of the vagus (dmnV), rostral ventrolateral medulla (RVLM) and the nucleus tractus solitarii (NTS), and retrofacial nucleus (RFN) of the dorsal respiratory and ventral respiratory groups (DRG and VRG), respectively. Many locomotor-activated neurons in the PPR and NRM were positive for 5-HT. Few *Fos*+ neurons were observed in the control animal. Scale bar: 20 μm **(A–C)**; 10 μm **(D)**.

DISCUSSION

General Observations and Limitations of the Study

In the present experiments we have documented the location of brainstem neurons activated during MLR-evoked locomotion in the precollicular–postmammillary decerebrate cat and examined their correspondence to serotonergic, noradrenergic, and cholinergic phenotypes. Fictive locomotion experiments were conducted to determine the activation pattern produced from centrally driven locomotor pathways. Due to the nature of these experiments, most of the data presented in this study is on individual animals, with some minor differences seen between animals; however, the differences demonstrated between

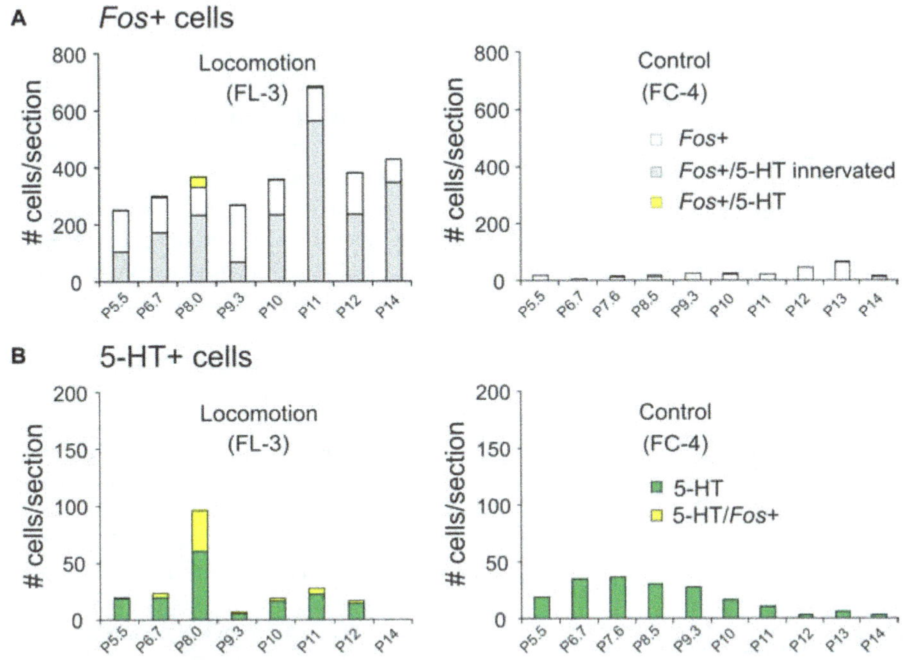

FIGURE 11 | Distribution of *Fos*+ neurons with or without co-labeling with 5-HT in the pons/medulla following bilateral stimulation of the MLR. **(A)** The number of *Fos*-labeled cells increased tremendously compared to the non-locomotor control animal. A small number of *Fos*+ neurons were serotonergic. **(B)** Comparison of serotonergic neurons with or without *Fos* expression in the locomotor and control animals. Most serotonergic neurons within the PPR were positive for *Fos*. Numeration includes all labeled cells from single sections at the indicated levels.

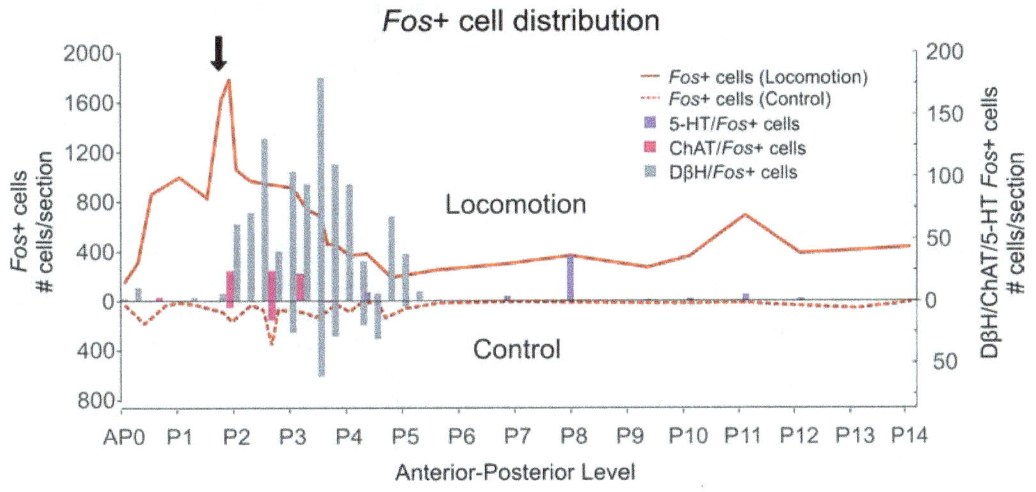

FIGURE 12 | *Fos*+ cell distribution within brainstem following MLR-evoked fictive locomotion. Numeration includes all labeled cells from single sections at the indicated AP levels. The numbers of activated neurons in locomotor and control animals are indicated above and below the *X*-axis, respectively. Scale bar for noradrenergic, cholinergic, and serotonergic neurons indicated on right side of diagram. MLR stimulation level is indicated by *arrow*. Data from FL-3 and FC-4.

MLR-stimulated and control animals was strongly significant. The results provide evidence in support of the idea that the anatomical equivalent of the MLR is the CnF and/or SubCnF region rather than the cholinergic PPT (Jordan, 1998; Takakusaki et al., 2016). Furthermore, it shows that MLR stimulation activates both reticular and monoaminergic neurons in parallel, providing anatomical and functional validation for centrally mediated monoaminergic neuromodulation of spinal locomotor circuitry during evoked locomotion (Noga et al., 2009, 2011, 2017). Lastly, the results also show that MLR stimulation activates neurons within vestibular, cardiovascular, and respiratory areas. Overall, these results demonstrate a complex neuromodulation

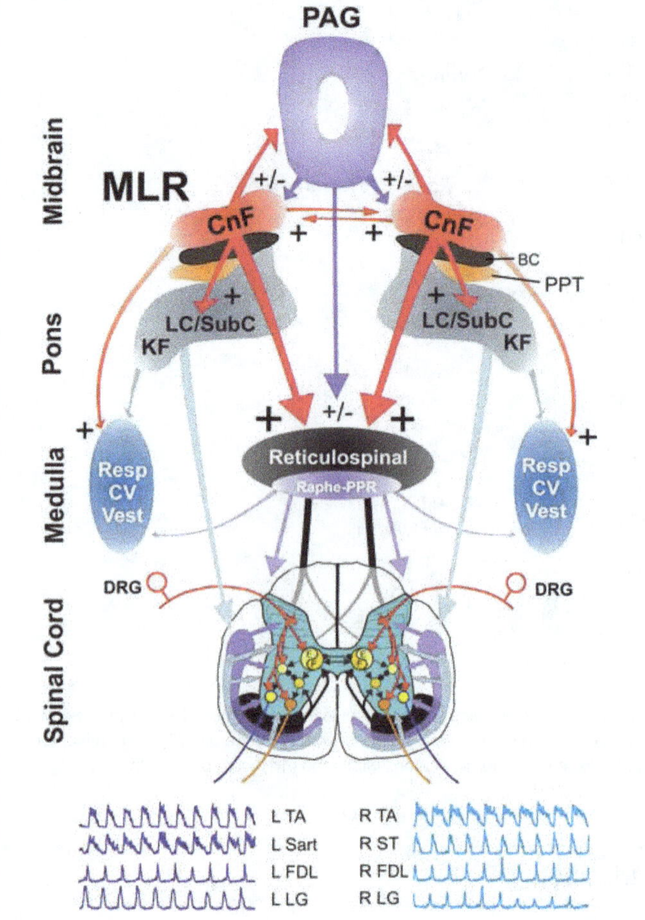

FIGURE 13 | Model of brainstem pathways for initiation of locomotion in the cat. Relationships between the various components of the pathway activated by the MLR, the spinal central pattern generator for locomotion (CPG), and their output motoneurons for bilateral hindlimb locomotion. The model incorporates parallel activation of descending RS and neuromodulatory pathways originating in the catecholaminergic and serotonergic nuclei of the pons and medulla, in addition to the facilitation of cardiorespiratory and vestibular centers during locomotion. Glutamatergic neurons within the CnF and SubCnF region form the primary phenotype for initiation and control of locomotion (Caggiano et al., 2018; Josset et al., 2018). Glutamatergic PPT neurons may contribute to the initiation of low speed locomotion (Caggiano et al., 2018) although this is disputed (Josset et al., 2018). Cholinergic neurons do not initiate locomotion but may play a modulatory role for ongoing locomotion (Roseberry et al., 2016; Caggiano et al., 2018; Josset et al., 2018) possibly by their effects on other brainstem output neurons. RS neurons of the magnocellular reticular formation, which form the final common motor pathway of the brainstem, relay the central command for initiation of locomotion to the spinal locomotor central pattern generator ultimately activating hindlimb motoneurons (Shefchyk et al., 1984; Noga et al., 2003; Jordan et al., 2008). The model also incorporates known projections between CnF/MLR nuclei on each side of the midbrain (Edwards, 1975; Steeves and Jordan, 1984). At the spinal level, flexor (F) and extensor (E) components of the locomotor pattern generator are activated/modulated by descending bilateral RS and monoaminergic projections as well as by crossed excitatory (▶) and inhibitory (●) segmental projections from the generator opposite to it. Details of the rhythm and pattern components of the locomotor generator are omitted to emphasize general interconnections between them and their target neurons. Electroneurograms: FDL, flexor digitorum longus; LG, lateral gastrocnemius; Sart, sartorius; ST, semitendinosus; TA, tibialis anterior. R, right; L, left.

pattern of brainstem neurons that integrate the kinematic, dynamic, and metabolic facets of locomotor activity induced by electrical stimulation.

Mesencephalic Locomotor Region

Historically, two adjacent nuclei, the CnF and the PPT, have been proposed as putative structural correlates of the MLR and two schools of thought have emerged in support of one or the other nucleus. Much of the preclinical literature, including Shik et al. (1966) original description, has supported the more dorsally located CnF, where electrical mapping studies consistently show it to promote locomotion (Takakusaki et al., 2003). Others have favored the more ventral, cholinergic cell-containing PPT (Garcia-Rill et al., 1986, 1987, 2011), despite its more varied electrical mapping results (Takakusaki et al., 2003, 2016). Data from the present study are discussed below with respect to this and other recent studies of this area of the midbrain.

Cuneiform Nucleus and the Sub-Cuneiform Region

The lowest electrical threshold sites for initiation of locomotion in the present study were found within the boundaries of the CnF nucleus and SubCnF region, thereby defining the MLR (see also Takakusaki, 2008, 2013; Takakusaki et al., 2016). Extensive labeling of neurons in these sites was observed, the majority of which are likely glutamatergic (Mena-Segovia et al., 2009; Wang and Morales, 2009). Cells in these areas are consistently labeled in studies examining locomotor activated neurons with *Fos* IHC (e.g., Silveira et al., 1995; Brudzynski and Wang, 1996; Iwamoto et al., 1996; Lamprea et al., 2002; Ferreira-Netto et al., 2005). Recent optogenetic studies show that glutamatergic CnF neurons are capable of initiating locomotion at short latencies, through a range of gait patterns and speeds (Roseberry et al., 2016; Capelli et al., 2017; Caggiano et al., 2018; Josset et al., 2018). Importantly, it is glutamatergic mesencephalic reticular formation neurons, including regions of the CnF, SubCnF, and PPT, that are activated during treadmill locomotion and which may code for locomotor speed (Roseberry et al., 2016; Caggiano et al., 2018). Cholinergic neurons, in contrast are characterized by repetitive, slow firing (Takakusaki et al., 1996). In non-human primates, rhythmically active cells are preferentially located in more dorsal CnF and SubCnF locations than tonically activated ones (Goetz et al., 2016). These latter cells are located within a region with higher densities of choline acetyl transferase labeled (cholinergic) neurons, corresponding to the PPT. GABAergic CnF neurons (Mena-Segovia et al., 2009; Wang and Morales, 2009) cannot initiate locomotion and rather, block locomotion when activated (Roseberry et al., 2016). If they were activated by electrical stimulation in the present study, their influence was overcome by activation of other neurons.

Pedunculopontine Tegmental Nucleus and Other Cholinergic Nuclei

The classically defined cholinergic PPT nucleus has long been considered a component of the MLR (Garcia-Rill et al., 1986, 1987, 2011) but the role of cholinergic PPT neurons in locomotion is controversial. In the present study, we examined neuronal *Fos* expression in the area encompassing the PPT and the adjacent cholinergic nucleus, LDT. Cholinergic neurons of the PPT and LDT were distributed within the mesopontine tegmentum as described previously (Jones and Beaudet, 1987). These neurons were not co-extensive with the low threshold locomotor producing sites within the CnF and SubCnF. Based on the known anatomical projections of the CnF and SubCnF (Steeves and Jordan, 1984; Caggiano et al., 2018) and on anticipated but limited current spread, stimulation of these low threshold MLR sites would be expected to activate some cells within this area of the tegmentum. However, relatively few cholinergic PPT/LDT neurons were activated compared to non-cholinergic *Fos+* neurons (**Figures 8E, 9**). Overall, this data support the growing body of evidence that cholinergic neuron activation does not play a principal role in MLR-evoked locomotion. This is consistent with our study showing that cholinergic antagonists fail to block MLR-evoked locomotion in decerebrate cats (Jordan et al., 2014) and data from Takakusaki et al. (2016) showing that electrical stimulation of PPT results in a muscarinic-sensitive motor inhibition. Selective deletion of the vesicular acetylcholine transporter also does not abolish open field locomotion nor affect locomotor coordination but may result in hyperactivity and balance problems in mature animals (Janickova et al., 2017). The results are also consistent with recent studies in rodents which show that optogenetic stimulation of cholinergic PPT neurons does not elicit locomotion in stationary animals (Roseberry et al., 2016; Caggiano et al., 2018; Josset et al., 2018). Cholinergic neurons may, however, modulate ongoing locomotion, producing accelerating (Roseberry et al., 2016) or decelerating effects on locomotor speed (Caggiano et al., 2018; Josset et al., 2018). This modulation is unlikely to result from co-release of glutamate or GABA (Roseberry et al., 2016; see also Wang and Morales, 2009) and could be the result of cholinergic action on neurons of the substantia nigra pars compacta (SNc) and VTA (see the section "Ascending Pathways") (Dautan et al., 2016; Xiao et al., 2016), CnF (Jin et al., 2016), and/or reticular formation (Tebēcis, 1973; Shiromani et al., 1990; Smetana et al., 2010). Within the LDT, a small, but similar number of cholinergic neurons also stained positive for *Fos* (**Figures 8A,B,E**). The LDT is thought to play a role in arousal, eye movements, learning and reward, visual orienting, and sensory-motor patterns, possibly via projections to the VTA and SNc (Wang and Morales, 2009; for review, see Martinez-Gonzalez et al., 2011).

Non-cholinergic neurons within the PPT, LDT, and adjacent area (Jones and Beaudet, 1987; Usunoff et al., 2003; Wang and Morales, 2009) were also activated by electrical stimulation of the MLR. Photo-activation of glutamatergic PPT neurons is reported to induce low-speed locomotion from rest in a subset of trials ($\sim$50%), but with long onset latency and requiring high frequency (50 Hz) stimulation (Caggiano et al., 2018). This has led to the suggestion that glutamatergic PPT neurons may be involved in explorative locomotor behavior (Caggiano et al., 2018). In support of this suggestion, these authors have shown that both the CnF and the PPT glutamatergic neurons project predominantly ipsilaterally, to locomotor areas of the MedRF (Noga et al., 2003). In a different study, however, glutamatergic PPT cell activation not only failed to initiate locomotion, it also decelerated and stopped ongoing locomotion (Josset et al., 2018; see also Takakusaki et al., 2016). Partial or complete lesions of the PPT (affecting all neuronal types) also fail to result in gait deficits (Gut and Winn, 2015) indicating that such modulatory effects on locomotion are likely compensated for by other modulatory systems. Further careful electrophysiological studies are needed to establish the role for the PPT.

Although more concentrated within the rostral pole of the PPT (Pienaar et al., 2017), GABAergic PPT neurons cannot initiate locomotion and rather, block locomotion when activated (Roseberry et al., 2016; Caggiano et al., 2018). If they were activated by electrical stimulation in the present study, their influence was minimal.

Ascending Pathways

Fos expression was elevated in the ipsilateral PAG (**Figure 4A**), an important mediator of defensive behavior including escape locomotion (Koutsikou et al., 2017). More ventrally, labeling was observed within the FTC, FF, and VTA in a sagittaly continuous band of activated neurons. Bilateral MLR stimulation produced symmetrical *Fos* expression (**Figures 6E, 8E**) within the PAG and FTC, and may be the activation pattern for rectilinear locomotion with balanced bilateral MLR activity (Noga and Opris, 2017b; see the section "Asymmetry in Brainstem Circuits"). This functional connectivity is consistent with anterograde tracer studies targeting the MLR and/or the CnF nucleus (Edwards, 1975; Edwards and de Olmos, 1976; Steeves and Jordan, 1984; Sotnichenko, 1985). The strong interconnection of the CnF, PAG (Edwards and de Olmos, 1976; Mantyh, 1983; Steeves and Jordan, 1984; Sotnichenko, 1985; Ferreira-Netto et al., 2005; Dampney et al., 2013; Caggiano et al., 2018), and the limbic system (see Koutsikou et al., 2017) indicates that the MLR plays an important role in the integration of complex motor behaviors related to defensive behavior (Sinnamon, 1993; Jordan, 1998).

Neurons within the VTA showed increased *Fos* activity (**Figure 4A**). The VTA contains dopaminergic neurons involved in goal-directed behavior and reinforcement-learning (Wise, 2004). It receives a direct input from non-catecholaminergic neurons of the PAG (Suckow et al., 2013) and from cholinergic and glutamatergic neurons of the PPT and LDT (Mena-Segovia and Bolam, 2017). Stimulation of cholinergic PPT terminals within the VTA activates dopaminergic neurons and transiently increases locomotor activity (Dautan et al., 2016). In contrast, LDT cholinergic neuron activation decreases locomotion (Dautan et al., 2016) and results in reward reinforcement (Xiao et al., 2016). These differential effects are likely due to actions on different neurons within the VTA. PPT glutamatergic neurons also increase arousal and drive motivated behavior via ascending projections, in part to the VTA (Kroeger et al., 2017; Yoo et al., 2017).

Descending Pathways

Reticular Formation

The major output pathway of the brainstem for activation of locomotor circuits is the RS pathway originating in the rostral medulla (Orlovskii, 1970; Garcia-Rill et al., 1983; Shefchyk et al., 1984; Steeves and Jordan, 1984; Garcia-Rill and Skinner, 1987; Noga et al., 1988, 1991, 2003). In the present study, neurons in the nucleus reticularis magnocellularis (FTM) were the primary reticular neurons activated in this region, dorsal to the TB and pyramids. Relatively few neurons were labeled in the FTG, although more posteriorly we observed labeling within the FTL (**Figure 10**; P9.3) which gradually merged with areas corresponding to the cardiorespiratory regions of the caudal medulla (see the section "Coupling of Neuronal Networks"). An asymmetrical activation pattern was observed with unilateral stimulation of the MLR (**Figures 3–5**), mirroring the anatomical projection pattern of the MLR (Steeves and Jordan, 1984). The implications of this pattern are discussed below (see the section "Asymmetry in Brainstem Circuits").

One candidate RS neuron mediating MLR-evoked locomotion is the Lhx3/Chx10-expressing neuron in the mouse (Bretzner and Brownstone, 2013). These neurons are glutamatergic, are targets of MLR (CnF) projections, support tonic repetitive firing, project to the spinal cord, and are activated (express *Fos*) during wheel running or treadmill locomotion. They are found in the ventral and α (FTM in the cat) parts of the gigantocellular reticular nuclei (together termed α/vGRN or GiA/GiV). Optogenetic studies in mice have shown that activation of glutamatergic neurons within the LPGi, a caudal subgroup of the magnocellular nucleus, can also trigger continuous locomotion (Capelli et al., 2017). Neurons in this area harbor terminals of MLR (CnF/PPT) efferents and express *Fos* after locomotion (Capelli et al., 2017). Some neurons in this lateral subdivision of the FTM caudal to 7M were also labeled in the present study. However, MLR (CnF) projections in the cat do not extend much more caudally than 7M (Steeves and Jordan, 1984), indicating that activation of reticular neurons at more caudal levels may be indirect, via local circuits within the brainstem (Shimamura et al., 1980). Further studies are needed to clarify whether there are species differences that may account for these discrepancies (see also Caggiano et al., 2018).

Interestingly, a large percentage of the MedRF neurons were innervated by serotonergic fibers. Such innervation of variously sized cells in the reticular formation has been described before (Kobayashi et al., 1994; see also Gao and Mason, 1997; Viana Di Prisco) as well as for vestibular (Halberstadt and Balaban, 2003) and cardio-respiratory neurons (see the section "Coupling of Neuronal Networks"). The serotonergic innervation of RS neurons may thus provide the basis for a neuromodulatory influence of 5-HT on brainstem circuits (Takakusaki et al., 1993), in addition to its effects on spinal circuits for locomotion (see Schmidt and Jordan, 2000).

Monoaminergic Neurons

As discussed in the section "Introduction," monoamines play a key role in the activation of spinal locomotor networks. The present study now confirms that monoaminergic neurons are activated during MLR-evoked locomotion (**Figures 6, 10**), with increased activity-dependent labeling of both catecholaminergic neurons of the LC, SubC, and KF nuclei and serotonergic neurons of the NRM and PPR. These nuclei are the primary source of the monoaminergic innervation of the spinal cord (Westlund et al., 1982; Clark and Proudfit, 1991a,b; Jones and Light, 1992). Monoaminergic neurons are likely activated by direct projections from the CnF and/or MLR (Edwards, 1975; Steeves and Jordan, 1984; Sotnichenko, 1985). Furthermore, both cerulear (Rasmussen et al., 1986) and raphe neurons are rhythmically active during overground locomotion (Veasey et al., 1995; Jacobs et al., 2002) and stimulation of the PPR in the neonatal rat also produces serotonergic receptor-dependent locomotor-like activity (Liu and Jordan, 2005). Taken together with our observation that stimulation of the MLR results in the spinal release of 5-HT and NE (Noga et al., 2017), these results provide the anatomical basis for the central control of locomotor activity by 5-HT and NE, in the absence of peripheral afferent feedback from moving limbs. Thus, in addition to RS command neurons (see the section "Reticular Formation"), monoaminergic neurons comprise a major component of the central descending pathways controlling locomotion.

Coupling of Neuronal Networks

Cells in other brainstem nuclei show increased activity-dependent labeling following MLR-evoked locomotion. These include nuclei of cardiovascular, respiratory, and vestibular systems (**Figure 10**). Several studies have demonstrated that locomotor and respiratory rhythms are centrally coupled (DiMarco et al., 1983; Millhorn et al., 1987; Perségol et al., 1988; Kawahara et al., 1989, 1993; Ezure and Tanaka, 1997). Respiratory and cardiovascular networks are also coupled through peripheral feedback (Iwamoto et al., 1996) and/or central interconnections between the different pattern generators (Dick et al., 2009; Le Gal et al., 2014). Here we present functional and anatomical evidence for a central coupling of locomotor, respiratory, and cardiovascular networks (DiMarco et al., 1983; Eldgridge et al., 1985; Bell, 2006; Wienecke et al., 2015) as well as activation of neurons within the medial VLN following stimulation of the MLR. While most of the nuclei of the cardiovascular, respiratory, and vestibular systems in the cat are not directly innervated by the CnF/MLR (Edwards, 1975; Steeves and Jordan, 1984), other nuclei receiving projections from the MLR (e.g., monoaminergic system, see below) may act as intermediaries to modulate their activity.

Respiratory Nuclei

In the present study, stimulation of the MLR increased *Fos* expression in nuclei involved in respiratory control, including neurons in the NTS, RFN, and LRN of the dorsal and VRGs. Other nuclei that may modulate respiratory activity under specific conditions also showed increased *Fos* expression in the present study. These included neurons within the raphe/PPR region, LC, SubC, KF, PPT, and PAG. Although respiratory responses to MLR stimulation were not monitored in these animals, previous work has shown that stimulation of the hypothalamic and MLRs facilitate respiration (Eldgridge et al., 1981; DiMarco et al., 1983; Millhorn et al., 1987; Kawahara et al., 1989; Ezure and Tanaka, 1997). Serotonergic neurons from the raphe nuclei and parapyramidal region project to the dorsal (Voss et al., 1990) and ventral respiratory column and may also contribute to central chemoreception and respiratory control (Ribas-Salgueiro et al., 2005; DePuy et al., 2011; Morinaga et al., 2019). Evidence of their involvement in control of breathing in the present study comes from the observation that serotonin-immunoreactive boutons were found in close apposition to many of these neurons (see also Voss et al., 1990). LC and KF nuclei are also involved in the control of breathing (Dutschmann and Herbert, 2006; Gargaglioni et al., 2010; Dutschmann and Dick, 2012; Barnett et al., 2018). Effects are likely mediated by noradrenergic (Magalhães et al., 2018) or glutamatergic projections (in the case of the KF) (Herbert et al., 1990; Ezure and Tanaka, 2006; Yokota et al., 2007; Geerling et al., 2017). The major source of cholinergic innervation of the brainstem regions controlling breathing is from the PPT and LDT (Kubin and Fenik, 2004) and neurons from these nuclei may thus have contributed to the activation of medullary respiratory-related neurons in the present experiments (Chatonnet et al., 2003). Lastly, respiratory activity may be modulated by the PAG; indirectly through its projections to the CnF (from the dlPAG); or directly by projections to the parabrachial complex, midline medulla, and VRG (from the dmPAG, lPAG, and vlPAG; see Dampney et al., 2013).

Cardiovascular Nuclei

Stimulation of the MLR invariably increased blood pressure (**Figure 2**) and *Fos* expression in nuclei associated with cardiovascular regulation (**Figure 10**). Consistent with this observation, stimulation of the CnF in the anesthetized rat increases arterial blood pressure in the absence of locomotion. The effect on blood pressure may be mediated by activation of sympathoexcitatory neurons in the RVLM (Verberne, 1995), catecholaminergic neurons of the KF/parabrachial complex and LC (Lam et al., 1996; Shafei and Nasimi, 2011), the dorsal PAG (Lam et al., 1996), and/or serotonergic neurons of the caudal raphe nuclei (Lam and Verberne, 1997; DePuy et al., 2011). Neurons within the parapyramidal region also project to cardiovascular-related nuclei (NTS) and may increase mean arterial blood pressure, independent of the RVLM (Helke et al., 1989). Interestingly, cholinergic systems may counteract the pressor effect of CnF stimulation by acting directly on nuclei known to produce hypotension (Shafei et al., 2013). Lastly, a role of the dorsolateral (sympathoexcitatory) and ventrolateral (inhibitory) PAG in the regulation of cardiovascular function has also been demonstrated (e.g., Carrive and Bandler, 1991; Lovick, 1992; Subramanian and Holstege, 2014) possibly via the FTM, raphe nuclei (Gao et al., 1997; Hermann et al., 1997), RVLM, or CnF (see Dampney et al., 2013).

Vestibular Nuclei

Vestibular signals are important in the regulation of balance (Shinoda et al., 2006) and contribute to cardiovascular and respiratory regulation during movement (McCall et al., 2017). In the present study, *Fos* labeling was observed in the VMN and VIN, areas important for stabilization of the head during movement (Cullen, 2012). Relatively few neurons within the lateral VLN were labeled. Orientation and movement of the head in the walking cat are active processes but reflexes appear to play only a partial role in determining head movement during walking, indicating that signals from the centrally generated locomotor synergy must be the main drivers for head movements (Zubair et al., 2016). In contrast, although vestibulospinal neurons within the VLN are rhythmically active during locomotion (Orlovsky, 1972; Matsuyama and Drew, 2000), their rhythmic activity likely reflects hindlimb and labyrinthine inputs during walking (Arshian et al., 2014) rather than centrally generated activity. Supporting this, bilateral lesions of the VLN in decerebrate cats do not interrupt MLR-evoked locomotion (Jell et al., 1985). The VLN are not directly innervated by projections of the MLR (Steeves and Jordan, 1984). Possible sources of activation of these nuclei (reviewed by McCall et al., 2017) in the reduced paralyzed preparation may include cerebellar (fastigial) nuclei (Takakusaki et al., 2016) or spinal interneurons (Noga et al., 2009, 2011) signaling locomotor activity. Interestingly, afferent inputs that may contribute to the vestibulo-cardiovascular and respiratory reflex relayed through the VMN and VIN originate in the medullary and pontine reticular formation, LRN, and raphe nuclei (Jian et al., 2005) and it is possible that activity in these nuclei from centrally driven locomotor inputs (this study; Zubair et al., 2016) could, via the VLN, further enhance cardiovascular and respiratory center activation (Stocker et al., 1997) in addition to those nuclei described above.

Asymmetry in Brainstem Circuits

As revealed in the present study, unilateral stimulation of the MLR produced an asymmetrical activation of brainstem neurons with *Fos* expression more commonly observed on the side of stimulation (**Figures 3–5**) even though bilateral locomotor activity was observed. This distribution reflects the anatomical projections of the MLR which are mostly uncrossed through the parabrachial region to the MedRF (Steeves and Jordan, 1984; see also Edwards, 1975; Sotnichenko, 1985). The results are consistent with the functional asymmetry of the RS output revealed by localized reversible cooling of the spinal cord in the decerebrate cat during fictive locomotion (Noga et al., 1995). Furthermore, they are consistent with electrophysiological studies which show that the majority of activated RS neurons project through the ventral funiculus on the same side as the stimulated MLR (Garcia-Rill and Skinner, 1987) to terminate on ipsilateral lumbar spinal neurons in the intermediate zone and ventral horn (Holstege and Kuypers, 1982; Capelli et al., 2017). Although fewer, projections from the MLR to the contralateral reticular formation (Steeves and Jordan, 1984; Capelli et al., 2017) and contralaterally/bilaterally projecting RS neurons (Peterson et al., 1975; Garcia-Rill and Skinner, 1987) likely account for the activation of RS neurons on the side opposite to stimulation [this study; Noga et al., 1995; see Humphries et al. (2006, 2007) for a discussion of intrinsic reticular network connections]. Finally, crossed spinal (Holstege and Kuypers, 1982; Kausz, 1991) or segmental pathways (Jankowska and Noga, 1990; Kjaerulff and Kiehn, 1997;

Kremer and Lev-Tov, 1997; Matsuyama et al., 2004a) likely also contribute to the generation of bilateral locomotor activity with unilateral stimulation of the MLR. In such a way, secondary projection systems compensate for the anatomical asymmetry of the primary MLR projection. Thus, the spinal activation pattern produced by unilateral MLR stimulation is essentially symmetrical (Dai et al., 2005). While this experimental situation reveals the complex projections within brainstem and spinal cord, spontaneous locomotion likely would provide a more balanced descending output to the spinal locomotor centers (Noga and Opris, 2017b), reflective of the pattern of activation observed within the brainstem (**Figures 6, 8, 10**) and spinal cord (Noga et al., 2009, 2011) produced with bilateral MLR stimulation. In this situation, forward or rectilinear locomotion likely occurs through bilaterally symmetric commands transmitted by the MLR and RS pathways. In contrast, during turning movements, an asymmetric command may be generated and transmitted along RS pathways to modulate CPGs on one side. Such a command would need to overwhelm compensatory mechanisms from contralaterally projecting RS neurons and segmental commissural neurons (Noga et al., 2003; Matsuyama et al., 2004a). A theoretical model in mammals for symmetry breaking of rectilinear locomotion by adjusting the level of activity of components of the descending locomotor pathway has been presented (Noga and Opris, 2017b). In that model, steering of locomotor activity may be achieved by temporarily adjusting the balance of MLR and/or RS outputs - in essence, creating an asymmetrical drive on either side of the brainstem. Evidence in favor of such an organization at the RS level for steering of locomotor activity has recently been presented (Oueghlani et al., 2018).

Descending Pathway for Initiation of Locomotion

A new model of the descending pathway for the control of locomotion (after Noga et al., 2017) is presented in **Figure 13**, with the MLR representing a central node in the control of locomotion by higher brain centers. Data presented in the present study indicate that the anatomical locus of the MLR is the CnF/SubCnF region of the midbrain. Little evidence is found to support the participation of cholinergic neurons in the initiation of locomotion by electrical stimulation of this region, although a modulatory role of locomotor activity is possible (Roseberry et al., 2016; Caggiano et al., 2018; Josset et al., 2018). This is consistent with recent optogenetic studies that show that initiation of locomotor activity is primarily, if not exclusively, the result of activation of glutamatergic neurons within the CnF and SubCnf (Roseberry et al., 2016; Caggiano et al., 2018; Josset et al., 2018). The MLR is reciprocally connected with the contralateral MLR (Steeves and Jordan, 1984; Bayev et al., 1988) possibly facilitating/coordinating descending signal output on both sides of the brainstem, and with the PAG (Mantyh, 1983; Bayev et al., 1988; Sandner et al., 1992; Ferreira-Netto et al., 2005; Dampney et al., 2013; Caggiano et al., 2018) which may be important for the mediation of rapid defensive decision making or the mediation of locomotion during pursuit. Electrical stimulation of the MLR activates three primary brainstem targets affecting locomotor circuits within the spinal cord: RS, ceruleospinal and raphespinal. RS neurons located within the MedRF (FTM) comprise the primary "command pathway" for the initiation of locomotion (Shik et al., 1966, 1967; Orlovskii, 1970; Jordan, 1991; Noga et al., 2003). Glutamatergic RS neurons in this region activate spinal locomotor neurons (e.g., Douglas et al., 1993; Hägglund et al., 2010; Bretzner and Brownstone, 2013; Capelli et al., 2017). Activation of noradrenergic (LC, SubC, and KF) and serotonergic (NRM and PPR) neurons within the pons and medulla results in the rapid, widespread release of the neuromodulators NE and 5-HT in the spinal cord during locomotion (Noga et al., 2017). Central respiratory (Resp), cardiovascular (CV), and vestibular (Vest) neurons are also activated by MLR stimulation, either directly or indirectly (Voss et al., 1990; Nasimi et al., 2012; Damasceno et al., 2014), likely in anticipation of the increased metabolic and postural demands associated with locomotion. Additionally, MLR stimulation activates neurons within the PAG, an area important for mediating defensive behaviors (Deng et al., 2016).

The RS neurons of the MedRF (FTM) also have multiple inputs in addition to the MLR (Steeves and Jordan, 1984; Garcia-Rill and Skinner, 1987; Bretzner and Brownstone, 2013). They are innervated by the ipsilateral SLR (Sinnamon and Stopford, 1987; Takakusaki et al., 2016), the contralateral cerebellar locomotor region (Mori et al., 1998), the PAG (Mantyh, 1983; Dampney et al., 2013), the motor cortex via corticoreticular pathways (Matsuyama et al., 2004b), as well as various sensory systems (e.g., visual, auditory, and vestibular) (Furigo et al., 2010; Miller et al., 2017). Thus locomotion may be initiated by activation of the RF directly, bypassing the MLR (Shik et al., 1966; Noga et al., 1988; Mori et al., 1998; Bretzner and Brownstone, 2013; Capelli et al., 2017) or modulated by activation of sensory or neuromodulatory inputs to the RF (Antri et al., 2008; Smetana et al., 2010; Noga and Opris, 2017a,b; Oueghlani et al., 2018). The neuronal circuit selected for goal-directed locomotion may depend upon the behavioral context (Sinnamon, 1993), whether locomotion is required for either exploration, foraging, or defense (see Jordan, 1998; Takakusaki, 2008).

AUTHOR CONTRIBUTIONS

BN and LJ: conceptualization, supervision, and funding acquisition. BN, LJ, DJ, XD, and LV: methodology. BN, DJ, and XD: investigation. XD, IO, DJ, FS, LV, CL-H, and SX: formal analysis. BN, XD, IO, and LV: visualization. BN, XD, IO, and SC: writing – original draft. BN, LJ, IO, and SC: writing – review and editing.

FUNDING

This work was supported by the National Institutes of Health (NIH) Grants R01 NS046404 and R56NS46404-6A1 to BN, the State of Florida and the Miami Project to Cure Paralysis, and a Medical Research Council Grant to LJ, a Rick Hansen Man in Motion Legacy Fund Studentship to XD, and a research fellowship from the Neurosurgery Research and Education Foundation (NREF) to SC (GR010471).

ACKNOWLEDGMENTS

The authors would like to thank B. Frydel for assistance in the use of StereoInvestigator and Neurolucida Systems and M. Riesgo, J. R. Douglas, and A. Pinzon for assistance during some of the experiments.

REFERENCES

Antri, M., Auclair, F., Albrecht, J., Djeudjang, N., and Dubuc, R. (2008). Serotonergic modulation of sensory transmission to brainstem reticulospinal cells. *Eur. J. Neurosci.* 28, 655–667. doi: 10.1111/j.1460-9568.2008.06368.x

Antri, M., Orsal, D., and Barthe, J.-Y. (2002). Locomotor recovery in the chronic spinal rat: effects of long-term treatment with a 5-HT2 agonist. *Eur. J. Neurosci.* 16, 467–476. doi: 10.1046/j.1460-9568.2002.02088.x

Arshian, M. S., Hobson, C. E., Catanzaro, M. F., Miller, D. J., Puterbaugh, S. R., Cotter, L. A., et al. (2014). Vestibular nucleus neurons respond to hindlimb movement in the decerebrate cat. *J. Neurophysiol.* 111, 2423–2432. doi: 10.1152/jn.00855.2013

Barbeau, H., and Rossignol, S. (1991). Initiation and modulation of the locomotor pattern in the adult chronic spinal cat by noradrenergic, serotonergic and dopaminergic drugs. *Brain Res.* 546, 250–260. doi: 10.1016/0006-8993(91)91489-n

Barnett, W. H., Jenkin, K. S. E., Milsom, W. K., Paton, J. F., Abdala, A. P., Molkov, Y. I, et al. (2018). The Kölliker–Fuse nucleus orchestrates the timing of expiratory abdominal nerve bursting. *J. Neurophysiol.* 119, 401–412. doi: 10.1152/jn.00499.2017

Bayev, K. V., Beresovskii, V. K., Kebkalo, T. G., and Savoskina, L. A. (1988). Afferent and efferent connections of brainstem locomotor regions: study by means of horseradish peroxidase transport technique. *Neuroscience* 26, 871–891. doi: 10.1016/0306-4522(88)90106-6

Bell, H. J. (2006). Respiratory control at exercise onset: an integrated systems perspective. *Resp. Physiol. Neurobiol.* 152, 1–15. doi: 10.1016/j.resp.2006.02.005

Berman, A. (1968). *The Brainstem of the Cat.* Madison, WI: The University of Wisconsin press.

Bretzner, F., and Brownstone, R. M. (2013). Lhx3-Chx10 reticulospinal neurons in locomotor circuits. *J. Neurosci.* 33, 14681–14692. doi: 10.1523/jneurosci.5231-12.2013

Brudzynski, S. M., and Wang, D. (1996). C-fos immunohistochemical localization of neurons in the mesencephalic locomotor region in the rat brain. *Neuroscience* 75, 793–803. doi: 10.1016/0306-4522(96)00284-9

Caggiano, V., Leiras, R., Goñi-Erro, H., Masini, D., Bellardita, C., Bouvie, R. J., et al. (2018). Midbrain circuits that set locomotor speed and gait selection. *Nature* 553, 455–460. doi: 10.1038/nature25448

Capelli, P., Pivetta, C., Esposito, M. S., and Arber, S. (2017). Locomotor speed control circuits in the caudal brainstem. *Nature* 551, 373–377. doi: 10.1038/nature24064

Carrive, P., and Bandler, R. (1991). Control of extracranial and hindlimb blood flow by the midbrain periaqueductal grey of the cat. *Exp. Brain Res.* 84, 599–606. doi: 10.1007/BF00230972

Cazalets, J. R., Sqalli-Houssaini, Y., and Clarac, F. (1992). Activation of the central pattern generators for locomotion by serotonin and excitatory amino acids in neonatal rat. *J. Physiol.* 455, 187–204. doi: 10.1113/jphysiol.1992.sp019296

Chatonnet, F., Boudinot, E., Chatonnet, A., Taysse, L., Daulon, S., Champagnat, J., et al. (2003). Respiratory survival mechanisms in acetylcholinesterase knockout mouse. *Eur. J. Neurosci.* 18, 1419–1427. doi: 10.1046/j.1460-9568.2003.02867

Christie, K. J., and Whelan, P. J. (2005). Monoaminergic establishment of rostrocaudal gradients of rhythmicity in the neonatal mouse spinal cord. *J. Neurophysiol.* 94, 1554–1564. doi: 10.1152/jn.00299.2005

Clark, F. M., and Proudfit, H. K. (1991a). The projection of locus coeruleus neurons to the spinal cord in the rat determined by anterograde tracing combined with immunocytochemistry. *Brain Res.* 538, 231–245. doi: 10.1016/0006-8993(91)90435-x

Clark, F. M., and Proudfit, H. K. (1991b). The projection of noradrenergic neurons in the A7 catecholamine cell group to the spinal cord in the rat demonstrated by anterograde tracing combined with immunocytochemistry. *Brain Res.* 547, 279–288. doi: 10.1016/0006-8993(91)90972-x

Cullen, K. E. (2012). The vestibular system: multimodal integration and encoding of self-motion for motor control. *Trends Neurosci.* 35, 185–196. doi: 10.1016/j.tins.2011.12.001

Dai, X., Noga, B. R., Douglas, J. R., and Jordan, L. M. (2005). Localization of spinal neurons activated during locomotion using the *c-fos* immunohistochemical method. *J. Neurophysiol.* 93, 3442–3452. doi: 10.1152/jn.00578.2004

Damasceno, R. S., Takakura, A. C., and Moreira, T. S. (2014). Regulation of the chemosensory control of breathing by kölliker–Fuse neurons. *Am. J. Physiol. Regul. Integr. Comp. Physiol.* 307, R57–R67. doi: 10.1152/ajpregu.00024.2014

Dampney, R. A. L., Furlong, T. M., Horiuchi, J., and Iigaya, K. (2013). Role of dorsolateral periaqueductal grey in the coordinated regulation of cardiovascular and respiratory function. *Auton. Neurosci.* 175, 17–25. doi: 10.1016/j.autneu.2012.12.008

Dautan, D., Souza, A. S., Huerta-Ocampo, I., Valencia, M., Assous, M., Witten, I. B., et al. (2016). Segregated cholinergic transmission modulates dopamine neurons integrated in distinct functional circuits. *Nat. Neurosci.* 19, 1025–1033. doi: 10.1038/nn.4335

Deng, H., Xiao, X., and Wang, Z. (2016). Periaqueductal gray neuronal activities underlie different aspects of defensive behaviors. *J. Neurosci.* 36, 7580–7588. doi: 10.1523/JNEUROSCI.4425-15.2016

DePuy, S. D., Kanbar, R., Coates, M. B., Stornetta, R. L., and Guyenet, G. (2011). Control of breathing by raphe obscurus serotonergic neurons in mice. *J. Neurosci.* 31, 1981–1990. doi: 10.1523/JNEUROSCI.4639-10.2011

Di Prisco, G. V., Dubuc, R., and Grillner, S. (1994). 5-HT innervation of reticulospinal neurons and other brainstem structures in lamprey. *J. Comp. Neurol.* 342, 23–34. doi: 10.1002/cne.903420104

Dick, T. E., Baekey, D. M., Paton, J. F. R., Lindsey, B. G., and Morris, K. F. (2009). Cardio-respiratory coupling depends on the pons. *Resp. Physiol. Neurobiol.* 168, 76–85. doi: 10.1016/j.resp.2009.07.009

DiMarco, A. F., Romaniuk, J. R., Von Euler, C., and Yamamoto, Y. (1983). Immediate changes in ventilation and respiratory pattern associated with onset and cessation of locomotion in the cat. *J. Physiol.* 343, 1–16. doi: 10.1113/jphysiol.1983.sp014878

Douglas, J. R., Noga, B. R., Dai, X., and Jordan, L. M. (1993). The effects of intrathecal administration of excitatory amino acid agonists and antagonists on the initiation of locomotion in the adult cat. *J. Neurosci.* 13, 990–1000. doi: 10.1523/JNEUROSCI.13-03-00990.1993

Dutschmann, M., and Dick, T. E. (2012). Pontine mechanisms of respiratory control. *Compr. Physiol.* 2, 2443–2469. doi: 10.1002/cphy.c100015

Dutschmann, M., and Herbert, H. (2006). The Kölliker–Fuse nucleus gates the postinspiratory phase of the respiratory cycle to control inspiratory off-switch and upper airway resistance in rat. *Eur. J. Neurosci.* 24, 1071–1084. doi: 10.1111/j.1460-9568.2006.04981.x

Edwards, S. B. (1975). Autoradiographic studies of the projections of the midbrain reticular formation: descending projections of nucleus cuneiformis. *J. Comp. Neurol.* 161, 341–358. doi: 10.1002/cne.901610306

Edwards, S. B., and de Olmos, J. S. (1976). Autoradiographic studies of the projections of the midbrain reticular formation: ascending projections of nucleus cuneiformis. *J. Comp. Neurol.* 165, 417–432. doi: 10.1002/cne.901650403

Eldgridge, F. L., Millhorn, D. E., Kiley, J. P., and Waldrop, T. G. (1985). Stimulation by central command of locomotion, respiration and circulation during exercise. *Resp. Physiol.* 59, 313–337. doi: 10.1016/0034-5687(85)90136-7

Eldgridge, F. L., Millhorn, D. E., and Waldrop, T. G. (1981). Exercise hyperpnea and locomotion: parallel activation from the hypothalamus. *Science* 211, 844–846. doi: 10.1126/science.7466362

Ezure, K., and Tanaka, I. (1997). Convergence of central respiratory and locomotor rhythms onto single neurons of the lateral reticular nucleus. *Exp. Brain Res.* 113, 230–242. doi: 10.1007/BF02450321

Ezure, K., and Tanaka, I. (2006). Distribution and medullary projection of respiratory neurons in the dorsolateral pons of the rat. *Neuroscience* 141, 1011–1023. doi: 10.1016/j.neuroscience.2006.04.020

Feraboli-Lohnherr, D., Barthe, J. Y., and Orsal, D. (1999). Serotonin-induced activation of the network for locomotion in adult spinal rats. *J. Neurosci. Res.* 55, 87–98. doi: 10.1002/(SICI)1097-4547(19990101)55

Ferreira-Netto, C., Borelli, K. G., and Brandão, M. L. (2005). Neural segregation of Fos-protein distribution in the brain following freezing and escape behaviors induced by injections of either glutamate or NMDA into the dorsal periaqueductal gray of rats. *Brain Res.* 1031, 151–163. doi: 10.1016/j.brainres.2004.10.044

Furigo, I. C., De Oliveira, W. F., De Oliveira, A. R., Colmoli, E., Baldo, M. V. C., Mota-Ortiz, S. R., et al. (2010). The role of the superior colliculus in predatory hunting. *Neuroscience* 165, 1–15. doi: 10.1016/j.neuroscience.2009.10.004

Gao, K., Kim, Y.-H. H., and Mason, P. (1997). Serotonergic pontomedullary neurons are not activated by antinociceptive stimulation in the paeriaqueductal gray. *J. Neurosci.* 17, 3285–3292. doi: 10.1523/JNEUROSCI.17-09-03285.1997

Gao, K., and Mason, P. (1997). Somatodendritic and axonal anatomy of intracellularly labeled serotonergic neurons in the rat medulla. *J. Comp. Neurol.* 389, 309–328. doi: 10.1002/(sici)1096-9861(19971215)389:2<309::aid-cne9>3.3.co;2-d

Garcia-Rill, E., Houser, C. R., Skinner, R. D., Smith, W., and Woodward, D. J. (1987). Locomotion-inducing sites in the vicinity of the pedunculopontine nucleus. *Brain Res. Bull.* 18, 731–738. doi: 10.1016/0361-9230(87)90208-5

Garcia-Rill, E., Simon, C., Smith, K., Kezunovic, N., and Hyde, J. (2011). The pedunculopontine tegmental nucleus: from basic neuroscience to neurosurgical applications: arousal from slices to humans: implications for DBS. *J. Neural Transm.* 118, 1397–1407. doi: 10.1007/s00702-010-0500-x

Garcia-Rill, E., and Skinner, R. D. (1987). The mesencephalic locomotor region. II. Projections to reticulospinal neurons. *Brain Res.* 411, 13-20. doi: 10.1016/0006-8993(87)90676-7

Garcia-Rill, E., Skinner, R. D., Conrad, C., Mosley, D., and Campbell, C. (1986). Projections of the mesencephalic locomotor region in the rat. *Brain Res. Bull.* 17, 33–40. doi: 10.1016/0361-9230(86)90158-9

Garcia-Rill, E., Skinner, R. D., and Fitzgerald, J. A. (1983). Activity in the mesencephalic locomotor region during locomotion. *Exp. Neurol.* 82, 609-622. doi: 10.1016/0014-4886(83)90084-5

Gargaglioni, L. H., Hartzler, L. K., and Putnam, R. W. (2010). The locus coeruleus and central chemosensitivity. *Respir. Physiol. Neurobiol.* 173, 264–273. doi: 10.1016/j.resp.2010.04.024

Geerling, J. C., Yokota, S., Rukhadze, I., Roe, D., and Chamberlin, N. L. (2017). Kölliker–Fuse GABAergic and glutamatergic neurons project to distinct targets. *J. Comp. Neurol.* 525, 1844–1860. doi: 10.1002/cne.24164

Goetz, L., Piallat, B., Bhattacharjee, M., Mathieu, H., David, O., and Chabardès, S. (2016). On the role of the pedunculopontine nucleus and mesencephalic reticular formation in locomotion in nonhuman primates. *J. Neurosci.* 36, 4917–4929. doi: 10.1523/JNEUROSCI.2514-15.2016

Grillner, S., Georgopoulos, A. P., and Jordan, L. M. (1997). "Selection and initiation of motor behavior," in *Neurons, Network and Motor Behavior*, eds P. S. G. Stein, A. I. Selverston, and D. G. Stuart, (Cambridge, MA: MIT Press), 3–19.

Grillner, S., and Shik, M. L. (1973). On the descending control of the lumbosacral spinal cord from the "mesencephalic locomotor region". *Acta Physiol. Scand.* 87, 320–333. doi: 10.1111/j.1748-1716.1973.tb05396.x

Grillner, S., Wallén, P., Saitoh, K., Kozlov, A., and Robertson, B. (2008). Neural bases of goal-directed locomotion in vertebrates – an overview. *Brain Res. Rev.* 57, 2–12. doi: 10.1016/j.brainresrev.2007.06.027

Gut, N. K., and Winn, P. (2015). Deep brain stimulation of different pedunculopontine targets in a novel rodent model of Parkinsonism. *J. Neurosci.* 35, 4792–4803. doi: 10.1523/jneurosci.3646-14.2015

Hägglund, M., Borgius, L., Dougherty, K. J., and Kiehn, O. (2010). Activation of groups of excitatory neurons in the mammalian spinal cord or hindbrain evokes locomotion. *Nat. Neurosci.* 13, 246–252. doi: 10.1038/nn.2482

Halberstadt, A. L., and Balaban, C. D. (2003). Organization of projections from the raphe nuclei to the vestibular nuclei in rats. *Neuroscience* 120, 573–594. doi: 10.1016/S0306-4522(02)00952-1

Helke, C. J., Thor, K. B., and Sasek, C. A. (1989). Chemical neuroanatomy of the parapyramidal region of the ventral medulla in the rat. *Prog. Brain Res.* 81, 17–28. doi: 10.1016/S0079-6123(08)61997-4

Herbert, H., Moga, M. M., and Saper, C. B. (1990). Connections of the parabrachial nucleus with the nucleus of the solitary tract and the medullary reticular formation in the rat. *J. Comp. Neurol.* 293, 540–580. doi: 10.1002/cne.902930404

Herdegen, T., and Leah, J. D. (1998). Inducible and constitutive transcription factors in the mammalian nervous system: control of gene expression by Jun, Fos, and Krox, and CREB/ATF proteins. *Brain Res. Rev.* 28, 370–490. doi: 10.1016/s0165-0173(98)00018-6

Hermann, D. M., Luppi, P.-H., Peyron, C., Hinckel, P., and Jouvet, M. (1997). Afferent projections to the rat nuclei raphe magnus, raphe pallidus and reticularis gigantocellularis pars α demonstrated by iontophoretic application of choleratoxin (subunit b). *J. Chem. Neuroanat.* 13, 1–21. doi: 10.1016/S0891-0618(97)00019-7

Holstege, G., and Kuypers, H. G. (1982). The anatomy of the brain stem pathways to the spinal cord in a cat. A labelled amino acid tracing study. *Prog. Brain Res.* 57, 145–175. doi: 10.1016/S0079-6123(08)64128-X

Huang, A., Noga, B. R., Carr, P. A., Fedirchuk, B., and Jordan, L. M. (2000). Spinal cholinergic neurons activated during locomotion: localization and electrophysiological characterization. *J. Neurophysiol.* 83, 3537–3547. doi: 10.1152/jn.2000.83.6.3537

Humphries, M. D., Gurney, K., and Prescott, T. J. (2006). The brainstem reticular formation is a small-world, not scale-free, network. *Proc. R. Soc. B Biol. Sci.* 273, 503–511. doi: 10.1098/rspb.2005.3354

Humphries, M. D., Gurney, K., and Prescott, T. J. (2007). Is there a brainstem substrate for action selection? *Philos. Trans. R. Soc. Lond. Ser. B Biol. Sci.* 362, 1627–1639. doi: 10.1098/rstb.2007.2057

Iwamoto, G. A., Wappel, S. M., Fox, G. M., Buetow, K. A., and Waldrop, T. G. (1996). Identification of diencephalic and brainstem cardiorespiratory areas activated during exercise. *Brain Res.* 726, 109–122. doi: 10.1016/0006-8993(96)00303-4

Jacobs, B. L., Martín-Cora, F. J., and Fornal, C. A. (2002). Activity of medullary serotonergic neurons in freely moving animals. *Brain Res. Rev.* 40, 45–52. doi: 10.1016/S0165-0173(02)00187-X

Janickova, H., Rosborough, K., Al-Onaizi, M., Kljakic, O., Guzman, M. S., Gros, R., et al. (2017). Deletion of the vesicular acetylcholine transporter from pedunculopontine/laterodorsal tegmental neurons modifies gait. *J. Neurochem.* 140, 787–798. doi: 10.1111/jnc.139.10

Jankowska, E., Jukes, M. G. M., Lund, S., and Lundberg, A. (1967). The effect of DOPA on the spinal cord. VI. Half-centre organization of interneurons transmitting effects from the flexor reflex afferents. *Acta Physiol. Scand.* 70, 389–402. doi: 10.1111/j.1748-1716.1967.tb03637.x

Jankowska, E., and Noga, B. R. (1990). Contralaterally projecting lamina VIII interneurons in middle lumbar segments in the cat. *Brain Res.* 535, 327–330. doi: 10.1016/0006-8993(90)91618-Q

Jell, R. M., Elliot, C., and Jordan, L. M. (1985). Initiation of locomotion from the mesenecephalic locomotor region: effects of selective brainstem lesions. *Brain Res.* 328, 121–128. doi: 10.1016/0006-8993(85)91330-7

Jian, B. J., Acernese, A. W., Lorenzo, J., Card, J. P., and Yates, B. J. (2005). Afferent pathways to the region of the vestibular nuclei that participates in cardiovascular and respiratory control. *Brain Res.* 1044, 241–250. doi: 10.1016/j.brainres.2005.03.010

Jin, X., Schwabe, K., Krauss, J. K., and Alam, M. (2016). The anterior and posterior pedunculopontine tegmental nucleus are involved in behavior and neuronal activity of the cuneiform and entopeduncular nuclei. *Neuroscience* 322, 39–53. doi: 10.1016/j.neuroscience.2016.02.016

Jones, B. E., and Beaudet, A. (1987). Distribution of acetylcholine and catecholamine neurons in the cat brainstem: a choline acetyltransferase and tyrosine hydroxylase immunohistochemical study. *J. Comp. Neurol.* 261, 15–32. doi: 10.1002/cne.902610103

Jones, S. L., and Light, A. R. (1992). Serotonergic medullary raphespinal projection to the lumbar spinal cord in the rat: a retrograde immunohistochemical study. *J. Comp. Neurol.* 322, 599–610. doi: 10.1002/cne.903220413

Jordan, L. M. (1991). "Brainstem and spinal cord mechanisms for the initiation of locomotion," in *Neurobiological Basis of Human Locomotion*, eds M. Shimamura, S. Grillner, and V. R. Edgerton, (Tokyo: Japan Scientific Societies Press), 3–20.

Jordan, L. M. (1998). Initiation of locomotion in mammals. *Ann. N. Y. Acad. Sci.* 860, 83–93. doi: 10.1111/j.1749-6632.1998.tb09040.x

Jordan, L. M., Liu, J., Hedlund, P. B., Akay, T., and Pearson, K. G. (2008). Descending command systems for the initiation of locomotion in mammals. *Brain Res. Rev.* 57, 183–191. doi: 10.1016/j.brainresrev.2007.07.019

Jordan, L. M., McVagh, J. R., Noga, B. R., Cabaj, A. M., Majczyński, H., Sławińska, U., et al. (2014). Cholinergic mechanisms in spinal locomotion – potential target for rehabilitation approaches. *Front. Neural Circuits* 8:132. doi: 10.3389/fncir.2014.00132

Jordan, L. M. J., and Sławińska, U. (2014). "The brain and spinal cord networks controlling locomotion," in *Neuronal Networks in Brain Function, CNS Disorders, and Therapeutics*, eds C. L. Faingold, and H. Blumenfeld, (Amsterdam: Elsevier Inc.), 215–233. doi: 10.1016/b978-0-12-415804-7.00017-4

Josset, N., Roussel, M., Lemieux, M., Lafrance-Zoubga, D., Rastqar, A., and Bretzner, F. (2018). Distinct contributions of mesencephalic locomotor region nuclei to locomotor control in the freely behaving mouse. *Curr. Biol.* 28, 884–901. doi: 10.1016/j.cub.2018.02.007

Kausz, M. (1991). Arrangement of neurons in the medullary reticular formation and raphe nuclei projecting to thoracic, lumbar and sacral segments of the spinal cord in the cat. *Anat. Embryol.* 183, 151–163. doi: 10.1007/BF00174396

Kawahara, K., Nakazono, Y., Yamauchi, Y., and Miyamoto, Y. (1989). Coupling between respiratory and locomotor rhythms during fictive locomotion in decerebrate cats. *Neurosci. Lett.* 103, 326–330. doi: 10.1016/0304-3940(89)90121-3

Kawahara, K., Yoshioka, T., Yamauchi, Y., and Niizeki, K. (1993). Heart beat fluctuation during fictive locomotion in decerebrate cats: locomotor-cardiac coupling of central origin. *Neurosci. Lett.* 150, 200–202. doi: 10.1016/0304-3940(93)90535-S

Kiehn, O., Hultborn, H., and Conway, B. A. (1992). Spinal locomotor activity in acutely spinalized cats induced by intrathecal application of noradrenaline. *Neurosci. Lett.* 143, 243–246. doi: 10.1016/0304-3940(92)90274-b

Kiehn, O., and Kjærulff, O. (1996). Spatiotemporal characteristics of 5-HT and dopamine-induced rhythmic hindlimb activity in the *in vitro* neonatal rat. *J. Neurophysiol.* 75, 1472–1482. doi: 10.1152/jn.1996.75.4.1472

Kjaerulff, O., and Kiehn, O. (1997). Crossed rhythmic synaptic input to motoneurons during selective activation of the contralateral spinal locomotor network. *J. Neurosci.* 17, 9433–9447. doi: 10.1523/JNEUROSCI.17-24-09433.1997

Kobayashi, Y., Matsuyama, K., and Mori, S. (1994). Distribution of serotonin cells projecting to the pontomedullary reticular formation in the cat. *Neurosci. Res.* 20, 43–55. doi: 10.1016/0168-0102(94)90021-3

Koutsikou, S., Apps, R., and Lumb, B. M. (2017). Top down control of spinal sensorimotor circuits essential for survival. *J. Physiol.* 595, 4151–4158. doi: 10.1113/JP273360

Kremer, E., and Lev-Tov, A. (1997). Localization of the spinal network associated with generation of hindlimb locomotion in the neonatal rat and organization of its transverse coupling system. *J. Neurophysiol.* 77, 1155–1170. doi: 10.1152/jn.1997.77.3.1155

Kroeger, D., Ferrari, L. L., Petit, G., Mahoney, C. E., Fuller, P. M., Arrigoni, E., et al. (2017). Cholinergic, glutamatergic, and GABAergic neurons of the pedunculopontine tegmental nucleus have distinct effects on sleep/wake behavior in mice. *J. Neurosci.* 37, 1352–1366. doi: 10.1523/JNEUROSCI.1405-16.2016

Kubin, L., and Fenik, V. (2004). Pontine cholinergic mechanisms and their impact on respiratory regulation. *Resp. Physiol. Neurobiol.* 143, 235–249. doi: 10.1016/j.resp.2004.04.017

Lam, W., Gundlach, A. L., and Verberne, A. J. (1996). Increased nerve growth factor inducible-A gene and c-fos messenger RNA levels in the rat midbrain and hindbrain associated with the cardiovascular response to electrical stimulation of the mesencephalic cuneiform nucleus. *Neuroscience* 71, 193–211. doi: 10.1016/0306-4522(95)00450-5

Lam, W., and Verberne, A. J. M. (1997). Cuneiform nucleus stimulation-induced sympathoexcitation: role of adrenoceptors, excitatory amino acid and serotonin receptors in rat spinal cord. *Brain Res.* 757, 191–201. doi: 10.1016/S0006-8993(97)00201-1

Lamprea, M. R., Cardenas, F. P., Vianna, D. M., Castilho, V. M., Cruz-Morales, S. E., and Brandão, M. L. (2002). The distribution of fos immunoreactivity in rat brain following freezing and escape responses elicited by electrical stimulation of the inferior colliculus. *Brain Res.* 950, 186–194. doi: 10.1016/s0006-8993(02)03036-6

Le Gal, J. P., Juvin, L., Cardoit, L., Thoby-Brisson, M., and Morin, D. (2014). Remote control of respiratory neural network by spinal locomotor generators. *PLoS One* 9:e89670. doi: 10.1371/journal.pone.0089670

Lee, A. M., Hoy, J. L., Bonci, A., Wilbrecht, L., Stryker, M. P., and Niell, C. M. (2014). Identification of a brainstem circuit regulating visual cortical state in parallel with locomotion. *Neuron* 83, 455–466. doi: 10.1016/j.neuron.2014.06.031

Liu, J., and Jordan, L. M. (2005). Stimulation of the parapyramidal region of the neonatal rat bran stem produces locomotor-like activity involving spinal 5-HT7 and 5-HT2A receptors. *J. Neurophysiol.* 94, 1392–1404. doi: 10.1152/jn.00136.2005

Lovick, T. A. (1992). Inhibitory modulation of the cardiovascular defense response by the ventrolateral periaqueductal grey matter in rats. *Exp. Brain Res.* 89, 133–139. doi: 10.1007/BF00229010

Magalhães, K. S., Spiller, P. F., da Silva, M. P., Kuntze, L. B., Paton, J. F. R., Machado, B. H., et al. (2018). Locus Coeruleus as a vigilance centre for active inspiration and expiration in rats. *Sci. Rep.* 8:15654. doi: 10.1038/s41598-018-34047-w

Mantyh, P. W. (1983). Connections of midbrain periaqueductal gray in the monkey. II. Descending efferent projections. *J. Neurophysiol.* 49, 582–594. doi: 10.1152/jn.1983.49.3.582

Marcoux, J., and Rossignol, S. (2000). Initiating or blocking locomotion in spinal cats by applying noradrenergic drugs to restricted lumbar spinal segments. *J. Neurosci.* 20, 8577–8585. doi: 10.1523/JNEUROSCI.20-22-08577.2000

Martinez-Gonzalez, C., Bolam, J. P., and Mena-Segovia, J. (2011). Topographical organization of the pedunculopontine nucleus. *Front. Neuroanat.* 5:22. doi: 10.3389/fnana.2011.00022

Matsuyama, K., and Drew, T. (2000). Vestibulospinal and reticulospinal neuronal activity during locomotion in the intact cat. I. Walking on a level surface. *J. Neurophysiol.* 84, 2237–2256. doi: 10.1152/jn.2000.84.5.2237

Matsuyama, K., Kakajima, K., Mori, F., Aoki, M., and Mori, S. (2004a). Lumbar commissural interneurons with reticulospinal inputs in the cat: morphology and discharge patterns during fictive locomotion. *J. Comp. Neurol.* 474, 546–561. doi: 10.1002/cne.20131

Matsuyama, K., Mori, F., Nakajima, K., Drew, T., Aoki, M., and Mori, S. (2004b). Locomotor role of the corticoreticular-reticulopinal-spinal interneuronal system. *Prog. Brain Res.* 143, 239–249. doi: 10.1016/S0079-6123(03)43024-0

McCall, A. A., Miller, D. M., and Yates, B. J. (2017). Descending influences on vestibulospinal and vestibulosympathetic reflexes. *Front. Neurol.* 27:8. doi: 10.3389/fneur.2017.00112

Mena-Segovia, J., and Bolam, J. P. (2017). Rethinking the pedunculopontine nucleus: from cellular organization to function. *Neuron* 94, 7–18. doi: 10.1016/j.neuron.2017.02.027

Mena-Segovia, J., Micklem, B. R., Nair-Roberts, R. G., Ungless, M. A., and Bolam, J. P. (2009). GABAergic neuron distribution in the pedunculopontine nucleus defines functional subterritories. *J. Comp. Neurol.* 515, 397–408. doi: 10.1002/cne.22065

Miller, D. M., DeMayo, W. M., Bourdages, G. H., Wittman, S. R., Yates, B. J., and McCall, A. A. (2017). Neurons in the pontomedullary reticular formation receive converging inputs from the hindlimb and labyrinth. *Exp. Brain Res.* 235, 1195–1207. doi: 10.1007/s00221-017-4875-x

Millhorn, D. E., Eldridge, F. L., Waldrop, T. G., and Kiley, J. P. (1987). Diencephalic regulation of respiration and arterial pressure during actual and fictive locomotion in cat. *Circ. Res.* 61, I53–I59.

Mori, S., Matsui, T., Kuze, B., Asanome, M., Nakajima, K., and Matsuyama, K. (1998). Cerebellar-induced locomotion: reticulospinal control of spinal rhythm generating mechanism in cats. *Ann. N. Y. Acad. Sci.* 860, 94–105. doi: 10.1111/j.1749-6632.1998.tb09041.x

Mori, S., Matsuyama, K., Kohyama, J., Kobayashi, Y., and Takakusaki, K. (1992). Neuronal constituents of postural and locomotor control systems and their interactions in cats. *Brain Dev.* 14, S109–S120.

Mori, S., Sakamoto, T., Ohta, Y., Takakusaki, K., and Matsuyama, K. (1989). Site-specific postural and locomotor changes evoked in awake, freely moving intact cats by stimulating the brainstem. *Brain Res.* 505, 66–74. doi: 10.1016/0006-8993(89)90116-9

Morinaga, R., Nakamuta, N., and Yamamoto, Y. (2019). Serotonergic projections to the ventral respiratory column from raphe nuclei in rats. *Neurosci. Res.* 143, 20–30. doi: 10.1016/j.neures.2018.05.004

Nasimi, A., Shafei, M. N., and Alaei, H. (2012). Glutamate injection into the cuneiform nucleus in rat, produces correlated single unit activities in the Kolliker–Fuse nucleus and cardiovascular responses. *Neuroscience* 223, 439–446.

Noga, B. R., Fortier, P. A., Kriellaars, D. J., Dai, X., Detillieux, G. R., and Jordan, L. M. (1995). Field potential mapping of neurons in the lumbar spinal cord activated following stimulation of the mesencephalic locomotor region. *J. Neurosci.* 15, 2203–2217. doi: 10.1523/JNEUROSCI.15-03-02203.1995

Noga, B. R., Johnson, D. M. G., Riesgo, M. I., and Pinzon, A. (2009). Locomotor-activated neurons of the cat. I. Serotonergic innervation and co-localization of 5-HT7, 5-HT2A and 5-HT1A receptors in the thoraco-lumbar spinal cord. *J. Neurophysiol.* 102, 1560–1576. doi: 10.1152/jn.91179.2008

Noga, B. R., Johnson, D. M. G., Riesgo, M. I., and Pinzon, A. (2011). Locomotor-activated neurons of the cat. II. Noradrenergic innervation and co-localization with NEα1A or NEα2B receptors in the thoraco-lumbar spinal cord. *J. Neurophysiol.* 105, 1835–1849. doi: 10.1152/jn.00342.2010

Noga, B. R., Kettler, J., and Jordan, L. M. (1988). Locomotion produced in mesencephalic cats by injections of putative transmitter substances and antagonists into the medial reticular formation and the pontomedullary locomotor strip. *J. Neurosci.* 8, 2074–2086. doi: 10.1523/JNEUROSCI.08-06-02074.1988

Noga, B. R., Kriellaars, D. J., Brownstone, R. M., and Jordan, L. M. (2003). Mechanism for activation of locomotor centers in the spinal cord by stimulation of the mesencephalic locomotor region. *J. Neurophysiol.* 90, 1464–1478. doi: 10.1152/jn.00034.2003

Noga, B. R., Kriellaars, D. J., and Jordan, L. M. (1991). The effect of selective brainstem or spinal cord lesions on treadmill locomotion evoked by stimulation of the mesencephalic or pontomedullary locomotor regions. *J. Neurosci.* 11, 1691–1700. doi: 10.1523/JNEUROSCI.11-06-01691.1991

Noga, B. R., and Opris, I. (2017a). "The hierarchical circuit for executive control of movement (Chapter 5),". in *Physics of the Mind and Brain Disorders: Integrated Neural Circuits Supporting the Emergence of Mind*, eds I. Opris, and M. R. Casanova (New York, NY: Springer Series in Cognitive and Neural Systems).

Noga, B. R., and Opris, I. (2017b). "From symmetry to symmetry-breaking in locomotion (Chapter 8)," in *Physics of the Mind and Brain Disorders: Integrated Neural Circuits Supporting the Emergence of Mind*, eds I. Opris, and M. R. Cassanova (New York, NY: Springer Series in Cognitive and Neural Systems), 155–174. doi: 10.1007/978-3-319-29674-6_7

Noga, B. R., Turkson, R. P., Xie, S., Taberner, A., Pinzon, A., and Hentall, I. D. (2017). Monoamine release in the cat lumbar spinal cord during fictive locomotion evoked by the mesencephalic locomotor region. *Front. Neural Circuits* 11:59. doi: 10.3389/fncir.2017.00059

Noga, B. R., Xie, S., Sanchez, F. J., and Blythe, A. D. (2008). Activity-dependent labelling of brainstem monoaminergic and non-monoaminergic neurons during mesencephalic locomotor region evoked fictive locomotion in the cat. *Soc. Neurosci. Abstr.* 34:576.

Orlovskii, G. N. (1970). Relations between reticulospinal neurons and locomotor regions of the brainstem. *Biofizika* 15, 171–177.

Orlovsky, G. N. (1972). Activity of vestibulospinal neurons during locomotion. *Brain Res.* 46, 85–98. doi: 10.1016/0006-8993(72)90007-8

Oueghlani, Z., Simonnet, C., Cardoit, L., Courtland, G., Cazalets, J.-R., Morin, D., et al. (2018). Brainstem steering of locomotor activity in the newborn rat. *J. Neurosci.* 38, 7725–7740. doi: 10.1523/JNEUROSCI.1074-18.2018

Perségol, L., Jordan, M., Viala, D., and Fernandez, C. (1988). Evidence for central entrainment of the medullary respiratory pattern by the locomotor pattern in the rabbit. *Exp. Brain Res.* 71, 153–162. doi: 10.1007/BF00247530

Peterson, B. W., Maunz, R. A., Pitts, N. G., and Mackel, R. (1975). Patterns of projection and branching of reticulospinal neurons. *Exp. Brain Res.* 23, 333–351. doi: 10.1007/BF00238019

Pienaar, I. S., Vernon, A., and Winn, P. (2017). The cellular diversity of the pedunculopontine nucleus: relevance to behavior in health and aspects of Parkinson's disease. *Neuroscientist* 23, 415–431. doi: 10.1177/1073858416682471

Rasmussen, K., Morilak, D. A., and Jacobs, B. L. (1986). Single unit activity of locus coeruleus neurons in the freely moving cat. I. During naturalistic behaviors and in response to simple and complex stimuli. *Brain Res.* 371, 324–334. doi: 10.1016/0006-8993(86)90370-7

Ribas-Salgueiro, J. L., Gaytán, S. P., Ribas, J., and Pásaro, R. (2005). Characterization of efferent projections of chemosensitive neurons in the caudal parapyramidal area of the rat brain. *Brain Res. Bull.* 66, 235–248. doi: 10.1016/j.brainresbull.2005.05.014

Roseberry, T. K., Lee, A. M., Lalive, A. L., Wilbrecht, L., Bonci, A., and Kreitzer, A. C. (2016). Cell-type-specific control of brainstem locomotor circuits by basal ganglia. *Cell* 164, 526–537. doi: 10.1016/j.cell.2015.12.037

Sandner, G., Di Scala, G., Rocha, B., and Angst, M. J. (1992). C-fos immunoreactivity in the brain following unilateral electrical stimulation of the dorsal periaqueductal gray in freely moving rats. *Brain Res.* 573, 276–283. doi: 10.1016/0006-8993(92)90773-3

Schmidt, B. J., and Jordan, L. M. (2000). The role of serotonin in reflex modulation and locomotor rhythm production in the mammalian spinal cord. *Brain Res. Bull.* 53, 689–710. doi: 10.1016/s0361-9230(00)00402-0

Shafei, M. N., and Nasimi, A. (2011). Effect of glutamate stimulation of the cuneiform nucleus on cardiovascular regulation in anesthetized rats: role of the pontine Kolliker–Fuse nucleus. *Brain Res.* 1385, 135–143. doi: 10.1016/j.brainres.2011.02.046

Shafei, M. N., Niazmand, S., Enayatfard, L., Hosseini, M., and Daloee, M. H. (2013). Pharmacological study of cholinergic system on cardiovascular regulation in the cuneiform nucleus of rat. *Neurosci. Lett.* 549, 12–17. doi: 10.1016/j.neulet.2013.05.046

Shefchyk, S. J., Jell, R. M., and Jordan, L. M. (1984). Reversible cooling of the brainstem reveals areas required for mesencephalic locomotor region evoked treadmill locomotion. *Exp. Brain Res.* 56, 257–262. doi: 10.1007/BF00236281

Shik, M. L., Severin, F. V., and Orlovskii, G. N. (1966). Control of walking and running by means of electrical stimulation of the mid-brain. *Biofizika* 11, 659–666.

Shik, M. L., Severin, F. V., and Orlovskii, G. N. (1967). Structures of the brain stem responsible for evoked locomotion. *Fiziol. Zh. SSSR I M Sechenova* 53, 1125–1132.

Shimamura, M., Kogure, I., and Wada, S. (1980). Three types of reticular neurons involved in the spinobulbo-spinal reflex of cats. *Brain Res.* 186, 99–113. doi: 10.1016/0006-8993(80)90258-9

Shinoda, Y., Sugiuchi, Y., Izawa, Y., and Hata, Y. (2006). Long descending motor tract axons and their control of neck and axial muscles. *Prog. Brain Res.* 151, 527–563. doi: 10.1016/s0079-6123(05)51017-3

Shiromani, P. J., Lai, Y. Y., and Siegel, J. M. (1990). Descending projections from the dorsolateral pontine tegmentum to the paramedian reticular nucleus of the caudal medulla in the cat. *Brain Res.* 517, 224–228. doi: 10.1016/0006-8993(90)91030-K

Silveira, M. C. L., Sandner, G., Di Scala, G., and Graeff, F. G. (1995). C-fos immunoreactivity in the brain following electrical or chemical stimulation of the medial hypothalamus. *Brain Res.* 674, 265–274. doi: 10.1016/0006-8993(94)01451-m

Sinnamon, H. M. (1993). Preoptic and hypothalamic neurons and the initiation of locomotion in the anesthetized rat. *Prog. Neurobiol.* 41, 323–344. doi: 10.1016/0301-0082(93)90003-B

Sinnamon, H. M., and Stopford, C. K. (1987). Locomotion elicited by lateral hypothalamic stimulation in the anesthetized rat does not require the dorsal midbrain. *Brain Res.* 402, 78–86. doi: 10.1016/0006-8993(87)91049-3

Smetana, R., Juvin, L., Dubuc, R., and Alford, S. (2010).). A parallel cholinergic brainstem pathway for enhancing locomotor drive. *Nat. Neurosci.* 13, 731–738. doi: 10.1038/nn.2548

Sotnichenko, T. S. (1985). Differentiation of efferent projections of the medial (cuneiform nucleus) and lateral regions of the reticular formation in cat midbrain. *Neurophysiology* 17, 466–471. doi: 10.1007/bf01052183

Sqalli-Houssaini, Y., and Cazalets, J.-R. (2000). Noradrenergic control of locomotor networks in the in vitro spinal cord of the neonatal rat. *Brain Res.* 852, 100–109. doi: 10.1016/s0006-8993(99)02219-2

Steeves, J. D., and Jordan, L. M. (1980). Localization of a descending pathway in the spinal cord which is necessary for controlled treadmill locomotion. *Neurosci. Lett.* 20, 283-288. doi: 10.1016/0304-3940(80)90161-5

Steeves, J. D., and Jordan, L. M. (1984). Autoradiographic demonstration of the projections from the mesencephalic locomotor region. *Brain Res.* 307, 263-276. doi: 10.1016/0006-8993(84)90480-3

Steeves, J. D., Jordan, L. M., and Lake, N. (1976). The close proximity of catecholamine containing cells to the 'mesencephalic locomotor region' (MLR). *Brain Res.* 100, 663–670. doi: 10.1016/0006-8993(75)90166-3

Steeves, J. D., Schmidt, B. J., Skovgaard, B. J., and Jordan, L. M. (1980). The effect of noradrenaline and 5-hydroxytryptamine depletion on locomotion in the cat. *Brain Res.* 185, 349–362. doi: 10.1016/0006-8993(80)91073-2

Stocker, S. D., Steinbacher, B. C., Balaban, C. D., and Yates, B. J. (1997). Connections of the caudal ventrolateral medullary reticular formation in the cat brainstem. *Exp. Brain Res.* 116, 270–282. doi: 10.1007/PL00005755

Subramanian, H. H., and Holstege, G. (2014). Chapter 17 - The midbrain periaqueductal gray changes the eupneic respiratory rhythm into a breathing pattern necessary for survival of the individual and of the species. *Prog. Brain Res.* 212, 351–384. doi: 10.1016/B978-0-444-63488-7.00017-3

Suckow, S. K., Deichsel, E. L., Ingram, S. I., Morgan, M. M., and Aicher, S. A. (2013). Columnar distribution of catecholaminergic neurons in the ventrolateral periaqueductal gray and their relationship to efferent pathways. *Synapse* 67, 94–108. doi: 10.1002/syn.21624

Takakusaki, K. (2008). Forebrain control of locomotor behaviors. *Brain Res. Rev.* 57, 192–198. doi: 10.1016/j.brainresrev.2007.06.024

Takakusaki, K. (2013). Neurophysiology of gait: from the spinal cord to the frontal lobe. *Mov. Disord.* 28, 1483–1491. doi: 10.1002/mds.25669

Takakusaki, K., Chiba, R., Nozu, T., and Okumura, T. (2016). Brainstem control of locomotion and muscle tone with special reference to the role of the mesopontine tegmentum and medullary reticulospinal systems. *J. Neural Transm.* 123, 695–729. doi: 10.1007/s00702-015-1475-4

Takakusaki, K., Habaguchi, T., Ohtinata-Sugimoto, J., Saitoh, K., and Sakamoto, T. (2003). Basal ganglia efferents to the brainstem centers controlling postural muscle tone and locomotion: a new concept for understanding motor disorders in basal ganglia dysfunction. *Neuroscience* 119, 293–308. doi: 10.1016/S0306-4522(03)00095-2

Takakusaki, K., Kohyama, J., Masuyama, K., and Mori, S. (1993). Synaptic mechanisms acting on lumbar motoneurons during postural augmentation induced by serotonin injection into the rostral pontine reticular formation in decerebrate cats. *Exp. Brain Res.* 93, 471–482. doi: 10.1007/bf00229662

Takakusaki, K., Shiroyama, T., Yamamoto, T., and Kitai, S. T. (1996). Cholinergic and noncholinergic tegmental pedunculopontine projection neurons in rats revealed by intracellular labeling. *J. Comp. Neurol.* 371, 345–361. doi: 10.1002/(sici)1096-9861(19960729)371:3<345::aid-cne1>3.0.co;2-2

Tebēcis, A. K. (1973). Transmitters and reticulospinal neurons. *Exp. Neurol.* 40, 297–308. doi: 10.1016/0014-4886(73)90075-7

Usunoff, K. G., Itzev, D. E., Lolov, S. R., and Wree, A. (2003). Pedunculopontine tegmental nucleus. Part 1: cytoarchitecture, transmitters, development and connections. *Biomed. Rev.* 14, 95–120. doi: 10.14748/bmr.v14.111

Veasey, S. C., Fornal, C. A., Metzler, C. W., and Jacobs, B. L. (1995). Response of serotonergic caudal raphe neurons in relation to specific motor activities in freely moving cats. *J. Neurosci.* 15, 5346–5359. doi: 10.1523/JNEUROSCI.15-07-05346.1995

Verberne, A. J. M. (1995). Cuneiform nucleus stimulation produces activation of medullary sympathoexcitatory neurons in rats. *Am. J. Physiol.* 268, R752–R758. doi: 10.1152/ajpregu.1995.268.3.R752

Viala, D., and Buser, P. (1969). The effects of DOPA and 5-HTP on rhythmic efferent discharges in hind limb nerves in the rabbit. *Brain Res.* 12, 437–443. doi: 10.1016/0006-8993(69)90011-0

Voss, M. D., de Castro, D., Lipski, J., Pilowski, P. M., and Jiang, C. (1990). Serotonin immunoreactive boutons form close appositions with respiratory neurons of the dorsal respiratory group in the cat. *J. Comp. Neurol.* 295, 208–218. doi: 10.1002/cne.902950205

Wang, H. L., and Morales, M. (2009). Pedunculopontine and laterodorsal tegmental nuclei contain distinct populations of cholinergic, glutamatergic and GABAergic neurons in the rat. *Eur. J. Neurosci.* 29, 340–358. doi: 10.1111/j.1460-9568.2008.06576.x

Westlund, K. N., Bowker, R. M., Ziegler, M. G., and Coulter, J. D. (1982). Descending noradrenergic projections and their spinal terminations. *Prog. Brain Res.* 57:1982. doi: 10.1016/S0079-6123(08)64131-X

Wienecke, J., Enriquez Denton, M., Stecina, K., Kirkwood, P. A., and Hultborn, H. (2015). Modulation of spontaneous locomotor and respiratory drives to hindlimb motoneurons temporally related to sympathetic drives as revealed by Mayer waves. *Front. Neural Circ.* 9:1. doi: 10.3389/fncir.2015.00001

Wise, R. A. (2004). Dopamine, learning and motivation. *Nat. Rev. Neurosci.* 5, 483–494. doi: 10.1038/nrn1406

Xiao, C., Cho, J. R., Zhou, C., Treweek, J. B., Chan, K., McKinney, S. L., et al. (2016). Cholinergic mesopontine signals govern locomotion and reward through dissociable midbrain pathways. *Neuron* 90, 333–347. doi: 10.1111/jnc.13910

Yokota, S., Oka, T., Tsumori, T., Nakamura, S., and Yasui, Y. (2007). Glutamatergic neurons in the Kölliker–Fuse nucleus project to the rostral ventral respiratory group and phrenic nucleus: a combined retrograde tracing and in situ hybridization study in the rat. *Neurosci. Res.* 59, 341–346. doi: 10.1016/j.neures.2007.08.004

Yoo, J. H., Zell, V., Wu, J., Punta, C., Ramajayam, N., Shen, X., et al. (2017). Activation of pedunculopontine glutamate neurons is reinforcing. *J. Neurosci.* 37, 38–46. doi: 10.1523/JNEUROSCI.3082-16.2016

Zubair, H. N., Beloozerova, I. N., Sun, H., and Marlinski, V. (2016). Head movement during walking in the cat. *Neuroscience* 332, 101–120. doi: 10.1016/j.neuroscience.2016.06.031

Effect of Different Movement Speed Modes on Human Action Observation: An EEG Study

*Tian-jian Luo, Jitu Lv, Fei Chao and Changle Zhou**

Fujian Provincal Key Lab of Brain-Inspired Computing, Department of Cognitive Science, School of Informatics, Xiamen University, Xiamen, China

Correspondence:
Changle Zhou
dozero@xmu.edu.cn

Action observation (AO) generates event-related desynchronization (ERD) suppressions in the human brain by activating partial regions of the human mirror neuron system (hMNS). The activation of the hMNS response to AO remains controversial for several reasons. Therefore, this study investigated the activation of the hMNS response to a speed factor of AO by controlling the movement speed modes of a humanoid robot's arm movements. Since hMNS activation is reflected by ERD suppressions, electroencephalography (EEG) with BCI analysis methods for ERD suppressions were used as the recording and analysis modalities. Six healthy individuals were asked to participate in experiments comprising five different conditions. Four incremental-speed AO tasks and a motor imagery (MI) task involving imaging of the same movement were presented to the individuals. Occipital and sensorimotor regions were selected for BCI analyses. The experimental results showed that hMNS activation was higher in the occipital region but more robust in the sensorimotor region. Since the attended information impacts the activations of the hMNS during AO, the pattern of hMNS activations first rises and subsequently falls to a stable level during incremental-speed modes of AO. The discipline curves suggested that a moderate speed within a decent inter-stimulus interval (ISI) range produced the highest hMNS activations. Since a brain computer/machine interface (BCI) builds a path-way between human and computer/mahcine, the discipline curves will help to construct BCIs made by patterns of action observation (AO-BCI). Furthermore, a new method for constructing non-invasive brain machine brain interfaces (BMBIs) with moderate AO-BCI and motor imagery BCI (MI-BCI) was inspired by this paper.

Keywords: action observation, different speed modes, hMNS activations, ERD suppressions, BCI

1. INTRODUCTION

Human mirror neuron system (hMNS) components activate the sensorimotor, parietal, and occipital cortices when a human performs, observes, or imitates an action (Rizzolatti, 2005; Tanji et al., 2015). Initial studies of the hMNS focused on motor imitation and learning, as well as action understanding and observation (Rizzolatti and Sinigaglia, 2010; Pineda et al., 2013). Furthermore, the hMNS has gradually come to be regarded as crucial for social skills such as understanding the intensions and emotional states of others (Blakemore and Decety, 2001; Schulte-Rüther et al., 2007). Action observation (AO) was considered one of the primary ways of inducing hMNS activations in early studies (Caspers et al., 2010; Mukamel et al., 2010; Rozzi and Fogassi, 2017). The modulation of hMNS recruitments by AO has positive effects on cognitive psychology and sport rehabilitation for creating scientific recovery strategies (Franceschini et al., 2012). hMNS activations by AO also provide another way to construct a brain computer/machine interface (BCI) for mechanical control and medical auxiliary purposes (Neuper et al., 2009). A BCI constructs an alternative method for communicating between human and computers/machines. In BCIs, the motor related BCI was constructed by the variation patterns in mu (8–12 Hz) and beta (18–25 Hz) bands power extracted by electroencephalography (EEG) when a human image, observer, or execute limb/leg movements. Variations in band power in the two rhythms are referred to as event-related desynchronization (ERD) suppression. Hence, the ERD suppression will be caused by motor imagery (MI) and AO. In fact, the definitions of AO tasks influence the degree of ERD suppression. However, the relationships between action definitions for AO and hMNS activations are still unknown from a scientific view.

In general, in the movements designing of an AO therapy for stroke patients or a BCI system, the parameters and affecting factors will influence the performance of therapy or BCI accuracy. In fact, the affecting factors will be controlled if we explore the disciplines of the relationships between movements for AO and the hMNS activations. Hence, the the research of the affecting factors of movements for action observation will do favor for designing a AO therapy scheme or an AO-BCI system. Most prior studies offer different hypotheses regarding the relationships between movements for AO and the hMNS activations (Iacoboni et al., 2005; Filimon et al., 2007; Newman-Norlund et al., 2007). Since many AO studies are based in cognitive psychology and sports psychology, while few are based in rehabilitation and BCI research, the distribution and degree of hMNS activations remain controversial with respect to several features of AO (Perry et al., 2010; Vogt et al., 2013). The mode of AO movements is the main factor that limits hMNS and motor system activation. Several neurophysiological studies indicate that ongoing movement plays an important role in triggering hMNS responses when activations are induced by AO (Maranesi et al., 2013). Aside from the condition of ongoing movements, other studies hypothesize that the manifestations of actions in AO tasks influence hMNS activations. In a study of action meaning (Agnew et al., 2012), compared with meaningless movements, meaningful movements caused higher hMNS activations. For example, lipreading of speech is one of the meaningful movements. Researches on lipreading showed lipreading will enhance speech perception and speech recognition (Summerfield, 1992; Silsbee and Bovik, 1996). Lipreading enhancement in young deaf children will help auditory speech perception (Geers, 1994). Lipreading and audiovisual speech integration are used in therapy of autism (Smith and Bennetto, 2007). Hence, the researches on action meaning will be useful for the therapy, rehabilitation, and neuroscience. In addition, the degree of movement complexity in an mode of AO movement has also been found to affecting hMNS activations (Biagi et al., 2010; Gatti et al., 2017). Moreover, additional variables that modulate hMNS activation and ERD suppression, such as experience and familiarity, have also been studied (Calvo-Merino et al., 2006; Bello et al., 2014).

Although the factors affecting the relationships between movements for AO and hMNS activation have been explored by the above studies, hMNS specificity and its full significance remain uncertain. The definitions of AO tasks clearly influence the degree of ERD suppression (Orgs et al., 2008). Furthermore, the manifestations of AO tasks and their stimuli affect attentional resources and hMNS activation (Oberman et al., 2007). Since the majority of affecting factors are related to the modes of AO movements, explorations of the relationships between movements for AO and hMNS activation are translated into the relationships between movement modes and the degree of ERD suppressions. Speed, complexity, magnitude, and individual proficiency are well-characterized factors known to affect movement modes, and have been explored in previous studies (Abdi and Williams, 2010; Biagi et al., 2010; Agnew et al., 2012; Maranesi et al., 2013; Bello et al., 2014). However, to the best of our knowledge, the present study is the first to investigate the effect of speed during AO. If the speed affecting factor is well-explored for AO among individuals, the designing for therapy scheme and AO-BCI will be more accurate for individuals. In addition, since the parameters and affecting factors will be well controlled in designing AO-BCI, but not in designing MI-BCI, the performance of AO-BCI will be better than MI-BCI. Furthermore, based on BCI system, the brain computer/machine brain interfaces (BMBIs) are capable of bidirectional communication with the brain. The interfaces consist of efferent and afferent modules. The efferent modules decode motor intentions by the variation patterns in mu and beta bands power, like conventional BCIs. The afferent modules encode feedback about the interactions of the machine through patterns of intracortical microstimulation. In general, the efferent modules are always designed by patterns of motor imagery. Meanwhile, the afferent modules can't be designed by patterns of MI. However, the afferent modules will be designed by patterns of action observation. When the efferent modules by MI drive a machine performing movements, the feedback by observation to activate hMNS will cause ERD suppression to design afferent modules. Today's BMBIs are constructed without considering the affecting factors of movements, so the performance is bad. However, if the speed and other affecting factors are considered for designing BMBIs, the performance will be better.

EEG (Lei et al., 2015; Abbott, 2016) has been widely used to construct BCI systems for exploring hMNS activations due to its high temporal resolution. In our study, the experimental movements were made by a humanoid robot at four different speed modes for AO tasks. A humanoid robot platform provides identical appearance, background and complexity to eliminate other effects. All four speed modes, slow (0.25 Hz), moderate (1.25 Hz), fast (2.75 Hz), and finalistic (4 Hz), were defined by questionnaires administered to 26 participants. Another six subjects were asked to attend AO experiments and an MI experiment for comparison. All eight stimuli (left movement and right movement at four speed modes) were randomly presented to all subjects in AO experiments, and another two stimuli were randomly presented to the same subjects in MI experiments. Both experiments are designed by a BCI form to validate the relationships between speed mode of AO and the hMNS activations. Due to the high temporal resolution, quantitative EEG (Lei et al., 2015; Abbott, 2016) is used as a convenient and cheap method to explore hMNS activations by measuring ERD suppressions (Oberman et al., 2007; Orgs et al., 2008). The ERD suppressions in EEG data are analyzed using a series of BCI methods and spatio-spectral-temporal characteristics. The following three main points are analyzed and discussed in this study:

(1) The brain regions involved in AO, such as the sensorimotor and occipital regions, are compared since studies on activation regions for AO have paradoxical conclusions (Perry et al., 2010; Frenkel-Toledo et al., 2013).
(2) The patterns of the relationships between AO speed modes and hMNS activations. If the patterns are clearly explored by experiments, individual rehabilitation strategies with specific optimal speeds will be precisely designed for individuals.
(3) Application to brain machine brain interface (BMBI). The average pattern of all individuals will show optimal speed ranges that are best suited to constructing AO-BCIs. Moreover, a well-established non-invasive AO-BCI with a high rate of accuracy and information transfer rate (ITR) will help to build BMBIs.

2. MATERIALS AND METHODS

2.1. Ethics Statement

This study was carried out in accordance with the recommendations of the guideline of EEG experiment, Xiamen University ethics committee with written informed consent from all subjects. All subjects gave written informed consent in accordance with the Declaration of Helsinki. The protocol was approved by the Xiamen University ethics committee.

2.2. Participants

Six right-handed healthy human subjects (five male and one female, mean age: 24.6 years, $SD = 1.46$) were invited to participate in AO and MI experiments with payment. All subjects had no history of neurological disease and either normal or corrected-to-normal vision. Subjects also did not have any professional experience with AO or MI experiments. In accordance with the principles of the Helsinki Declaration, all subjects provided written informed consent approved by the Xiamen University.

2.3. Stimuli Design

As shown in **Figure 1**, stimuli for AO in different speed modes were performed by a humanoid robot. AO stimuli were presented to all subjects in 12 sessions as experiment 1. Afterwards, an MI comparison experiment in which two guidance arrows were presented to the same subjects in three sessions was performed as experiment 2.

2.3.1. Experiment 1:AO Experiments in Different Speed Modes

In previous studies, AO experimental paradigms were designed with sequential video clips of human arm, hand, or finger movements presented to subjects (Frenkel-Toledo et al., 2014; Gatti et al., 2017). However, our experiments were designed to explore speed factor during AO. Because human movements feature unconstant speed, angle, and magnitude across repetitive experiments, the inconsistency of the variables will introduce confounding factors that disturb the analyses of hMNS activations. To eliminate such confounding factors, a fine-tuning parameter-setting paradigm must be incorporated into the design. Based on the anthropomorphic and relevant AO studies (Press, 2011), the hMNS is strongly activated by observations of both human and non-human agents (e.g., humanoid robots). Human or non-human agents do not differ significantly in their ability to activate the hMNS in AO studies involving humans and humanoid robots. Since the robot platform features an operating system for controlling all movement parameters, a humanoid robot platform was used in the design of our AO experimental paradigms.

Based on the "NAO Choregraphe 1.14 platform" (Pot et al., 2009), periodic-swinging movements of the robot's left/right arm

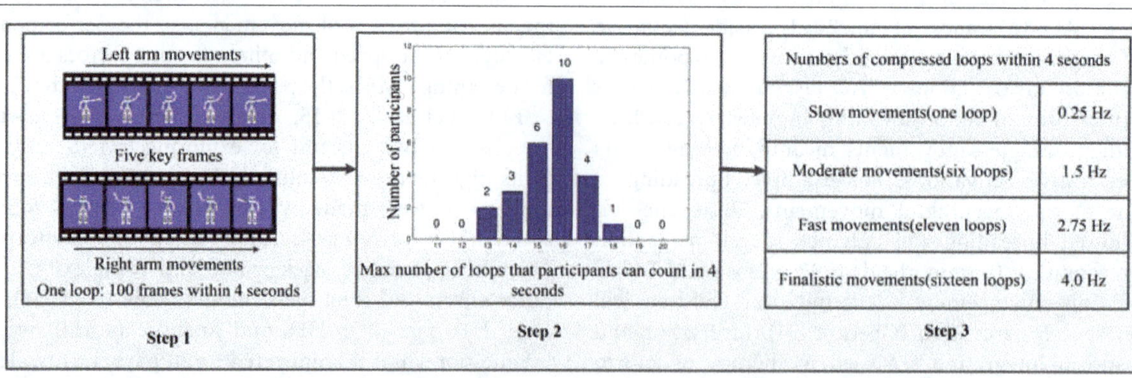

FIGURE 1 | Stimuli design of AO in different speed modes. The Step 1 contains one loop of periodic-swinging arm movement includes 100 frames over four seconds because the platform has a fixed frame rate of 25 fps. The Step 2 summarizes the results of the correct maximum loop number counted by each participant. The Step 3 defines the role of speed modes in the pattern of relationships between AO tasks and hMNS activations. As well as for simplicity and convenience, four different loops with a constant interval were constructed. Step 1: One loop for AO at standard speed. Step 2: Twenty-six participants count loops at higher speed modes to determine the max (16 loops). Step 3: Select four speed modes for experiments by equi-partition.

were utilized as AO tasks in experiment 1. As shown in **Figure 1** (Step 1), one loop of periodic-swinging arm movement includes 100 frames over 4 s because the platform has a fixed frame rate of 25 fps. Five key frames for both the left and right arms show the same procedure of the periodic movements. The robot stretches its arm at the beginning of the loop and waves its arm up to the head during half of the loop. The remainder of the loop consists of the same procedure in the opposite direction. The platform ensures that the robot's left/right-arm movements maintain a constant speed, angle, and magnitude. The entity body of the robot was presented to subjects in order to distinguish left-arm or right-arm movements during AO using EEG-based BCI analysis methods (Bauer and Gharabaghi, 2015). The robot's arms are dynamic, while the other parts of the robot remain static to keep the speed variable clear and unique.

Theoretically, more speed modes will be better for the results. However, due to the limitation of participants and the experimental platform, we only explore the rough pattern of the factor affections for simplicity and convenience. Four different loops with a constant interval were constructed as shown in **Figure 1** (Step 3). For simplicity, the four incremental speed movements are defined as "slow movement," "moderate movement," "fast movement," and "finalistic movement." In **Figure 1** (Step 1), one loop of 100 frames over 4 s is defined as "slow movement." Due to time duration in AO experiments (4 s per trial), we obtain higher movement speed modes by adding number of loops, and compressing multi-loops within 4 s. To identify a robust and suitable number of multi-loops for "finalistic movement," 26 participants were invited to watch 10 different looped (11–20) video clips that were compressed into 4 s. Participants were asked to count the number of loop in each video clip. The results from all participants were then compared with ground truth to identify the maximum loop number for each participant. **Figure 1** (Step 2) summarizes the results of the correct maximum loop number counted by each participant. The results show that 16 loops was the maximum loop number for all of the participants. Therefore, "finalistic movement" was defined as 16 loops compressed into 4 s. "Moderate movement" was set to six loops, and "fast movement" was set to 11 loops, by the principle of equipartition. In all, experiment 1 gives four different speed modes of AO to explore the role of speed. All four speed modes were presented to subjects during AO in experiment 1.

2.3.2. Experiment 2: Relevant MI Experiment

After experiment 1, all six healthy human subjects were asked to attend experiment 2. The MI experiment was compared with the AO experiment. Following the design criteria of MI experimental paradigms (Tangermann et al., 2012), two guidance arrows were defined in experiment 2 to guide the imagined movement direction. In experiment 2, the subjects were asked to imagine his/her-self as performing the same movement as the humanoid robot in experiment 1. Both MI guidance arrows used in experiment 2 were presented to all subjects after experiment 1.

2.4. Experimental Procedures

As shown in **Figure 2**, the experimental procedures for AO in different speed modes and MI were divided into trials and sessions. EEG recordings were set for both AO and MI experiments.

2.4.1. Trial Procedures

Influenced by conventional AO/MI experimental trial setups (Calvo-Merino et al., 2004; Wang et al., 2012), the presentation of a trial is shown in **Figure 2A**. In each trial, initial instructions guided subjects to simply observe the robot's movements (experiment 1) or guidance arrows (experiment 2) on the screen and a manually respond as rapidly as possible whenever the catch trial static robot (experiment 1) or blank (experiment 2) is presented. Subjects were also asked to minimize eye movements and keep their eyes fixed on the monitor when observing the stimuli. Manual responses to the catch trial were input by pressing the "SPACE" button. Each trial started with a fixation cross presented in the middle of a gray screen. The duration of the fixation cross was 2,000 ms. After presentation of the fixation cross, stimuli were presented in the middle of the gray screen for 4,000 ms to investigate participants' ERD suppressions via EEG recordings and were followed by a 2,000-ms pause as a break. If the presentation was an AO stimulus (experiment 1), subjects were asked to focus on the moving arm of the robot; otherwise, when the presentation was an MI stimulus (experiment 2), subjects were asked to imagine him/her-self moving like the robot by following the guidance arrows. Subsequent trials followed the same procedure for both experiment 1 and experiment 2.

2.4.2. Session Procedures

In experiment 1, each subject completed 12 AO sessions within 6 days, whereas in experiment 2, each subject completed three MI sessions within 2 days. Data recordings for one session occurred in the morning, with another session taking place later in the afternoon the same day. As shown in **Figure 2D**, each session comprised two tasks, and each task was divided into 40 trials. A relaxation time to prevent fatigue was determined by subjects between the two tasks. Experiment 1 comprised eight AO stimuli and one catch trial stimulus, which are described in **Figure 2B**. Each of the eight AO stimuli (left and right in four speed modes) was randomly presented four times, and the catch trial stimulus was randomly presented eight times within one session (See **Figure 2D**). Experiment 2 comprised two MI stimulus arrows and one blank catch trial stimulus, which are described in **Figure 2C**. Each of the two MI stimuli (left and right) was randomly presented four times, and the catch trial stimulus was randomly presented eight times within one session (See **Figure 2D**). Response times to the catch trial stimulus were recorded for both experiments 1 and 2 because the response times help confirm attentional states during AO and MI experiments.

2.4.3. EEG Recordings

Each subject was seated individually in a comfortable arm chair in front of a computer monitor in a dimly lit, sound-attenuated room and asked to read the instructions carefully on the screen. AO stimuli (experiment 1) and MI stimuli (experiment 2) were displayed on a DELL P2314H LCD monitor with a refresh rate of 60 frames/s. Displays were controlled by the psychology software tool "E-Prime 2.0." The distances between monitor and the subjects were set at 100 cm by following the BCI experimental criterion to prevent other confounding factors in the hMNS activation (Onishi et al., 2017). During the entire run of both experiments, a spatially homogeneous gray background with a luminance of 38 cd/m2 was enabled. EEG recordings for all subjects were performed on a "NeuroScan SynAmps2" device with a "Neuroscan QuikCap international 10–20 system." EEG signals were referenced to the nose, grounded at the frontal position (Fpz), and sampled at 250 Hz. After data acquisition, the preprocessing operations on the signals for notch filtering and bandpass filtering were 48–52 and 0.1–100 Hz, respectively. All 64 electrode impedances in QuikCap were kept below 5kω during the experiment. Moreover, the horizontal and vertical EOG signals were recorded. The EOG signals were used to correct for the influence of blinking and eyeball movements.

2.5. Analysis Methods

As shown in **Figure 3**, three main EEG data analyses procedures were utilized in this study. **Figure 3** (Step 1) illustrates the preprocessing procedure. Raw EEGs from six subjects were first corrected for EOG artifacts via blind component separation. Then, a band filter ranging from 0.15 to 30 Hz was adopted

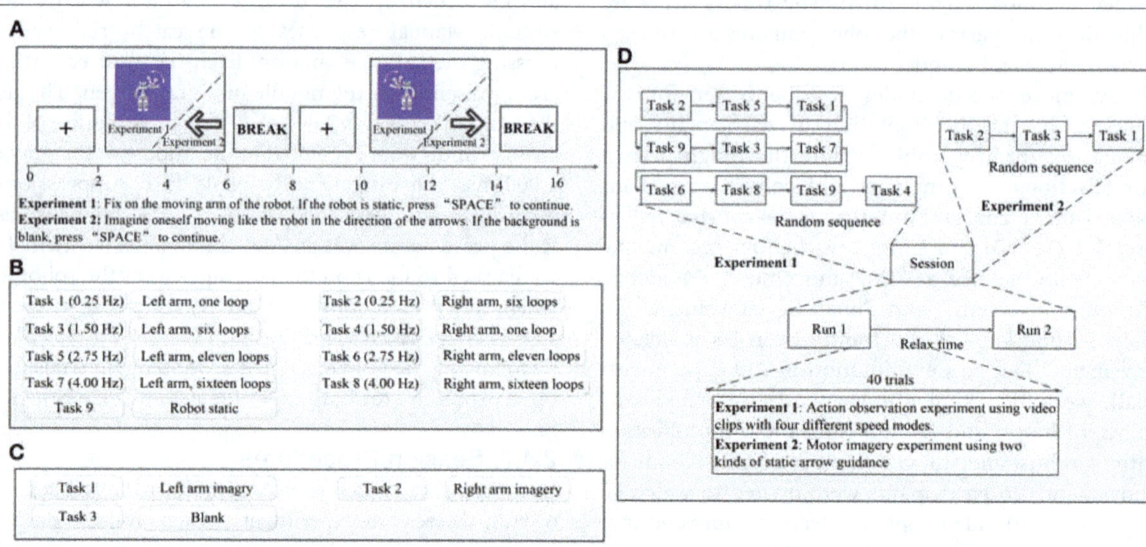

FIGURE 2 | Experimental procedures. In each trial, initial instructions guided subjects to simply observe the robot's movements (experiment 1) or guidance arrows (experiment 2) on the screen and a manually respond as rapidly as possible whenever the catch trial static robot (experiment 1) or blank (experiment 2) is presented. Each trial started with a fixation cross presented in the middle of a gray screen. The duration of the fixation cross was 2,000 ms. After presentation of the fixation cross, stimuli were presented in the middle of the gray screen for 4,000 ms to investigate participants' ERD suppressions via EEG recordings and were followed by a 2,000-ms pause as a break. Each of the eight AO stimuli (left and right in four speed modes) was randomly presented four times, and the catch trial stimulus was randomly presented eight times within one session in Experiment 1. Each of the two MI stimuli (left and right) was randomly presented four times, and the catch trial stimulus was randomly presented eight times within one session in Experiment 2. **(A)** Example trial sequence for experiment 1 and experiment 2. **(B)** Task descriptions for experiment 1. **(C)** Task descriptions for experiment 2. **(D)** Example session sequence for experiment 1 and experiment 2.

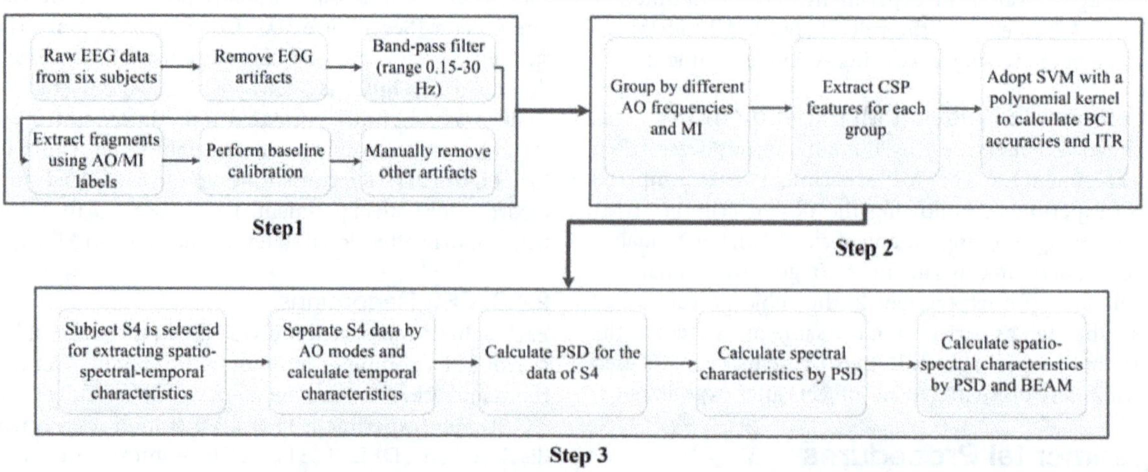

FIGURE 3 | EEG data analysis procedures. Step 1: Pre-processing. Step 2: BCI analyses. Step 3: Extracting spatio-spectral-temporal characteristics.

for EEG data, since the effective parts are above 0.15 Hz and under 30 Hz. By using AO (experiment 1) and MI (experiment 2) labels recorded in "NeuroScan," fragments of each experimental condition were extracted for all subjects. After fragment extraction, a baseline calibration method to prevent deviation and a manual removal method to reducing artifacts were performed on all fragments.

Recent studies first found that hMNS activations initially occurs in the sensorimotor region of the brain during AO (Perry et al., 2010). The ERD suppressions in the sensorimotor region then extend to attentional resources, which cause more intense hMNS activations in the occipital region (Frenkel-Toledo et al., 2013). Likewise, ERD suppressions caused by MI are first found in the sensorimotor region and then extend to global cerebral activity. To explore the affected regions of the brain during AO, the patterns of relationships between AO speed modes and hMNS activations, as well as to compare AO and MI to construct a BMBI, the sensorimotor, occipital and "sensorimotor + occipital" regions were adopted for BCI analyses of both AO and MI experiments. Potentials covering central-parietal regions C3, C1, Cz, C2, C4, P3, P1, Pz, P2, and P4 were chosen for the sensorimotor region, while potentials covering parietal-occipital regions PO5, PO3, POz, PO4, PO6, O1, Oz, and O2 were chosen for the occipital region. The "sensorimotor + occipital" region included both sets of potentials.

As illustrated in **Figure 3** (Step 2), the procedure for BCI analyses comprised four steps. First, left fragments and right fragments were grouped by identical AO speed (experiment 1). Second, all groups of fragments were presented to extract filter bank common spatial pattern (FB-CSP) features (Ang et al., 2012). Since ERD suppressions are modulated by the power variations of the left and right cerebral hemispheres, an FB-CSP algorithm was adopted to extract power variations using a bank of filters and an optimization method. The optimal CSP eigenvectors were set to $S = 4$ based on experience. Third, the principal component analysis (PCA) algorithm of a linear dimensionality reduction technique was adopted to reduce feature dimensions (Abdi and Williams, 2010). Because of the high sampling rate in EEG recordings, FB-CSP features have a high number of dimensions that are hard to classify by machine-learning models. The PCA algorithm looks for the highest variability in FB-CSP features by projecting original features to lower dimensions. The optimal PCA was set to $M = 10$ for the regulation of "99%" of the variability. Finally, the dimension-reduced FB-CSP features were incorporated into the support vector machine (SVM) classifier for BCI classification (Sardouie and Shamsollahi, 2012). The SVM classifier is a common BCI classifier with excellent generalizability by searching for the largest margin of a decision hyperplane that will strictly classify the unseen test data. The reductive features were incorporated into SVM classifiers with a polynomial kernel. A 6*6 cross-validation strategy was applied to train the SVM classifiers for all five groups. Since each group has 392 trials of effective EEG fragments with a random order for left and right, 320 trials were provided as training data, and the remaining 64 trials as evaluation data in one loop of evaluation.

Figure 3 (Step 3) displays the procedure for extracting spatio-spectral-temporal characteristics. Subject 4, who had the best BCI accuracies, was chosen for the analyses of these characteristics. The temporal characteristics were first extracted by calculating mean voltages of EEG fragments among four different speed AO modes (both for left and right). Then, a power spectral density (PSD) (Demandt et al., 2012) algorithm with parameters of specific rhythm ranges was used for each average fragment to obtain spectral characteristics. The spectral characteristics were drawn by the "eeglab 14.1.1" tool as "ERD images" (Delorme and Makeig, 2004). Brain electrical activity maps (BEAMs) (Duffy et al., 1979) were imported to obtain the positions of the potentials, and the spatio-spectral characteristics were drawn by the "eeglab 14.1.1" tool.

In addition, the response times of catch trial stimuli as feedback behavioral data were analyzed by statistical analyses. Mean time values for all 15 sessions (Sessions 1–12 for experiment 1 and sessions 13–15 for experiment 2) were calculated for all subjects to obtain the attentional conditions of all sessions by calculating mean values and standard deviations among all sessions.

3. RESULTS

3.1. Feedback Behavioral Data

Catch trial stimuli appear 16 times in each session, and we have recorded the response times for all catch trial stimuli in each session. **Tables 1, 2** illustrate the mean response times within one session for experiment 1 and experiment 2, respectively. The mean time and standard deviations among all sessions in both experiments are also presented.

As shown in **Table 1**, the average response times among all sessions of experiment 1 were within 2,000 ms, and the corresponding standard deviations were within 100–200 ms. These results demonstrate that all subjects exhibited focused attention during AO experiments and EEG recordings. Therefore, EEG recordings in experiment 1 were free from attention artifacts. The standard deviations of all subjects were within a similar range, indicating that the responses to stimuli were stable. The response times of Subjects 2 and 3 had lower averages and standard deviations, which may be related to their younger age, as this tends to be related to faster response times. Since our behavioral data conform to experimental principles, the EEG data of experiment 1 were considered objective and appropriate for analyses. Similarly, as illustrated in **Table 2**, the average response time among all sessions of experiment 2 were within 300 ms, and the corresponding standard deviations were within 10 and 20 ms. These results conform with the response times of MI experiments, indicating that the EEG recordings in experiment 2 were objective and appropriate for analyses. Compared with **Tables 1, 2**, the blank catch trial stimuli was easier to recognize than a static robot, and the individual differences in the response times of younger subjects has less influence on the MI experiments.

3.2. BCI Analyses of AO and MI Experiments

After preprocessing, the EEG fragments (left and right) of four speed AO modes and MI modes were used for BCI analyses. In

FB-CSP feature extraction, the bank of bank filters following a previous study are shown in **Table 3**. **Table 3** illustrates the BCI analysis results for three regions in four AO speed modes and MI mode. The average accuracies and standard deviations of BCI classification and ITR were calculated. To display the comparison of the results, **Figure 4** shows the average accuracies of all modes in all regions.

From the BCI analysis results in **Table 4** and **Figure 4**, we see four findings:

(1) For the accuracies in the occipital region, the results were AO-0.25 Hz (71.44%), AO-1.5 Hz (74.78%), AO-2.75 Hz (58.42%), and AO-4 Hz (59.29%). However, the results were AO-0.25 Hz (61.76%), AO-1.5 Hz (69.27%), AO-2.75 Hz (56.29%), and AO-4 Hz (55.99%) in the sensorimotor region. Similarity, the accuracies of the "sensorimotor+occipital" were AO-0.25 Hz (62.07%), AO-1.5 Hz (68.92%), AO-2.75 Hz (56.81%), and AO-4 Hz (56.33%). Considering the results across all regions, the BCI accuracies from increasing speed modes of AO presented a pattern of initially increasing and then decreasing to a stable level.

(2) Comparing AO-BCI accuracies between occipital and sensorimotor regions, the results were 71.44 and 61.76% at AO-0.25 Hz, 74.78 and 69.27% at AO-1.5 Hz, 58.42 and 56.29% at AO-2.75 Hz, and 59.29 and 55.99% at AO-4 Hz. AO in any speed mode had a more significant BCI accuracy in the occipital region than in the sensorimotor region. However, the accuracies of MI-BCI were 57.72% in the occipital region and 61.35% in the sensorimotor region. MI mode had a more significant BCI accuracy in the sensorimotor region than in the occipital region.

(3) The BCI accuracies in the "sensorimotor+occipital" region were at a similar level to those in the sensorimotor region. The results were 62.07 and 61.76% at AO-0.25 Hz, 68.92 and 69.27% at AO-1.5 Hz, 56.81 and 56.29% at AO-2.75 Hz, and 56.33 and 55.99% at AO-4 Hz. However, a large difference was detected between the "sensorimotor+occipital" and occipital regions. The results were 62.07 and 71.44% at AO-0.25 Hz, 68.92 and 74.78% at AO-1.5 Hz, 56.81 and 58.42% at AO-2.75 Hz, and 56.33 and 55.99% at AO-4 Hz. These results suggested the BCI accuracy was more robust in the sensorimotor region and was resistant the influence of other regions. Moreover, the higher BCI accuracies in the occipital region may be influenced by factors other than hMNS activations.

(4) Because the standard deviations of all experimental modes in all regions were within the range of [0, 10], AO in different speed modes and MI mode have similar robustness. The average standard deviations in all regions between AO modes showed that AO-0.25 Hz (5.69) and AO-1.5 Hz (5.80) have lower robustness than AO-2.75 Hz (2.98) and AO-4 Hz (2.13). Since ITR presents the efficiency of BCI, the average results of ITR in all regions showed that AO-1.5 Hz (2.01) had a significantly higher efficiency than AO-0.25 Hz (1.10), AO-2.75 Hz (0.23), AO-4 Hz (0.24), and MI (0.43). AO in moderate-speed mode was more suitable for the design of BCIs.

(5) The average accuracies have the same pattern of initially increasing and then decreasing to a stable level. In the results between subjects, subjects "S1, S3, S4" correspond to the average pattern, but subjects "S2 and S5" not correspond to the average pattern from AO-0.25 Hz to AO-4 Hz. However, subjects "S2 and S5" have approximate accuracies in AO-0.25

TABLE 1 | Statistical analyses of response times for Experiment 1 (ms).

Sessions	Subject 1	Subject 2	Subject 3	Subject 4	Subject 5	Subject 6
Session 1	1760.53	868.97	868.97	1521.47	1716.25	1007.38
Session 2	1087.91	912.84	696.41	1411.47	1254.91	1706.56
Session 3	1201.75	993.75	621.06	1031.94	1695.63	1436.28
Session 4	1141.13	890.38	642.44	1102.09	1783.66	1093.78
Session 5	1243.38	943.69	518.03	1052.81	1644.91	1306.13
Session 6	1175.63	1047.78	749.00	1625.84	1701.25	1577.13
Session 7	1115.03	853.84	829.81	1306.88	1304.25	1420.00
Session 8	1417.50	818.72	777.56	1367.94	1562.38	1513.63
Session 9	1417.50	699.81	763.16	1655.03	1301.03	1268.88
Session 10	1392.31	660.88	759.81	1509.13	1284.75	1204.16
Session 11	1339.03	557.09	828.41	1509.13	1450.06	1181.03
Session 12	1582.00	656.63	790.31	1348.56	1526.16	1181.09
Average	1310.30	825.37	727.84	1370.19	1518.77	1324.67
Standard	201.81	150.67	92.55	213.45	194.04	208.90

The average accuracies and standard deviations of response times were calculated for experiment 1.

TABLE 2 | Statistical analyses of response times for Experiment 2 (ms).

Sessions	Subject 1	Subject 2	Subject 3	Subject 4	Subject 5	Subject 6
Session 13	234.44	238.09	183.81	298.13	286.75	193.63
Session 14	284.31	282.72	219.16	307.94	317.06	221.09
Session 15	258.03	262.84	204.41	287.88	262.31	237.88
Average	258.93	261.22	202.46	297.98	288.71	217.53
Standard	24.95	22.36	17.76	10.03	27.43	22.34

The average accuracies and standard deviations of response times were calculated for experiment 2.

TABLE 3 | The subbands of band-pass filters in FB-CSP feature extraction.

Subbands	fb_1	fb_2	fb_3	fb_4	fb_5	fb_6	fb_7	fb_8	fb_9	fb_{10}
Frequency(Hz)	[0, 4]	[4, 8]	[8, 12]	[12, 16]	[16, 20]	[20, 24]	[24, 28]	[28, 32]	[32, 36]	[36, 40]

A bank of 10 band-pass filters from 0 to 40 Hz without overlaps are set.

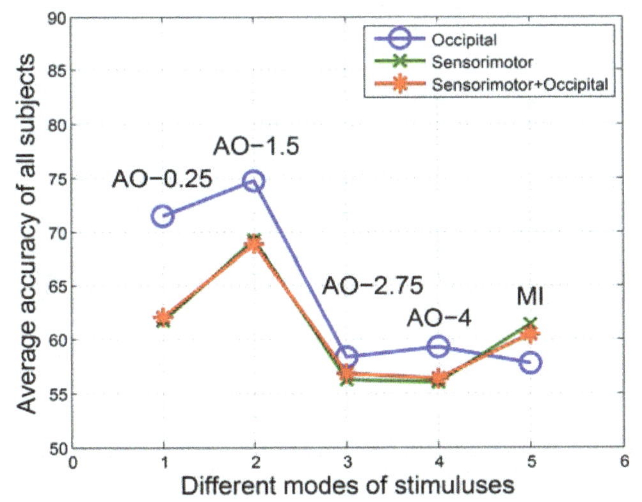

FIGURE 4 | The average accuracies of all modes in all regions. Potentials covering central-parietal regions C3, C1, Cz, C2, C4, P3, P1, Pz, P2, and P4 were chosen for the sensorimotor region, while potentials covering parietal-occipital regions PO5, PO3, POz, PO4, PO6, O1, Oz, and O2 were chosen for the occipital region. The "sensorimotor + occipital" region included both sets of potentials.

Hz and AO-4 Hz. This because different individuals have different patterns of speed modes, and our study was researched on rough speeds due to limitations of device and platform.

These five findings will help us understand affected regions in the brain during AO and the patterns of relationships between AO speed modes and hMNS activations. By selecting the optimal speed mode of AO, we also solved the problem of BMBI. These findings and conclusions are discussed below.

TABLE 4 | The BCI analysis results for three regions for four AO modes and MI modes.

Subjects	AO-0.25 Hz	AO-1.5 Hz	AO-2.75 Hz	AO-4.0 Hz	MI
OCCIPITAL REGION					
S1	69.27	79.17	54.43	59.38	60.16
S2	77.08	69.79	59.11	59.38	59.90
S3	69.01	76.30	54.95	62.24	57.03
S4	69.27	81.77	68.75	61.46	57.29
S5	67.71	65.36	56.25	54.43	58.85
S6	76.30	76.30	57.03	58.85	53.13
Average	71.44	74.78	58.42	59.29	57.72
Standard	4.12	6.10	5.33	2.73	2.60
ITR (bits/min)	2.06	2.78	0.31	0.38	0.26
SENSORIMOTOR REGION					
S1	69.01	75.52	56.77	56.77	55.47
S2	72.14	68.49	57.03	57.29	57.03
S3	56.77	67.45	58.33	55.47	54.69
S4	54.69	67.19	56.51	52.60	54.69
S5	60.42	70.83	55.21	56.77	67.97
S6	57.55	66.15	53.91	57.03	78.29
Average	61.76	69.27	56.29	55.99	61.35
Standard	7.14	3.45	1.54	1.77	9.72
ITR (bits/min)	0.61	1.65	0.17	0.16	0.56
"OCCIPITAL + SENSORIMOTOR" REGION					
S1	55.21	73.96	56.25	56.25	55.47
S2	71.61	69.53	60.68	58.85	55.21
S3	65.10	59.11	54.43	58.33	56.25
S4	58.33	81.25	56.77	54.17	55.47
S5	62.76	64.32	56.77	55.47	61.72
S6	59.38	65.36	55.99	54.95	78.39
Average 62.07	68.92	56.81	56.33	60.42	
Standard	5.82	7.84	2.08	1.88	9.14
ITR (bits/min)	0.64	1.59	0.20	0.17	0.47

Potentials covering central-parietal regions C3, C1, Cz, C2, C4, P3, P1, Pz, P2, and P4 were chosen for the sensorimotor region, while potentials covering parietal-occipital regions PO5, PO3, POz, PO4, PO6, O1, Oz, and O2 were chosen for the occipital region. The "sensorimotor + occipital" region included both sets of potentials. The average accuracies and standard deviations of BCI classification and ITR were calculated.

3.3. Spatio-Spectral-Temporal Characteristics of AO Experiments

To further analyse the detailed characteristics, the best-performing data, S4, was chosen to extract the spatio-spectral-temporal characteristics of AO modes.

3.3.1. Temporal Characteristics

The average microvolt of C3 and C4 are drawn on left movements and right movements, respectively. The difference of "C3-C4" in left movements and "C4-C3" in right movements are drawn for temporal characteristics in **Figure 5**. Two key sites, C3 and C4 from the sensorimotor region, were chosen to analyse temporal characteristics.

Three key findings from the results in **Figure 5** are as follows:

(1) Look from the overall, the average microvolt variations of C4 sites are higher than C3 sites on left movements, while the average microvolt variations of C3 sites are higher than C4 sites on right movements. These findings demonstrate the brain's hemisphere lateralization effect during AO.

(2) Look from the difference average microvolt variations of (C3-C4) in left movements and (C4-C3) in right movements, the differences of AO-0.25 Hz and AO-1.5 Hz are significantly higher than AO-2.75 Hz and AO-4 Hz for both left movements and right movements. These results confirm that variations during AO captured a pattern of increases with slow-speed movements and decreases with fast-speed movements.

(3) In fact, we have calculated the average of difference variations from 1,000 samples for both four different speed modes on left movements and right movements. The results are 0.958 (AO-0.25 Hz), 0.974 (AO-1.5 Hz), 0.048 (AO-2.75 Hz), and 0.112 (AO-4 Hz) on left movements, and 0.907 (AO-0.25

Hz), 0.988 (AO-1.5 Hz), 0.821 (AO-2.75 Hz), and 0.5865 (AO-4 Hz) on right movements. These results suggest some relationships between speed and stimulus direction.

3.3.2. Spectral Characteristics

Figure 6 shows the spectral characteristics of AO in four different speed modes. Four key potentials, C3 and C4 for the

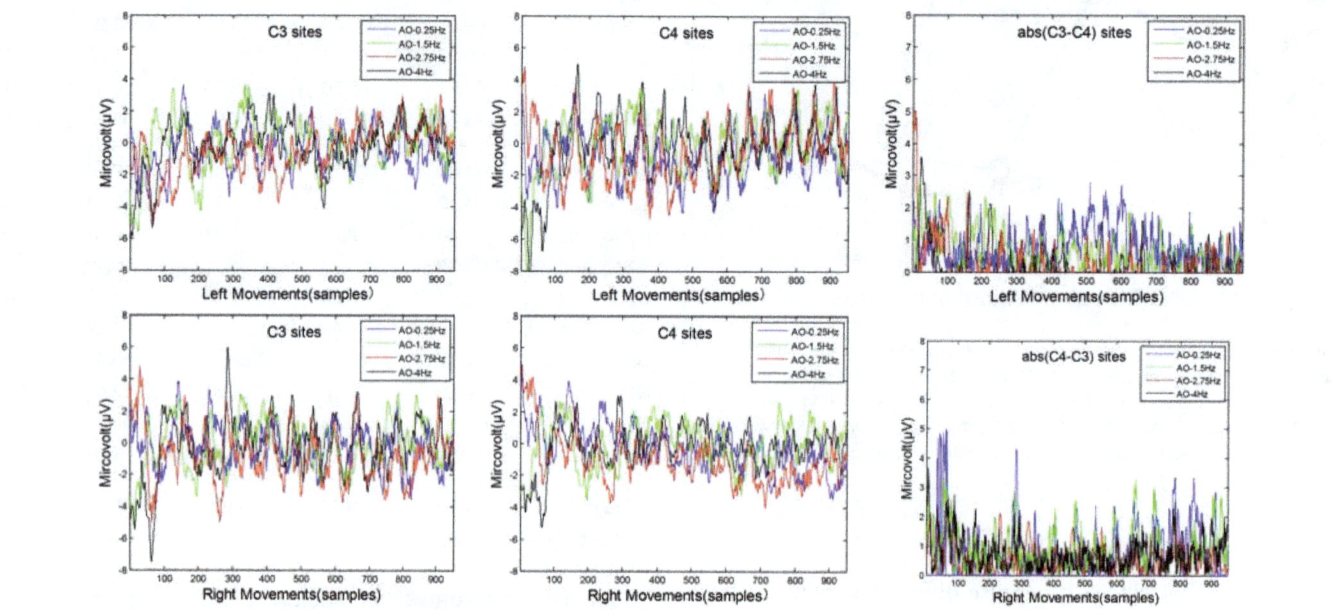

FIGURE 5 | The temporal characteristics of AO in four different speed modes. Two key sites, C3 and C4 from the sensorimotor region, were chosen to analyse temporal characteristics. The average microvolt of C3 and C4 are drawn on left movements and right movements, respectively. The difference of "C3–C4" in left movements and "C4–C3" in right movements are also drawn for temporal characteristics.

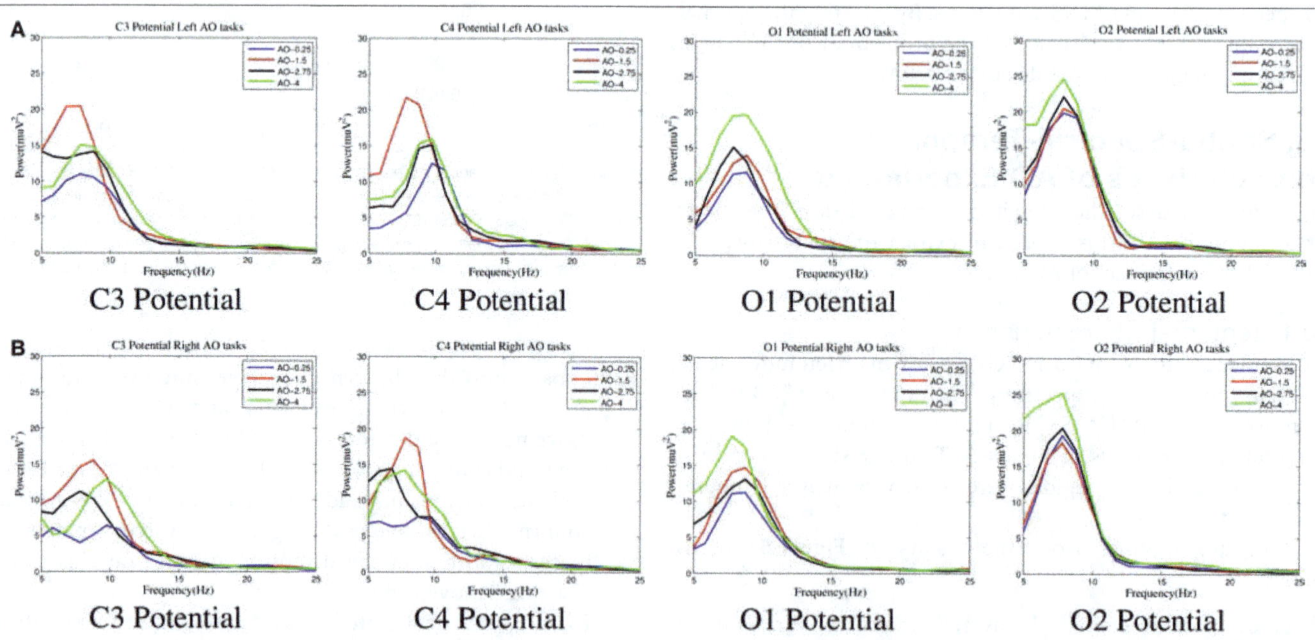

FIGURE 6 | The spectral characteristics of AO in four different speed modes. Four key potentials, C3 and C4 for the sensorimotor region and O1 and O2 for the occipital region, were chosen to analyse the spectral characteristics. The curves for all four AO modes (left movements and right movements) are drawn by "MATLAB R2012a." **(A)** Left movements of AO. **(B)** Right movements of AO.

sensorimotor region and O1 and O2 for the occipital region, were chosen to analyse the spectral characteristics.

Three important findings from **Figure 6** are as follows:

(1) In all of the AO modes, the power varied significantly in the mu range (8–12 Hz) at all C3/C4/O1/O2 potentials, but the variation in the beta range (18–25 Hz) was lower. These results show that the mu range is more sensitive in hMNS during AO.

(2) Regardless of whether left or right movements were examined, the power captured variation in the sensorimotor region (C3/C4) with a pattern where the largest was in AO-1.5 Hz, moderate was in AO-2.75 Hz and AO-4 Hz, and the smallest as in AO-0.25 Hz. However, the power captured variation in the occipital region (O1/O2) had an entirely different pattern in which the largest was in AO-4 Hz and the smallest was AO-1.5 Hz, AO-2.75 Hz, and AO-0.25 Hz with no obvious differences. These results suggest that the sensorimotor region was significantly activated at AO-1.5 Hz, whereas the occipital region was significantly activated at AO-4 Hz.

(3) Regardless of whether left or right movements were examined, the hemisphere effect of the power difference was prominent in the occipital region (O1/O2) but was not obvious in the sensorimotor region (C3/C4). These results demonstrate that the occipital region is more activated than the sensorimotor region.

3.3.3. Spatio-Spectral Characteristics

Figure 7 shows the spatio-spectral characteristics of AO in four different speed modes. The key rhythms, 8, 12, 18, and 25 Hz, were chosen to extract spatio-spectral characteristics from 64 potentials, since the ERD suppressions were induced in the mu (8–12 Hz) and beta (18–25 Hz) ranges.

From the results in **Figure 7**, we find that:

(1) In all eight AO modes, the BEAMs showed that the power in the mu range (8–12 Hz) was higher than that in the beta range (18–25 Hz) in the occipital region. These results demonstrate that the mu range plays a predominant role in hMNS activations.

(2) In contrast to the ERD suppressions during the four different AO speed modes, the ERD suppressions were stronger at AO-0.25 Hz and AO-1.5 Hz than at AO-2.75 Hz and AO-4 Hz in the sensorimotor region. These findings demonstrate that in the sensorimotor region, slow-speed movements cause greater hMNS activation than fast-speed movements during AO.

(3) Comparing left and right movements in one AO mode, the left movements produced more obvious ERD suppressions in the right hemisphere of the brain, whereas the right movements produced more obvious ERD suppressions in the left hemisphere of the brain. These results are due to the mirror effect from the hMNS. However, the movements that subjects observed were also mirror movements. Therefore,

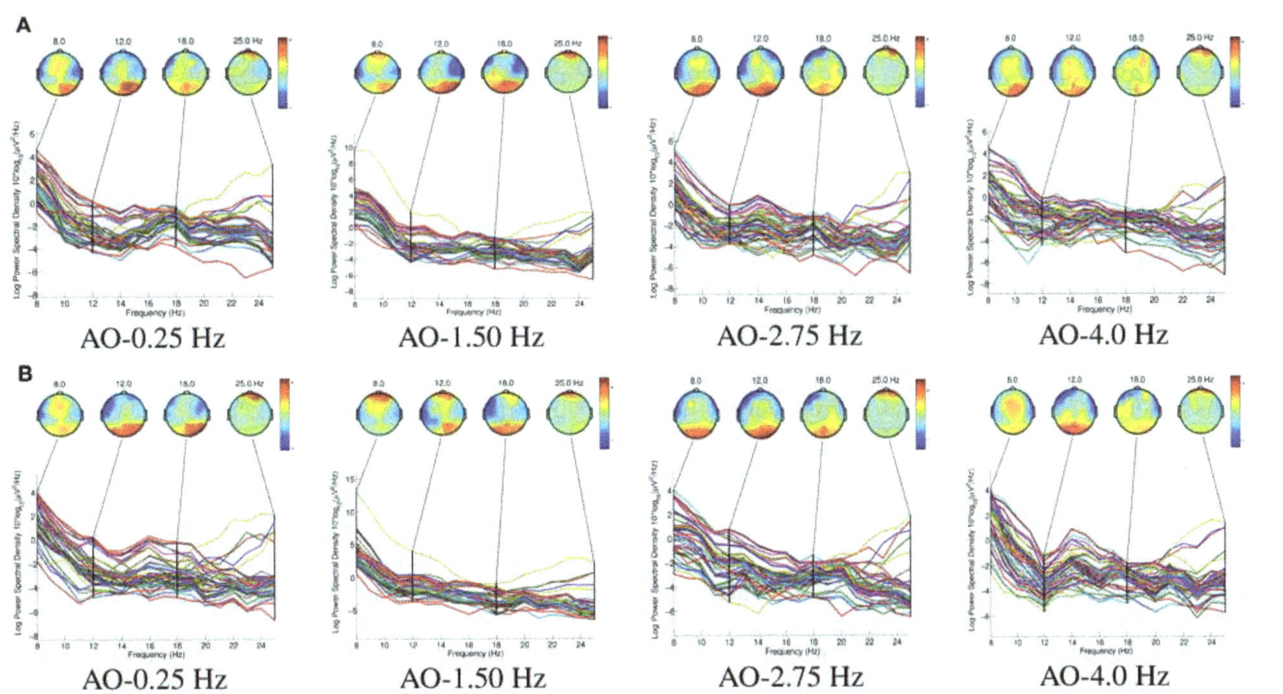

FIGURE 7 | The spatio-spectral characteristics of AO in four different speed modes. The key rhythms, 8, 12, 18, and 25 Hz, were chosen to extract spatio-spectral characteristics from 64 potentials, since the ERD suppressions were induced in the mu (8–12 Hz) and beta (18–25 Hz) ranges. The "BEAM" for all four AO modes(left and right movements) are drawn by "eeglab 14.1.1." **(A)** Left movements of AO. **(B)** Right movements of AO.

the ERD suppressions occurred in the ipsilateral region of the subject's brain relative to the movements of the robot.

4. DISCUSSION

This study further explored the brain regions affected during AO, the patterns of relationships between AO speed modes and hMNS activations, and the comparison of AO and MI for constructing BMBIs. AO experiments with different speed modes (experiment 1) and an MI mode (experiment) were explored at the central nervous system level since hMNS activation caused by AO are reflected by ERD suppressions, which are measured via EEG recording. BCI analyses and spatio-spectral-temporal characteristics were used to explore the variations in ERD suppressions. Based on our results, we were able to draw three major conclusions, which are discussed below:

(1) The occipital region exhibits higher hMNS activation than the sensorimotor region during AO, but the sensorimotor region shows more robust hMNS activations than the occipital region.
(2) hMNS activations initially rise and then fall to a stable level during incremental AO speed modes. A moderate-speed AO produced the best hMNS activations in our results.
(3) The BCI accuracy and ITR of moderate-speed AO-BCI produced the same level of MI-BCI as training experience, suggesting a new method for constructing non-invasive BMBIs in healthy individuals.

4.1. The Affected Regions of the Brain During AO

According to a statistical study (Molenberghs et al., 2012), the support of mirror neurons, the connections across regions, and the strong mirror properties in the hMNS produce mirror properties in the sensorimotor and occipital regions during AO. In fact, the sensorimotor region is related to action imitation and action presentation. Processing of the subjects' action preparation and spatial orientation for a specific action depend on the sensorimotor region. The occipital region is part of the lateral occipitotemporal cortex (LOTC) (Barton et al., 1996; Kable and Chatterjee, 2006). The LOTC is a set of regions that are thought to function in integrating information and determining the purpose of an action. Several previous studies have found that the LOTC region forms direct and indirect connections with hMNS regions (Weiner and Grill-Spector, 2011; Lingnau and Downing, 2015). Therefore, the occipital, sensorimotor, and "sensorimotor+occipital" regions were adopted for BCI analyses and the extraction of spatio-spectral-temporal characteristic from EEG data during AO in this study.

The accuracies of BCI show that the occipital region exhibits higher ERD suppressions than the sensorimotor region (see **Figure 4**). Similar results were also found in the BEAMs (see **Figure 7**). The differences in affected regions during AO found in our study support a previous model of hMNS activation affecting multiple regions (Perry et al., 2010; Frenkel-Toledo et al., 2013). Two main reasons may account for the differences in hMNS activations between the two regions: First, AO paradigms are visually evoked stimuli (Wieser et al., 2016; Park, 2017). Therefore, the visually relevant occipital region first generates power variations (Pegado et al., 2014). After recognition of stimuli, hMNS activations generate power variations in the sensorimotor region (Oberman et al., 2005, 2008). Since the occipital region undergoes rapid and prolonged activation in response to visual stimuli, the degree of activation in the occipital region must be higher than that in the sensorimotor region. Second, the arm movements of the robot turn into attended information during the presentation of AO stimuli (Hwang et al., 2018). Recent studies suggest that attended information increases the activation of mu rhythms (8–12 Hz) in the occipital region during the presentation of visually evoked stimuli (Gray et al., 2015; Sprague et al., 2015). However, distracting information will suppress the activation of the alpha rhythm in the occipital region (Händel et al., 2011; Klimesch, 2012; Zumer et al., 2014). In addition, spectral characteristics and spatio-spatial characteristics suggest that the mu range plays a prominent role in hMNS activations (See **Figures 5**, **6**). Therefore, the attended information provided by the left/right-arm movements of the robot cause more intense power differences in the occipital region than in the sensorimotor region.

Comparing the accuracies of BCI in the three explored regions, the results reflect the robustness of hMNS activation in these regions. The accuracies of BCI in the "sensorimotor+occipital" region remained the same as the sensorimotor region but were significantly different in the occipital region (See **Figure 4**). Since the activation of the sensorimotor region is caused by ERD suppressions, whereas the activation of the occipital region is caused by both ERD suppressions and attended information, ERD suppressions play a dominant role in the activation of the "sensorimotor+occipital" region. In fact, a large number of sessions must be presented over several days. Therefore, the attended information will change during all sessions. As time passes, the activation of the mu range caused by attended information will gradually reduce due to visual fatigue (Lambooij et al., 2009). However, ERD suppressions remain steady during the presentation of stimuli without influence from visual fatigue (Nam et al., 2011). Therefore, the sensorimotor region is more robust for hMNS activations than the occipital region during AO. The findings in our study of hMNS activations conform to the affected regions and formation principles during AO and support further studies on the hMNS.

4.2. The Patterns of hMNS Activations Affected by AO Speed Modes

We found that the patterns of hMNS activations first rise and then fall to a stable level during incremental-speed modes of AO (See **Figure 4**). Relationships between speed modes and left/right movements were also found in spatio-spatial characteristics (See **Figure 7**). The patterns were appropriate for both the sensorimotor region and the occipital region. The reasons why the curves reveal these patterns are as follows. Since AO stimuli in different speed modes were presented in a periodic way in experiment 1, the refractory period of visual stimuli must be considered during the presentation (Huettel and McCarthy, 2000). Previous studies suggest that the inter-stimulus intervals (ISIs) in the refractory period are within 360–2,000 ms for auditory and visual senses (Coch et al., 2005; Brisson and Jolicœur, 2007). Other studies demonstrate that the ISIs of repetitive contents are within 500 ms (Davis et al., 1972; Johannsen and Röder, 2014). In fact, the ISIs in our experiments were 4,000 ms (slow movement), 666.7 ms (moderate movement), 363.6 ms (fast movement), and 250 ms (finalistic movement). Comparing the ISIs of the four speed modes, the fast and finalistic movements exceeded the repetitive content limits of ISI. Therefore, a visual refractory period will appear during the presentation of fast- and finalistic-movement AO tasks. Since the ERD suppressions are also affected by the visual refractory period during AO (Luck et al., 2000; Caravaglios et al., 2015), the hemisphere effects of ERD suppressions will be reduced by the visual refractory period. In other words, increased speed modes of AO within the limits of ISI will promote hMNS activations that benefit from the absence of a visual refractory period.

The patterns suggested that different speed modes of AO define the extent and distribution of hMNS activations. The purpose of our study was to explore the patterns of relationships between AO speed modes and hMNS activations, since the AO speed modes affect action imitation and action presentation during AO. Meanwhile, the speed modes of AO also play important roles in action information integration and the purpose of action in previous studies (Rizzolatti, 2005; Hobson and Bishop, 2016). Therefore, the speed factor must be considered in relevant studies and applications related to action, such as cognitive psychology, rehabilitation treatment, and BCI. The patterns in our study suggest that periodic actions performed at a moderate speed within decent ISI ranges as visual stimuli for observation will contribute to optimized rehabilitation treatment setups for healthy or unhealthy individuals. AO stimuli of moderate speed within decent ISI will also improve the performance of AO-BCI.

Recently, neurological diseases have been remedied by AO strategies, which are good at ameliorating motor recovery (Buccino et al., 2011). For healthy individuals, AO strategies are good at facilitating motor learning and increasing force (Stefan et al., 2005). Actions performed at a suitable speed mode for observation may enhance action motivation and optimize the recruitment of motor function (Porro et al., 2007). Current treatments for chronic stroke and motor impairment patients construct action execution (AE) strategies based on ecological values (Buccino, 2014), which are valid for improving motor function and ameliorating autonomy, such as grasping cups or cleaning the floor (Ertelt et al., 2007). However, since individual patients with neurological diseases usually have clinical impairments, these patients cannot accomplish such AE assignments in daily treatment without help. The limits for individual patients in AE will be remitted by an optimal AO strategy design. Because the AO assignments are visual stimuli, which need patients to focus their attention, AO assignments are easier to accomplish in daily treatment than AE assignments. In addition, regardless of whether AE or AO assignments are used, the treatment strategies of the medical rehabilitative field must be tailored to satisfy the individual needs of each subject. Treatment strategies should be designed with due consideration of environmental, social, and economic factors, as well as the pathology and characteristics of the subject. Our study suggests that an individually tailored speed within a decent ISI range must be considered when constructing rehabilitation AO treatments for individual subjects.

4.3. The Construction of BMBI Based on AO-BCI and MI-BCI

Our study suggests a new way to construct AO-BCI on a humanoid robot platform. Experimental paradigms are defined by parameters such that confounding factors are eliminated by precise settings. Compared with MI-BCI, AO-BCI offers a number of advantages. Typically, MI-BCI is constructed on the self-imaged spontaneous potential of ERD suppressions. Subjects may imagine self-motion, others-motion, wrist movement, arm movement, or hand movement without specific instruction. In addition, the familiarity factor also affects MI-BCI performance, since MI-BCI performance significantly increases for fully fledged subjects (Schroeder and Chestek, 2016; Subramanian et al., 2016). However, AO-BCI, as a visually evoked stimulus, eliminates the uncertainties of spontaneous MI-BCI. Moreover, familiarity in the BCI is controlled by the stimulus design. In experiments 1 and 2, none of the subjects had previous training experience. However, the BCI results of experiment 1 significantly outperformed those of experiment 2 for slow and moderate movements (See **Figure 4**). A comparison of the results demonstrated that fixed AO modes were less influenced by the subjects' experience, which is another advantage of constructing AO-BCIs.

The performance of AO-BCI and MI-BCI are mismatched in this study since the subjects for MI-BCI lacked MI training. With enough training in MI-BCI, the average accuracy and ITR among subjects can reach 75% and 1.8 bits/min for two classes of MI-BCI (Park et al., 2013). Due to confounding factors, achieving the same level of average accuracy and ITR in AO-BCI has thus far proven difficult. However, by adopting fine-tuned stimuli in AO, as in the present study, the average accuracy and ITR of AO-BCI reached 70% and 1.65 bits/min, which are similar to those of a well-trained MI-BCI (See **Figure 4**). These findings prompted us to construct a BMBI in healthy subjects using the stimulus paradigms of AO and well-trained MI. In recent studies, the majority of BMBIs were based on invasive signal processing technology and used animal carriers (Tessadori et al., 2012). However, BMBIs are rarely based on healthy human brains given the requirement for non-invasive signal processing techniques. As a system of bi-directional transmission, the BMBI must be built on two kinds of stimulators. The accuracy of performance and the ITR of efficiency must achieve the same level for both transmissions. Designing BMBIs that are influenced by variables remains a meaningful but difficult problem. The construction of BMBIs based on AO-BCI and MI-BCI in our study was based on EEG recordings, which will satisfy the requirement for a non-invasive method in healthy individual subjects.

5. CONCLUSION

Our experimental results suggest that the occipital region exhibits higher but less robust hMNS activations than the sensorimotor region. In addition, the patterns of hMNS activations first rise and then fall to a stable level during incremental-speed modes of AO. Moreover, the creation of an AO-BCI provides a novel means of building BMBI systems in healthy individuals with well-trained MI-BCI. However, as time passes, the subjects' refractory period, fatigue and pressure for waiting will lead limit the EEG recordings. Thus, our results provide only rough patterns of the relationships between AO speed modes and hMNS activations. Further studies with larger experimental trials are needed to explore the exact patterns. More modes of AO are also needed to explore confounding factors. Only then can accurate patterns of AO be completed to study the human brain.

AUTHOR CONTRIBUTIONS

CZ, TL, and JL designed the experiments; TL and JL completed the experiments; TL analyzed the EEG data; CZ, FC, and TL wrote the paper.

ACKNOWLEDGMENTS

This work was supported by the National Natural Science Foundation of China (No.61673322 and 61673326), the Major State Basic Research Development Program of China (973 Program) (No. 2013CB329502), the Fundamental Research Funds for the Central Universities (No. 20720160126), and Natural Science Foundation of Fujian Province of China (No. 2017J01128 and 2017J01129).

REFERENCES

Abbott, D. F. (2016). Probing the human brain functional connectome with simultaneous EEG and fMRI. *Front. Neurosci.* 10:302. doi: 10.3389/fnins.2016.00302

Abdi, H., and Williams, L. J. (2010). Principal component analysis. *Wiley Interdisc. Rev. Comput. Stat.* 2, 433–459. doi: 10.1002/wics.101

Agnew, Z. K., Wise, R. J., and Leech, R. (2012). Dissociating object directed and non-object directed action in the human mirror system; implications for theories of motor simulation. *PLoS ONE* 7:e32517. doi: 10.1371/journal.pone.0032517

Ang, K. K., Chin, Z. Y., Wang, C., Guan, C., and Zhang, H. (2012). Filter bank common spatial pattern algorithm on BCI competition IV datasets 2a and 2b. *Front. Neurosci.* 6:39. doi: 10.3389/fnins.2012.00039

Barton, J. J., Simpson, T., Kiriakopoulos, E., Stewart, C., Crawley, A., Guthrie, B., et al. (1996). Functional MRI of lateral occipitotemporal cortex during pursuit and motion perception. *Ann. Neurol.* 40, 387–398.

Bauer, R., and Gharabaghi, A. (2015). Reinforcement learning for adaptive threshold control of restorative brain-computer interfaces: a Bayesian simulation. *Front. Neurosci.* 9:36. doi: 10.3389/fnins.2015.00036

Bello, J. P., Modroño, C., Marcano, F., and González-Mora, J. (2014). The mirror neuron system and motor dexterity: what happens? *Neuroscience* 275, 285–295. doi: 10.1016/j.neuroscience.2014.06.010

Biagi, L., Cioni, G., Fogassi, L., Guzzetta, A., and Tosetti, M. (2010). Anterior intraparietal cortex codes complexity of observed hand movements. *Brain Res. Bull.* 81, 434–440. doi: 10.1016/j.brainresbull.2009.12.002

Blakemore, S.-J., and Decety, J. (2001). From the perception of action to the understanding of intention. *Nat. Rev. Neurosci.* 2, 561–567. doi: 10.1038/35086023

Brisson, B., and Jolicœur, P. (2007). A psychological refractory period in access to visual short-term memory and the deployment of visual-spatial attention: multitasking processing deficits revealed by event-related potentials. *Psychophysiology* 44, 323–333. doi: 10.1111/j.1469-8986.2007.00503.x

Buccino, G. (2014). Action observation treatment: a novel tool in neurorehabilitation. *Philos. Trans. R. Soc. Lond. B Biol. Sci.* 369:20130185. doi: 10.1098/rstb.2013.0185

Buccino, G., Gatti, R., Giusti, M. C., Negrotti, A., Rossi, A., Calzetti, S., et al. (2011). Action observation treatment improves autonomy in daily activities in Parkinson's disease patients: results from a pilot study. *Mov. Disord.* 26, 1963–1964. doi: 10.1002/mds.23745

Calvo-Merino, B., Glaser, D. E., Grèzes, J., Passingham, R. E., and Haggard, P. (2004). Action observation and acquired motor skills: an fMRI study with expert dancers. *Cereb. Cortex* 15, 1243–1249. doi: 10.1093/cercor/bhi007

Calvo-Merino, B., Grèzes, J., Glaser, D. E., Passingham, R. E., and Haggard, P. (2006). Seeing or doing? Influence of visual and motor familiarity in action observation. *Curr. Biol.* 16, 1905–1910. doi: 10.1016/j.cub.2006.07.065

Caravaglios, G., Muscoso, E. G., Di Maria, G., and Costanzo, E. (2015). Patients with mild cognitive impairment have an abnormal upper-alpha event-related desynchronization/synchronization (ERD/ERS) during a task of temporal attention. *J. Neural Transm.* 122, 441–453. doi: 10.1007/s00702-014-1262-7

Caspers, S., Zilles, K., Laird, A. R., and Eickhoff, S. B. (2010). ALE meta-analysis of action observation and imitation in the human brain. *Neuroimage* 50, 1148–1167. doi: 10.1016/j.neuroimage.2009.12.112

Coch, D., Skendzel, W., and Neville, H. J. (2005). Auditory and visual refractory period effects in children and adults: an ERP study. *Clin. Neurophysiol.* 116, 2184–2203. doi: 10.1016/j.clinph.2005.06.005

Davis, H., Osterhammel, P., Wier, C., and Gjerdingen, D. (1972). Slow vertex potentials: interactions among auditory, tactile, electric and visual stimuli. *Electroencephalogr. Clin. Neurophysiol.* 33, 537–545.

Delorme, A., and Makeig, S. (2004). EEGLAB: an open source toolbox for analysis of single-trial EEG dynamics including independent component analysis. *J. Neurosci. Methods* 134, 9–21. doi: 10.1016/j.jneumeth.2003.10.009

Demandt, E., Mehring, C., Vogt, K., Schulze-Bonhage, A., Aertsen, A., and Ball, T. (2012). Reaching movement onset-and end-related characteristics of EEG spectral power modulations. *Front. Neurosci.* 6:65. doi: 10.3389/fnins.2012.00065

Duffy, F. H., Burchfiel, J. L., and Lombroso, C. T. (1979). Brain electrical activity mapping (beam): a method for extending the clinical utility of EEG and evoked potential data. *Ann. Neurol.* 5, 309–321.

Ertelt, D., Small, S., Solodkin, A., Dettmers, C., McNamara, A., Binkofski, F., et al. (2007). Action observation has a positive impact on rehabilitation of motor deficits after stroke. *Neuroimage* 36, T164–T173. doi: 10.1016/j.neuroimage.2007.03.043

Filimon, F., Nelson, J. D., Hagler, D. J., and Sereno, M. I. (2007). Human cortical representations for reaching: mirror neurons for execution, observation, and imagery. *Neuroimage* 37, 1315–1328. doi: 10.1016/j.neuroimage.2007.06.008

Franceschini, M., Ceravolo, M. G., Agosti, M., Cavallini, P., Bonassi, S., Dall'Armi, V., et al. (2012). Clinical relevance of action observation in upper-limb stroke rehabilitation: a possible role in recovery of functional dexterity. a randomized clinical trial. *Neurorehabil. Neural Repair* 26, 456–462. doi: 10.1177/1545968311427406

Frenkel-Toledo, S., Bentin, S., Perry, A., Liebermann, D. G., and Soroker, N. (2013). Dynamics of the EEG power in the frequency and spatial domains during observation and execution of manual movements. *Brain Res.* 1509, 43–57. doi: 10.1016/j.brainres.2013.03.004

Frenkel-Toledo, S., Bentin, S., Perry, A., Liebermann, D. G., and Soroker, N. (2014). Mirror-neuron system recruitment by action observation: effects of focal brain damage on mu suppression. *Neuroimage* 87, 127–137. doi: 10.1016/j.neuroimage.2013.10.019

Gatti, R., Rocca, M. A., Fumagalli, S., Cattrysse, E., Kerckhofs, E., Falini, A., et al. (2017). The effect of action observation/execution on mirror neuron system recruitment: an fMRI study in healthy individuals. *Brain Imaging Behav.* 11, 565–576. doi: 10.1007/s11682-016-9536-3

Geers, A. (1994). Techniques for assessing auditory speech perception and lipreading enhancement in young deaf children. *Volta Rev.* 96, 85–96.

Gray, M. J., Frey, H.-P., Wilson, T. J., and Foxe, J. J. (2015). Oscillatory recruitment of bilateral visual cortex during spatial attention to competing rhythmic inputs. *J. Neurosci.* 35, 5489–5503. doi: 10.1523/JNEUROSCI.2891-14.2015

Händel, B. F., Haarmeier, T., and Jensen, O. (2011). Alpha oscillations correlate with the successful inhibition of unattended stimuli. *J. Cogn. Neurosci.* 23, 2494-2502. doi: 10.1162/jocn.2010.21557

Hobson, H. M., and Bishop, D. V. (2016). Mu suppression–a good measure of the human mirror neuron system? *Cortex* 82, 290–310. doi: 10.1016/j.cortex.2016.03.019

Huettel, S. A., and McCarthy, G. (2000). Evidence for a refractory period in the hemodynamic response to visual stimuli as measured by MRI. *Neuroimage* 11, 547–553. doi: 10.1006/nimg.2000.0553

Hwang, K., Shine, J. M., and D'Esposito, M. (2018). Frontoparietal activity interacts with task-evoked changes in functional connectivity. *Cereb. Cortex.* doi: 10.1093/cercor/bhy011. [Epub ahead of print].

Iacoboni, M., Molnar-Szakacs, I., Gallese, V., Buccino, G., Mazziotta, J. C., and Rizzolatti, G. (2005). Grasping the intentions of others with one's own mirror neuron system. *PLoS Biol.* 3:e79. doi: 10.1371/journal.pbio.0030079

Johannsen, J., and Röder, B. (2014). Uni-and crossmodal refractory period effects of event-related potentials provide insights into the development of multisensory processing. *Front. Hum. Neurosci.* 8:552. doi: 10.3389/fnhum.2014.00552

Kable, J. W., and Chatterjee, A. (2006). Specificity of action representations in the lateral occipitotemporal cortex. *J. Cogn. Neurosci.* 18, 1498–1517. doi: 10.1162/jocn.2006.18.9.1498

Klimesch, W. (2012). α-band oscillations, attention, and controlled access to stored information. *Trends Cogn. Sci.* 16, 606–617. doi: 10.1016/j.tics.2012.10.007

Lambooij, M., Fortuin, M., Heynderickx, I., and IJsselsteijn, W. (2009). Visual discomfort and visual fatigue of stereoscopic displays: a review. *J. Imaging Sci. Technol.* 53, 1–14. doi: 10.2352/J.ImagingSci.Technol.2009.53.3.030201

Lei, X., Wu, T., and Valdes-Sosa, P. A. (2015). Incorporating priors for EEG source imaging and connectivity analysis. *Front. Neurosci.* 9:284. doi: 10.3389/fnins.2015.00284

Lingnau, A., and Downing, P. E. (2015). The lateral occipitotemporal cortex in action. *Trends Cogn. Sci.* 19, 268–277. doi: 10.1016/j.tics.2015.03.006

Luck, S. J., Woodman, G. F., and Vogel, E. K. (2000). Event-related potential studies of attention. *Trends Cogn. Sci.* 4, 432–440. doi: 10.1016/S1364-6613(00)01545-X

Maranesi, M., Ugolotti Serventi, F., Bruni, S., Bimbi, M., Fogassi, L., and Bonini, L. (2013). Monkey gaze behaviour during action observation and its relationship to mirror neuron activity. *Eur. J. Neurosci.* 38, 3721–3730. doi: 10.1111/ejn.12376

Molenberghs, P., Cunnington, R., and Mattingley, J. B. (2012). Brain regions with mirror properties: a meta-analysis of 125 human fmri studies. *Neurosci. Biobehav. Rev.* 36, 341–349. doi: 10.1016/j.neubiorev.2011.07.004

Mukamel, R., Ekstrom, A. D., Kaplan, J., Iacoboni, M., and Fried, I. (2010). Single-neuron responses in humans during execution and observation of actions. *Curr. Biol.* 20, 750–756. doi: 10.1016/j.cub.2010.02.045

Nam, C. S., Jeon, Y., Kim, Y.-J., Lee, I., and Park, K. (2011). Movement imagery-related lateralization of event-related (de) synchronization (ERD/ERS): Motor-imagery duration effects. *Clin. Neurophysiol.* 122, 567–577. doi: 10.1016/j.clinph.2010.08.002

Neuper, C., Scherer, R., Wriessnegger, S., and Pfurtscheller, G. (2009). Motor imagery and action observation: modulation of sensorimotor brain rhythms during mental control of a brain–computer interface. *Clin. Neurophysiol.* 120, 239–247. doi: 10.1016/j.clinph.2008.11.015

Newman-Norlund, R. D., van Schie, H. T., van Zuijlen, A. M., and Bekkering, H. (2007). The mirror neuron system is more active during complementary compared with imitative action. *Nat. Neurosci.* 10:nn1911. doi: 10.1038/nn1911

Oberman, L. M., Hubbard, E. M., McCleery, J. P., Altschuler, E. L., Ramachandran, V. S., and Pineda, J. A. (2005). EEG evidence for mirror neuron dysfunction in autism spectrum disorders. *Brain Res. Cogn. Brain Res.* 24, 190–198. doi: 10.1016/j.cogbrainres.2005.01.014

Oberman, L. M., Pineda, J. A., and Ramachandran, V. S. (2007). The human mirror neuron system: a link between action observation and social skills. *Soc. Cogn. Affect. Neurosci.* 2, 62–66. doi: 10.1093/scan/nsl022

Oberman, L. M., Ramachandran, V. S., and Pineda, J. A. (2008). Modulation of mu suppression in children with autism spectrum disorders in response to familiar or unfamiliar stimuli: the mirror neuron hypothesis. *Neuropsychologia* 46, 1558–1565. doi: 10.1016/j.neuropsychologia.2008.01.010

Onishi, A., Takano, K., Kawase, T., Ora, H., and Kansaku, K. (2017). Affective stimuli for an auditory p300 brain-computer interface. *Front. Neurosci.* 11:522. doi: 10.3389/fnins.2017.00522

Orgs, G., Dombrowski, J.-H., Heil, M., and Jansen-Osmann, P. (2008). Expertise in dance modulates alpha/beta event-related desynchronization during action observation. *Eur. J. Neurosci.* 27, 3380–3384. doi: 10.1111/j.1460-9568.2008.06271

Park, C., Looney, D., ur Rehman, N., Ahrabian, A., and Mandic, D. P. (2013). Classification of motor imagery BCI using multivariate empirical mode decomposition. *IEEE Trans. Neural Syst. Rehabil. Eng.* 21, 10–22. doi: 10.1109/TNSRE.2012.2229296

Park, J. (2017). A neural basis for the visual sense of number and its development: a steady-state visual evoked potential study in children and adults. *Dev. Cogn. Neurosci.* doi: 10.1016/j.dcn.2017.02.011. [Epub ahead of print].

Pegado, F., Comerlato, E., Ventura, F., Jobert, A., Nakamura, K., Buiatti, M., et al. (2014). Timing the impact of literacy on visual processing. *Proc. Natl. Acad. Sci. U.S.A.* 111, E5233–E5242. doi: 10.1073/pnas.1417347111

Perry, A., Bentin, S., Shalev, I., Israel, S., Uzefovsky, F., Bar-On, D., et al. (2010). Intranasal oxytocin modulates EEG mu/alpha and beta rhythms during perception of biological motion. *Psychoneuroendocrinology* 35, 1446–1453. doi: 10.1016/j.psyneuen.2010.04.011

Pineda, J. A., Grichanik, M., Williams, V., Trieu, M., Chang, H., and Keysers, C. (2013). EEG sensorimotor correlates of translating sounds into actions. *Front. Neurosci.* 7:203. doi: 10.3389/fnins.2013.00203

Porro, C. A., Facchin, P., Fusi, S., Dri, G., and Fadiga, L. (2007). Enhancement of force after action observation: behavioural and neurophysiological studies. *Neuropsychologia* 45, 3114–3121. doi: 10.1016/j.neuropsychologia.2007.06.016

Pot, E., Monceaux, J., Gelin, R., and Maisonnier, B. (2009). "Choregraphe: a graphical tool for humanoid robot programming," in *The 18th IEEE International Symposium on Robot and Human Interactive Communication* (Toyama), 46–51.

Press, C. (2011). Action observation and robotic agents: learning and anthropomorphism. *Neurosci. Biobehav. Rev.* 35, 1410–1418. doi: 10.1016/j.neubiorev.2011.03.004

Rizzolatti, G. (2005). The mirror neuron system and its function in humans. *Anat. Embryol.* 210, 419–421. doi: 10.1007/s00429-005-0039-z

Rizzolatti, G., and Sinigaglia, C. (2010). The functional role of the parieto-frontal mirror circuit: interpretations and misinterpretations. *Nat. Rev. Neurosci.* 11, 264–274. doi: 10.1038/nrn2805

Rozzi, S., and Fogassi, L. (2017). Neural coding for action execution and action observation in the prefrontal cortex and its role in the organization of socially driven behavior. *Front. Neurosci.* 11:492. doi: 10.3389/fnins.2017.00492

Sardouie, S. H., and Shamsollahi, M. B. (2012). Selection of efficient features for discrimination of hand movements from meg using a BCI competition IV data set. *Front. Neurosci.* 6:42. doi: 10.3389/fnins.2012.00042

Schroeder, K. E., and Chestek, C. A. (2016). Intracortical brain-machine interfaces advance sensorimotor neuroscience. *Front. Neurosci.* 10:291. doi: 10.3389/fnins.2016.00291

Schulte-Rüther, M., Markowitsch, H. J., Fink, G. R., and Piefke, M. (2007). Mirror neuron and theory of mind mechanisms involved in face-to-face interactions: a functional magnetic resonance imaging approach to empathy. *J. Cogn. Neurosci.* 19, 1354–1372. doi: 10.1162/jocn.2007.19.8.1354

Silsbee, P. L., and Bovik, A. C. (1996). Computer lipreading for improved accuracy in automatic speech recognition. *IEEE Trans. Speech Audio Process.* 4, 337–351.

Smith, E. G., and Bennetto, L. (2007). Audiovisual speech integration and lipreading in autism. *J. Child Psychol. Psychiatry* 48, 813–821. doi: 10.1111/j.1469-7610.2007.01766.x

Sprague, T. C., Saproo, S., and Serences, J. T. (2015). Visual attention mitigates information loss in small-and large-scale neural codes. *Trends Cogn. Sci.* 19, 215–226. doi: 10.1016/j.tics.2015.02.005

Stefan, K., Cohen, L. G., Duque, J., Mazzocchio, R., Celnik, P., Sawaki, L., et al. (2005). Formation of a motor memory by action observation. *J. Neurosci.* 25, 9339–9346. doi: 10.1523/JNEUROSCI.2282-05.2005

Subramanian, L., Morris, M. B., Brosnan, M., Turner, D. L., Morris, H. R., and Linden, D. E. (2016). Functional magnetic resonance imaging neurofeedback-guided motor imagery training and motor training for Parkinson's disease: randomized trial. *Front. Behav. Neurosci.* 10:111. doi: 10.3389/fnbeh.2016.00111

Summerfield, Q. (1992). Lipreading and audio-visual speech perception. *Philos. Trans. R. Soc. Lond. B Biol. Sci.* 335, 71–78.

Tangermann, M., Müller, K.-R., Aertsen, A., Birbaumer, N., Braun, C., Brunner, C., et al. (2012). Review of the BCI competition IV. *Front. Neurosci.* 6:55. doi: 10.3389/fnins.2012.00055

Tanji, K., Sakurada, K., Funiu, H., Matsuda, K., Kayama, T., Ito, S., et al. (2015). Functional significance of the electrocorticographic auditory responses in the premotor cortex. *Front. Neurosci.* 9:78. doi: 10.3389/fnins.2015.00078

Tessadori, J., Bisio, M., Martinoia, S., and Chiappalone, M. (2012). Modular neuronal assemblies embodied in a closed-loop environment: toward future integration of brains and machines. *Front. Neural Circ.* 6:99. doi: 10.3389/fncir.2012.00099

Vogt, S., Di Rienzo, F., Collet, C., Collins, A., and Guillot, A. (2013). Multiple roles of motor imagery during action observation. *Front. Hum. Neurosci.* 7:807. doi: 10.3389/fnhum.2013.00807

Wang, D., Miao, D., and Blohm, G. (2012). Multi-class motor imagery EEG decoding for brain-computer interfaces. *Front. Neurosci.* 6:151. doi: 10.3389/fnins.2012.00151

Weiner, K. S., and Grill-Spector, K. (2011). Not one extrastriate body area: using anatomical landmarks, hMT+, and visual field maps to parcellate limb-selective activations in human lateral occipitotemporal cortex. *Neuroimage* 56, 2183–2199. doi: 10.1016/j.neuroimage.2011.03.041

Wieser, M. J., Reicherts, P., Juravle, G., and von Leupoldt, A. (2016). Attention mechanisms during predictable and unpredictable threat-a steady-state visual evoked potential approach. *Neuroimage* 139, 167–175. doi: 10.1016/j.neuroimage.2016.06.026

Zumer, J. M., Scheeringa, R., Schoffelen, J.-M., Norris, D. G., and Jensen, O. (2014). Occipital alpha activity during stimulus processing gates the information flow to object-selective cortex. *PLoS Biol.* 12:e1001965. doi: 10.1371/journal.pbio.1001965

4

The Role of Long Noncoding RNAs in Central Nervous System and Neurodegenerative Diseases

*Chang-Wei Wei, Ting Luo, Shan-Shan Zou and An-Shi Wu**

Department of Anesthesiology, Beijing Chao-Yang Hospital, Capital Medical University, Beijing, China

***Correspondence:**
An-Shi Wu
wuanshi880923@163.com

Long noncoding RNAs (lncRNAs) refer to a group of noncoding RNAs (ncRNAs) that has a transcript of more than 200 nucleotides in length in eukaryotic cells. The lncRNAs regulate gene expression at epigenetic, transcriptional, and post-transcriptional levels by multiple action modes. In this review, we describe the diverse roles reported for lncRNAs, and discuss how they could mechanistically be involved in the development of central nervous system (CNS) and neurodegenerative diseases. Further studies on the function of lncRNAs and their mechanism will help deepen our understanding of the development, function, and diseases of the CNS, and provide new ideas for the design and development of some therapeutic drugs.

Keywords: long noncoding RNAs, central nervous system, neurodegenerative diseases, regulatory mechanism, gene expression

INTRODUCTION

Over the past decade, the extensive applications of second-generation sequencing technology have led to the discovery of tens of thousands of RNA transcripts that have similar properties to mRNAs, but are not translated into proteins. Long noncoding RNA (lncRNA) is a kind of noncoding RNA (ncRNA), with a length of longer than 200 nucleotides, that lacks a significant open reading frame (ORF) encoding a protein (Sun and Kraus, 2015). The central nervous system (CNS) is the most highly evolved and sophisticated biological system. The development of the CNS is a complex arrangement of stem cells, growth/differentiation factors, transcription factors, and epigenetic control. It consists of a large number of neuronal and glial cell subtypes distributed in rigorous and precise regions, forming a dynamic neural network that responds to internal signals and external stimuli and then is responsible for mediating the complex functional repertoire of the CNS including performing higher level functions, for example, cognition and behavior (Graff and Mansuy, 2008). As one of the most abundant ncRNA classes, lncRNAs are derived from different locations in the genome for transcription and are highly expressed in the brain (Mercer et al., 2008; Qureshi et al., 2010). The role of lncRNAs has been validated in brain development, neuronal function, maintenance, and differentiation.

Neurodegenerative diseases are associated with multiple clinical manifestations, brain pathologies, and health consequences (Quan et al., 2017). They include relatively well-known conditions like Alzheimer's disease (AD), Parkinson's disease (PD), and Huntington's disease (HD). In particular, AD and PD are a group of typically late-onset, progressive disorders that lead to cognitive and/or movement disorders (Peden and Ironside, 2012). Although drug therapy and/or surgery can delay the progression of these diseases, most neurodegenerative diseases remain untreatable. In addition, neurodegenerative diseases represent an increasing financial burden on health care systems, which attempt to respond to an aging population. Therefore, there is an urgent need to develop methods for preventing or curing neurodegenerative diseases. Some efforts carried out by the scientific community revealed important insights into the molecular bases of these disease, but the specific mechanism remains unknown. Increasing evidence has suggested that lncRNAs are involved in the pathogenesis of neurodegenerative diseases (Johnson, 2012; Briggs et al., 2015; Riva et al., 2016). This review summarizes data on lncRNA expression in the central nervous system (CNS) and neurodegenerative diseases and focuses on the role of some specific lncRNAs, which may provide new insights into our understanding of the etiology and pathophysiology of the neurodegenerative diseases.

BIOLOGY OF lncRNAs

Definition of lncRNAs

Genomewide analysis of the eukaryotic transcriptome revealed that up to 90% of the human genome IS transcribed. However, the GENCODE-annotated exon of the protein-encoding gene covers only 2.94% of the genome, while the rest are ncRNAs (Djebali et al., 2012). Noncoding transcripts are further divided into house-keeping ncRNAs and regulatory ncRNAs. House-keeping ncRNAs include ribosomes, metastasis, small nuclei, and small nucleolar RNA. Regulatory ncRNAs are generally divided into two classes based on nucleotide length. Those <200 nucleotides are commonly referred to as short/small ncRNAs, including microRNAs (miRNAs), small interfering RNAs, and Piwi-related RNAs, and those >200 nucleotides are known as lncRNAs (Nagano and Fraser, 2011).

The lncRNA transcripts are partially similar to messenger RNAs (mRNAs) as they are frequently transcribed by RNA polymerase II, contain classical splice sites (GU/AG), have an mRNA-like structure that contains intron and exon structures, exhibit alternative splicing, no open reading frame (ORF) in the sequence, and are associated with the same types of histone modifications as protein-coding genes (PCGs)(Ponting et al., 2009). They also have a specific secondary structure that provides multiple sites for protein binding or the specific binding between DNA and RNA by the principle of base pair complementarity. The main sources of lncRNAs are from PCG-related regions (Magistri et al., 2012), gene regulatory regions (Hung et al., 2011; Mercer et al., 2011), and specific chromosomal regions (Azzalin et al., 2007). The lncRNA was originally thought to be the "noise" of genomic transcription and as not having biological functions. However, recent studies have shown that lncRNAs can regulate gene expression at epigenetic, transcriptional, and post-transcriptional levels, and participate in X-chromosome silencing, genome imprinting, and chromatin modification, transcriptional activation, and many other important biological processes (Singh and Prasanth, 2013; Goff and Rinn, 2015; Kazemzadeh et al., 2015). Until now, only very few lncRNAs have been validated by experiment, while most of the lncRNAs have been annotated via bioinformatics and still need further experimental verification.

Expression and Sequence Conservation of lncRNAs

In 2002, Japanese scientists revealed that in large-scale sequencing of a mouse full-length complementary DNA (cDNA) library, a large number of ncRNA transcripts were identified (Okazaki et al., 2002). However, due to lack of functional annotation, these RNA transcripts did not attract the attention of researchers during subsequent periods. Not until 2007 did the situation change. Rinn et al. in Stanford University reported a 2.2-Kb functional lncRNA gene (Hox transcript antisense intergenic RNA, *HOTAIR*) (Rinn et al., 2007). It was found that *HOTAIR* could interact with the protein complex polycomb, which can modify chromatin, inhibit the transcription of the *Hox* gene, and regulate the growth and development of organisms. In 2008, Mercer et al. used *in situ* hybridization to identify the expression of a large amount of lncRNAs in mouse brain (Mercer et al., 2008). The expression levels of these lncRNAs are associated with specific neuroanatomical locations, cell types, and subcellular locations. For example, *Evf2* is mainly expressed in the ventral forebrain. The tissue-specific expression of lncRNAs also includes *Hox* transcript antisense intergenic RNA myeloid1 (*HOTAIRM1*), which is specifically expressed in the bone marrow (Zhang et al., 2009) and *Msx1* antisense RNA (*Msx1-AS* RNA), which is expressed only in differentiated teeth and bone cells (Coudert et al., 2005). The expression level of *Msx1-AS* RNA is negatively correlated with the content of Msx1 protein (Babajko et al., 2009).

The lncRNAs can appear in different subcellular structures, and the proportion of those lncRNAs located in the nucleus is the largest. For example, lncRNA *MEN* ε/β is mainly located in the nucleus, and is an important component of nuclear substructure paraspeckles (Sasaki et al., 2009; Sunwoo et al., 2009). Furthermore, metastasis-associated lung adenocarcinoma transcript 1 (*MALAT-1*) and nuclear-enriched abundant transcript 1 (*Neat1*) are localized mainly in the nuclear speckle of the nucleus, and are associated with the cleavage of RNA precursors (Hutchinson et al., 2007; Tripathi et al., 2010). In addition, Cesana et al. reported that *linc-MD1* is mainly expressed in the cytoplasm of differentiated muscle cells, and regulates the differentiation of skeletal muscles as a competing endogenous RNA (ceRNA) (Cesana et al., 2011). In 2011, Rackham et al. first identified three lncRNAs (*lncND5*, *lncND6*, and *lncCytb*) encoded by mitochondrial genome DNA in the analysis of high-throughput sequencing data (Rackham et al., 2011). This shows that lncRNAs may exist in many subcellular structures. Hence, special subcellular localization plays an important role in the biological function of lncRNAs.

The sequence conservation of lncRNAs is low. The sequence similarity is close to the intron region of the PCG, lower than 70% in humans and mice, and slightly lower than that in the 5′UTR or 3′UTR of genes (Pang et al., 2006). It was revealed in some studies that low sequence conservation did not affect the functional conservation of lncRNAs. Illustrated by the examples of *Xist* and *HOTAIR* expressed in mammals, although they are not highly conservative in sequence, the roles in X chromosome dosage compensation and epigenetic silencing are the same (Braidotti et al., 2004; Pauler et al., 2005). In addition, some lncRNAs with high sequence homology have also been found such as *MALAT1* and *Neat1* (Nakagawa et al., 2012; Zhang et al., 2012).

THE lncRNAs IN CNS DEVELOPMENT

The CNS development is a complex and stereotyped process that requires the precise spatiotemporal regulation of pluripotent stem cell proliferation and differentiation. Neurons are able to change their set of synaptic connections and the relative strength of each of these connections over time in response to sensory experience and other environmental cues. The dynamic expression of lncRNAs plays an important role in controlling these processes (**Table 1**).

Molecular Mechanisms of lncRNAs in Cell Proliferation and Differentiation

A study has revealed that approximately 40% of lncRNAs are distributed in the CNS (equivalent to 4,000–20,000 lncRNA genes) (Briggs et al., 2015). It may be that brain complexity requires more regulatory RNA to maintain normal brain development and function. The lncRNAs are involved in the regulation of the proliferation and development of the nervous system, and enable the nervous system to proliferate and differentiate according to normal time and spatial orders (Amaral et al., 2013).

The lncRNAs are involved in the differentiation of embryonic cells into neural cells during the embryonic period (Klattenhoff et al., 2013). A genetic analysis of the embryo revealed that lncRNAs are closely associated with the coding genes involved in neuronal differentiation and cell morphological maintenance, such as brain-derived neurotrophic factor (*BDNF*), developing brain homeobox 1 (*DBX1*), neuron–glia-related cell-adhesion molecule (*Nrcam*), etc. (Lv et al., 2013). Studies on neural stem cells revealed that lncRNAs are involved in regulating the differentiation of stem cells into neural cells (Ng et al., 2012; Antoniou et al., 2014; Ramos et al., 2016). For example, Ng *et al.* revealed that *lncRNA-ES1*, *lncRNA-ES2,* and *lncRNA-ES* are associated with the maintenance and differentiation of neural stem cells. Guttman et al. discovered at least 1,000 conserved intergenic lncRNAs genes by analyzing the chromatin of mouse neurons (including neural precursor cells) in 2009; they also primarily hypothesized and verified the role of lncRNAs in the maintenance of embryonic stem cells (Guttman et al., 2009). Subsequently, functional genomic analysis revealed that these intergenic lncRNA genes were not only involved the differentiation of mouse ventral forebrain-derived neural stem cells, but also in brain aging, mouse hippocampal development, differentiation of gamma aminobutyric acid (GABA)-ergic neurons, oligodendrocyte myelination, and the calcineurin-dependent signaling pathway, by regulating the expression of some important genes (Mercer et al., 2010).

A recent study has revealed that lncRNAs are associated with PCGs in neural development and play an important role in maintaining the intrinsic morphology and characteristics of neurons (Roberts et al., 2014). For example, the sex-determining region Y-box 2 (*Sox2*) is an important regulator of neural stem cell differentiation and nerve growth. *Sox2OT* encodes a sense-orientation transcript that overlaps with the *Sox2.* The genomic proximity of *Sox2OT* and *Sox2* suggested a possible regulatory role for *Sox2OT* in the neural stem cell differentiation and regeneration of neural cells.

The lncRNAs and Synaptic Plasticity

Synaptic plasticity is the basis of learning and memory and plays a key role in maintaining the stability of the nerve pathway. Some studies found that many lncRNAs might be involved in the regulation of synaptic plasticity (Leal et al., 2014; Panja and Bramham, 2014; Maag et al., 2015). Angelman syndrome (AS) is caused by the deletion of or an inactivating mutation in the maternal E3 ubiquitin ligase (*UBE3A*) gene and is characterized by intellectual disability, severe developmental delays, and speech impairment (Mabb et al., 2011). Furthermore, due to the expression of lncRNA *UBE3A-ATS*, the paternal allele of *UBE3A* undergoes silencing. A study found that hippocampal long-term potentiation (LTP) is defective in the AS-mutant mouse model (Jiang et al., 1998). Similar plasticity deficits may be the cause of learning disabilities observed in AS patients. This important role of *UBE3A-ATS* in neuronal function highlights the possible role of lncRNA in memory formation, while further studies on the role of other lncRNAs in these processes are necessary. The normal development of gamma-aminobutyric acid-ergic (GABAergic) inhibitory interneurons in the hippocampus is the key to learning in embryonic and adult brains. The *Evf-2* lncRNA, which transcribed from the Dlx-5/6 ultraconserved region, is essential for GABAergic neuron development. The *Evf-2* acts through the Dlx-2 transcriptional coactivator to increase the transcriptional activity of Dlx-5/6 and glutamate decarboxylase 1 (Gad1 required for the conversion of glutamate to GABA) (Colasante et al., 2008), and then regulates the gene expression of GABAergic interneurons in the developing mouse brain. The *Evf-2* silencing leads to abnormal synaptic activity in mice through abnormal formation of GABAergic circuits in the hippocampus and dentate gyrus (Bond et al., 2009).

In neurons, local protein synthesis in synaptodendritic microdomains has been implicated in the growth and plasticity of synapses. The lncRNA brain cytoplasmic 200 (*BC200*) is selectively located in the dendrites of postsynaptic neurons, and regulates local protein synthesis by blocking transcription initiation, thereby, controlling signal transduction (Kondrashov et al., 2005). In addition, *BC1* is an lncRNA located in the dendrites of neurons, which is a specific repressor of translation. Experimental use of internal ribosome entry mechanisms and sucrose density gradient centrifugation showed that BC1-mediated repression targets translation at the level of initiation. Specifically, *BC1* RNA inhibited formation of the 48S preinitiation complex, i.e., recruitment of the small ribosomal subunit to the mRNA (Wang et al., 2002). After that, the authors demonstrated that the lack of *BC1* could induce nerve overexcitation (Wang et al., 2005).

Neurons can change their connections when they face changes in the environment. Alterations in components of ion channels or signal proteins may affect neuronal excitability or neuronal

TABLE 1 | Molecular mechanisms of lncRNA in neuronal differentiation and synaptogenesis.

lncRNAs	Biological function	Molecular mechanisms	References
RMST	Promotes neuronal differentiation	The RMST interacts with *SOX2* to regulate neurogenic genes including *ASCL1* and *DLX1*	Ng et al., 2013; Lee et al., 2017
Linc-Brn1b	Specifies cortical NSPC fate and regulates area patterning and layer formation of mouse neocortex	Deletion of the linc-*Brn1b* locus leads to significant decrease in Brn1 expression	Sauvageau et al., 2013; Wang et al., 2017
Tuna	Regulates pluripotency and neural differentiation of ESCs	*TUNA* formed a complex with three pluripotency-related RNA-binding proteins, PTBP1, hnRNP-K, and NCL	Lin et al., 2014
Gomafu	Controls retinal development; Dysregulated in schizophrenia	*Gomafu/Miat* regulates splicing of neuronal genes, including *DISC1*, *ERRB4*, and *WNT7B*, probably via association with splicing factors SF1, SRSF1, and QKI	Briggs et al., 2015; Wang et al., 2017
KCNA2-AS	Regulates neuronal firing properties	It dynamically downregulates expression of the *KCNA2* potassium channel subunit	Zhao et al., 2013
BDNF-AS	Depletion of BDNF-AS promotes neuronal outgrowth adult neurogenesis; BDNF-AS modulates synaptic function	*BDNF-AS* negatively regulates BDNF expression by recruiting EZH2 (a PRC2 core component) in response to neuronal depolarization	Modarresi et al., 2012
Malat1	Promotes dendrite maturation and synaptogenesis in cultured hippocampal neurons	*Malat1* associates with SR family splicing factors to control expression of synaptic molecules including Nlgn1 and SynCAM1	Wang et al., 2017
BC1/BC200	Regulates synaptic excitability	Controls the translational repression of specific target mRNAs within synapses through a mechanism involving direct recruitment of translational machineries	Zhong et al., 2009

RMST, rhabdomyosarcoma 2 associated transcript; ASCL1, achaete-scute family bHLH transcription factor 1; DLX1, distal-less homeobox 1; Tuna, TCL1 upstream neural differentiation-associated RNA; PTBP1, polypyrimidine tract binding protein 1; hnRNP-K, heterogeneous nuclear ribonucleoprotein K; NCL, nucleolin; DISC1, disrupted in schizophrenia 1; EZH2, enhancer of zeste 2 polycomb repressive complex 2 subunit; PRC2, proteasome component 2.

function. For example, the magnitude of the action potential can be affected by changing the subunit stoichiometry of potassium channels. Potassium voltage-gated channel subfamily A member 2 (*KCNA2*) is a major potassium channel subunit, and its expression is regulated by overlapping antisense RNA when facing peripheral nerve injury or neuralgia. In a healthy rat model, *KCNA2* antisense (*KCNA2-AS*) is expressed in few dorsal root ganglia (DRG) neurons (<20% of DRG), and *KCNA2* is expressed in most DRG neurons. However, in the face of peripheral nerve injury, a large amount of *KCNA2-AS* is induced by transcription factor myeloid zinc finger 1 in DRG neurons. *In vivo* and *in vitro* experiments have revealed that the overexpression of *KCNA2-AS* could decrease KCNA2 mRNA and protein content. The mechanism may be that it binds with competing DNA- or RNA-binding factors, thereby, regulating the expression of *KCNA2* (Zhao et al., 2013). This regulation alters the function of DRG neurons. Therefore, *KCNA2-AS* can respond to peripheral nerve damage by altering synaptic plasticity. The lncRNA *NEAT1* provides a scaffolding function in the nucleus that releases regulatory proteins after neuronal activation to finetune excitatory responses and correlate with pathological seizure states. In addition, downregulation of lncRNA *NEAT1* results in changes in the expression of multiple gene transcripts involved in ion channel function following neuronal activation (Barry et al., 2017).

The BDNF is a class of secreted growth factors that are essential for neuronal growth, synaptic plasticity, and participation in learning and memory processes (Leal et al., 2014; Ninan, 2014; Zagrebelsky and Korte, 2014). The BDNF is an important growth factor, not only being regulated by miRNA, but also regulated by lncRNA. Dissection of the human BDNF locus revealed that antisense transcription of the *BDNF* gene from anti-BDNF (*BDNF-AS*, also annotated as *BDNF-OS*) in the brain takes place to form dsRNA duplexes with BDNF mRNA. Inhibition of *BDNF-AS* by antagoNAT *in vivo* or siRNA *in vitro* both resulted in increased *BDNF* mRNA and protein levels, which promoted neurite outgrowth and maturation, suggesting that anti-BDNF plays an important role in *BDNF* function (Lipovich et al., 2012; Modarresi et al., 2012). Further studies revealed that *BDNF-AS* inhibits *BDNF* transcription by recruiting the zeste homolog 2 (EZH2) and polycomb suppression complex 2 (PRC2) enhancers to the *BDNF* promoter region (Pruunsild et al., 2007).

The lncRNA *Gomafu* is widely expressed in the brain, (Mercer et al., 2008) and has recently been shown to modulate alternative splicing of the schizophrenia-associated genes *DISC1* and *ERBB4* (Barry et al., 2014). Since deletion of *Erbb4* in mice enhances LTP in the hippocampus, it is important to determine whether *Gomafu*-regulated splice isoforms affect normal synaptic plasticity (Pitcher et al., 2008; Shamir et al., 2012). In addition, lncRNA *MALAT1* mediates spinal cord maturation and synapse formation by recruiting splicing factors. In cultured hippocampal neurons, knock-down of Malat1 reduces synaptic density, whereas overexpression leads to autonomous increase in cells at synaptic density (Bernard et al., 2010).

These findings suggest that lncRNAs can regulate the synaptic plasticity, and thus, the fidelity of cognitive and memory processes by dynamically monitoring and integrating multiple transcriptional and post-transcriptional events.

THE ROLE OF LNCRNAS IN NEURODEGENERATIVE DISEASES

The lncRNAs have broad-spectrum functions in the normal brain development and function maintenance. It is not surprising that dysregulation of lncRNAs might play a pivotal role in neurodegenerative diseases. This view has been reinforced by the identification of a growing number of lncRNAs that directly regulate the expression of genes associated with neurodegenerative disorders, including AD, PD, HD, respectively.

The Correlation of lncRNAs and Alzheimer's Disease

The AD is a neurodegenerative disease with cognitive decline as the main clinical manifestation. Its pathological mechanism has not been completely understood to date. The main pathological characteristic of AD is the progressive disease of neurons accompanied by the loss of neurons, senile plaques (SPs), and neurofibrillary tangles (Dewachter et al., 2000; Ghosal et al., 2009). Senile plaques mainly consist of β-amyloid (Aβ). Amyloid precursor protein was abnormally cleaved by β-amyloid precursor protein cleaving enzyme 1 (BACE1) to produce Aβ. The excessive accumulation of Aβ produces neurotoxicity. The *BACE1-AS* is an lncRNA transcribed from the antisense strand of the *BACE1* gene, which is highly expressed in the brain of patients with AD. A study revealed that the expression of *BACE1-AS* was significantly increased under extracellular stimulation, such as $Aβ_{42}$ (Faghihi et al., 2008). However, *BACE1-AS* does not inhibit the transcription of mRNA by forming dimers through binding with the coding genes as general natural antisense transcripts (NATs). In contrast, *BACE1-AS* covers the binding site of *miR-485-5p* on *BACE1* mRNA, thereby, silencing the inhibition of *miR-485-5p* on BACE1 mRNA and increasing the stability of *BACE1* mRNA (Faghihi et al., 2010). This leads to the production of more $Aβ_{42}$ and an increase in the formation of SPs in the brain in AD patients, aggravating the development of the disease. Feng et al. found that the level of the *BACE1* is increased in the plasma of AD patients and that it has a high specificity (88%) for AD, indicating *BACE1* may be a potential candidate biomarker to predict AD (Feng et al., 2018). Recently, Yang et al., investigated the hippocampal expression patterns of dysregulated lncRNAs in a rat model of AD through microarray (Yang et al., 2017). The authors identified a total of 315 lncRNAs and 311 mRNAs significantly dysregulated in the AD model, such as *BC158567, MRAK050857, Mrak033976*, etc. These differentially expressed genes are involved in synaptic transmission regulation, cholinergic regulation, and CNS neuron differentiation, all of which are important in learning and memory, as well as the development of AD. Furthermore, the dysregulated lncRNAs in the AD group are involved in the neuroactive ligand–receptor interaction, the renin–angiotensin system, axon guidance, and the PI3K–Akt, MAPK, and mTOR signaling pathways. Among these, the PI3K–Akt, MAPK, and mTOR signaling pathways play important roles in long-term learning and memory.

The BC200 RNA is selectively located in neuronal synapses, which regulates the synthesis of proteins surrounding the postsynaptic membrane. Mus et al. revealed that the expression of *BC200* RNA was significantly downregulated in the prefrontal cortical area in normal elderly subjects (49–86 years old, by autopsy), and was significantly increased in the brain of AD patients. Further studies have revealed that the distribution of *BC200* RNA in the brain of AD patients has changed. The *BC200* RNA in the brain of AD patients is located in the perinuclear area in the cluster, instead of the synaptic terminals. Hence, it loses its regulatory function on proteins surrounding the postsynaptic membrane. The overexpression and error spatial localization of *BC200* RNA may excessively inhibit the synthesis of cytoplasmic proteins, thereby, aggravating the pathological changes of AD (Mus et al., 2007).

The *17A* is also an lncRNA that has been recently discovered. It is located in intron 3 of the G protein-coupled receptor-51 (*GRP51*) gene, regulates the production of *GRP51* variable transcript, and inhibits the canonical transcription of GAGA(B2) receptors, thereby, significantly affecting the GABA-B signaling pathway. The inflammatory reaction in the brain in AD patients can activate the expression of *17A*. This increases the secretion of Aβ and the Aβ42/Aβ40 ratio, aggravating the progress of the disease (Massone et al., 2011). Another lncRNA *51A* overlapping with *SORL1* (antisense) was also shown to affect Aβ formation and upregulated in AD (Ciarlo et al., 2013).

In addition, neurotrophic factors (NTFs) play an important role in maintaining nervous system function. The expression level of *BDNF* is significantly changed in neurodegenerative diseases, psychosis, and neurodevelopmental disorders (Lu et al., 2013, 2014; Song et al., 2015). The inhibition of *BDNF-AS* expression can increase the expression of BDNF in the brain, which has a wide prospect for the treatment of neurodegenerative diseases. Glial cell-derived neurotrophic factor opposite strand (*GDNFOS*) is transcribed from the antisense strand of the GDNF gene. A study revealed that there was a difference in the expression of GDNFOS subunit in AD brains compared with normal brains, but the underlying mechanisms remain unknown at present (Airavaara et al., 2011). Furthermore, another study found that *Sox2OT* and *1810014B01Rik* could serve as biomarkers in the early and late stages of neurodegenerative diseases (Arisi et al., 2011). Tremendous efforts have been put into their translational applications by identifying specific lncRNAs that are changed in Alzheimer's disease in order to provide biomarkers and better illustrate molecular pathways.

The Correlation Between lncRNAs and Parkinson's Disease

Parkinson's disease (PD) is a neurodegenerative disease that commonly occurs in the elderly. Its pathological characteristic is the degeneration of dopaminergic neurons in the substantia nigra-striatum system, which decreases dopamine secretion, resulting in a series of extrapyramidal responses. The maintenance of mitochondrial homeostasis plays an important role in the progression of PD (Moreira et al., 2010; Jin et al., 2014; Luo et al., 2015). Gene studies revealed that PD family-related genes such as *α-synuclein, parkin*, PTEN-induced putative kinase 1 (*PINK1*), *DJ-1*, and leucine-rich repeat kinase 2 (*LRRK2*) were closely related to mitochondrial function (Puspita et al., 2017). Endogenous *PINK1* is localized in the mitochondrial membrane and plays an important role in energy metabolism in neurons and muscle cells. In addition, *PINK1* can also inhibit the release of cytochrome C from mitochondria and decrease the occurrence of apoptosis. The inhibition or overexpression of *PINK1* can lead to abnormal mitochondrial morphology and affect the release of dopamine, resulting in behavior defects (Petit et al., 2005). Study found that lncRNA *NEAT1* was significantly upregulated in the midbrain of PD mice, and that lncRNA *NEAT1* promoted MPTP-induced autophagy in PD by stabilizing PINK1 protein (Yan et al., 2018). Noncoding antisense PTEN-induced putative kinase 1 (*naPINK1*) is an lncRNA transcribed from the antisense strand of the *PINK1* gene, which can stabilize the expression of the *PINK1* variable transcript *svPINK1*. The silencing of *naPINK1* leads to the decrease in *svPINK1* in neurons. This suggests that the PD process can be improved by regulating the *PINK1* locus (Scheele et al., 2007).

Ubiquitin carboxy-terminal hydrolase L1 (*Uchl1*) is a neuron-restricted protein acting as a de-ubiquitinating enzyme or a monoubiquitin stabilizer. The *UCHL1* gene mutations have been discovered to be related to familial PD and the oxidative inactivation of Uchl1 protein has been reported in PD and AD brains (Choi et al., 2004). The *Uchl1-AS* is a nuclear-enriched lncRNA that is transcribed antisense to the mouse *Uchl1*. The *Uchl1-AS* increases the protein synthesis of UCHL1 at the post-transcriptional level and then regulates the progression of PD (Carrieri et al., 2015). Furthermore, the activity of *Uchl1-AS* is controlled by the signaling pathway. The *Uchl1* mRNA is mainly localized in the cytoplasm, while *Uchl1-AS* is abundant in the nucleus of dopaminergic neurons. Interestingly, the mTOR inhibitor-Rapamycin treatment resulted in the induction of Uchl1 protein by association of shuttling *Uchl1-AS* from the nucleus to the cytoplasm, suggesting that the interaction between Uchl1–ncRNA–mTOR may be critical for PD development (Carrieri et al., 2012; Vucićević et al., 2014).

Correlation Between lncRNAs and Huntington's Disease

Huntington's disease (HD) is a rare autosomal dominant inherited neurodegenerative disease. Its pathological change is the loss of neurons in the striatum and cortex in brain. There is a CAG repetitive sequence in exon 1 of its pathogenic gene huntingtin (*HTT*), which encodes polyglutamine. The excessive repeat amplification of CAG in the gene-coding region induces the prolongation of the polyglutamine chain in protein, thereby inducing lesions (Aziz et al., 2011; De Souza and Leavitt, 2015). The *HTT* can regulate the nuclear translocation of transcription inhibiting factor RE-1 silencing transcription factor (REST), which is also known as neuron-restrictive silencer factor (NRSF)(Shimojo, 2008). Mutation in HTT leads to the abnormal nuclear/interstitial translocation of REST/NRSF, thereby, inducing the abnormal expression of the downstream target gene of REST/NRSF, including PCGs and ncRNA. Through studies on the expression profile of brain tissue in HD patients, Johnson et al. revealed that the expression of *HAR1* lncRNA in striatum decreased significantly, and the main cause was that REST inhibited *HAR1* transcription by locating in the *HAR1* locus *via* the specific DNA regulatory element (Johnson et al., 2010). Chung et al. discovered an lncRNA-*HTTAS* transcribed from the antisense strand of *HTT*. This has two types of transcripts: *HTTAS-v1* (exons 1 and 3) and *HTTAS-v2* (exons 2 and 3), where exon 1 contains repeated gene loci. Cell level verification results revealed that the overexpression of *HTTAS-v1* could significantly decrease the transcription level of *HTT*, while *HTT* transcription level significantly increased after *HTTAS-v1* was disrupted by siRNA. Furthermore, *HTTAS-v1* expression was found to be downregulated in frontal cortex of HD patients, and this strongly suggests that the change in *HTTAS* may play a certain role in the progress of HD (Chung et al., 2011).

The lncRNA *TUG1* has been shown to be a direct downstream target of p53, which is known to be upregulated in HD itself. Therefore, *TUG1* appears to be a pro-survival factor in neurons. The upregulation we observed in HD - probably through p53 activation–actually acts against mutHTT cytotoxicity (Khalil et al., 2009). The *NEAT1* is a nuclear-enrich lncRNA that is essential for the formation and maintenance of paraspeckles, which are subnuclear bodies found in mammalian cells (Clemson et al., 2009). Sunwoo et al. found that the levels of *NEAT1* were increased in R6/2 mice and HD patients. In order to determine the biological effects of *NEAT1* on neuronal survival, the authors transfected neuro2A cells with the *NEAT1* short isotype vector and subjected them to H2O2-induced damage. The *NEAT1* transfected cells showed enhanced viability under oxidative stress, confirming that upregulation of *NEAT1* contributes to neuroprotective mechanisms against neuronal damage rather than pathology of neurodegenerative diseases (Sunwoo et al., 2017). It has been reported that *MEG3* is a REST target and is dynamically expressed during neurodevelopment and associated with PRC2 chromatin regulators. This supporting *MEG3* might be participating in chromatin regulation, noncoding transcription, and neurodevelopment in HD (Johnson, 2012). Although functional studies on *DGCR5* have not been performed, the fact that this neuro-specific disease-related transcript is directly targeted by REST suggests that it has important functions in the human nervous system (Sutherland et al., 1996; Johnson, 2012).

Summary of lncRNAs in Neurodegenerative Diseases

An increasing number of studies report on lncRNAs as being implicated in neurodegenerative diseases, including AD, PD, and HD (**Table 2**).

The roles of *BACE1-AS* lncRNA have been widely defined in AD. The *BACE1-AS* levels are upregulated in AD brains,

TABLE 2 | Dysregulated lncRNAs in neurodegenerative diseases.

lncRNAs	Direction of change	Relative disease	Biological function	References
Sox2OT	Up	AD, PD	Regulate cotranscribed *Sox2* gene expression to down neurogenesis.	Arisi et al., 2011; Shimozaki, 2014
BC200	up(Soma) down(Dentritic)	AD, PD	Modulate local proteins in postsynaptic dendritic micro-domains to maintenance of long-term synaptic plasticity.	Lukiw et al., 1992; Mus et al., 2007; Vucićević et al., 2014; Luo and Chen, 2016
BACE1-AS	up	AD	Increase *BACE1* mRNA stability resulting in additional Aβ42 generation through a post-transcriptional feed-forward mechanism.	Faghihi et al., 2008; Liu et al., 2014
NAT-Rad18	up	AD	Down the expression of DNA repair protein Rad18 resulting in the neuron being more sensitive to apoptosis.	Parenti et al., 2007
NDM29	up	AD	Promotes Aβ secretion with increased Aβ42/ Aβ40 ratio, expression induced by inflammatory processes.	Massone et al., 2012
51A	up	AD	Promotes the alternative splicing of *SORL1* and increases Aβ formation.	Ciarlo et al., 2013; Tan et al., 2013; Luo and Chen, 2016
17A	up	AD	Impair GABAB signaling pathway by decreasing *GABAB R2* transcription.	Massone et al., 2011
GDNFOS	Dysregulated/ differences in tissue expression patterns	AD	Modulate the expression of endogenous *GDNF* in human brain.	Airavaara et al., 2011
naPINK1	up	PD	Stabilize the *svPINK1*, resulting in disturbed mitochondrial respiratory chain, and then increase the sensitivity to apoptosis.	Chiba et al., 2009; Sai et al., 2012
PINK1-AS	-	PD	Positively regulates the stability of *svPINK1* transcript.	Scheele et al., 2007
UCHL1-AS	-	PD	Positively regulates *UCHL1* mRNA translation.	Carrieri et al., 2012, 2015
HAR1	down	HD	Necessary for retinal development, the function with HD not be mentioned.	Johnson et al., 2010; Johnson, 2012
HTT-AS	down	HD	*HTTAS-v1* specifically reduces endogenous *HTT* transcript levels.	Chung et al., 2011
MEG3	down	HD	Binds the PCR2 epigenetic silencing complex.	Johnson, 2012

AD, Alzheimer's disease; PD, Parkinson's disease; HD, Huntington's disease; Sox2OT, Sox2 overlapping transcript; BACE1-AS, β-site amyloid precursor protein cleaving enzyme 1 antisense; GDNFOS, glial cell derived neurotrophic factor opposite strand; HAR1, human accelerated region 1; HTT-AS, Huntingtin antisense; PINK1-AS, PTEN induced putative kinase 1 antisense; UCHL1-AS, ubiquitin C-terminal hydrolase L1 antisense; MEG3, maternally expressed 3; NDM29, Neuroblastoma Differentiation Marker 29.

where *BACE1-AS* acts by stabilizing BACE1 mRNA, thereby, increasing BACE1 protein content and Aβ42 formation. While lncRNA *BC200, 17A, BC158567, MRAK050857, Mrak033976, BDNF-AS, Sox2OT,* and *1810014B01Rik* are also involved in AD. In PD, the lncRNA *UCHL1-AS1* acts by directly promoting translation of UCHL1 protein leading to perturbation of the ubiquitin–proteasome system. Different lncRNAs, such as *naPINK1, NEAT1 PINK1-AS, BC200,* and *Sox2OT,* were found to be dysregulated in their expression also in PD. Several studies reported altered expression levels of known lncRNAs *HTT-AS, TUG1, NEAT1, MEG3,* and *DGCR5* in the brains of HD patients. The emerging role of lncRNAs in neurodegenerative diseases suggests that their dysregulation may trigger neuronal death through an unexplored RNA-based regulatory mechanism that needs to be further investigated.

CHALLENGES AND PERSPECTIVES

With the continuous deepening of gene regulation research and the emergence of more biological methods, lncRNA function and mechanism will be further elucidated.

This relatively poorly characterized class of RNAs, with little or no coding capacity, has been implicated in the growth and development of the nervous system, the differentiation of neurons, synaptic plasticity, and the occurrence and progress of many diseases. Although many studies have been performed in clinical patients using various disease models, the exact role and impact of lncRNAs in disease pathogenesis still remain obscure. At present, there are still challenges for our understanding of lncRNAs.

Our lack of understanding of the molecular mechanisms of lncRNA action makes it particularly difficult for us to recognize the biological function of lncRNA. As we move forward from the annotation of lncRNAs to more emphasis on molecular function and biology, we still do not fully understand the biological significance of lncRNAs as a group. We need better tools to track lncRNA localization across the genome, monitor lncRNA interactions with proteins and nucleic acids, and determine the structure and elucidate the key structure–function relationships of lncRNAs, especially how they interact with proteins. Furthermore, unlike PCGs with systemic functional annotation systems, the lack of an annotation system for lncRNA function makes it difficult to evaluate computational algorithms for functional prediction. Finally, is it useful to find lncRNAs in neurodegenerative diseases? Two major long-term challenges in disease research are (a) the development of noninvasive diagnostic methods for monitoring the progression of neurodegenerative diseases, and (b) the development of treatments to cure and reverse disease processes.

In fact, more and more attention has been paid to lncRNAs as potential targets for disease biomarkers or therapeutic strategies. Indeed, several commercial entities targeting lncRNAs (such as OPKO-CURNA and RaNA therapeutic agents) have been developed to design and develop oligonucleotide therapeutics for the treatment of neurodegenerative diseases (Qureshi and Mehler, 2013). Hereby, further investigation into the role of lncRNAs will provide a better understanding of how the brain functions and how diseases develop, and lead to greater insights into further therapeutic development for neurodegenerative diseases based on manipulations of lncRNA functions.

AUTHOR CONTRIBUTIONS

C-WW substantial contributions to the conception and design of the work, the acquisition, analysis, interpretation of data for the work. C-WW drafting the work and revising it critically for important intellectual content. A-SW final approval of the version to be published. TL and S-SZ agreement to be accountable for all aspects of the work in ensuring that questions related to the accuracy and integrity of any part of the work are appropriately investigated and resolved.

FUNDING

This work was supported by the National Natural Science Foundation of China (No. 81371199, 81771139).

REFERENCES

Airavaara, M., Pletnikova, O., Doyle, M. E., Zhang, Y. E., Troncoso, J. C., and Liu, Q. R. (2011). Identification of novel GDNF isoforms and cis-antisense GDNFOS gene and their regulation in human middle temporal gyrus of Alzheimer disease. *J. Biol. Chem.* 286, 45093–45102. doi: 10.1074/jbc.M111.310250

Amaral, P. P., Dinger, M. E., and Mattick, J. S. (2013). Non-coding RNAs in homeostasis, disease and stress responses: an evolutionary perspective. *Brief. Funct. Genomics* 12, 254–278. doi: 10.1093/bfgp/elt016

Antoniou, D., Stergiopoulos, A., and Politis, P. K. (2014). Recent advances in the involvement of long non-coding RNAs in neural stem cell biology and brain pathophysiology. *Front. Physiol.* 5: 155. doi: 10.3389/fphys.2014.00155

Arisi, I., D'Onofrio, M., Brandi, R., Felsani, A., Capsoni, S., Drovandi, G., et al. (2011). Gene expression biomarkers in the brain of a mouse model for Alzheimer's disease: mining of microarray data by logic classification and feature selection. *Biochim. Biophys. Acta* 24, 721–738. doi: 10.3233/JAD-2011-101881

Aziz, N. A., van Belzen, M. J., Coops, I. D., Belfroid, R. D., and Roos, R. A. (2011). Parent-of-origin differences of mutant HTT CAG repeat instability in Huntington's disease. *Eur. J. Med. Genet.* 54, e413–e418. doi: 10.1016/j.ejmg.2011.04.002

Azzalin, C. M., Reichenbach, P., Khoriauli, L., Giulotto, E., and Lingner, J. (2007). Telomeric repeat containing RNA and RNA surveillance factors at mammalian chromosome ends. *Science* 318, 798–801. doi: 10.1126/science.1147182

Babajko, S., Petit, S., Fernandes, I., Meary, F., LeBihan, J., Pibouin, L., et al. (2009). Msx1 expression regulation by its own antisense RNA: consequence on tooth development and bone regeneration. *Cells Tissues Organs* 189, 115–121. doi: 10.1159/000151748

Barry, G., Briggs, J. A., Hwang, D. W., Nayler, S. P., Fortuna, P. R., Jonkhout, N., et al. (2017). The long non-coding RNA NEAT1 is responsive to neuronal activity and is associated with hyperexcitability states. *Sci. Rep.* 7:40127. doi: 10.1038/srep40127

Barry, G., Briggs, J. A., Vanichkina, D. P., Poth, E. M., Beveridge, N. J., Ratnu, V. S., et al. (2014). The long non-coding RNA Gomafu is acutely regulated in response to neuronal activation and involved in schizophrenia-associated alternative splicing. *Mol. Psychiatry* 19, 486–494. doi: 10.1038/mp.2013.45

Bernard, D., Prasanth, K. V., Tripathi, V., Colasse, S., Nakamura, T., Xuan, Z., et al. (2010). A long nuclear-retained non-coding RNA regulates synaptogenesis by modulating gene expression. *EMBO J.* 29, 3082–3093. doi: 10.1038/emboj.2010.199

Bond, A. M., Vangompel, M. J., Sametsky, E. A., Clark, M. F., Savage, J. C., Disterhoft, J. F., et al. (2009). Balanced gene regulation by an embryonic brain ncRNA is critical for adult hippocampal GABA circuitry. *Nat. Neurosci.* 12, 1020–1027. doi: 10.1038/nn.2371

Braidotti, G., Baubec, T., Pauler, F., Seidl, C., Smrzka, O., Stricker, S., et al. (2004). The Air noncoding RNA: an imprinted cis-silencing transcript. *Cold Spring Harb. Symp. Quant. Biol.* 69, 55–66. doi: 10.1101/sqb.2004.69.55

Briggs, J. A., Wolvetang, E. J., Mattick, J. S., Rinn, J. L., and Barry, G. (2015). Mechanisms of long non-coding RNAs in mammalian nervous system development, plasticity, disease, and evolution. *Neuron* 88, 861–877. doi: 10.1016/j.neuron.2015.09.045

Carrieri, C., Cimatti, L., Biagioli, M., Beugnet, A., Zucchelli, S., Fedele, S., et al. (2012). Long non-coding antisense RNA controls Uchl1 translation through an embedded SINEB2 repeat. *Nature* 491, 454–457. doi: 10.1038/nature11508

Carrieri, C., Forrest, A. R., Santoro, C., Persichetti, F., Carninci, P., Zucchelli, S., et al. (2015). Expression analysis of the long non-coding RNA antisense to Uchl1 (AS Uchl1) during dopaminergic cells' differentiation *in vitro* and in neurochemical models of Parkinson's disease. *Front. Cell. Neurosci.* 9:114. doi: 10.3389/fncel.2015.00114

Cesana, M., Cacchiarelli, D., Legnini, I., Santini, T., Sthandier, O., Chinappi, M., et al. (2011). A long noncoding RNA controls muscle differentiation by functioning as a competing endogenous RNA. *Cell* 147, 358–369. doi: 10.1016/j.cell.2011.09.028

Chiba, M., Kiyosawa, H., Hiraiwa, N., Ohkohchi, N., and Yasue, H. (2009). Existence of Pink1 antisense RNAs in mouse and their localization. *Cytogenet. Genome Res.* 126, 259–270. doi: 10.1159/000251963

Choi, J., Levey, A. I., Weintraub, S. T., Rees, H. D., Gearing, M., Chin, L. S., et al. (2004). Oxidative modifications and down-regulation of ubiquitin carboxyl-terminal hydrolase L1 associated with idiopathic Parkinson's and Alzheimer's diseases. *J. Biol. Chem.* 279, 13256–13264. doi: 10.1074/jbc.M314124200

Chung, D. W., Rudnicki, D. D., Yu, L., and Margolis, R. L. (2011). A natural antisense transcript at the Huntington's disease repeat locus regulates HTT expression. *Hum. Mol. Genet.* 20, 3467–3477. doi: 10.1093/hmg/ddr263

Ciarlo, E., Massone, S., Penna, I., Nizzari, M., Gigoni, A., Dieci, G., et al. (2013). An intronic ncRNA-dependent regulation of SORL1 expression affecting Abeta formation is upregulated in post-mortem Alzheimer's disease brain samples. *Dis. Model. Mech.* 6, 424–433. doi: 10.1242/dmm.009761

Clemson, C. M., Hutchinson, J. N., Sara, S. A., Ensminger, A. W., Fox, A. H., Chess, A., et al. (2009). An architectural role for a nuclear noncoding RNA: NEAT1 RNA is essential for the structure of paraspeckles. *Mol. Cell* 33, 717–726. doi: 10.1016/j.molcel.2009.01.026

Colasante, G., Collombat, P., Raimondi, V., Bonanomi, D., Ferrai, C., Maira, M., et al. (2008). Arx is a direct target of Dlx2 and thereby contributes to the tangential migration of GABAergic interneurons. *J. Neurosci.* 28, 10674–10686. doi: 10.1523/JNEUROSCI.1283-08.2008

Coudert, A. E., Pibouin, L., Vi-Fane, B., Thomas, B. L., Macdougall, M., Choudhury, A., et al. (2005). Expression and regulation of the Msx1 natural antisense transcript during development. *Nucleic Acids Res.* 33, 5208–5218. doi: 10.1093/nar/gki831

De Souza, R. A., and Leavitt, B. R. (2015). Neurobiology of Huntington's disease. *Curr. Top. Behav. Neurosci.* 22: 81–100. doi: 10.1007/7854_2014_353

Dewachter, I., van Dorpe, J., Spittaels, K., Tesseur, I., Van Den Haute, C., Moechars, D., et al. (2000). Modeling Alzheimer's disease in transgenic mice: effect of age and of presenilin1 on amyloid biochemistry and pathology in APP/London mice. *Exp. Gerontol.* 35, 831–841. doi: 10.1016/S0531-5565(00)00149-2

Djebali, S., Davis, C. A., Merkel, A., Dobin, A., Lassmann, T., Mortazavi, A., et al. (2012). Landscape of transcription in human cells. *Nature* 489, 101–108. doi: 10.1038/nature11233

Faghihi, M. A., Modarresi, F., Khalil, A. M., Wood, D. E., Sahagan, B. G., Morgan, T. E., et al. (2008). Expression of a noncoding RNA is elevated in Alzheimer's disease and drives rapid feed-forward regulation of beta-secretase. *Nat. Med.* 14, 723–730. doi: 10.1038/nm1784

Faghihi, M. A., Zhang, M., Huang, J., Modarresi, F., Van der Brug, M. P., Nalls, M. A., et al. (2010). Evidence for natural antisense transcript-mediated inhibition of microRNA function. *Genome Biol.* 11:R56. doi: 10.1186/gb-2010-11-5-r56

Feng, L., Liao, Y. T., He, J. C., Xie, C. L., Chen, S. Y., Fan, H. H., et al. (2018). Plasma long non-coding RNA BACE1 as a novel biomarker for diagnosis of Alzheimer disease. *BMC Neurol.* 18:4. doi: 10.1186/s12883-017-1008-x

Ghosal, K., Vogt, D. L., Liang, M., Shen, Y., Lamb, B. T., and Pimplikar, S. W. (2009). Alzheimer's disease-like pathological features in transgenic mice expressing the APP intracellular domain. *Proc. Natl. Acad. Sci. U.S.A.* 106, 18367–18372. doi: 10.1073/pnas.0907652106

Goff, L. A., and Rinn, J. L. (2015). Linking RNA biology to lncRNAs. *Genome Res.* 25, 1456–1465. doi: 10.1101/gr.191122.115

Graff, J., and Mansuy, I. M. (2008). Epigenetic codes in cognition and behaviour. *Behav. Brain Res.* 192, 70–87. doi: 10.1016/j.bbr.2008.01.021

Guttman, M., Amit, I., Garber, M., French, C., Lin, M. F., Feldser, D., et al. (2009). Chromatin signature reveals over a thousand highly conserved large non-coding RNAs in mammals. *Nature* 458, 223–227. doi: 10.1038/nature07672

Hung, T., Wang, Y., Lin, M. F., Koegel, A. K., Kotake, Y., Grant, G. D., et al. (2011). Extensive and coordinated transcription of noncoding RNAs within cell-cycle promoters. *Nat. Genet.* 43, 621–629. doi: 10.1038/ng.848

Hutchinson, J. N., Ensminger, A. W., Clemson, C. M., Lynch, C. R., Lawrence, J. B., and Chess, A. (2007). A screen for nuclear transcripts identifies two linked noncoding RNAs associated with SC35 splicing domains. *BMC Genomics* 8:39. doi: 10.1186/1471-2164-8-39

Jiang, Y. H., Armstrong, D., Albrecht, U., Atkins, C. M., Noebels, J. L., Eichele, G., et al. (1998). Mutation of the Angelman ubiquitin ligase in mice causes increased cytoplasmic p53 and deficits of contextual learning and long-term potentiation. *Neuron* 21, 799–811. doi: 10.1016/S0896-6273(00)80596-6

Jin, H., Kanthasamy, A., Ghosh, A., Anantharam, V., Kalyanaraman, B., and Kanthasamy, A. G. (2014). Mitochondria-targeted antioxidants for treatment of Parkinson's disease: preclinical and clinical outcomes. *Biochim. Biophys. Acta* 1842, 1282–1294. doi: 10.1016/j.bbadis.2013.09.007

Johnson, R. (2012). Long non-coding RNAs in Huntington's disease neurodegeneration. *Neurobiol. Dis.* 46, 245–254. doi: 10.1016/j.nbd.2011.12.006

Johnson, R., Richter, N., Jauch, R., Gaughwin, P. M., Zuccato, C., Cattaneo, E., et al. (2010). Human accelerated region 1 noncoding RNA is repressed by REST in Huntington's disease. *Physiol. Genomics* 41, 269–274. doi: 10.1152/physiolgenomics.00019.2010

Kazemzadeh, M., Safaralizadeh, R., and Orang, A. V. (2015). LncRNAs: emerging players in gene regulation and disease pathogenesis. *J. Genet.* 94, 771–784. doi: 10.1007/s12041-015-0561-6

Khalil, A. M., Guttman, M., Huarte, M., Garber, M., Raj, A., Rivea Morales, D., et al. (2009). Many human large intergenic noncoding RNAs associate with chromatin-modifying complexes and affect gene expression. *Proc. Natl. Acad. Sci. U.S.A.* 106, 11667–11672. doi: 10.1073/pnas.0904715106

Klattenhoff, C. A., Scheuermann, J. C., Surface, L. E., Bradley, R. K., Fields, P. A., Steinhauser, M. L., et al. (2013). Braveheart, a long noncoding RNA required for cardiovascular lineage commitment. *Cell* 152, 570–583. doi: 10.1016/j.cell.2013.01.003

Kondrashov, A. V., Kiefmann, M., Ebnet, K., Khanam, T., Muddashetty, R. S., and Brosius, J. (2005). Inhibitory effect of naked neural BC1 RNA or BC200 RNA on eukaryotic *in vitro* translation systems is reversed by poly(A)-binding protein (PABP). *J. Mol. Biol.* 353, 88–103. doi: 10.1016/j.jmb.2005.07.049

Leal, G., Comprido, D., and Duarte, C. B. (2014). BDNF-induced local protein synthesis and synaptic plasticity. *Neuropharmacology* 76(Pt C), 639–656. doi: 10.1016/j.neuropharm.2013.04.005

Lee, S., Seo, H. H., Lee, C. Y., Lee, J., Shin, S., Kim, S. W., et al. (2017). Human long noncoding RNA regulation of stem cell potency and differentiation. *Stem Cells Int.* 2017: 6374504. doi: 10.1155/2017/6374504

Lin, N., Chang, K. Y., Li, Z., Gates, K., Rana, Z. A., Dang, J., et al. (2014). An evolutionarily conserved long noncoding RNA TUNA controls pluripotency and neural lineage commitment. *Mol. Cell* 53, 1005–1019. doi: 10.1016/j.molcel.2014.01.021

Lipovich, L., Dachet, F., Cai, J., Bagla, S., Balan, K., Jia, H., et al. (2012). Activity-dependent human brain coding/noncoding gene regulatory networks. *Genetics* 192, 1133–1148. doi: 10.1534/genetics.112.145128

Liu, T., Huang, Y., Chen, J., Chi, H., Yu, Z., Wang, J., et al. (2014). Attenuated ability of BACE1 to cleave the amyloid precursor protein via silencing long noncoding RNA BACE1AS expression. *Mol. Med. Rep.* 10, 1275–1281. doi: 10.3892/mmr.2014.2351

Lu, B., Nagappan, G., Guan, X., Nathan, P. J., and Wren, P. (2013). BDNF-based synaptic repair as a disease-modifying strategy for neurodegenerative diseases. *Nat. Rev. Neurosci.* 14, 401–416. doi: 10.1038/nrn3505

Lu, B., Nagappan, G., and Lu, Y. (2014). BDNF and synaptic plasticity, cognitive function, and dysfunction. *Handb. Exp. Pharmacol.* 220: 223–250. doi: 10.1007/978-3-642-45106-5_9

Lukiw, W. J., Handley, P., Wong, L., and Crapper McLachlan, D. R. (1992). BC200 RNA in normal human neocortex, non-Alzheimer dementia (NAD), and senile dementia of the Alzheimer type (AD). *Neurochem. Res.* 17, 591–597. doi: 10.1007/BF00968788

Luo, Q., and Chen, Y. (2016). Long noncoding RNAs and Alzheimer's disease. *Clin. Interv. Aging* 11: 867–872. doi: 10.2147/CIA.S107037

Luo, Y., Hoffer, A., Hoffer, B., and Qi, X. (2015). Mitochondria: a therapeutic target for Parkinson's disease?. *Int. J. Mol. Sci.* 16, 20704–20730. doi: 10.3390/ijms160920704

Lv, J., Liu, H., Huang, Z., Su, J., He, H., Xiu, Y., et al. (2013). Long non-coding RNA identification over mouse brain development by integrative modeling of chromatin and genomic features. *Nucleic Acids Res.* 41, 10044–10061. doi: 10.1093/nar/gkt818

Maag, J. L., Panja, D., Sporild, I., Patil, S., Kaczorowski, D. C., Bramham, C. R., et al. (2015). Dynamic expression of long noncoding RNAs and repeat elements in synaptic plasticity. *Front. Neurosci.* 9: 351. doi: 10.3389/fnins.2015.00351

Mabb, A. M., Judson, M. C., Zylka, M. J., and Philpot, B. D. (2011). Angelman syndrome: insights into genomic imprinting and neurodevelopmental phenotypes. *Trends Neurosci.* 34, 293–303. doi: 10.1016/j.tins.2011.04.001

Magistri, M., Faghihi, M. A., St Laurent, G. III., and Wahlestedt, C. (2012). Regulation of chromatin structure by long noncoding RNAs: focus on natural antisense transcripts. *Trends Genet.* 28, 389–396. doi: 10.1016/j.tig.2012.03.013

Massone, S., Ciarlo, E., Vella, S., Nizzari, M., Florio, T., Russo, C., et al. (2012). NDM29, a RNA polymerase III-dependent non coding RNA, promotes amyloidogenic processing of APP and amyloid beta secretion. *Biochim. Biophys. Acta* 1823, 1170–1177. doi: 10.1016/j.bbamcr.2012.05.001

Massone, S., Vassallo, I., Fiorino, G., Castelnuovo, M., Barbieri, F., Borghi, R., et al. (2011). 17A, a novel non-coding RNA, regulates GABA B alternative splicing and signaling in response to inflammatory stimuli and in Alzheimer disease. *Neurobiol. Dis.* 41, 308–317. doi: 10.1016/j.nbd.2010.09.019

Mercer, T. R., Dinger, M. E., Sunkin, S. M., Mehler, M. F., and Mattick, J. S. (2008). Specific expression of long noncoding RNAs in the mouse brain. *Proc. Natl. Acad. Sci. U.S.A.* 105, 716–721. doi: 10.1073/pnas.0706729105

Mercer, T. R., Qureshi, I. A., Gokhan, S., Dinger, M. E., Li, G., Mattick, J. S., et al. (2010). Long noncoding RNAs in neuronal-glial fate specification and oligodendrocyte lineage maturation. *BMC Neurosci.* 11:14. doi: 10.1186/1471-2202-11-14

Mercer, T. R., Wilhelm, D., Dinger, M. E., Solda, G., Korbie, D. J., Glazov, E. A., et al. (2011). Expression of distinct RNAs from 3' untranslated regions. *Nucleic Acids Res.* 39, 2393–2403. doi: 10.1093/nar/gkq1158

Modarresi, F., Faghihi, M. A., Lopez-Toledano, M. A., Fatemi, R. P., Magistri, M., Brothers, S. P., et al. (2012). Inhibition of natural antisense transcripts *in vivo* results in gene-specific transcriptional upregulation. *Nat. Biotechnol.* 30, 453–459. doi: 10.1038/nbt.2158

Moreira, P. I., Zhu, X., Wang, X., Lee, H. G., Nunomura, A., Petersen, R. B., et al. (2010). Mitochondria: a therapeutic target in neurodegeneration. *Biochim. Biophys. Acta* 1802, 212–220. doi: 10.1016/j.bbadis.2009.10.007

Mus, E., Hof, P. R., and Tiedge, H. (2007). Dendritic BC200 RNA in aging and in Alzheimer's disease. *Proc. Natl. Acad. Sci. U.S.A.* 104, 10679–10684. doi: 10.1073/pnas.0701532104

Nagano, T., and Fraser, P. (2011). No-nonsense functions for long noncoding RNAs. *Cell* 145, 178–181. doi: 10.1016/j.cell.2011.03.014

Nakagawa, S., Ip, J. Y., Shioi, G., Tripathi, V., Zong, X., Hirose, T., et al. (2012). Malat1 is not an essential component of nuclear speckles in mice. *RNA* 18, 1487–1499. doi: 10.1261/rna.033217.112

Ng, S. Y., Bogu, G. K., Soh, B. S., and Stanton, L. W. (2013). The long noncoding RNA RMST interacts with SOX2 to regulate neurogenesis. *Mol. Cell* 51, 349–359. doi: 10.1016/j.molcel.2013.07.017

Ng, S. Y., Johnson, R., and Stanton, L. W. (2012). Human long non-coding RNAs promote pluripotency and neuronal differentiation by association with chromatin modifiers and transcription factors. *EMBO J.* 31, 522–533. doi: 10.1038/emboj.2011.459

Ninan, I. (2014). Synaptic regulation of affective behaviors; role of BDNF. *Neuropharmacology* 76(Pt C), 684–695. doi: 10.1016/j.neuropharm.2013.04.011

Okazaki, Y., Furuno, M., Kasukawa, T., Adachi, J., Bono, H., Kondo, S., et al. (2002). Analysis of the mouse transcriptome based on functional annotation of 60,770 full-length cDNAs. *Nature* 420, 563–573. doi: 10.1038/nature 01266

Pang, K. C., Frith, M. C., and Mattick, J. S. (2006). Rapid evolution of noncoding RNAs: lack of conservation does not mean lack of function. *Trends Genet.* 22, 1–5. doi: 10.1016/j.tig.2005.10.003

Panja, D., and Bramham, C. R. (2014). BDNF mechanisms in late LTP formation: a synthesis and breakdown. *Neuropharmacology* 76(Pt C), 664–676. doi: 10.1016/j.neuropharm.2013.06.024

Parenti, R., Paratore, S., Torrisi, A., and Cavallaro, S. (2007). A natural antisense transcript against Rad18, specifically expressed in neurons and upregulated during beta-amyloid-induced apoptosis. *Eur. J. Neurosci.* 26, 2444–2457. doi: 10.1111/j.1460-9568.2007.05864.x

Pauler, F. M., Stricker, S. H., Warczok, K. E., and Barlow, D. P. (2005). Long-range DNase I hypersensitivity mapping reveals the imprinted Igf2r and Air promoters share cis-regulatory elements. *Genome Res.* 15, 1379–1387. doi: 10.1101/gr.3783805

Peden, A. H., and Ironside, J. W. (2012). Molecular pathology in neurodegenerative diseases. *Curr. Drug Targets* 13, 1548–1559. doi: 10.2174/138945012803530134

Petit, A., Kawarai, T., Paitel, E., Sanjo, N., Maj, M., Scheid, M., et al. (2005). Wild-type PINK1 prevents basal and induced neuronal apoptosis, a protective effect abrogated by Parkinson disease-related mutations. *J. Biol. Chem.* 280, 34025–34032. doi: 10.1074/jbc.M505143200

Pitcher, G. M., Beggs, S., Woo, R. S., Mei, L., and Salter, M. W. (2008). ErbB4 is a suppressor of long-term potentiation in the adult hippocampus. *Neuroreport* 19, 139–143. doi: 10.1097/WNR.0b013e3282f3da10

Ponting, C. P., Oliver, P. L., and Reik, W. (2009). Evolution and functions of long noncoding RNAs. *Cell* 136, 629–641. doi: 10.1016/j.cell.2009.02.006

Pruunsild, P., Kazantseva, A., Aid, T., Palm, K., and Timmusk, T. (2007). Dissecting the human BDNF locus: bidirectional transcription, complex splicing, and multiple promoters. *Genomics* 90, 397–406. doi: 10.1016/j.ygeno.2007.05.004

Puspita, L., Chung, S. Y., and Shim, J. W. (2017). Oxidative stress and cellular pathologies in Parkinson's disease. *Mol. Brain* 10:53. doi: 10.1186/s13041-017-0340-9

Quan, Z., Zheng, D., and Qing, H. (2017). Regulatory roles of long non-coding RNAs in the central nervous system and associated neurodegenerative diseases. *Front. Cell. Neurosci.* 11:175. doi: 10.3389/fncel.2017.00175

Qureshi, I. A., Mattick, J. S., and Mehler, M. F. (2010). Long non-coding RNAs in nervous system function and disease. *Brain Res.* 1338c, 20–35. doi: 10.1016/j.brainres.2010.03.110

Qureshi, I. A., and Mehler, M. F. (2013). Long non-coding RNAs: novel targets for nervous system disease diagnosis and therapy. *Neurotherapeutics* 10, 632–646. doi: 10.1007/s13311-013-0199-0

Rackham, O., Shearwood, A. M., Mercer, T. R., Davies, S. M., Mattick, J. S., and Filipovska, A. (2011). Long noncoding RNAs are generated from the mitochondrial genome and regulated by nuclear-encoded proteins. *RNA* 17, 2085–2093. doi: 10.1261/rna.029405.111

Ramos, A. D., Attenello, F. J., and Lim, D. A. (2016). Uncovering the roles of long noncoding RNAs in neural development and glioma progression. *Neurosci. Lett.* 625, 70–79. doi: 10.1016/j.neulet.2015.12.025

Rinn, J. L., Kertesz, M., Wang, J. K., Squazzo, S. L., Xu, X., Brugmann, S. A., et al. (2007). Functional demarcation of active and silent chromatin domains in human HOX loci by noncoding RNAs. *Cell* 129, 1311–1323. doi: 10.1016/j.cell.2007.05.022

Riva, P., Ratti, A., and Venturin, M. (2016). The Long Non-coding RNAs in neurodegenerative diseases: novel mechanisms of pathogenesis. *Curr. Alzheimer Res.* 13, 1219–1231. doi: 10.2174/15672050136661606221 12234

Roberts, T. C., Morris, K. V., and Wood, M. J. (2014). The role of long non-coding RNAs in neurodevelopment, brain function and neurological disease. *Philos. Trans. R. Soc. Lond. B Biol. Sci.* 369:20130507. doi: 10.1098/rstb.2013.0507

Sai, Y., Zou, Z., Peng, K., and Dong, Z. (2012). The Parkinson's disease-related genes act in mitochondrial homeostasis. *Neurosci. Biobehav. Rev.* 36, 2034–2043. doi: 10.1016/j.neubiorev.2012.06.007

Sasaki, Y. T., Ideue, T., Sano, M., Mituyama, T., and Hirose, T. (2009). MENepsilon/beta noncoding RNAs are essential for structural integrity of nuclear paraspeckles. *Proc. Natl. Acad. Sci. U.S.A.* 106, 2525–2530. doi: 10.1073/pnas.0807899106

Sauvageau, M., Goff, L. A., Lodato, S., Bonev, B., Groff, A. F., Gerhardinger, C., et al. (2013). Multiple knockout mouse models reveal lincRNAs are required for life and brain development. *Elife* 2: e01749. doi: 10.7554/eLife.01749

Scheele, C., Petrovic, N., Faghihi, M. A., Lassmann, T., Fredriksson, K., Rooyackers, O., et al. (2007). The human PINK1 locus is regulated *in vivo* by a non-coding natural antisense RNA during modulation of mitochondrial function. *BMC Genomics* 8:74. doi: 10.1186/1471-2164-8-74

Shamir, A., Kwon, O. B., Karavanova, I., Vullhorst, D., Leiva-Salcedo, E., Janssen, M. J., et al. (2012). The importance of the NRG-1/ErbB4 pathway for synaptic plasticity and behaviors associated with psychiatric disorders. *J. Neurosci.* 32, 2988–2997. doi: 10.1523/JNEUROSCI.1899-11.2012

Shimojo, M. (2008). Huntingtin regulates RE1-silencing transcription factor/neuron-restrictive silencer factor (REST/NRSF) nuclear trafficking indirectly through a complex with REST/NRSF-interacting LIM domain protein (RILP) and dynactin p150 Glued. *J. Biol. Chem.* 283, 34880–34886. doi: 10.1074/jbc.M804183200

Shimozaki, K. (2014). Sox2 transcription network acts as a molecular switch to regulate properties of neural stem cells. *World J. Stem Cells* 6, 485–490. doi: 10.4252/wjsc.v6.i4.485

Singh, D. K., and Prasanth, K. V. (2013). Functional insights into the role of nuclear-retained long noncoding RNAs in gene expression control in mammalian cells. *Chromosome Res.* 21, 695–711. doi: 10.1007/s10577-013-9391-7

Song, J. H., Yu, J. T., and Tan, L. (2015). Brain-derived neurotrophic factor in Alzheimer's disease: risk, mechanisms, and therapy. *Mol. Neurobiol.* 52, 1477–1493. doi: 10.1007/s12035-014-8958-4

Sun, M., and Kraus, W. L. (2015). From discovery to function: the expanding roles of long noncoding RNAs in physiology and disease. *Endocr. Rev.* 36, 25–64. doi: 10.1210/er.2014-1034

Sunwoo, H., Dinger, M. E., Wilusz, J. E., Amaral, P. P., Mattick, J. S., and Spector, D. L. (2009). MEN epsilon/beta nuclear-retained non-coding RNAs are up-regulated upon muscle differentiation and are essential components of paraspeckles. *Genome Res.* 19, 347–359. doi: 10.1101/gr.087775.108

Sunwoo, J. S., Lee, S. T., Im, W., Lee, M., Byun, J. I., Jung, K. H., et al. (2017). Altered expression of the long noncoding RNA NEAT1 in Huntington's disease. *Mol. Neurobiol.* 54, 1577–1586. doi: 10.1007/s12035-016-9928-9

Sutherland, H. F., Wadey, R., McKie, J. M., Taylor, C., Atif, U., Johnstone, K. A., et al. (1996). Identification of a novel transcript disrupted by a balanced translocation associated with DiGeorge syndrome. *Am. J. Hum. Genet.* 59, 23–31.

Tan, L., Yu, J. T., Hu, N., and Tan, L. (2013). Non-coding RNAs in Alzheimer's disease. *Mol. Neurobiol.* 47, 382–393. doi: 10.1007/s12035-012-8359-5

Tripathi, V., Ellis, J. D., Shen, Z., Song, D. Y., Pan, Q., Watt, A. T., et al. (2010). The nuclear-retained noncoding RNA MALAT1 regulates alternative splicing by modulating SR splicing factor phosphorylation. *Mol. Cell* 39, 925–938. doi: 10.1016/j.molcel.2010.08.011

Vucićević, D., Schrewe, H., and Orom, U. A. (2014). Molecular mechanisms of long ncRNAs in neurological disorders. *Front. Genet.* 5:48. doi: 10.3389/fgene.2014.00048

Wang, A., Wang, J., Liu, Y., and Zhou, Y. (2017). Mechanisms of long non-coding RNAs in the assembly and plasticity of neural circuitry. *Front. Neural Circuits* 11:76. doi: 10.3389/fncir.2017.00076

Wang, H., Iacoangeli, A., Lin, D., Williams, K., Denman, R. B., Hellen, C. U., et al. (2005). Dendritic BC1 RNA in translational control mechanisms. *J. Cell Biol.* 171, 811–821. doi: 10.1083/jcb.200506006

Wang, H., Iacoangeli, A., Popp, S., Muslimov, I. A., Imataka, H., Sonenberg, N., et al. (2002). Dendritic BC1 RNA: functional role in regulation of translation initiation. *J. Neurosci.* 22, 10232–10241. doi: 10.1523/JNEUROSCI.22-23-10232.2002

Yan, W., Chen, Z. Y., Chen, J. Q., and Chen, H. M. (2018). LncRNA NEAT1 promotes autophagy in MPTP-induced Parkinson's disease through stabilizing PINK1 protein. *Biochem. Biophys. Res. Commun.* 496, 1019–1024. doi: 10.1016/j.bbrc.2017.12.149

Yang, B., Xia, Z. A., Zhong, B., Xiong, X., Sheng, C., Wang, Y., et al. (2017). Distinct hippocampal expression profiles of long non-coding RNAs in an Alzheimer's disease model. *Mol. Neurobiol.* 54, 4833–4846. doi: 10.1007/s12035-016-0038-5

Zagrebelsky, M., and Korte, M. (2014). Form follows function: BDNF and its involvement in sculpting the function and structure of synapses. *Neuropharmacology* 76(Pt C), 628–638. doi: 10.1016/j.neuropharm.2013.05.029

Zhang, B., Arun, G., Mao, Y. S., Lazar, Z., Hung, G., Bhattacharjee, G., et al. (2012). The lncRNA Malat1 is dispensable for mouse development but its transcription plays a cis-regulatory role in the adult. *Cell Rep.* 2, 111–123. doi: 10.1016/j.celrep.2012.06.003

Zhang, X., Lian, Z., Padden, C., Gerstein, M. B., Rozowsky, J., Snyder, M., et al. (2009). A myelopoiesis-associated regulatory intergenic noncoding RNA transcript within the human HOXA cluster. *Blood* 113, 2526–2534. doi: 10.1182/blood-2008-06-162164

Zhao, X., Tang, Z., Zhang, H., Atianjoh, F. E., Zhao, J. Y., Liang, L., et al. (2013). A long noncoding RNA contributes to neuropathic pain by silencing Kcna2 in primary afferent neurons. *Nat. Neurosci.* 16, 1024–1031. doi: 10.1038/nn.3438

Zhong, J., Chuang, S. C., Bianchi, R., Zhao, W., Lee, H., Fenton, A. A., et al. (2009). BC1 regulation of metabotropic glutamate receptor-mediated neuronal excitability. *J. Neurosci.* 29, 9977–9986. doi: 10.1523/JNEUROSCI.3893-08.2009

5

Non-Invasive High Frequency Median Nerve Stimulation Effectively Suppresses Olfactory Intensity Perception in Healthy Males

Ashim Maharjan[1]*, Mei Peng*[2] *and Yusuf O. Cakmak*[1,3,4]*

[1]*Department of Anatomy, School of Biomedical Sciences, University of Otago, Dunedin, New Zealand,* [2]*Department of Food Science, University of Otago, Dunedin, New Zealand,* [3]*Brain Health Research Centre, Division of Sciences, University of Otago, Dunedin, New Zealand,* [4]*Medical Technologies Centre of Research Excellence, Auckland, New Zealand*

***Correspondence:**
Yusuf O. Cakmak
yusuf.cakmak@otago.ac.nz

Median nerve stimulation (MNS) had been performed in the existing literature to alleviate symptoms of nausea and vomiting. The observed facilitative effects are thought to be mediated by the vagal pathways, particularly the vagus nerve (VN) brainstem nuclei of the dorsal motor nucleus of vagus and nucleus tractus solitarius (DMV-NTS). Sense of smell is one of the major sensory modalities for inducing vomiting and nausea as a primary defense against potentially harmful intake of material. This study aimed to test effects of non-invasive, high and low frequency MNS on human olfactory functioning, with supplementary exploration of the orbitofrontal cortex (OFC) using near-infrared spectroscopy (NIRS). Twenty healthy, male, adults performed supra-threshold odor intensity tests (labeled magnitude scale, LMS) for four food-related odorant samples (presented in three different concentrations) before and after receiving high-, low frequency MNS and placebo (no stimulation), while cortical activities in the OFC was monitored by the NIRS. Data of the NIRS and LMS test of separate stimulation parameters were statistically analyzed using mixed-model analysis of variance (ANOVA). Only the high frequency MNS showed effects for suppressing the intensity perception of the moderate concentration of Amyl Acetate (p:0.042) and strong concentration of Isovaleric Acid (p:0.004) and 1-Octen-3-ol (p:0.006). These behavioral changes were coupled with significant changes in the NIRS recordings of the left (p:0.000) and right (p:0.003) hemispheric orbitofrontal cortices. This is the first study that applied non-invasive, high frequency MNS to suppress the supra-threshold odor ratings of specific concentrations of odors. The vagal networks are potential relays of MNS to influence OFC. Results from the current article implore further research into non-invasive, high frequency MNS in the investigation of its modulatory effects on olfactory function, given its potential to be used for ameliorating nausea and malnutrition associated with various health conditions.

Keywords: median nerve stimulation, near-infrared spectroscopy, orbitofrontal cortex, olfaction, labeled magnitude scale, non-invasive electrostimulation, nausea and vomiting

INTRODUCTION

Sense of smell, in combination with vision and taste, are essential contributors to inducing nausea or vomiting as the primary defense against dangerous or contaminated food (Andrews, 1992). The link between odor and nausea even dates back to the Roman empire where invaders were thought to give off a nauseating odor, caused by the use of rancid butter as hair ointment (Classen et al., 1994). Nausea and vomiting are one of the most frequently reported symptoms in clinical settings due to the wide range of conditions including medications, motion sickness, infections, hormonal disorders, pregnancy, central nervous system disorders, psychiatric disorders, anesthesia, and cardiovascular dysfunctions (Andrews, 1992; Babic and Browning, 2014; Lee and Fan, 2015). Furthermore, nausea and vomiting often coincide with a loss of appetite. For those who suffer from this cluster of symptoms for a long term, such as patients who undergo chemotherapy treatment, their quality of life can be substantially affected (Guerdoux-Ninot et al., 2016). Despite its high prevalence and numerous causes, the treatment options for nausea with medication are not highly effective and can also have side effects (Lee and Fan, 2015). Median nerve stimulation (MNS) is one of the alternative approaches that are being explored in the current literature to reduce nausea and vomiting.

MNS was initially performed using manual acupuncture on the median nerve (MN) [a traditional Chinese method using Neiguan acupuncture point (pericardium meridian of acupuncture point 6; PC-6)]. Over the past couple of decades, MNS has advanced from manual acupuncture techniques (Napadow et al., 2009; Bai et al., 2010; Lee and Fan, 2015) to electroacupuncture (EA) which is a modification of the acupuncture technique using electrical current (Spiegel et al., 1999; Chen et al., 2003; Tatewaki et al., 2005; Lee and Fan, 2015). A popular form of MNS in the current literature is the use of transcutaneous electrical nerve stimulation (TENS; Zatorre et al., 1992; Urasaki et al., 1998; Ferretti et al., 2007; Lee and Fan, 2015). In the current literature, MNS is used to treat gastrointestinal diseases (Diehl, 1999; Wang et al., 2000; Chang et al., 2001; Takahashi, 2006; Xu et al., 2006) and alleviating symptoms of nausea and vomiting in clinical settings that includes post-surgery/chemotherapy, pregnancy or motion sickness (Xu et al., 2006; Dhond et al., 2008; Ren et al., 2010; Zotelli et al., 2014).

In the existing literature, MNS has been used to alleviate symptoms of nausea and vomiting, effects that are thought to occur through the vagal pathways (Chen et al., 2003; Tada et al., 2003; Tatewaki et al., 2005; Xu et al., 2006; Bai et al., 2010; Ren et al., 2010; Takahashi, 2011; Zotelli et al., 2014; Lee and Fan, 2015). The use of low frequency (10–25 Hz) MNS has also demonstrated a positive control of gastric mobility *via* increased gastric emptying and the ability to regulate gastric dysthymia (Chen et al., 2003; Tatewaki et al., 2005; Xu et al., 2006). As the vagus nerve (VN) is recognized as the sole contributor to the control of gastric acid secretion and mobility, this tantalizes VN and MNS interactions. In both animal models and human studies, MNS has displayed the ability to modulate the VN (Ouyang et al., 2002; Chen et al., 2003; Xu et al., 2006; Takahashi, 2011). In a previous article by Ouyang et al. (2002), low frequency MNS accelerated gastric emptying of liquids and improved gastric slow-wave rhythmicity. Modulation of gastric function using MNS was also absent after vagotomy in animal models (Noguchi and Hayashi, 1996; Xu et al., 2006). This supports the notion that the potential pathway of MNS on gastric functions are through the dorsal motor nucleus of vagus-Nucleus Tractus Solitarius (DMV-NTS), both of which are VN brainstem nuclei (Ruggiero et al., 1998; Cakmak, 2006; Imai et al., 2008).

In a previous article by our group (Maharjan et al., 2018), non-invasive and high frequency auricular VN electrostimulation improved olfactory performance in the supra-threshold test. However, to date, the MNS' potential effects on olfactory function *via* its interactions with vagal nerve networks has not been explored yet. Therefore, this study aimed to observe the effects of non-invasive MNS on olfactory sensory function using a labeled magnitude scale (LMS) test in healthy, male, adults under high and low frequencies of electrostimulation with supplementary exploration of the orbitofrontal cortex (OFC) using near-infrared spectroscopy (NIRS).

METHODS

Participants

Twenty Caucasian-male, healthy, non-smokers (age range = 22–32 years, mean: 25.05 years, standard deviation: 2.36 years) participated in the current study. Prior to the study, each participant was asked not to consume any food or non-water beverages for 2 h prior to the experiments. They were also instructed to refrain from applying any fragrance product/s on the day of the experiment. All participants gave an informed, written consent to participate in the experiment, in accordance with the Declaration of Helsinki and met the exclusion criteria set for the experiment (non-smoker, in a healthy condition and were of NZ-European descent). The experiment was approved by the Otago Human Participants Ethics Committee (Reference: H16/148) and registered to the Australian New Zealand clinical trials registry (ANZCTR; registration ID: ACTRN12617000034336, Clinical trial name: MODOLF).

Labeled Magnitude Scale (LMS) Test

The LMS test is a widely-used psychophysical scaling method for quantifying intensity perception of sensory stimuli (Green et al., 1993, 1996). The LMS is composed of seven verbal labels arranged according to the geometric means of their rated magnitude which ranges from 0 to 100 ("no sensation"-0, "barely detectable"-1.4, "weak"-6.1, "moderate"-17.2, "strong"-35.4, "very strong"-53.3, "strongest imaginable"-100). Following previous protocols (Green et al., 1993, 1996; Kalva et al., 2014), the current study tested responses to four different odors—two "pleasant" odors [Citral (CAS number: 5392-40-5; purity: 99%, Sigma-Aldrich, St. Louis, MO, USA)—commonly described as citrus and Amyl Acetate (CAS number: 628-63-7;

purity: 99%, Sigma-Aldrich, St. Louis, MO, USA)—commonly described as banana] and two "unpleasant" odors [Isovaleric Acid (CAS number: 503-74-2; purity: 99%, Sigma-Aldrich, St. Louis, MO, USA)—commonly described as cheese and 1-Octen-3-ol (CAS number: 3391-86-4; purity: 99%, Sigma-Aldrich, St. Louis, MO, USA)—commonly described as mushroom]—with three different concentrations for each odor. Specifically, these odors included Citral (2 ppm, 20 ppm, 200 ppm), 1-Octen-3-ol (3 ppm, 18 ppm, 108 ppm), Amyl Acetate (1.5 ppm, 15 ppm, 150 ppm) and Isovaleric acid (4 ppm, 28 ppm, 196 ppm). All odors were diluted in distilled water. The selection of these concentrations underwent four stages of bench-top testing (n = 6–10) which were performed to differentiate three concentrations (weak, moderate and strong) for each odorant. Participants used the LMS scale to rate each concentration of each odor in the bench-top testing stages. After four stages of bench-top testing, the use of specific concentrations for each odor matched the ratings (weak, moderate and strong) in the LMS to a satisfactory level. All results of bench-top testing are provided in **Supplementary Table S1**.

An additional screening criterion used in the initial studies of the LMS test (Green et al., 1996) was also included to ensure that each participant could differentiate weak, moderate and strong concentrations of each odor (Citral, Amyl Acetate, Isovaleric Acid, 1-Octen-3-ol). In this instance, we used Ethyl-butyrate (CAS number: 105-54-4; purity: 99%, Sigma-Aldrich, St. Louis, MO, USA) using 1.25 ppm as weak concentration, 13.69 ppm as moderate concentration and 150 ppm as strong concentration. These concentrations of Ethyl-butyrate also underwent four stages of bench-top testing (**Supplementary Table S1**). This odor was chosen as it was distinct from the odors used in the testing phase of the current study. Before the start of the pre-stimulation and post-stimulation LMS, each participant was given a separate set of glass lidded bottles with an example of a weak and strong concentration of an independent odor distinct to the testing odors (Ethyl-butyrate: weak-1.25 ppm and strong-150 ppm). Each concentration of all four odors was presented in a 240-ml glass lidded bottles. To sample an odorant, the subject was asked to place the glass bottle approximately 2 cm away from the nose and inhale within a 2–3 s window. Separate sets of randomized numeral labeled bottles were used for pre-stimulation and post-stimulation LMS. Each concentration was presented once (in both pre-stimulation LMS and post-stimulation LMS), in a randomized order that was counterbalanced for each stage (pre- and post-stimulation LMS) across all participants. 30 s inter-stimulus interval was present between the presentation of each odor. The participants' response on the LMS was measured using the software "Compusense" (Compusense Cloud, Version 8.8.6766.17069, Compusense Inc., Guelph, ON, Canada).

Application of Median Nerve Stimulation (MNS)

Non-invasive MNS was applied to the participant using "TENS ECO-2" (SCHWA-MEDICO, 35630 Ehringshausen, Germany) by the experimenter, using TENS for all three different parameters—high frequency MNS (80 Hz), low frequency MNS (10 Hz) and placebo (no stimulation but the electrodes were still attached). TENS in the current experiment was performed with the use of two pairs of disposable rubber electrode-pads, placed on the MN region of the left forearm, with the cathode being 3 cm proximal to the anode (**Figure 1b**), similar to previous studies using MNS with TENS (Urasaki et al., 1998; Ferretti et al., 2007). The TENS intensity was adjusted to obtain a tingling sensation over the MN territory of the palm and visible flexion response of index and/or middle finger (and/or thumb). This indicated the stimulation of the sensory and motor fibers of the MN in each stimulation session. In addition, the stimulation intensity was also kept to a comfortable range for the participant to ensure there was no perception of pain. The strength of the MNS (amplitude) was between 8 mA and 15 mA and the pulse bandwidth was 180 μS width bipolar square waveform.

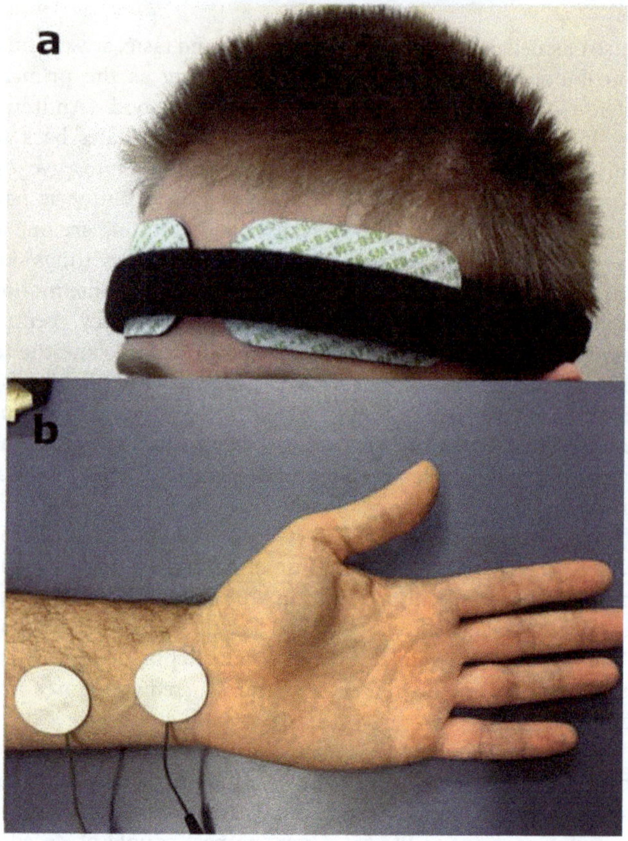

FIGURE 1 | (a) Near-infrared spectroscopy (NIRS) electrodes set up on the forehead of the participant. **(b)** The location of the non-invasive median nerve stimulation (MNS) using the pair of disposable rubber electrode-pads on the MN region of the left forearm. Written informed consent was obtained from the participant for the publication of this image (**Supplementary Figure S1**).

Procedure

Each participant was given a brief introduction to all the stages of the experiment and were instructed to attend three, 30–45-min sessions with at least 24-h apart. The experimental room was an isolated environment with air conditioning, allowing for a consistent temperature (23 ± 1°C) in the absence of any olfactory or visual stimuli representing food or distractions. The participants were instructed not to sniff during the olfactory tests to eliminate the potential effects of sniffing itself during the olfactory tests and NIRS recordings. The participant was seated directly opposite to the experimenter. A consent form and exclusion criteria sheet were signed to qualify the participants for the study. A brief explanation of the full experimental process and the olfactory test (LMS) were given to the participant. Pre-stimulation, LMS was performed for 10–15 min, followed directly by the allocated stimulation parameter for 10 min (high frequency MNS, low frequency MNS or placebo) that was delegated randomly for each participant. Lastly, post-stimulation, LMS (10–15 min) was performed directly after the allocated stimulation parameter (**Figure 2**). This study followed a double-blind design.

Figure 2 details the experimental design of the current study. A within-participant design was enforced. In each session, participants were randomly assigned to one of the three experimental conditions: high frequency MNS, low frequency MNS or placebo. The order of experimental conditions was counterbalanced across the participants. In addition to the exclusion criteria put in place to ensure that all participants were in healthy condition for the experiment, University of Pennsylvania Smell Identification Test (UPSIT) odor identification test (OIT; Sensonics International, Haddon Heights, NJ, USA) and odor discrimination/memory test (ODMT; Sensonics International, Haddon Heights, NJ, USA) were performed by each participant, after the placebo session. The results from these olfactory tests were compared to that of previous studies (Doty et al., 1984, 1995; Choudhury et al., 2003) to ensure that all participants met the standard for normative, healthy response in healthy, adult, male subjects.

Near-Infrared Spectroscopy (NIRS)

NIRS (COVIDIEN INVOS OXIMETER, Model 5100C-PA, Mansfield, MA, USA) was performed in the current study to measure participants' activity from the OFC. This INVOS (*in vivo* Optical Spectroscopy)-NIRS model is a clinically validated and FDA approved device, used in over 600 peer-reviewed articles and three randomized controlled trials

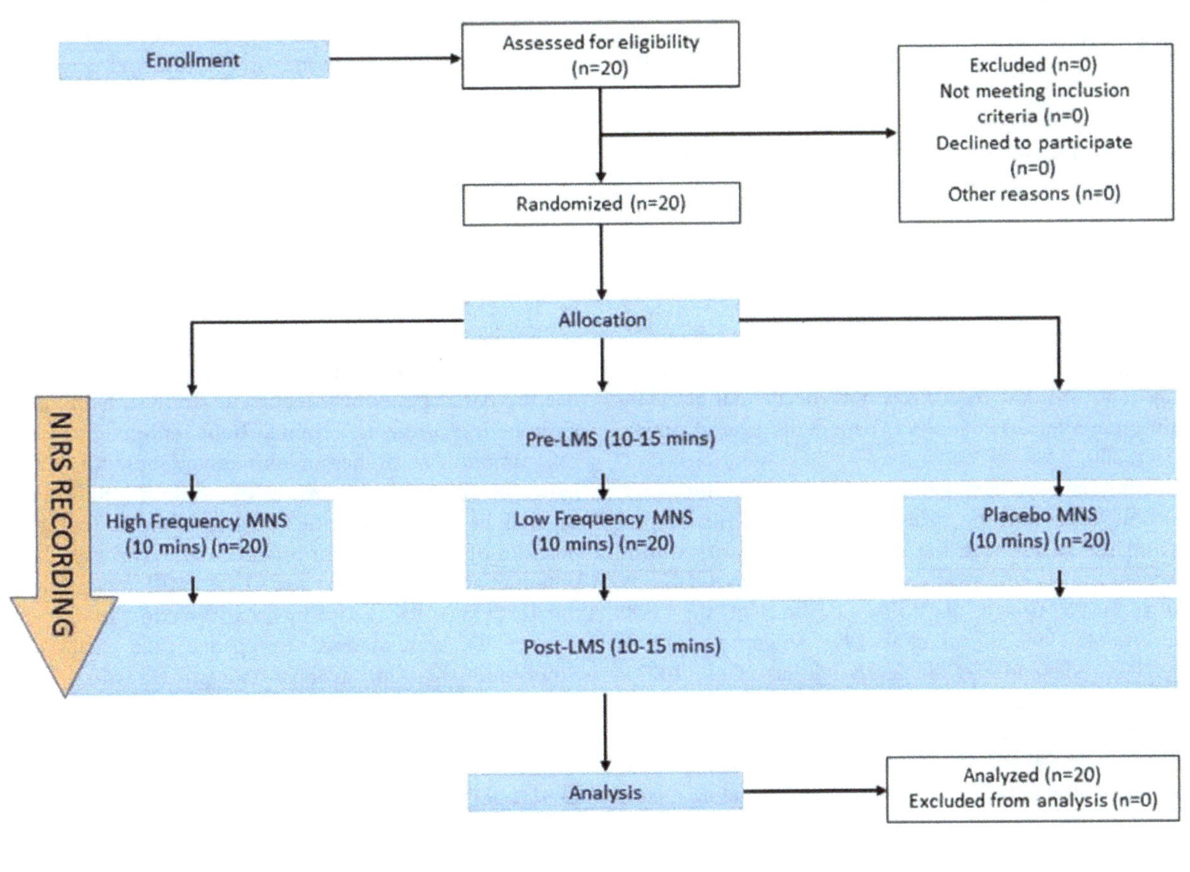

FIGURE 2 | Schematic sequence of each stage of the current study. The sequence of the experimental stages includes pre-stimulation labeled magnitude scale (Pre-LMS), allocated stimulation parameter (high frequency MNS, low frequency MNS, placebo) and post-stimulation (Post-LMS). A brief 5-min introduction, prior to the experiment comprised of obtaining participant's consent and device set up. MNS, LMS, NIRS recordings from both hemispheres of the orbitofrontal cortex (OFC) were recorded simultaneously across all stages of the experiment (Pre-LMS, allocated stimulation parameter, Post-LMS) for all participants.

(Harrer et al., 2010; Edmonds et al., 2016, 2017). The setup of this device is shown in **Figure 1a**. In the existing literature, several studies have demonstrated the efficiency of the NIRS in monitoring the activation of the OFC under olfactory stimulus (Hongo et al., 1995; Cho et al., 1998; Edmonds et al., 1998; Ishimaru et al., 2004; Harada et al., 2006; Kobayashi et al., 2012). With the aid of fMRI localization, olfactory expression was understood to be present in the lateral and anterior orbito-frontal gyri of the frontal lobe. With this knowledge, several studies have recorded from the orbito-frontal region using NIRS techniques and found that oxygenated hemoglobin (HbO_2) concentration increased only over the orbito-frontal region during olfactory stimulation (Ishimaru et al., 2004; Harada et al., 2006; Kobayashi et al., 2012).

INVOS-NIRS facilitates non-invasive method of monitoring regional tissue oxygenation (oxy- and deoxyhemoglobin) by using the modified Beer-Lambert law for light attenuation changes through the illuminated tissue (relating to optical density to chromophore concentration). INVOS-NIRS measures the red pigment of hemoglobin molecules within the red blood cells which is understood to have the highest light absorption of the wavelengths (730 and 810 nm; Edmonds et al., 2004; Covidien, 2013). The INVOS-NIRS system sensors used two near-infrared light sources at two different wavelengths (730 and 810 nm) and two photodiode detectors at a distance to observe the oxygen-hemoglobin saturation of the tissues beneath the sensors. The sensor's light emitting diode sends light to either a proximal or distal detector in a parabolic path, which allows the processing of separate data of shallow and deep optical signals. With the use of an algorithm of subtraction of the short vs. long travel distance of the light, INVOS-NIRS enables high spatial resolution (effective localization of the area of measurement) and enables the elimination of skin and scalp data (Hongo et al., 1995; Edmonds et al., 2004; Covidien, 2013). With the wavelengths of 730–810 nm, it is worth mentioning that melanin and water also behave as chromophores, but fortunately, INVOS-NIRS has shown in the existing literature that recordings have been unaffected by normal skin pigmentation in adults (Misra et al., 1998; Damian and Schlosser, 2007).

By measuring regional hemoglobin oxygen saturation (rSO_2), the INVOS-NIRS system provides absolute, real time data accuracy from the cortex with the use of multi-sensors within the same sensor and is empirically validated in human subjects (Hongo et al., 1995; Cho et al., 1998; Edmonds et al., 1998, 2004; Roberts et al., 1998; Higami et al., 1999; Singer et al., 1999; Yao et al., 2001; Alexander et al., 2002; Iglesias et al., 2003). rSO_2 reflects the balance between cerebral oxygen supply and demand, measuring the continuous local brain oxygen balance in a non-invasive approach (Cho et al., 1998; Edmonds et al., 1998, 2004; Blas et al., 1999; Janelle et al., 2002; Prabhune et al., 2002; Casati et al., 2005; Harada et al., 2006).

Unlike other systems that only assesses venous or arterial blood, the current study used the clinically validated and FDA approved INVOS-NIRS, which measures a 3:1 ratio of venous and arterial blood. This algorithm was calibrated using blood samples with the assumption that 25% of the blood within the sample volume being arterial while 75% of the blood within the sample volume was venous (Edmonds et al., 2004) This represented a venous-blood saturation (venous-weighted percent of rSO_2-$VWrSO_2$%) which can be used to provide real-time data about the balance (or imbalance) of oxygen supply/demand. Thus, this reflects venous oxygen reserve (VOR; oxygen remaining from extraction of associated tissues and vital organs) providing accurate measurement of site-specific tissue oxygenation (Blas et al., 1999; Janelle et al., 2002; Prabhune et al., 2002; Casati et al., 2005). In the current literature, reduction in VOR is considered a warning sign of developing pathology or deteriorating patient condition with reports of 20%–25% from baseline or rSO_2 of 40–50 considered to be cause of concern in association with neurologic dysfunction and other adverse outcomes (Hongo et al., 1995; Cho et al., 1998; Edmonds et al., 1998, 2004; Roberts et al., 1998; Higami et al., 1999; Singer et al., 1999; Yao et al., 2001; Alexander et al., 2002; Iglesias et al., 2003; Murkin et al., 2007; Ballard et al., 2012; Vretzakis et al., 2013).

The current study also used disposable electrodes for each participant to ensure highest hygiene and data quality, in addition to using a rigid head band to stabilize the electrodes and the cables that are attached to the electrodes (**Figure 1a**). We measured from the forehead region (**Figure 1a**) to avoid issues regarding hair or hair follicles that can produce excessive photon scattering in INVOS-NIRS resulting in artificial low rSO_2 (Oriheula-Espina et al., 2010). Furthermore, this forehead region is the routine zone of cerebral oximetry monitoring by INVOS-NIRS and has FDA validated approval for the use of this device for cerebral monitoring (Prabhune et al., 2002; Casati et al., 2005; Edmonds et al., 2017). INVOS-NIRS system also provides a reliable signal strength index (SSI) for stable recordings with each channel showing a 5-unit bar scale system. Any signal over 1 bar indicates a stable recording to generate an accurate $VWrSO_2$ (%) recording [Chapter 6.4.16 and 11.7.4 in the INVOS-NIRS 5100c manual (Covidien, 2013)]. In the current study, we ensured that the SSI bar was at the highest signal (5/5 SSI) throughout all of the recordings. We only enrolled healthy participants in the current study to eliminate potential pathological artifacts (cranial bone anomalies, frontal sinus inflammation or dyshemoglobinemia; Gopinath et al., 1995; de Letter et al., 1998; Madsen et al., 2000; McRobb et al., 2011) as well as maintaining a consistent room temperature and position of participant throughout the experiment to avoid any potential anomalies with the INVOS-NIRS measurements. With the INVOS-NIRS recordings, each section of the experiment (**Figure 2**), was mapped to ensure that each stage of the experiment had an average (mean) recording of $VWrSO_2$ (representing VOR) for each participant from the left and the right hemispheres of the OFC.

Data Analysis

Data from the NIRS device was transferred to the INVOS software which accommodated data presentation. We used average (mean) recordings of $VWrSO_2$ (%) data of specific time periods marked for each segment of each session which was in line with the previous research (Cho et al., 1998; Murkin et al., 2007). To insure that the baseline

TABLE 1 | Pre-stimulation results of the repeated-measures analysis of variance (ANOVA) that assessed the potential difference (if any) of the labeled magnitude scale (LMS) test and the near-infrared spectroscopy (NIRS; VWrSO$_2$%) data in all stimulation parameters [high frequency median nerve stimulation (MNS), low frequency MNS and placebo].

Olfactory test and NIRS recordings (h = hemisphere)	Stimulation parameter (H-High, L-Low, P-Placebo)	Mean	SD	*F*-Value	*p*-value
Pre-S LMS Mod AA	H	16.2225	12.8618	0.910	0.411
	L	13.4375	9.7741		
	P	17.3500	12.3399		
Pre-S LMS Str VA	H	22.8375	16.9355	0.015	0.985
	L	22.2125	20.4004		
	P	22.7275	22.4596		
Pre-S LMS Str Octen	H	29.9650	23.4717	0.821	0.448
	L	27.8775	21.0517		
	P	32.3925	21.2645		
Left-h VWrSO$_2$ at Pre-S LMS	H	70.9675	9.3354	2.259	0.118
	L	70.8867	8.8145		
	P	72.7027	9.5207		
Right-h VWrSO$_2$ at Pre-S LMS	H	72.9550	7.5862	1.049	0.360
	L	71.2606	8.0289		
	P	72.7104	9.7302		

SD, standard deviation; LMS score ranges, 0–100; NIRS, 0–100%; H, high frequency MNS; L, low frequency MNS; P, placebo condition; left-h, left hemisphere; right-h, right hemisphere; mod AA, moderate concentration of Amyl Acetate; Str VA, Strong concentration of Isovaleric Acid; Str Octen, Strong concentration of 1-Octen-3-ol; Pre-S, Pre-Stimulation.

activity was consistent across all three different stimulation parameters for LMS and LMS-NIRS data, repeated-measures analysis of variance (ANOVA) was also applied to the data that was obtained at the pre-stimulation stage (**Table 1**). Mixed-model ANOVA was applied to data obtained from each stimulation parameters (i.e., high frequency MNS, low frequency MNS and placebo) for assessing VWrSO$_2$ (%) changes in separate hemispheric OFC (independent variable: left and right) across stages of the experiment (repeated-measures variable: pre-stimulation LMS, stimulation parameter and post-stimulation LMS). For the LMS data, mixed-model ANOVA (repeated-measures variable: pre-stimulation LMS, post-stimulation LMS; independent variables: stimulation, odor, concentration) were performed to assess differences between the scores before and after stimulation for all three parameters (high frequency MNS, low frequency MNS, and placebo). *Post hoc* test, based on simple effects tests with Bonferroni correction, was applied to understand any significance at *p*-value of 0.05. All the analyses were performed using SPSS (IBM SPSS Statistics, Ver. 20, St Leonards, NSW, Australia).

RESULTS

Pre-screening Olfactory Test Results—Odor Identification Test (OIT) and Odor Discrimination/Memory Tests (ODMT)

Half of the 20 participants displayed values of Mild Microsmia (30–33 out of 40 in OIT) while the other half of the participants displayed values of Normosmia (34–40 out of 40 in OIT). None of the participants in the current study displayed total anosmia which was the exclusion criteria for the current study and therefore, all participants presented olfactory performances in OIT to a standard held in line with the existing olfactory research (Doty et al., 1984, 1995). All participants scored between 8 and 12 out of 12 in the ODMT which corresponds to healthy ranges, in line with existing literature (Doty et al., 1984, 1995; Choudhury et al., 2003; Doty, 2003). In this context, all participants were qualified to take part in the current study.

Labeled Magnitude Scale (LMS) Test Results

Inspection of changes in LMS scores of all participants ($n = 20$) between the pre-stimulation and post-stimulation stages in all three stimulation parameters (high frequency MNS, low frequency MNS and placebo) suggested significant differences for only the high frequency MNS (**Figure 3**). Specifically, significant post-stimulation declines were evident for moderate concentration of Amyl Acetate (*post hoc* pair wise analysis with Bonferroni, pre-stimulation-post-stimulation, p:0.042, *Partial Eta Squared*: 0.006, low size effect), strong concentration of Isovaleric Acid (*post hoc* pairwise analysis with Bonferroni, pre-stimulation-post-stimulation, p:0.004, *Partial Eta Squared*: 0.012, low size effect) and strong concentration of 1-Octen-3-ol (*post hoc* pairwise analysis with Bonferroni, pre-stimulation-post-stimulation, p:0.006, *Partial Eta Squared*: 0.011, low size effect). Ratings for moderate concentration of Amyl Acetate, strong concentration of Isovaleric Acid and strong concentration of 1-Octen-3-ol were reduced in the post-stimulation LMS stage in comparison to the pre-stimulation LMS stage after high frequency MNS. Notably, there were no significant differences between the pre-stimulation and post-stimulation LMS stages in all concentrations of Citral, weak and strong concentrations of Amyl Acetate, and weak and moderate concentrations of Isovaleric Acid and 1-Octen-3-ol after high frequency MNS. Under low frequency MNS and placebo conditions, no significant changes were observed for

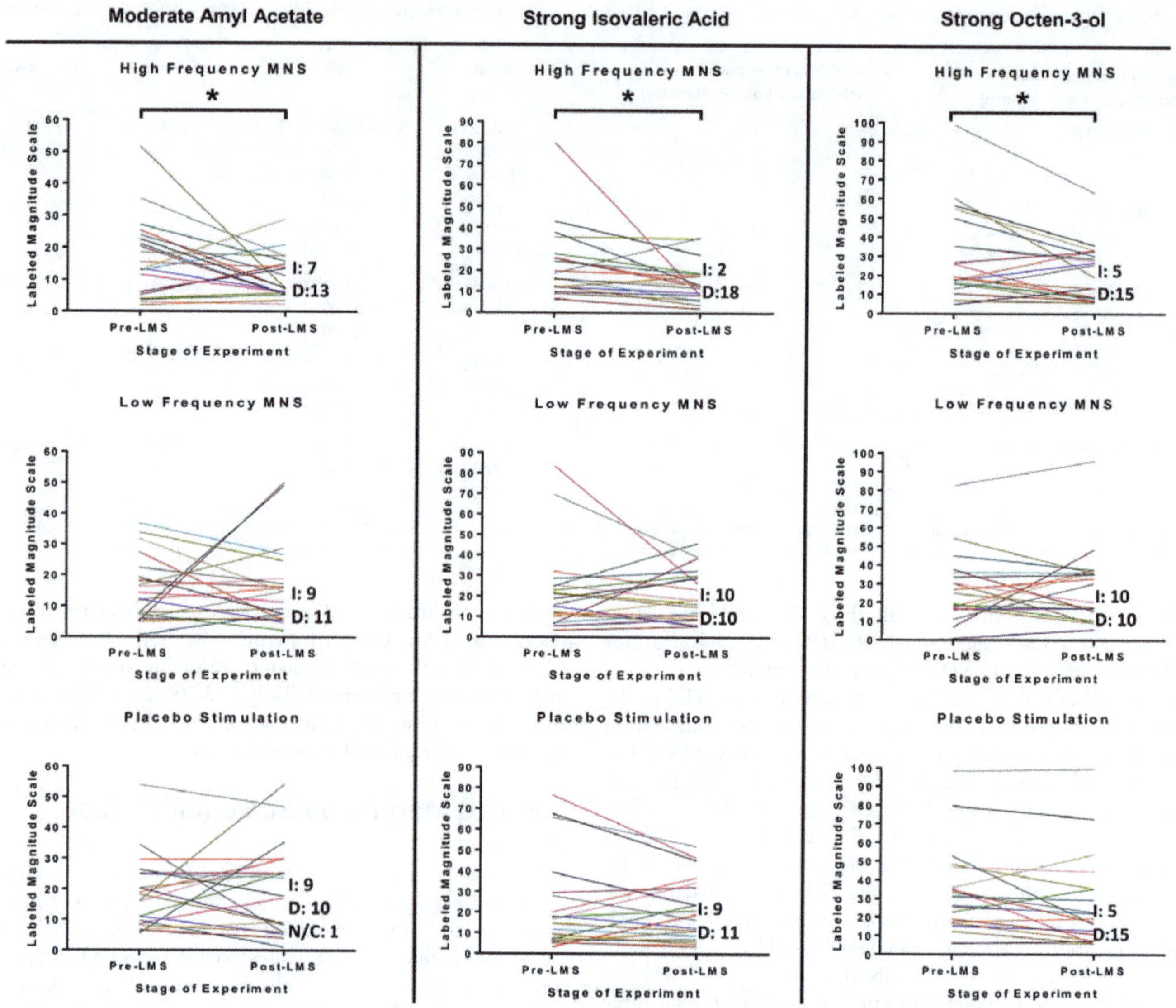

FIGURE 3 | LMS test results for moderate concentration of Amyl Acetate, strong concentration of Isovaleric Acid and strong concentration of 1-Octen-3-ol from each participant before and after each stimulation parameter (high frequency MNS, low frequency MNS and placebo). Each participant's scores, before (Pre-S LMS) and after (Post-S LMS) each of the stimulation parameters (high frequency MNS, low frequency MNS and placebo), for the LMS (LMS scores range = 0–100). Each colored line represents one case (total cases = 20). Letter "I" corresponds to cases that increased LMS test score in Post-S LMS in comparison to Pre-S LMS, letter "D" corresponds to cases that decreased LMS test score in Post-S LMS in comparison to Pre-S LMS and letters "N/C" corresponds to no change in LMS test score in Post-S LMS in comparison to Pre-S LMS. *Statistically significant ($p < 0.05$).

any odor in any of the different concentrations (**Supplementary Figures S2–S6**).

All Stage NIRS Data Analysis

Individual results from each participant's ($n = 20$) recording of $VWrSO_2$ (%) from the left and right hemispheres of the OFC is displayed in **Figure 4**. Significant differences across the three stages (pre-stimulation LMS, MNS/placebo, post-stimulation LMS) of $VWrSO_2$ (%) recordings were only present in the high frequency MNS parameter in both hemispheres of the OFC (left hemisphere: p:0.000, *Partial Eta Squared*: 0.463-large effect size; right hemisphere: p:0.003, *Partial Eta Squared*: 0.270-large effect size). *Post hoc* pairwise analysis with Bonferroni correction indicated that in the left and right hemispheres of the OFC, there were significant differences in $VWrSO_2$ (%) recordings between the pre-stimulation and stimulation stages (left hemisphere p:0.000; right hemisphere p:0.016) and pre-stimulation and post-stimulation stages (left hemisphere p:0.000; right hemisphere p:0.002). There were no significant differences between the left and the right hemispheric recordings of the OFC (p:0.592). The NIRS recordings of $VWrSO_2$ (%) increased in the stimulation and post-stimulation stages in comparison to the pre-stimulation stage in both hemispheres.

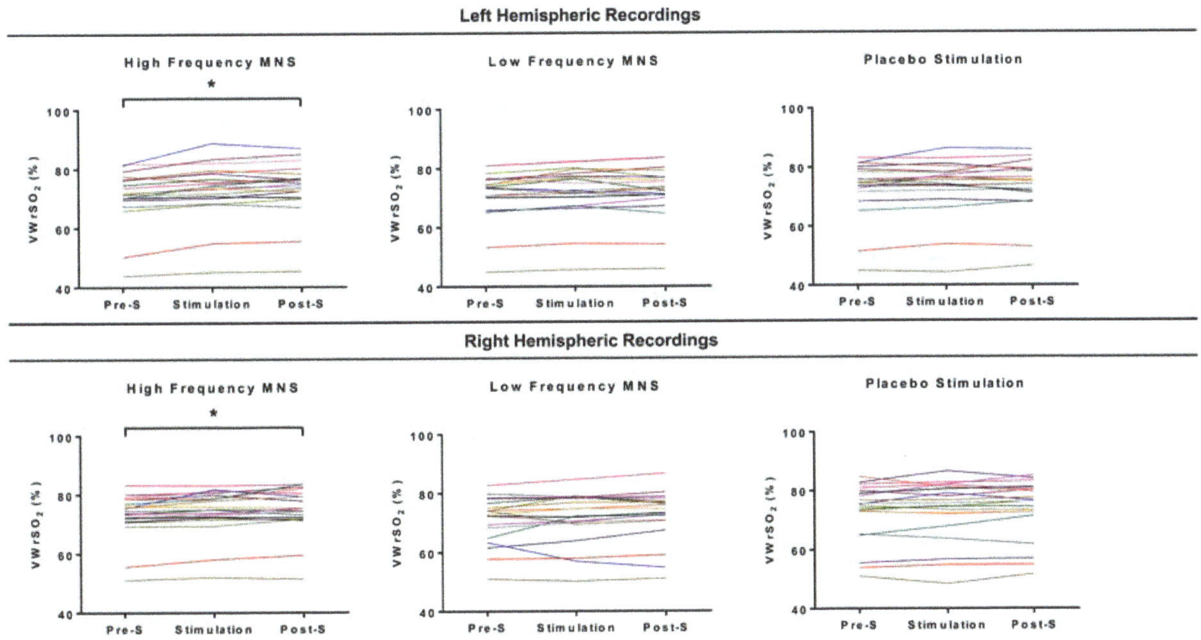

FIGURE 4 | Each of the participant's recordings for all three stages of the experiment (pre-stimulation LMS, stimulation parameter, post-stimulation LMS) for each stimulation parameter (high frequency MNS, low frequency MNS and placebo) from both the left and right hemispheres of the OFCs, measuring venous oxygen reserve (VWrSO$_2$%) using NIRS. Each colored line represents one case (total cases = 20). *Statistically significant ($p < 0.05$).

Pre-stimulation, Intergroup Differences of Labeled Magnitude Scale (LMS) and Respective Near-Infrared Spectroscopy (NIRS) Recordings From Orbitofrontal Cortices (OFC) Convergent and Divergent Co-transmission

Table 1 displays the results of the repeated-measures ANOVA that assessed the potential differences (if any were present) in the significant results from the LMS test (pre-stimulation vs. post-stimulation) and the NIRS recordings (VWrSO$_2$%) in all of the three different stimulation parameters (high frequency MNS, low frequency MNS, placebo) at the pre-stimulation stage of testing. As indicated in **Table 1**, there is no significant differences in the pre-stimulation stage for all significant results of the LMS test (moderate concentration of Amyl Acetate, strong concentration of Isovaleric Acid and strong concentration of 1-Octen-3-ol) and NIRS (VWrSO$_2$%) recordings under any of the stimulation parameters for both hemispheres of the OFC.

DISCUSSION

Studies of MNS in the existing literature have primarily focused on the cortical activation of primary (S-I) and secondary (S-II) somatosensory cortex (Spiegel et al., 1999; Nihashi et al., 2005; Napadow et al., 2009; Zhang et al., 2012; Zotelli et al., 2014), improvement of gastric function (Ouyang et al., 2002; Chen et al., 2003; Tatewaki et al., 2005; Xu et al., 2006; Takahashi, 2011) and alleviating symptoms associated with nausea and vomiting (Tatewaki et al., 2005; Xu et al., 2006; Bai et al., 2010; Takahashi, 2011; Zhang et al., 2012; Zotelli et al., 2014; Lee and Fan, 2015). As the VN is the key contributor towards gastric acid secretion and mobility, the modulation of gastric function by MNS addressed a potential interaction between MNS and VN. This interaction is supported in animal models and human studies (Ouyang et al., 2002; Chen et al., 2003; Xu et al., 2006; Takahashi, 2011). In the current literature, low frequency MNS has indicated several functions in regards to gastric mobility that includes accelerated gastric emptying of liquids and improved gastric slow-wave rhythmicity (Ouyang et al., 2002), effects absent after vagotomy (Noguchi and Hayashi, 1996; Xu et al., 2006). In a previous article by our group (Maharjan et al., 2018), non-invasive and high frequency auricular VN electrostimulation improved olfactory performance in the supra-threshold test. This indicated that high frequency, VN stimulation (VNS) can modulate olfactory function with its neural connections (**Figure 5**). In the context of modulation of olfactory function with high frequency VNS in our previous study and the existing literature on MNS' effects on changes in gastric mobility and secretion [which is also driven by the DMV and viscerosensory VN-NTS and subsequently to the insula-olfactory networks (**Figure 5**)] (Ruggiero et al., 1998; Cakmak, 2006; Imai et al., 2008; Mayer, 2011), we conceptualized that high frequency MNS may have a modulatory effect on olfactory function.

On the other hand, to date, MNS studies primarily used low frequencies (1.5–25 Hz). MNS with low frequencies (1.5–4.0 Hz) showed maximal activation of the S-I and S-II in animals models (Gyngell et al., 1996) and humans studies (Ibáñez et al., 1995)

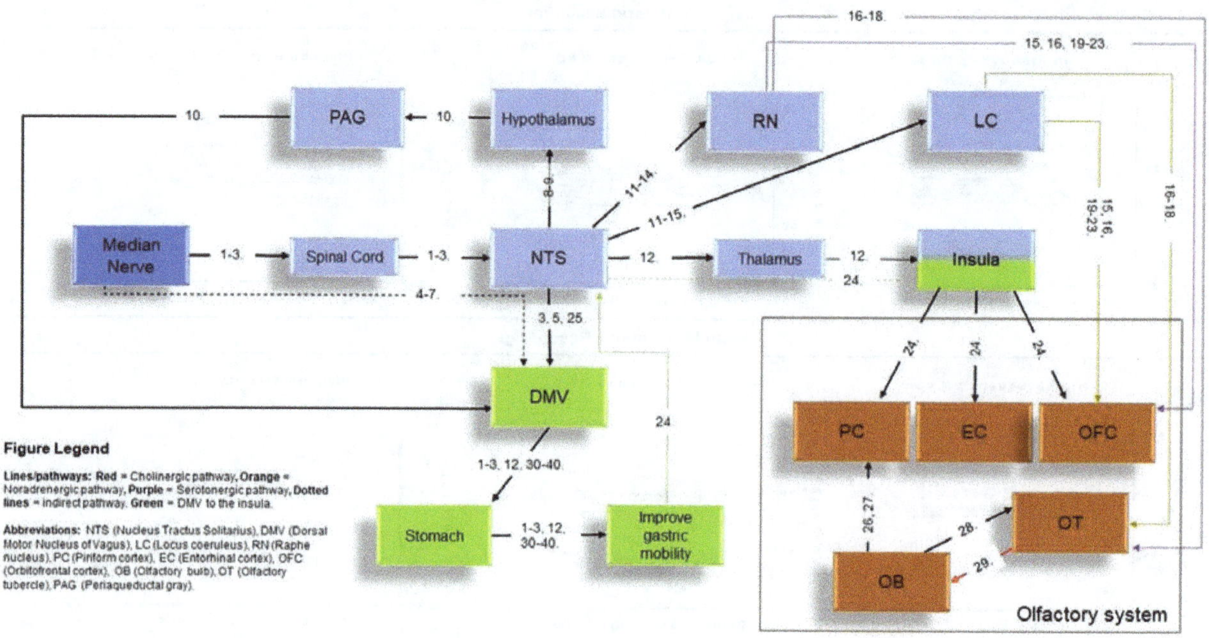

FIGURE 5 | The potential pathways to the olfactory network *via* MNS. Figure legend in the image indicates all abbreviations and the type of pathways (represented by different colors) present in the current diagram. Structures in color "blue" refer to the indirect stimulation of the vagus nerve (VN) pathway using MNS to the olfactory network while structures in color "green" refer to the stimulation of the Nucleus Tractus Solitarius-dorsal motor nucleus of vagus (NTS-DMV; VN brainstem nucleus) and subsequent interactions with the insula to the olfactory network *via* MNS. Orange structures represent the structures of the main olfactory system. Numbers in the figures represent references provided in a separate document in **Supplementary Table S2**. Abbreviations of structures are given in the Figure Legend on the bottom-left corner of the diagram.

while the use of 5 Hz resulted in an absence of activation in the S-I and the use of 15–30 Hz only had effects on some of the participants in the enrolled study (Puce et al., 1995). MNS using 0.5–1 Hz in conjunction with fMRI techniques in human subjects have found increased default network interconnectivity, greater connectivity between sensorimotor networks (Dhond et al., 2008) and increased activation of posterior insula, hypothalamus and cerebellum (Bai et al., 2010). Furthermore, low frequencies MNS of 10–25 Hz have been used on the modulation of gastric function (Noguchi and Hayashi, 1996; Ouyang et al., 2002; Xu et al., 2006; Imai et al., 2008). Low frequencies (1–25 Hz) have also been performed to alleviate symptoms of nausea and vomiting in animal models (Ouyang et al., 2002; Chen et al., 2003) and human studies (Xu et al., 2006; Bai et al., 2010). The use of MNS in higher frequencies (50 Hz) was only explored in a single study and resulted in reduced activation of the S-I in comparison to the use of lower frequencies of MNS (Davis et al., 1995). In the current study, the use of low frequency MNS (10 Hz) did not show any significant changes in the supra-threshold odor rating in the LMS test. This indicates that it is possible that the suppression of nausea and vomiting with MNS could be acting through different cortical structures that excludes the OFC and potentially separate mechanisms from the sense of smell for alleviating symptoms of nausea and vomiting. This requires further exploration in future research, coupled with the investigation of high frequency MNS in the alleviation of symptoms associated with nausea and vomiting as it could have stronger effects in comparison to low frequency MNS.

Results of the present study demonstrated that non-invasive high frequency MNS can reduce olfactory intensity ratings of the moderate concentration of Amyl Acetate, strong concentration of Isovaleric Acid and 1-Octen-3-ol in healthy participants. In contrast, non-invasive low frequency MNS and placebo groups did not show any effects on modulating olfactory sensory ratings in the LMS test. These results were also supported by statistically significant increase of $VWrSO_2$ (%) in the NIRS recordings in both hemispheres of the OFC only under high frequency MNS but not in the low frequency stimulation or placebo conditions. This is the first study that indicates that MNS under high frequency stimulation can suppress odor intensity ratings of specific concentrations of several odors in combination with the increased and simultaneous activation in the OFCs in both hemispheres. The previous study by our group (Maharjan et al., 2018) demonstrated that non-invasive high frequency (80 Hz) electrostimulation of the auricular VN can improve the performance of supra-threshold test in healthy, adult male participants. This improvement in supra-threshold olfactory function was also supported by a significant improvement of $VWrSO_2$ (%) in the NIRS recordings only in the right hemisphere (Maharjan et al., 2018). In the present study, high frequency electrostimulation (80 Hz) of the MN suppressed the supra-threshold function of odor intensity ratings in the healthy volunteers with the bilateral improvement of

VWrSO$_2$ (%) in the NIRS recordings in both hemispheres. Both studies' outcomes underlined the significance of high frequency (80 Hz) electrostimulation on modulating the olfactory function and also indicated the potential contribution of the OFC that accompanies the significant results from the supra-threshold olfactory tests in both studies with VWrSO$_2$ (%) recordings.

Although both electrostimulation techniques were capable of modulating olfactory supra-threshold function in healthy humans, use of 80 Hz electrostimulation on two different nerves modulated the supra-threshold olfactory function in opposite directions. In this context, it is worth to note the lateralization of the OFC for olfactory function. The right OFC, along with the right piriform cortex, is associated with increased activation during higher-order processing of smell sensation in comparison to the left hemispheric counterparts (Zatorre et al., 1992; Jones-Gotman and Zatorre, 1993; Hummel et al., 1995). This functional lateralization of OFC may explain the underlying mechanism of the opposite effects obtained with MNS vs. auricular VNS with high frequency (80 Hz) electrostimulation. The "smell image" may also be another factor that may contribute the suppression of olfactory function with high frequency MNS in the present study. It has been reported that each odor has been coded with its integrating senses in the brain. The smell image is described as an unconscious perception, influenced by multi-sensory inputs (including vision, sound, somatosensory-touch, taste and smell), contributing to our perception of smell that arises from the sub modalities of the somatosensory system (Shepherd, 2006). In the current study, use of high frequency MNS of 80 Hz may potentially decrease the activation of S-I (as a component of smell image) as in the reports of 50 Hz MNS study (Davis et al., 1995) and this may lead to the suppression of the smell image.

In the present study, weak, moderate and strong concentrations of 4 odors (Citral, Isovaleric Acid, Amyl Acetate and 1-Octen-3-ol) have been used. The results demonstrated that high frequency (80 Hz) MNS was capable of olfactory supra-threshold suppression for moderate concentration of Amyl Acetate, strong concentration of Isovaleric Acid and strong concentration of 1-Octen-3-ol. However, this effect was not present for the remainder. Effects on different concentrations of odors *via* MNS were not completely surprising as different odorants and different concentrations of each odorant can activate different sets of olfactory receptors (ORs; Kajiya et al., 2001; Buck, 2004). This suggests that effects of MNS could be as early as the encoding stage of olfactory processing. To confirm this hypothesis, future studies could use a combination of calcium imaging and electrophysiological techniques (Touhara, 2002) or single-cell reverse transcription-polymerase chain reaction techniques (Kajiya et al., 2001) in rodent models and explore if the specific ORs that are expressed under the concentrations of odors in the current study are suppressed after high frequency MNS. NIRS recording of the OFC was performed in the current study as it has been indicated in the existing literature that presentation of olfactory stimuli is represented in this region of the cortex (Ishimaru et al., 2004; Harada et al., 2006; Kobayashi et al., 2012). However, to understand how and what part of the neural olfactory system is affected by MNS (in this particular instance, high frequency MNS), investigations of the full neural circuitry of connections that MNS propagates to before reaching the OFC is necessary. This includes the potential pathways that MNS entails to reach the olfactory regions of the cortex/sub-cortex that is indicated in **Figure 5**. This could be performed in future investigations using magneto encephalography or fMRI, observing the neurocircuitry that is associated with MNS and specific olfactory tests. In particular, it would help address why high frequency MNS only had an effect on specific concentrations of odors in the present study.

The networks that relays the effects of MNS to the olfactory networks is potentially acting through the vagal brainstem nuclei. NTS is a recipient of direct neural inputs from the afferent (sensory) vagus as well as the direct and indirect inputs from the pharyngeal, glossopharyngeal and trigeminal nerves, the spinal tract, the area postrema, the hypothalamus, the cerebellum and vestibular/labyrinthine systems as well as the cerebral cortex, all of which play important roles in regulation of medullary reflexes controlling nausea and vomiting (Babic and Browning, 2014). These shared effects by all corresponding nerves is thought to intersect at the NTS, which is considered a focal point of neuroanatomical intersection center for pathways associated with the peripheral and cranial nerves of the scalp, face, auricular and body (van der Kooy et al., 1984; Ruggiero et al., 2000; Cakmak, 2006). MNS relays to the NTS (Noguchi and Hayashi, 1996; Zhang et al., 2002; Tada et al., 2003; Guan and Wu, 2005; Cakmak, 2006; Imai et al., 2008; Wang et al., 2015) where afferents for locus coeruleus (LC; Chandler et al., 2014) and raphe nucleus (RN) are present (Sawchenko, 1983; Ruggiero et al., 2000; Mello-Carpes and Izquierdo, 2013; Frangos et al., 2015). LC and RN, can innervate the olfactory tubercle (OT) using noradrenergic and serotonergic fibers respectively (Solano-Flores et al., 1980; Guevara-Guzman et al., 1991; Wesson and Wilson, 2011). Both of these structures can project to the OFC, directly or through the OT (Kannan and Yamashita, 1985; Mooney et al., 1987; Ikemoto, 2007; Price, 2010; Wesson and Wilson, 2011; Chandler et al., 2014; Zhou et al., 2015). LC and RN can also be stimulated through an indirect stimulation through the NTS using MNS (**Figure 5**). In addition, MNS could also follow the pathway from the NTS to the insula, which can activate the primary olfactory centers (piriform cortex-PC and entorhinal cortex-EC) and OFC (Mayer, 2011). Therefore, MNS could influence the OT, OFC and OB, *via* the LC, RN and insula (**Figure 5**).

In addition to the neuroanatomical insights, findings from the current study also give practical supports to use MNS as a way to ameliorate nausea symptoms in patients. Drawing evidence from interviews with cancer patients, it has been identified that some strong smells (e.g., shaving cream) and food-related smells (e.g., cooked meat, frying food) can trigger or aggravate nauseas, which aversively impact on patients' food intake (McGreevy et al., 2014; Olver et al., 2014). The current study found that MNS can effectively suppress the intensity perception of three of the four food-related odor compounds. Notably, two of these odorants are generally described by the population as unpleasant (i.e., cheese, mushroom; Ventanas et al., 2010; Mcrae et al., 2013). It is known from the previous literature that OFC is not only responsible for sensory integration, but also for assigning reward values to sensory stimulus (Rolls et al., 2003). The current finding indicates that the unpleasant odorants may be more susceptible to the modulatory effect of MNS. Although more research is needed to confirm whether MNS has differentiating effects on pleasant and unpleasant odor groups, its noticeable effects on Isovaleric Acid and 1-Octen-3-ol are promising for future investigations in the use of MNS on suppressing nausea-triggering olfactory perceptions. This non-invasive approach can particularly help cancer patients who commonly experience the cluster of symptoms associated with nausea, vomiting and loss of appetite (Guerdoux-Ninot et al., 2016).

The current study has some limitations. In the present study, only acute effects of high- and low frequency MNS were tested and chronic effects of MNS should also be investigated in future studies. The LMS test was selected for testing supra-threshold intensity perception due to its common applications in studying chemical senses. However, the LMS test procedure did not allow to observe odor-specific responses due to the presentation of stimuli without rigorous time controls. Future studies should replicate the current experimental design with different supra-threshold olfactory tests and with the use of a more accurate odor delivery system (such as a neuroimaging-compatible olfactometer). In addition, the use of NIRS techniques in the current experiment measured only the OFC (VWrSO_2%). fMRI or magneto encephalography approaches would be useful to clarify the modulation of olfactory networks by MNS. It should also be reiterated that the current study only included healthy male participants. Female participants were excluded from the study because olfactory functioning fluctuates across menstrual cycles, which could introduce biases with the current repeated-measures design. Building on the positive findings from the current study, future studies can examine effects on female cohorts incorporating calibration of menstrual cycles in the experimental design. The last but not the least, the significant results were obtained with the conservative approach of Bonferroni correction in the present study and we also provided the effect size analysis of significant results for future meta-analysis. The effect size analysis indicated low effect size for the significant LMS results and large effect size for the significant NIRS results. It's worth to note that low effect size for significant LMS results which are correlated with large effect size in NIRS (cortical data) do not clarify or indicate a weak or strong behavioral effect of MNS in the present study design. The clinical significance or clinical usability of MNS should be investigated in future studies with behavioral designs.

In conclusion, the present research investigated the potential role of MNS using high and low frequencies on olfactory intensity perception in healthy, adult, male participants, with supplementary exploration of the OFC. The present study indicated for the first time in human research that non-invasive high frequency MNS is able to modulate human olfactory functioning, accompanied by observation of increased activation in bilateral hemispheres of the OFC. Future studies should explore effects of MNS with high- and low frequencies on separate olfactory functioning, such as odor recognition, odor memory and odor identification, in combination with functional neuroimaging techniques, in order to understand the modulatory effect of MNS on specific olfactory-related neural circuitries.

AUTHOR CONTRIBUTIONS

YC: concept idea. YC and MP: project design. AM, YC and MP: performing experiments and data collection statistical analysis and preparation of final manuscript. MP and AM: interpretation of the results. YC and AM: draft manuscript.

FUNDING

This work was supported by the University of Otago, School of Biomedical Sciences, Dean's Bequest Fund.

REFERENCES

Alexander, J. C., Knonenfeld, M. A., and Dance, G. R. (2002). Reduced postoperative length of stay may result from using cerebral oximetry monitoring to guide treatment. *Annu. Thorac. Surg.* 73:s373. doi: 10.1016/s0003-4975(01)03537-8

Andrews, P. L. R. (1992). Physiology of nausea and vomiting. *Br. J. Anaesth.* 69, 2S–19S. doi: 10.1093/bja/69.supplement_1.2S

Babic, T., and Browning, K. N. (2014). The role of vagal neurocircuits in the regulation of nausea and vomiting. *Eur. J. Pharmacol.* 5, 38–47. doi: 10.1016/j.ejphar.2013.08.047

Bai, L., Yan, H., Li, N., Qin, W., Chen, P., Liu, P., et al. (2010). Neural specificity of acupuncture stimulation at pericardium 6: evidence from an fMRI study. *J. Magn. Reson. Imaging* 31, 71–77. doi: 10.1002/jmri.22006

Ballard, C., Jones, E., Gauge, N., Aarsland, D., Nilsen, O. B., Saxby, B. K., et al. (2012). Optimised anaesthesia to reduce post operative cognitive decline (POCD) in older patients undergoing elective surgery, a randomised controlled trial. *PLoS One* 7:e37410. doi: 10.1371/journal.pone.0037410

Blas, M. L., Lobato, E. B., and Martin, T. (1999). Noninvasive infrared spectroscopy as a monitor of retrograde cerebral perfusion during deep hypothermia. *J. Cardiothorac. Vasc. Anesth.* 13, 244–245. doi: 10.1016/s1053-0770(99)90114-3

Buck, L. B. (2004). Olfactory receptors and odor coding in mammals. *Nutr. Rev.* 62, S184–S188. doi: 10.1111/j.1753-4887.2004.tb00097.x

Cakmak, Y. O. (2006). Epilepsy, electroacupuncture and the nucleus of the solitary tract. *Acupunct. Med.* 24, 164–168. doi: 10.1136/aim.24.4.164

Casati, A., Fanelli, G., Pietropaoli, P., Proietti, R., Tufano, R., Danelli, G., et al. (2005). Continuous monitoring of cerebral oxygen saturation in elderly patients undergoing major abdominal surgery minimizes brain exposure to potential hypoxia. *Anaesth. Analg.* 101, 740–747. doi: 10.1213/01.ane.0000166974.96219.cd

Chandler, D. J., Gao, W.-J., and Waterhouse, B. D. (2014). Heterogeneous organization of the locus coeruleus projections to prefrontal and motor cortices. *Proc. Natl. Acad. Sci. U S A* 111, 6816–6821. doi: 10.1073/pnas.1320827111

Chang, X., Yan, J., Yi, S., Lin, Y., and Yang, R. (2001). The affects of acupuncture at sibai and neiting acupoints on gastric peristalsis. *J. Tradit. Chin. Med.* 21, 286–288.

Chen, J. D. Z., Qian, L., Ouyang, H., and Yin, J. (2003). Gastric electrical stimulation with short pulses reduces vomiting but not dysrhythmias in dogs. *Gastroenterology* 124, 401–409. doi: 10.1053/gast.2003.50048

Cho, H., Nemoto, E. M., Yonas, H., Balzer, J., and Sclabassi, R. J. (1998). Cerebral monitoring by means of oximetry and somatosensory evoked potentials during carotid endarterectomy. *J. Neurosurg.* 89, 533–538. doi: 10.3171/jns.1998.89.4.0533

Choudhury, E. S., Moberg, P., and Doty, R. L. (2003). Influences of age and sex on a microencapsulated odor memory test. *Chem. Senses* 28, 799–805. doi: 10.1093/chemse/bjg072

Classen, C., Howes, D., and Synnott, A. (1994). *Aroma: The Cultural History of Smell* 1st Edn. London: Routledge.

Covidien. (2013). *Operations Manual INVOS System, Model 5100C.* Mansfield, MA: 15 Hampshire Street.

Damian, M. S., and Schlosser, R. (2007). Bilateral near infrared spectroscopy in space-occupying middle cerebral artery stroke. *Neurocrit. Care* 6, 165–173. doi: 10.1007/s12028-007-0010-3

Davis, K. D., Wood, M. L., Crawley, A. P., and Mikulis, D. J. (1995). fMRI of human somatosensory and cingulate cortex during painful electrical nerve stimulation. *Neuroreport* 7, 321–325. doi: 10.1097/00001756-199512000-00077

de Letter, J. A., Sie, T. H., Moll, F. L., Algra, A., Eikelboom, B. C., and Ackerstaff, G. A. (1998). Transcranial cerebral oximetry during carotid endarterectomy: agreement between frontal and lateral probe measurements as compared with an electroencephalogram. *Cardiovasc. Surg.* 6, 373–377. doi: 10.1016/s0967-2109(98)00020-9

Dhond, R. P., Yeh, C., Park, K., Kettner, N., and Napadow, V. (2008). Acupuncture modulates resting state connectivity in default and sensorimotor brain networks. *Pain* 136, 407–418. doi: 10.1016/j.pain.2008.01.011

Diehl, D. L. (1999). Acupuncture for gastrointestinal and hepatobiliary disorders. *J. Altern. Complement. Med.* 5, 27–45. doi: 10.1089/acm.1999.5.27

Doty, R. L. (2003). *The Odor Discrimination/Memory TestTM Administration Manual.* 2nd Edn. Haddon Heights, NJ: Sensonics, Inc.

Doty, R. L., McKeown, D. A., Lee, W. W., and Shaman, P. (1995). A study of the test-retest reliability of 10 olfactory tests. *Chem. Senses* 20, 645–656. doi: 10.1093/chemse/20.6.645

Doty, R. L., Shaman, P., and Dann, M. (1984). Development of the university of pennsylvania smell identification test: a rapid quantitative olfactory function test for the clinic. *Physiol. Behav.* 32, 489–502. doi: 10.1016/0031-9384(84)90269-5

Edmonds, H. L. Jr., Gordon, E. K., and Levy, W. J. (2016). "Central nervous system monitoring," in *Kaplan's Cardiac Anesthesia*, 7th Edn. ed. J. A. Kaplan (Philadelphia: Elsevier Saunders), 466–495.

Edmonds, H. L. Jr., Ganzel, B. L., and Austin, E. H. III. (2004). Cerebral oximetry for cardiac and vascular surgery. *Semin. Cardiotorac. Vasc. Anesth.* 8, 147–166. doi: 10.1177/108925320400800208

Edmonds, H. L. Jr., Isley, M. R., and Balzer, J. (2017). "A guide to central nervous system near-infrared spectroscopic monitoring," in *Neuromonitoring for the Anesthesiologist and Other Health Care Providers*, 2nd Edn. eds. A. Koht, T. B. Sloan and R. Toleikis (New York, NY: Springer), 205–217.

Edmonds, H. L., Singer, I., Sehic, A., and Strickland, T. J. (1998). Multimodality neuromonitoring for neurocardiology. *J. Interv. Cardiol.* 11, 197–204. doi: 10.1111/j.1540-8183.1998.tb00119.x

Ferretti, A., Babiloni, C., Arienzo, D., Del Gratta, C., Rossini, P. M., Tartaro, A., et al. (2007). Cortical brain responses during passive nonpainful median nerve stimulation at low frequencies (0.5–4 Hz): an fMRI study. *Hum. Brain Mapp.* 28, 645–653. doi: 10.1002/hbm.20292

Frangos, E., Ellrich, J., and Komisaruk, B. R. (2015). Non-invasive access to the vagus nerve central projections via electrical stimulation of the external ear: fMRI evidence in humans. *Brain Stimul.* 8, 624–636. doi: 10.1016/j.brs.2014.11.018

Gopinath, S. P., Robertson, C. S., Contant, C. F., Narayan, R. K., Grossman, R. G., and Chance, B. (1995). Early detection of delayed traumatic intracranial hematomas using near-infrared spectroscopy. *J. Neurosurg.* 83, 438–444. doi: 10.3171/jns.1995.83.3.0438

Green, B. G., Dalton, P., Cowart, B., Shaffer, G., Rankin, K., and Higgins, J. (1996). Evaluating the 'labeled magnitude scale' for measuring sensations of taste and smell. *Chem. Senses* 21, 323–334. doi: 10.1093/chemse/21.3.323

Green, B. G., Shaffer, G. S., and Gilmore, M. M. (1993). Derivation and evaluation of a semantic scale of oral sensation magnitude with apparent ratio properties. *Chem. Senses* 18, 683–702. doi: 10.1093/chemse/18.6.683

Guan, Y. H., and Wu, X. P. (2005). The influence of electroacupunturing Neiguan on the content of ET, TXB2, and 6-Keto-PGF1a in acute myocardial ischemia rabbits. *Hu Bei Zhong Yi Xue Yuan Xue Bao* 7, 13–14.

Guerdoux-Ninot, E., Kilgour, R. D., Janiszewski, C., Jarlier, M., Meuric, J., Poirée, B., et al. (2016). Meal context and food preferences in cancer patients: results from a French self-report survey. *Springerplus* 5:810. doi: 10.1186/s40064-016-2538-1

Guevara-Guzman, R., Garcia-Diaz, D. E., Solano-Flores, L. P., Wayner, M. J., and Armstrong, D. L. (1991). Role of the paraventricular nucleus in the projection from the nucleus of the solitary tract to the olfactory bulb. *Brain Res. Bull.* 27, 447–450. doi: 10.1016/0361-9230(91)90140-f

Gyngell, M. L., Bock, C., Schmitz, B., Hoehn-Berlage, M., and Hossmann, K. A. (1996). Variation of functional MRI signal in response to frequency of somatosensory stimulation in α-chloralose anesthetized rats. *Magn. Reson. Med.* 36, 13–15. doi: 10.1002/mrm.1910360104

Harada, H., Tanaka, M., and Kato, T. (2006). Brain olfactory activation measured by near-infrared spectroscopy in humans. *J. Laryngol. Otol.* 120, 638–643. doi: 10.1017/s002221510600123x

Harrer, M., Waldenberger, F. R., Weiss, G., Folkmann, S., Gorlitzer, M., Moidl, R., et al. (2010). Aortic arch surgery using bilateral antegrade selective cerebral perfusion in combination with near-infrared spectroscopy. *Eur. J. Cardiothorac. Surg.* 38, 561–567. doi: 10.1016/j.ejcts.2010.03.016

Higami, T., Kozawa, S., Asada, T., Obo, H., Gan, K., Iwahashi, K., et al. (1999). Retrograde cerebral perfusion versus selective cerebral perfusion as evaluated by cerebral oxygen saturation during aortic arch reconstruction. *Annu. Thorac. Surg.* 67, 1091–1096. doi: 10.1016/s0003-4975(99)00135-6

Hongo, K., Kobayashi, S., Okudera, H., Hokama, M., and Nakagawa, F. (1995). Noninvasive cerebral optical spectroscopy: depth-resolved measurements of cerebral haemodynamics using indocyanine green. *Neurol. Res.* 17, 89–93. doi: 10.1080/01616412.1995.11740293

Hummel, T., Pauli, E., Schüler, P., Kettenmann, B., Stefan, H., and Kobal, G. (1995). Chemosensory event-related potentials in patients with temporal lobe epilepsy. *Epilepsia* 36, 79–85. doi: 10.1111/j.1528-1157.1995.tb01670.x

Ibáñez, V., Deiber, M. P., Sadato, N., Toro, C., Grissom, J., Woods, R. P., et al. (1995). Effects of stimulus rate on regional cerebral blood flow after median nerve stimulation. *Brain* 118, 1339–1351. doi: 10.1093/brain/118.5.1339

Iglesias, I., Murkin, J. W., Bainbridge, D., and Adams, S. (2003). Monitoring cerebral oxygen saturation significantly decreases postoperative length of stay: a prospective randomized blinded study. *Heart Surg. Forum* 6:204.

Ikemoto, S. (2007). Dopamine reward circuitry: two projection systems from the ventral midbrain to the nucleus accumbens-olfactory tubercle complex. *Brain Res. Rev.* 56, 27–78. doi: 10.1016/j.brainresrev.2007.05.004

Imai, K., Ariga, H., Chen, C., Mantyh, C., Pappas, T. N., and Takahashi, T. (2008). Effects of electroacupuncture on gastric motility and heart rate variability in conscious rats. *Auton. Neurosci.* 138, 91–98. doi: 10.1016/j.autneu.2007.11.003

Ishimaru, T., Yata, T., Horikawa, K., and Hatanaka, S. (2004). Near-infrared spectroscopy of the adult human olfactory cortex. *Acta Otolaryngologica. Suppl.* 6489, 95–98. doi: 10.1080/03655230410017751

Janelle, G. M., Mnookin, S., Gravenstein, N., Martin, T. D., and Urdaneta, F. (2002). Unilateral cerebral oxygen desaturation during emergent repair of a DeBakey type 1 aortic dissection: potential aversion of a major catastrophe. *Anesthesiology* 96, 1263–1265. doi: 10.1097/00000542-200205000-00033

Jones-Gotman, M., and Zatorre, R. J. (1993). ORMT in humans. *Brain Cogn.* 22, 182–198.

Kajiya, K., Inaki, K., Tanaka, M., Haga, T., Kataoka, H., and Touhara, K. (2001). Molecular bases of odor discrimination: reconstitution of olfactory receptors that recognize overlapping sets of odorants. *J. Neurosci.* 21, 6018–6025. doi: 10.1523/JNEUROSCI.21-16-06018.2001

Kalva, J. J., Sims, C. A., Puentes, L. A., Snyder, D. J., and Bartoshuk, L. M. (2014). Comparison of the hedonic general labeled magnitude scale with the hedonic 9-point scale. *J. Food Sci.* 79, S239–S245. doi: 10.1111/1750-3841.12342

Kannan, H., and Yamashita, H. (1985). Connections of neurons in the region of the nucleus tractus solitarius with the hypothalamic paraventricular nucleus: their possible involvement in neural control of the cardiovascular system in rats. *Brain Res.* 329, 205–212. doi: 10.1016/0006-8993(85)90526-8

Kobayashi, E., Karaki, M., Touge, T., Deguchi, K., Ikeda, K., Mori, N., et al. (2012). "Olfactory assessment using near-infrared spectroscopy," in *2012 ICME International Conference on Complex Medical Engineering (CME)* (Kobe, Japan: IEEE), 517–520.

Lee, A., and Fan, L. T. Y. (2015). Stimulation of the wrist acupuncture point PC6 postoperative nausea and vomiting. *Cochrane Database Syst. Rev.* 11:CD003281. doi: 10.1002/14651858.CD003281.pub4

Madsen, P. L., Skak, C., Rasmussen, A., and Secher, N. H. (2000). Interference of cerebral near-infrared oximetry in patients with icterus. *Anesth. Analg.* 90, 489–493. doi: 10.1213/00000539-200002000-00046

Maharjan, A., Wang, E., Peng, M., and Cakmak, Y. O. (2018). Improvement of olfactory function with high frequency non-invasive auricular electrostimulation in healthy humans. *Front. Neurosci.* 12:225. doi: 10.3389/fnins.2018.00225

Mayer, E. A. (2011). Gut feelings: the emerging biology of gut-brain communication. *Nat. Rev. Neurosci.* 12, 453–466. doi: 10.1038/nrn3071

McGreevy, J., Orrevall, Y., Belqaid, K., Wismer, W., Tishelman, C., and Bernhardson, B. M. (2014). Characteristics of taste and smell alterations reported by patients after starting treatment for lung Cancer. *Support. Care Cancer* 22, 2635–2644. doi: 10.1007/s00520-014-2215-2

Mcrae, J. F., Jaeger, S. R., Bava, C. M., Beresford, M. K., Hunter, D., Jia, Y., et al. (2013). Report identification of regions associated with variation in sensitivity to food-related odors in the human genome. *Curr. Biol.* 23, 1596–1600. doi: 10.1016/j.cub.2013.07.031

McRobb, C., Walczak, R., Lawson, S., Lodge, E., Lockhart, N., and Bandarenko, I. I. I. R. (2011). Carboxyhemoglobinemia in a pediatric cardiopulmonary bypass patient derived from a contaminated unit of allogenic blood. *Perfusion* 26, 302–307. doi: 10.1177/0267659111406993

Mello-Carpes, P. B., and Izquierdo, I. (2013). The nucleus of the solitary tract→nucleus paragigantocellularis→locus coeruleus→CA1 region of dorsal hippocampus pathway is important for consolidation of object recognition memory. *Neurobiol. Learn. Mem.* 100, 56–63. doi: 10.1016/j.nlm.2012.12.002

Misra, M., Stark, J., Dujovny, M., Wildman, R., and Ausman, J. I. (1998). Transcranial cerebral oximetry in random normal subjects. *Neurol. Res.* 20, 137–141. doi: 10.1080/01616412.1998.11740496

Mooney, K. E., Inokuchi, A., Snow, J. B. Jr., and Kimmelman, C. P. (1987). Projections from the ventral tegmental area to the olfactory tubercle in the rat. *Otolaryngol. Head Neck Surg.* 96, 151–157. doi: 10.1177/019459988709600207

Murkin, J. M., Adams, S. J., Novick, R. J., Quantz, M., Bainbridge, D., Iglesias, I., et al. (2007). Monitoring brain oxygen saturation during coronary bypass surgery: a randomized, prospective study. *Anesth. Analg.* 104, 51–58. doi: 10.1213/01.ane.0000246814.29362.f4

Napadow, V., Dhond, R. P., Kim, J., LaCount, L., Vangel, M., Harris, R. E., et al. (2009). Brain encoding of acupuncture sensation—coupling on-line rating with fMRI. *Neuroimage* 47, 1055–1065. doi: 10.1016/j.neuroimage.2009.05.079

Nihashi, T., Naganawa, S., Sato, C., Kawai, H., Nakamura, T., Fukatsu, H., et al. (2005). Contralateral and ipsilateral responses in primary somatosensory cortex following electrical median nerve stimulation—an fMRI study. *Clin. Neurophysiol.* 116, 842–848. doi: 10.1016/j.clinph.2004.10.011

Noguchi, E., and Hayashi, H. (1996). Increases in gastric acidity in response to EA stimulation of hindlimb of anesthetized rats. *Jpn. J. Physiol.* 46, 53–58. doi: 10.2170/jjphysiol.46.53

Olver, I. N., Eliott, J. A., and Koczwara, B. (2014). A qualitative study investigating chemotherapy-induced nausea as a symptom cluster. *Support. Care Cancer* 22, 2749–2756. doi: 10.1007/s00520-014-2276-2

Oriheula-Espina, F., Leff, D. R., James, D. R. C., Darzi, A. W., and Yang, G. Z. (2010). Quality control and assurance in functional near infrared spectroscopy (fNIRS) experimentation. *Phys. Med. Biol.* 55, 3701–3724. doi: 10.1088/0031-9155/55/13/009

Ouyang, H. U. I., Yin, J., Wang, Z., Pasricha, P. J., Chen, J. D. Z., Yin, J., et al. (2002). Electroacupuncture accelerates gastric emptying in association with changes in vagal activity. *Am. J. Gastroint. Liver Physiol.* 282, 390–396. doi: 10.1152/ajpgi.00272.2001

Prabhune, A., Sehic, A., Spence, P. A., Church, T., and Edmonds, H. L. Jr. (2002). Cerebral oximetry provides early warning of oxygen delivery failure during cardiopulmonary bypass. *J. Cardiothorac. Vasc. Anesth.* 16, 204–206. doi: 10.1053/jcan.2002.31069

Price, J. L. (2010). "Olfactory higher centers anatomy," in *Encyclopedia of Neuroscience*, ed. L. R. Squire (London: Elsevier Ltd), 129–136. doi: 10.1016/B978-008045046-9.01692-2

Puce, A., Constable, T., Luby, M. L., McCarthy, G., Nobre, A. C., Spencer, D. D., et al. (1995). Functional magnetic resonance imaging of sensory and motor cortex: comparison with electrophysiological localization. *J. Neurosurg.* 83, 262–270. doi: 10.3171/jns.1995.83.2.0262

Ren, Y., Bai, L., Feng, Y., Tian, J., and Li, K. (2010). Investigation of acupoint specificity by functional connectivity analysis based on graph theory. *Neurosci. Lett.* 482, 95–100. doi: 10.1016/j.neulet.2010.06.091

Roberts, K. W., Crnkowic, A. P., and Linneman, L. J. (1998). Nearinfrared spectroscopy detects critical cerebral hypoxia during carotid endarterectomy in awake patients. *Anesthesiology* 9:A933. doi: 10.1097/00000542-199809160-00038

Rolls, E. T., Kringelbach, M. L., and de Araujo, I. E. T. (2003). Different representations of pleasant and unpleasant odours in the human brain. *Eur. J. Neurosci.* 18, 695–703. doi: 10.1046/j.1460-9568.2003.02779.x

Ruggiero, D. A., Anwar, S., Kim, J., and Glickstein, S. B. (1998). Visceral afferent pathways to the thalamus and olfactory tubercle: behavioral implications. *Brain Res.* 799, 159–171. doi: 10.1016/s0006-8993(98)00442-9

Ruggiero, D. A., Underwood, M. D., Mann, J. J., Anwar, M., and Arango, V. (2000). The human nucleus of the solitary tract: visceral pathways revealed with an "*in vitro*" postmortem tracing method. *J. Auton. Nerv. Syst.* 79, 181–190. doi: 10.1016/s0165-1838(99)00097-1

Sawchenko, P. E. (1983). Central connections of the sensory and motor nuclei of the vagus nerve. *J. Auton. Nerv. Syst.* 9, 13–26. doi: 10.1016/0165-1838(83)90129-7

Shepherd, G. M. (2006). Smell images and the flavour system in the human brain. *Nature* 444, 316–321. doi: 10.1038/nature05405

Singer, I., Dawn, B., Edmonds, H. Jr., and Stickland, T. J. (1999). Syncope is predicted by neuromonitoring in patients with ICDs. *Pacing Clin. Electrophysiol.* 22, 216–222. doi: 10.1111/j.1540-8159.1999.tb00336.x

Solano-Flores, L. P., Aguilar-Baturoni, H. U., and Guevara-Aguilar, R. (1980). Locus coeruleus influences upon the olfactory tubercle. *Brain Res. Bull.* 5, 383–389. doi: 10.1016/s0361-9230(80)80008-6

Spiegel, J., Tintera, J., Gawehn, J., Stoeter, P., and Treede, R. D. (1999). Functional MRI of human primary somatosensory and motor cortex during median nerve stimulation. *Clin. Neurophysiol.* 110, 47–52. doi: 10.1016/s0168-5597(98)00043-4

Tada, H., Fujita, M., Harris, M., Tatewaki, M., Nakagawa, K., Yamamura, T., et al. (2003). Neural mechanism of acupuncture-induced gastric relaxations in rats. *Dig. Dis. Sci.* 48, 59–68. doi: 10.1023/A:1021730314068

Takahashi, T. (2006). Acupuncture for functional gastrointestinal disorders. *J. Gastroenterol.* 41, 408–417. doi: 10.1007/s00535-006-1773-6

Takahashi, T. (2011). Mechanism of acupuncture on neuromodulation in the gut—a review. *Neuromodulation* 14, 8–12. doi: 10.1111/j.1525-1403.2010.00295.x

Tatewaki, M., Strickland, C., Fukuda, H., Tsuchida, D., Hoshino, E., Pappas, T. N., et al. (2005). Effects of acupuncture on vasopressin-induced emesis in conscious dogs. *Am. J. Physiol. Regul. Integr. Comp. Physiol.* 288, 401–408. doi: 10.1152/ajpregu.00344.2004

Touhara, K. (2002). Odor discrimination by G protein-coupled olfactory receptors. *Microsc. Res. Tech.* 58, 135–141. doi: 10.1002/jemt.10131

Urasaki, E., Wada, S., Yasukouchi, H., and Yokota, A. (1998). Effect of transcutaneous electrical nerve stimulation (TENS) on central nervous system amplification of somatosensory input. *J. Neurol.* 245, 143–148. doi: 10.1007/s004150050194

van der Kooy, D., Koda, L. Y., McGinty, J. F., Gerfen, C. R., and Bloom, F. E. (1984). The organization of projections from the cortex, amygdala, and hypothalamus to the nucleus of the solitary tract in rat. *J. Comp. Neurol.* 224, 1–24. doi: 10.1002/cne.902240102

Ventanas, S., Mustonen, S., Puolanne, E., and Tuorila, H. (2010). Odour and flavour perception in flavoured model systems: influence of sodium chloride, umami compounds and serving temperature. *Food Qual. Prefer.* 21, 453–462. doi: 10.1016/j.foodqual.2009.11.003

Vretzakis, G., Georgopoulou, S., Stamoulis, K., Tassoudis, V., Mikroulis, D., Giannoukas, A., et al. (2013). Monitoring of brain oxygen saturation (INVOS) in a protocol to direct blood transfusions during cardiac surgery: a prospective randomized clinical trial. *J. Cardiothorac. Surg.* 8, 145–154. doi: 10.1186/1749-8090-8-145

Wang, S., Ren, L., Jia, L., Gu, Z., Fan, X., Chen, W., et al. (2015). Effect of acupuncture at Neiguan (PC 6) on cardiac function using echocardiography in myocardial ischemia rats induced by isoproter-enol. *J. Tradit. Chin. Med.* 35, 653–658. doi: 10.1016/s0254-6272(15)30155-2

Wang, Z., Qian, L., Ueno, T., and Chen, J. (2000). Mechanisms of various gastric electrical stimulations. *Gastroenterology* 118: A669. doi: 10.1016/S0016-5085(00)84814-3

Wesson, D. W., and Wilson, D. A. (2011). Sniffing out the contributions of the olfactory tubercle to the sense of smell: hedonics, sensory integration, and more? *Neurosci. Biobehav. Rev.* 35, 655–668. doi: 10.1016/j.neubiorev.2010.08.004

Xu, S., Hou, X., Zha, H., Gao, Z., Chen, Y., and Zhang, J. D. Z. (2006). Electroacupuncture accelerates solid gastric emptying and improves dyspeptic symptoms in patients with functional dyspepsia. *Dig. Dis. Sci.* 51, 2154–2159. doi: 10.1007/s10620-006-9412-x

Yao, F. S. F., Tseng, C. C., Woo, D., Huang, S. W., and Levin, S. K. (2001). Maintaining cerebral oxygen saturation during cardiac surgery decreased neurological complications. *Anesthesiology* 95:A152.

Zatorre, R. J., Jones-Gotman, M., Evans, A. C., and Meyer, E. (1992). Functional localization and lateralization of human olfactory cortex. *Nature* 360, 339–340. doi: 10.1038/360339a0

Zhang, G., Yin, H., Zhou, Y.-L., Han, H.-Y., Wu, Y.-H., Xing, W., et al. (2012). Capturing amplitude changes of low-frequency fluctuations in functional magnetic resonance imaging signal: a pilot acupuncture study on NeiGuan (PC6). *J. Altern. Complement. Med.* 18, 387–393. doi: 10.1089/acm.2010.0205

Zhang, F. B., Zhou, Y. P., Wang, Y. L., and Wang, K. M. (2002). Effect of electroacupuncture on blood free radicals, ET and CGRP contents in rats with acute myocardial ischemia. *Acupunct. Res.* 27, 192–196.

Zhou, J., Jia, C., Feng, Q., Bao, J., and Luo, M. (2015). Prospective coding of dorsal raphe reward signals by the orbitofrontal cortex. *J. Neurosci.* 35, 2717–2730. doi: 10.1523/JNEUROSCI.4017-14.2015

Zotelli, V. L. R., Grillio, C. M., and de Sousa Mda, L. (2014). Nausea control by needling at acupuncture point neiguan (PC6) during an intraoral impression-taking procedure. *J. Acupunct. Meridian Stud.* 7, 318–323. doi: 10.1016/j.jams.2014.04.009

6

Post-Stroke Hemiplegic Gait: New Perspective and Insights

Sheng Li [1,2], Gerard E. Francisco [1,2] and Ping Zhou [1,2,3]*

[1] Department of Physical Medicine and Rehabilitation, University of Texas Health Science Center, Houston, TX, United States, [2] TIRR Memorial Hermann Research Center, TIRR Memorial Hermann, Houston, TX, United States, [3] Guangdong Work Injury Rehabilitation Center, Guangzhou, China

***Correspondence:**
Sheng Li
sheng.li@uth.tmc.edu*

Walking dysfunction occurs at a very high prevalence in stroke survivors. Human walking is a phenomenon often taken for granted, but it is mediated by complicated neural control mechanisms. The automatic process includes the brainstem descending pathways (RST and VST) and the intraspinal locomotor network. It is known that leg muscles are organized into modules to serve subtasks for body support, posture and locomotion. Major kinematic mechanisms are recognized to minimize the center of gravity (COG) displacement. Stroke leads to damage to motor cortices and their descending corticospinal tracts and subsequent muscle weakness. On the other hand, brainstem descending pathways and the intraspinal motor network are disinhibited and become hyperexcitable. Recent advances suggest that they mediate post-stroke spasticity and diffuse spastic synergistic activation. As a result of such changes, existing modules are simplified and merged, thus leading to poor body support and walking performance. The wide range and hierarchy of post-stroke hemiplegic gait impairments is a reflection of mechanical consequences of muscle weakness, spasticity, abnormal synergistic activation and their interactions. Given the role of brainstem descending pathways in body support and locomotion and post-stroke spasticity, a new perspective of understanding post-stroke hemiplegic gait is proposed. Its clinical implications for management of hemiplegic gait are discussed. Two cases are presented as clinical application examples.

Keywords: gait, stroke, hemiparesis, spasticity, botulinum toxin, motor recovery

INTRODUCTION

Stroke is a leading cause of serious long-term disability (Benjamin et al., 2017). Walking dysfunction occurs in more than 80% of stroke survivors (Duncan et al., 2005). Despite of rehabilitation efforts, 25% of all stroke survivors have residual gait impairments that require full physical assistance before hospital discharge (Hendricks et al., 2002). Consequently, gait impairments cause difficulties in performing activities of daily living and mobility. Gait abnormality is characterized by a pronounced clinical presentation of gait asymmetry, as compared to healthy people (Olney and Richards, 1996; Richards and Olney, 1996). Stroke survivors usually have decreased stance phase and prolonged swing phase of the paretic side. Further, the walking speed is decreased and the stride length is shorter (Perry and Burnfield, 2010). These gait abnormalities along with muscle weakness place stroke survivors at a high risk of falls (Dobkin, 2005; Batchelor et al., 2012). Falls usually occur during walking in community-dwelling stroke survivors (Hyndman et al., 2002). Thus, improving walking safety and speed is the major goal for stroke survivors to prevent falls and to improve quality of life (Olney and Richards, 1996; Dobkin, 2005).

Walking is a phenomenon that is taken for granted by healthy individuals but requires an extremely complex process of neuromusculoskeletal control. Activation of muscles in lower limbs, trunk, and upper limbs in a certain spatiotemporal pattern is required to ensure appropriate joint positions to support and advance the body weight in different phases of gait cycles. In most situations, human walking at a comfortable speed on the level surface is primarily mediated by brainstem and spinal mechanisms (Dietz, 1996; Nielsen, 2003). However, supraspinal control adds complexity and flexibility of gait control and gait versatility to meet dynamic environmental needs and challenges (Dietz, 1996; Nielsen, 2003). Spasticity and paresis are main motor impairments after stroke (Li, 2017). In the context of spastic hemiparesis, muscles are weak and spastic and at different levels of impairments involving different regions of the upper limb, trunk and lower limb on one side. As a result, a wide spectrum of gait abnormalities is seen clinically.

In this article, major kinematic determinants and neural control of normal human gait are briefly reviewed from a historical perspective. Current findings of post-stroke hemiplegic gait as a result of altered neural control are then summarized. Based on recent advances on pathophysiology of muscle weakness and spasticity after stroke, a new perspective of understanding post-stroke hemiplegic gait is proposed. Its clinical implications for management of hemiplegic gait are discussed.

MAJOR KINEMATIC DETERMINANTS OF NORMAL HUMAN GAIT

For a biomechanical and kinesiological point of view, human walking can be described as progression of alternating weight-bearing limbs. As such, the displacement of the center of gravity (COG) of the whole-body is viewed as the end result of all muscle forces acting upon the body during the progression. During normal level walking, the body COG follows a smooth regular curve in the three-dimensional space. The peak-to-peak amplitudes are ~5 cm in the vertical and mediolateral planes, respectively Saunders et al. (1953). Using a hypothetical bipedal compass gait model and elementary geometrical arguments, Saunders et al. (1953) proposed six kinematic mechanisms that contribute to the efficient progress of the whole-body COG in the three dimensional space. These mechanisms are termed as six major determinants of human gait. They include pelvic rotation in the transverse plane, pelvic tilt in the coronal plan, knee flexion in the stance phase, foot and knee mechanisms and lateral displacement of the pelvis (hip adduction). This concept of major determinants was originally proposed to understand and manage pathological gait after orthopedic disorders, such as a fused hip joint (Saunders et al., 1953). From a historical perspective, major determinants of human gait are the fundamental concepts in understanding control of human gait and providing a foundation for clinical application of gait analysis. Although individual muscle activities (electromyography, EMG), joint kinematics, and ground reaction force were not available in the original "compass gait" model that permits only hip flexion and extension during walking, these determinants were able to explain the minimization of COG displacement well.

The conclusion of six determinants of human gait has been challenged in a number of studies (Gard and Childress, 1997, 1999; Croce et al., 2001; Kuo, 2007; Hayot et al., 2013). In the most recent study (Lin et al., 2014), Lin et al. quantitatively assessed the contribution of each determinant to the COG displacement over a gait cycle in young and healthy people. Using an "influence coefficient" concept, they found that hip flexion, stance knee flexion, and ankle-foot interaction significantly minimized the COG displacement in the sagittal plane; hip adduction and pelvic tilt are the main determinants of the mediolateral COG displacement in the coronal plane; however, pelvic rotation and pelvic tilt do not significantly affect the vertical COG displacement. Overall, there is general agreement between Saunders et al.'s classic article and this study with comprehensive quantitative kinematic data of individual joints. It is confirmatory that pelvic girdle movements (pelvic tilt, hip flexion, and adduction) contribute significantly to the displacement of COG in the three-dimensional space during walking.

NEURAL CONTROL OF NORMAL HUMAN GAIT

The above kinematic mechanisms are not able to account for a near perfect kinematic trajectory during human walking on a level surface, however. The distal part of the foot in the swing phase is lifted only 1–2 cm with <4 mm step-to-step variations (Winter, 1992). This displacement is enough to prevent stumbling, but not more than necessary. This remarkable precision of the foot position in the swing phase is determined by and the end result of coordinated activation of muscles from the lower extremities directly and of trunk and arm muscles indirectly. The number of different combinations of muscle activations that lead to the same foot position is almost infinite, i.e., the problem of motor redundancy (Bernstein, 1967). As suggested by Bernstein (1967), the brain may only control the endpoint, i.e., the foot position in this case, while allowing considerable flexibility for specific muscle activities. Using this fundamental approach, the muscle activities are not controlled individually. They are allowed to have a large range of flexibility as long as they are all scaled to each other to ensure the endpoint: the foot position within a desired range. These muscles are coordinated and organized into functional groups. They are often referred as muscle synergies or modules (Ting and McKay, 2007; Drew et al., 2008).

Different modules are described according to their biomechanical functions to the whole limb or the whole body during different types of locomotor functions, such as balance control or walking (Beyaert et al., 2015). There are five modules that are sufficient to perform sub-tasks of walking (Neptune et al., 2009). Module 1 includes gluteus medius, vasti, and rectus femoris muscles, primarily contributing to body support in early stance. Module 2 (soleus and gastrocnemius) is activated during both body support and propulsion in late stance. Module 3 (rectus femoris and tibialis anterior) acts to decelerate the leg in early and late swing, as well as to generate energy to the trunk throughout the swing phase. Module 4 mainly consists of the hamstring muscles. Activation of these muscles decelerates the ipsilateral leg prior to heel strike. Module 3 and Module 5 (iliopsoas) act together to accelerate the ipsilateral leg forward in early swing. These modules represent a general repertoire of motor actions that can be recruited in a variety of combinations and at different times for different locomotion and balance control needs, as well as for voluntary, rhythmic and reactive locomotor behaviors (McGowan et al., 2010; Allen and Neptune, 2012; Beyaert et al., 2015).

Extensive neural structures and pathways are involved in the process of gait control, including the spinal cord, brainstem, cerebellum, basal ganglia, limbic system, and cerebral cortex, as well as their interactions with the environment (see review Nielsen, 2003; Beyaert et al., 2015). Briefly, the above motor modules are largely controlled by the spinal cord and brainstem under regulating control of the cerebellum. More specifically, the pontine medullary reticular formation (PMRF) and vestibular nuclei provide body support and balance control, thus providing an upright posture against gravity by activating trunk and lower extremity extensor muscles. The additional neurons in the PMRF activate the spinal locomotor network under influence of the mesencephalic locomotor region and subthalamic locomotor region or cerebellum. Activation of this network allows rhythmic locomotor activity. These structures constitute automatic processes by simultaneously controlling body support, balance and rhythmic locomotor activity. However, locomotion occurs only when this automatic process is initiated "volitionally" or "emotionally." The volitional process involves the cerebral cortex while an emotional process involves the limbic system. The basal ganglia influence volitional, emotional and automatic processes through its interactions with the cerebral cortex, limbic system, and brainstem, respectively. Furthermore, real-time sensory feedback via visual signals, vestibular, and proprioceptive signals is crucial for locomotor adaptation. In summary, walking is mainly a result of automatic process, involving the spinal cord and brainstem mechanisms. It is usually achieved and maintained without conscious awareness and cognitive processing.

ALTERED NEURAL CONTROL AND PATHOMECHANICS OF POST-STROKE HEMIPLEGIC GAIT

Neural control mechanisms are altered in stroke survivors with walking dysfunction. As compared to normal healthy controls, stroke survivors have fewer modules during walking (Clark et al., 2010). In their study (Clark et al., 2010), Clark and colleagues analyzed modules based on EMG signals from eight leg muscles in 55 subjects with chronic stroke and in 20 controls. Most of affected legs had only just two or three modules. These modules were merged from the modules observed in control subjects, thus less independent neural control for affected leg. Furthermore, the authors reported that the number of simplified modules was correlated to preferred walking speed, speed modulation, step length asymmetry, and propulsive asymmetry. In other words, stroke survivors with fewer modules on the paretic limb walk more slowly and demonstrate more gait asymmetry (Routson et al., 2014).This modification of modular organization likely reflects the central nervous system's response to muscle weakness and lack of voluntary muscle control on the affected side to improve body support and locomotion. In addition to simplified modular organization, abnormal muscle synergies and spastic synergistic activation patterns are often resulted as well (Kline et al., 2007; Finley et al., 2008). For example, Finley et al. demonstrated a reflex-mediated coupling between hip flexion and knee extension in stroke survivors (Finley et al., 2008). As a result of abnormal patterns of muscle activation, joint positions are altered at rest and joint movements are coupled during walking.

A full spectrum of gait abnormality is observed clinically, depending on the level of muscle weakness, severity of spasticity, compensatory mechanisms, and their interactions. Primarily due to muscle strength on the paretic side, there is a hierarchy of gait impairments. According to walking speeds which correspond to muscle weakness, stroke survivors are classified into four groups with different features of gait impairments (Mulroy et al., 2003). They are: Fast walker, Moderate walker, Slow-Extended walker (circumductory gait), and Slow-Flexed walker.

In the Fast walker group, a stroke survivor has ~44% of a normal walking speed. There is a lack of heel rise in the terminal stance, due to inadequate plantarflexor (PF) muscle strength. Otherwise, discriminating gait events are within normal limits. Knee hyperextension in the stance phase is observed to compensate for lack of heel rise so that the body can roll forward onto the forefoot. As such, the step length is compromise secondary to lack of transition of momentum from the unaffected limb.

A typical Moderate walker has ~21% of a normal walking speed. The stroke survivor is able to walk without any assistance. The plantar flexor muscles on the paretic side are further weakened. There are some weakness in hip extensors (gluteus maximum) and knee extensors (quadriceps muscle). Along with weakness, Gluteus maximum muscles, quadriceps, and plantarflexors start to show spastic responses to quick stretch. As a result, excessive knee flexion and hip flexion occur at the mid stance phase. Due to the lack of pre-swing forward progression over the toe rocker, ankle plantar flexion, knee flexion, and heel-off are inadequate in the terminal stance. However, the survivor is still able to achieve a neutral foot position for clearance in the mid swing phase.

In the Slow-Extended walker group, quadriceps muscles are further weakened, and are not able to support the knee during the stance phase. Though weak, the gluteus maximus muscle is still strong enough to retract the femur into knee hyperextension to support the body. There are also some plantarflexors contracture and spasticity to provide necessary ankle stability. During the swing phase, there is persistent gluteus maximum and ankle plantarflexor spasticity. Hip hiking and leg circumduction occur for foot clearance. Stroke survivors in this group usually require assistive devices to walk. The walking speed is further decreased at ~11% of a normal speed.

In the Slow-Flexed walker group, the gluteus maximus muscle is weakened further to the extent that it is not able to retract the femur to stabilize the knee. Strength limitation across hip, knee and ankle joints leaves stroke survivors with the boardline walking ability. In the mid stance, there is excessive hip and knee flexion, ankle dorsiflexion, and trunk forward leaning. This posture persists in the swing phase with assistance. The assisted walking speed is at about 10% of a normal speed.

PATHOPHYSIOLOGY OF HEMIPARESIS AND SPASTICITY AFTER STROKE

Spasticity and muscle weakness (i.e., spastic paresis) are the primary motor impairments and impose significant challenges for patient care. Spasticity is estimated to be present in about 20–40% of stroke survivors (Zorowitz et al., 2013). Clinically, post-stroke spasticity is easily recognized as a phenomenon of velocity-dependent increase in tonic stretch reflexes ("muscle tone") with exaggerated tendon jerks, resulting from hyperexcitability of the stretch reflex (Lance, 1980). Based on decades of animal studies and recent human research (Brown, 1994; Gracies, 2005; Nielsen et al., 2007; Mukherjee and Chakravarty, 2010; Burke et al., 2013; Stecco et al., 2014; Li and Francisco, 2015), there are advances in understanding the pathophysiology of spasticity and its relation with paresis (Li and Francisco, 2015; Li, 2017). A brief summary is presented here. In a stroke survivor with spastic hemiplegia, damages occur to the motor cortices and their descending corticospinal tract (CST). These damages cause muscle weakness (usually hemiparesis) immediately after stroke, including upper extremity, trunk, and lower extremity muscles on the affected side. On the other hand, neuroplasticity occurs after stroke as well. Due to lesions of corticobulbar pathways accompanied with lesion of motor cortices and/or descending CST, bulbospinal hyperexcitability develops due to loss of supraspinal inhibition. This is mainly a phenomenon of disinhibition, or unmasking effects. There are several potential candidates, including reticulospinal (RST), vestibulospinal (VST), and rubrospinal projections (Miller et al., 2014; Li and Francisco, 2015; Owen et al., 2017). Medial RST hyperexcitability appears to be the most likely mechanism related to post-stroke spasticity (Li and Francisco, 2015). RST hyperexcitability provides unopposed excitatory descending inputs to spinal stretch reflex circuits, resulting in elevated excitability of spinal motor neurons. This adaptive change can account for most clinical findings on spasticity, for example, exaggerated stretch reflex, velocity-dependent resistance to stretch, muscle overactivity, or spontaneous firings of motor units. Spasticity usually leads to a synergistic pattern of activation during standing and walking, e.g., flexor synergy in the upper extremity and extensor synergy in the lower limb (Francisco and Li, 2016). The inter-limb activation coupling between upper and lower extremities is also reported (Kline et al., 2007).

A NEW PERSPECTIVE FOR UNDERSTANDING HEMIPLEGIC GAIT

These recent advances in understanding the pathophysiology of spasticity and its relations to muscle weakness can help us better understand hemiplegic gait in stroke survivors. Given the disinhibited brainstem descending pathways (RST and VST) are linked to post-stroke spasticity, reorganization of modular control, and spastic synergistic activation, a new perspective for understanding hemiplegic gait is schematically illustrated in **Figure 1**. Muscle weakness is primarily a result of damage to motor cortices and their descending CST after stroke. Muscle strength, especially knee extensor strength determines gait independence (Akazawa et al., 2017). Disinhibited brainstem descending pathways (RST and VST) are hyperexcitable. These descending projections are diffuse and the activated muscles are organized into fewer modules or motor synergies that provide body support and posture stability and locomotion (Nielsen, 2003; Beyaert et al., 2015). In addition, they also mediate spasticity and spastic synergistic patterns. The most commonly observed abnormal patterns include flexor synergies in the upper extremity and extensor synergies in the lower extremity. These spastic activations also lead to abnormal coupling within a limb (Finley et al., 2008) and between limbs (Kline et al., 2007). The interactions among muscle weakness, spasticity, and spastic activations act on the trunk, pelvis and the legs. Mechanical consequences of these interactions are the clinically observed gait impairments. They are exemplified in the stereotypical hemiplegic gait. It is usually described as hip extension, adduction, and medial rotation, knee extension, ankle plantar flexion, and inversion. The spastic muscles are synergistically activated into hip and knee extension during the stance phase of walking. The abnormal activation does not allow the hip and knee to flex for foot clearance. To compensate for these impairments, stroke survivors usually hike hip and circumduct the affected leg during the swing phase for foot clearance. As such it is known as a "circumductory gait." Depending on the severity of weakness and spasticity, and the degree of involvement (focal, regional, or extensive), a wide spectrum of gait impairments are clinically observed, as described above.

IMPLICATIONS FOR MANAGEMENT OF HEMIPLEGIC GAIT

Improving walking safety and speed is the major goal for gait rehabilitation for stroke survivors to prevent falls and subsequently to improve quality of life (Olney and Richards, 1996; Dobkin, 2005). A multi-modality interdisciplinary approach is usually employed and encouraged to bring the maximum clinical outcomes for stroke survivors. Gait rehabilitation programs include muscle strength training, task-specific gait training, treadmill training, electromechanical and robot-assisted gait training, functional electrical stimulations, ankle foot orthoses (AFOs), virtual reality, mental practice with motor imagery, and botulinum toxin injection of spastic muscles (Verma et al., 2012; Tenniglo et al., 2014; Beyaert et al., 2015;

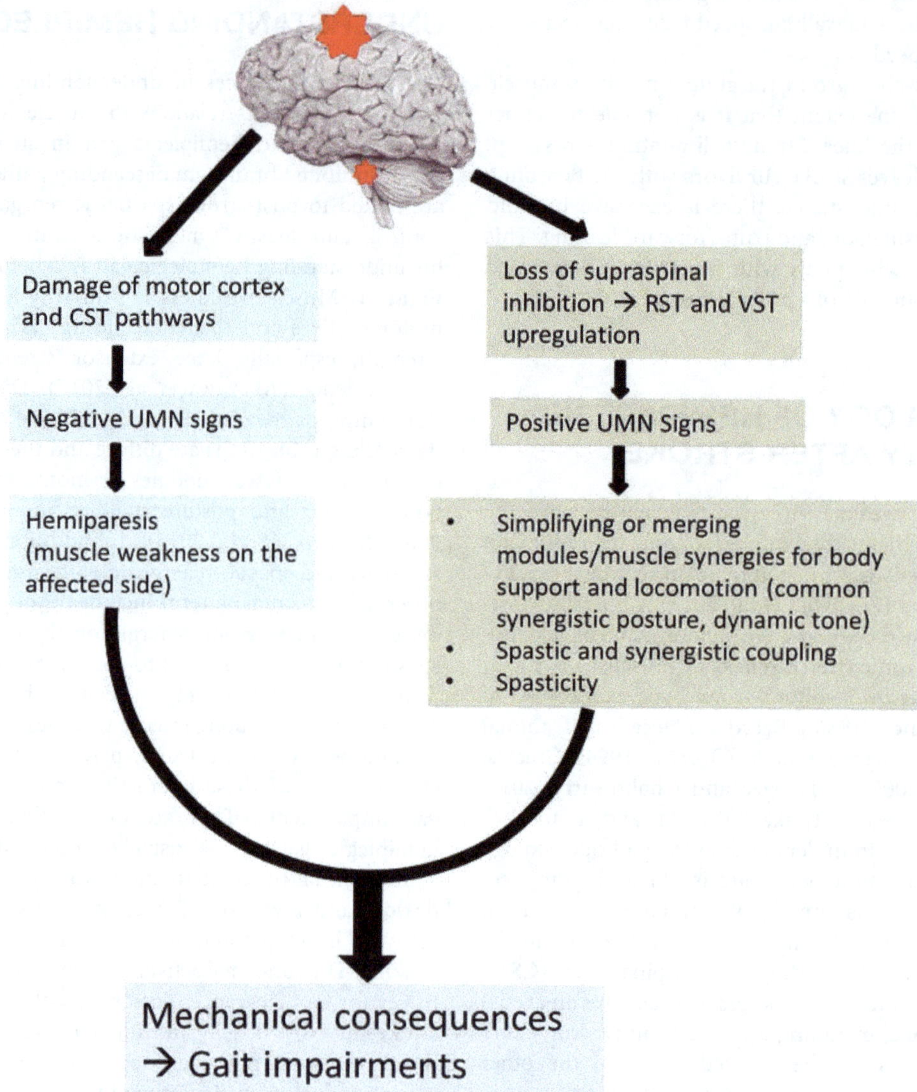

FIGURE 1 | Altered neural control for post-stroke gait. CST, corticospinal tract; RST, reticulospinal tract; VST, vestibulospinal tract.

Hsu et al., 2017; Jacinto and Reis Silva, 2018). The proposed new perspective also has clinical implications to improve management of hemiplegic gait. A few areas are discussed here as examples.

Spastic Kinetic Chain and Orthotic Management

As outlined above and in **Figure 1**, gait abnormality is a mechanical consequence of altered neural control after stroke. Abnormal joint posture during the stance phase represents the net result of interactions between ground reaction force and activation of spastic paretic muscles. For example, inadequate quadriceps support often results in a unique joint abnormality during the stance phase, i.e., greater knee flexion in the Moderate walker group. This knee position places the ground reaction force further anterior to the ankle joint, posterior to the knee joint, and anterior to the hip joint. In response to the increased moment imposed to each joint of the kinetic chain, spastic activation of gluteus muscles to assist hip extension, of quadriceps muscles to assist knee extension, and of ankle plantarflexors and invertors to assist ankle dorsiflexion and stabilization. For such a spastic kinetic chain, bracing with ankle-foot-orthosis to decrease ankle dorsiflexion angle is likely effective in changing the vector of ground reaction force (Owen, 2010). The forces required for maintaining joint position at each joint are reduced, and body support and joint stability are improved.

Muscle Selection for Botulinum Toxin Therapy

Botulinum toxin therapy is often used for spasticity management of leg muscles to improve gait (Esquenazi et al., 2015; Baker et al., 2016). Botulinum toxin (BoNT) acts to block presynaptic release of acetylcholine at the neuromuscular junction, therefore, intramuscular injection of BoNT can lead to spasticity reduction (Jahn, 2006). Due to this, BoNT injection also results in muscle weakness. As stated above, increased spasticity of quadriceps is likely to be part of synergistic activation for body support and posture stabilization. Quadriceps strength and support determines walking independence (Akazawa et al., 2017). Though quadriceps spasticity is often linked to knee joint stiffness, judicious consideration of treatment for spasticity is required because of the side effect of muscle weakness from BoNT. Another common observation is that stroke survivors have ankle plantarflexion and ankle inversion. Intramuscular EMG exams may detect spontaneous motor unit activation potentials (MUAPs) in most relevant muscles, such as tibialis posterior, gastrocnemius, soleus, tibialis anterior, extensor hallux longus muscles, i.e., spasticity (Mottram et al., 2009, 2010; Chang et al., 2013). It is not surprising to detect spasticity in all of these muscles, given diffused activation of brainstem descending pathways. The clinical presentation of ankle plantarflexion and ankle inversion suggests that this abnormality is primarily caused by tibialis posterior, gastrocnemius, and soleus, or spasticity of these muscles overrides spasticity of tibialis anterior and extensor halluces longus muscles. Not all muscles with spasticity need botulinum toxin injection in this case. Rather, selection of muscles is based on mechanical consequences of spastic muscles and their relation to ankle and foot positioning during walking.

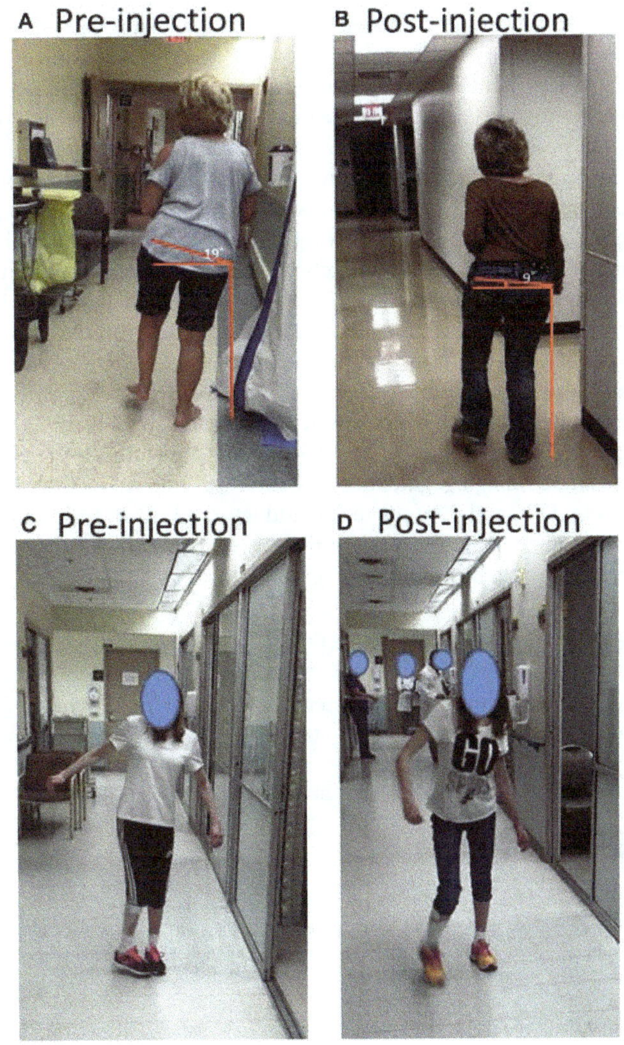

FIGURE 2 | (A,B) A stroke survivor with spasticity that resulted in dramatic trunk lateral flexion and hip hiking before and after botulinum toxin injections; **(C,D)** A stroke survivor with spasticity that resulted in dynamic hip adduction and pelvic anterior rotation before and after botulinum toxin injection. See text for details.

Muscles for Pelvis and Posture Control

Major kinematic determinants were originally proposed to explain contributions of individual joints (pelvic movement, hip, knee, and ankle joints) to minimize the COG displacement. The purpose was to understand human gait in general and to explain gait abnormality after orthopedic disorders in particular, such as hip joint fusion. As mentioned above, these kinematic determinants were in general validated by the modern instrumented gait analysis. Even though three out of six kinematic determinants involve pelvic movement, EMG studies are almost limited to leg muscles. Only one muscle (gluteus maximus) related to pelvic movement is commonly studied (Perry and Burnfield, 2010). The neural control mechanisms (brainstem-spinal network) involve trunk muscles and other pelvic movement related muscles as well. Post-stroke spastic hemiparesis could involve all muscles on the affected side. Depending on clinical presentations, these pelvic muscles could be the primary contributors of the gait impairments (**Figure 2**). Two cases are presented here to highlight the importance of spastic latissimus dorsi muscle and gluteus medius and tensor fasciae latae (TFL) muscles in post-stroke gait control. Written informed consent was obtained for scientific publication from both patients.

Case 1

A 62 year old right-handed female suffered right middle cerebral artery ischemic stroke 6 years ago with a residual left spastic hemiplegia. She was able to ambulate without any assistive device at a moderate walking speed. She presented with a mild circumductory gait. Lateral trunk flexion to the left side and her left hip hiking were prominent and constant during walking. According to its spread origin of latissimus dorsi muscle from inferior 3–4 ribs, low thoracic spine, lumbar spine and iliac crest, and its insertion to the intertubercular groove of the humerus, a spastic latissimus dorsi muscle was viewed to be responsible for this patient's abnormal posture during walking, including pelvic vertical elevation in the coronal plane, trunk lateral flexion, shoulder adduction, and internal rotation (**Figure 2A**). A total of 150 units of onabotulinumtoxin A were injected into this muscle under ultrasound imaging guidance. Trunk lateral flexion and pelvic elevation were much improved at 6 weeks after injection. As shown on **Figure 2B**, pelvic vertical elevation was decreased from 19 to 9° after injection.

Case 2

A 27 year old right handed female had a history of stroke after a traumatic brain injury 20 years ago which resulted in right spastic hemiplegia. She received botulinum toxin injections several times in the first 3 years after the accident. At a seated or supine position, she only had very mild muscle weakness in the right upper and lower extremities with minimum to negligible spasticity. The chief complaint was that her right toes were hitting the left toes during the mid-swing phase, i.e., problematic right hip internal rotation and adduction secondary to dynamic tone (**Figure 2C**). According to possible pathomechanics, dynamic spasticity in right anterior gluteus medius and TFL muscles could cause excessive anterior rotation of the pelvis in the transverse plane and hip internal rotation, while hip adductor spasticity contributes further to hip adduction. A total of 200 units of incobotulinumtoxin A were injected to these muscles under ultrasound imaging guidance (75 units to gluteus medius, 50 units to TFL, and 75 units to hip adductors). Improved walking posture in the follow up visit at 6 weeks after injection validated the pathomechanics analysis (**Figure 2D**).

CONCLUDING REMARKS

Given the disinhibited brainstem descending pathways (RST and VST) are linked to post-stroke spasticity, reorganization of modular control, and spastic synergistic activation, a new perspective for understanding hemiplegic gait is proposed. This new perspective highlights post-stroke hemiplegic gait impairments as mechanical consequences of altered neural control mechanisms of human gait. Hemiplegic gait is not a result of isolated skeletal muscular disorder, as often seen after orthopedic disorders. In clinical observational analysis, muscle weakness, spasticity, and spastic activation on the paretic arm, trunk and leg need to be taken into consideration. This new perspective also advances clinical management strategies as outlined above. However, these are examples and cases. They need to be validated in future laboratory and clinical studies.

AUTHOR CONTRIBUTIONS

SL developed the initial version of the manuscript and created the figures. GF and PZ critically revised the manuscript and contributed substantially to the manuscript development. All authors read and approved the final manuscript.

FUNDING

This study was supported in part by NIH NICHD/NCMRR R21HD087128, R21HD090453.

REFERENCES

Akazawa, N., Okawa, N., Tamura, K., and Moriyama, H. (2017). Determining the cut-off value for knee extensor strength for identifying independence in gait in chronic stroke survivors. *J. Rehabil. Med.* 49, 765–767. doi: 10.2340/16501977-2279

Allen, J. L., and Neptune, R. R. (2012). Three-dimensional modular control of human walking. *J. Biomech.* 45, 2157–2163. doi: 10.1016/j.jbiomech.2012.05.037

Baker, R., Esquenazi, A., Benedetti, M. G., and Desloovere, K. (2016). Gait analysis: clinical facts. *Eur. J. Phys. Rehabil. Med.* 52, 560–574.

Batchelor, F. A., MacKintosh, S. F., Said, C. M., and Hill, K. D. (2012). Falls after stroke. *Int. J. Stroke* 7, 482–490. doi: 10.1111/j.1747-4949.2012.00796.x

Benjamin, E. J., Blaha, M. J., Chiuve, S. E., Cushman, M., Das, S. R., Deo, R., et al. (2017). Heart disease and stroke statistics-2017 update: a report from the American Heart Association. *Circulation* 135, e146–e603. doi: 10.1161/CIR.0000000000000485

Bernstein, N. A. (1967). *The Co-ordination and Regulation of Movements.* Oxford: T. Pergamon Press.

Beyaert, C., Vasa, R., and Frykberg, G. E. (2015). Gait post-stroke: pathophysiology and rehabilitation strategies. *Neurophysiol. Clin.* 45, 335–355. doi: 10.1016/j.neucli.2015.09.005

Brown, P. (1994). Pathophysiology of spasticity. *J. Neurol. Neurosurg. Psychiatry* 57, 773–777. doi: 10.1136/jnnp.57.7.773

Burke, D., Wissel, J., and Donnan, G. A. (2013). Pathophysiology of spasticity in stroke. *Neurology* 80, S20–S26. doi: 10.1212/WNL.0b013e31827624a7

Chang, S. H., Francisco, G. E., Zhou, P., Rymer, W. Z., and Li, S. (2013). Spasticity, weakness, force variability, and sustained spontaneous motor unit discharges of resting spastic-paretic biceps brachii muscles in chronic stroke. *Muscle Nerve* 48, 85–92. doi: 10.1002/mus.23699

Clark, D. J., Ting, L. H., Zajac, F. E., Neptune, R. R., and Kautz, S. A. (2010). Merging of healthy motor modules predicts reduced locomotor performance and muscle coordination complexity post-stroke. *J. Neurophysiol.* 103, 844–857. doi: 10.1152/jn.00825.2009

Croce, U. D., Riley, P. O., Lelas, J. L., and Kerrigan, D. C. (2001). A refined view of the determinants of gait. *Gait Posture* 14, 79–84. doi: 10.1016/S0966-6362(01)00128-X

Dietz, V. (1996). Interaction between central programs and afferent input in the control of posture and locomotion. *J. Biomech.* 29, 841–844. doi: 10.1016/0021-9290(95)00175-1

Dobkin, B. H. (2005). Rehabilitation after Stroke. *N. Engl. J. Med.* 352, 1677–1684. doi: 10.1056/NEJMcp043511

Drew, T., Kalaska, J., and Krouchev, N. (2008). Muscle synergies during locomotion in the cat: a model for motor cortex control. *J. Physiol.* 586, 1239–1245. doi: 10.1113/jphysiol.2007.146605

Duncan, P. W., Zorowitz, R., Bates, B., Choi, J. Y., Glasberg, J. J., Graham, G. D., et al. (2005). Management of adult stroke rehabilitation care. a clinical practice guideline. *Stroke* 36, e100–e143. doi: 10.1161/01.STR.0000180861.54180.FF

Esquenazi, A., Moon, D., Wikoff, A., and Sale, P. (2015). Hemiparetic gait and changes in functional performance due to OnabotulinumtoxinA injection to lower limb muscles. *Toxicon* 107, 109–113. doi: 10.1016/j.toxicon.2015.08.004

Finley, J. M., Perreault, E. J., and Dhaher, Y. Y. (2008). Stretch reflex coupling between the hip and knee: implications for impaired gait following stroke. *Exp. Brain Res.* 188, 529–540. doi: 10.1007/s00221-008-1383-z

Francisco, G. E., and Li, S. (2016). *Spasticity. Physical Medicine and Rehabilitation, 5th Edn*, ed D. X. CIfu (Philadelphia, PA: Elsevier), 487–489.

Gard, S. A., and Childress, D. S. (1997). The effect of pelvic list on the vertical displacement of the trunk during normal walking. *Gait Posture* 5, 233–238. doi: 10.1016/S0966-6362(96)01089-2

Gard, S. A., and Childress, D. S. (1999). The influence of stance-phase knee flexion on the vertical displacement of the trunk during normal walking. *Arch. Phys. Med. Rehabil.* 80, 26–32. doi: 10.1016/S0003-9993(99)90303-9

Gracies, J. M. (2005). Pathophysiology of spastic paresis. II: Emergence of muscle overactivity. *Muscle Nerve* 31, 552–571. doi: 10.1002/mus.20285

Hayot, C., Sakka, S., and Lacouture, P. (2013). Contribution of the six major gait determinants on the vertical center of mass trajectory and the vertical ground reaction force. *Hum. Mov. Sci.* 32, 279–289. doi: 10.1016/j.humov.2012.10.003

Hendricks, H. T., van Limbeek, J., Geurts, A. C., and Zwarts, M. J. (2002). Motor recovery after stroke: a systematic review of the literature. *Arch. Phys. Med. Rehabil.* 83, 1629–1637. doi: 10.1053/apmr.2002.35473

Hsu, C. J., Kim, J., Roth, E. J., Rymer, W. Z., and Wu, M. (2017). Forced use of the paretic leg induced by a constraint force applied to the nonparetic leg in individuals poststroke during walking. *Neurorehabil. Neural Repair* 31, 1042–1052. doi: 10.1177/1545968317740972

Hyndman, D., Ashburn, A., and Stack, E. (2002). Fall events among people with stroke living in the community: circumstances of falls and characteristics of fallers. *Arch. Phys. Med. Rehabil.* 83, 165–170. doi: 10.1053/apmr.2002.28030

Jacinto, L. J., and Reis Silva, M. (2018). Gait analysis in the context of spasticity management. *Biosyst. Biorobot.* 19, 471–487. doi: 10.1007/978-3-319-72736-3_31

Jahn, R. (2006). Neuroscience. A neuronal receptor for botulinum toxin. *Science* 312, 540–541. doi: 10.1126/science.1127236

Kline, T. L., Schmit, B. D., and Kamper, D. G. (2007). Exaggerated interlimb neural coupling following stroke. *Brain* 130, 159–169. doi: 10.1093/brain/awl278

Kuo, A. D. (2007). The six determinants of gait and the inverted pendulum analogy: a dynamic walking perspective. *Hum. Mov. Sci.* 26, 617–656. doi: 10.1016/j.humov.2007.04.003

Lance, J. W. (1980). "Symposium synopsis," in *Spasticity: Disordered Motor Control*, eds R. G. Feldman, R. R. Young, and W. P. Koella (Chicago, IL: Year Book Medical Publishers), 485–494.

Li, S. (2017). Spasticity, motor recovery, and neural plasticity after stroke. *Front. Neurol.* 8:120. doi: 10.3389/fneur.2017.00120

Li, S., and Francisco, G. (2015). New insights into the pathophysiology of post-stroke spasticity. *Front. Hum. Neurosci.* 9:192. doi: 10.3389/fnhum.2015.00192

Lin, Y. C., Gfoehler, M., and Pandy, M. G. (2014). Quantitative evaluation of the major determinants of human gait. *J. Biomech.* 47, 1324–1331. doi: 10.1016/j.jbiomech.2014.02.002

McGowan, C. P., Neptune, R. R., Clark, D. J., and Kautz, S. A. (2010). Modular control of human walking: adaptations to altered mechanical demands. *J. Biomech.* 43, 412–419. doi: 10.1016/j.jbiomech.2009.10.009

Miller, D. M., Klein, C. S., Suresh, N. L., and Rymer, W. Z. (2014). Asymmetries in vestibular evoked myogenic potentials in chronic stroke survivors with spastic hypertonia: evidence for a vestibulospinal role. *Clin. Neurophysiol.* 125, 2070–2078. doi: 10.1016/j.clinph.2014.01.035

Mottram, C. J., Suresh, N. L., Heckman, C. J., Gorassini, M. A., and Rymer, W. Z. (2009). Origins of abnormal excitability in biceps brachii motoneurons of spastic-paretic stroke survivors. *J. Neurophysiol.* 102, 2026–2038. doi: 10.1152/jn.00151.2009

Mottram, C. J., Wallace, C. L., Chikando, C. N., and Rymer, W. Z. (2010). Origins of spontaneous firing of motor units in the spastic-paretic biceps brachii muscle of stroke survivors. *J. Neurophysiol.* 104, 3168–3179. doi: 10.1152/jn.00463.2010

Mukherjee, A., and Chakravarty, A. (2010). Spasticity mechanisms–for the clinician. *Front. Neurol.* 1:149. doi: 10.3389/fneur.2010.00149

Mulroy, S., Gronley, J., Weiss, W., Newsam, C., and Perry, J. (2003). Use of cluster analysis for gait pattern classification of patients in the early and late recovery phases following stroke. *Gait Posture* 18, 114–125. doi: 10.1016/S0966-6362(02)00165-0

Neptune, R. R., Clark, D. J., and Kautz, S. A. (2009). Modular control of human walking: a simulation study. *J. Biomech.* 42, 1282–1287. doi: 10.1016/j.jbiomech.2009.03.009

Nielsen, J. B. (2003). How we walk: central control of muscle activity during human walking. *Neuroscientist* 9, 195–204. doi: 10.1177/1073858403009003012

Nielsen, J. B., Crone, C., and Hultborn, H. (2007). The spinal pathophysiology of spasticity–from a basic science point of view. *Acta Physiol.* 189, 171–180. doi: 10.1111/j.1748-1716.2006.01652.x

Olney, S. J., and Richards, C. (1996). Hemiparetic gait following stroke. Part I: Characteristics. *Gait Posture* 4, 136–148. doi: 10.1016/0966-6362(96)01063-6

Owen, E. (2010). The importance of being earnest about shank and thigh kinematics especially when using ankle-foot orthoses. *Prosthet. Orthot. Int.* 34, 254–269. doi: 10.3109/03093646.2010.485597

Owen, M., Ingo, C., and Dewald, J. P. A. (2017). Upper extremity motor impairments and microstructural changes in bulbospinal pathways in chronic hemiparetic stroke. *Front. Neurol.* 8:257. doi: 10.3389/fneur.2017.00257

Perry, J., and Burnfield, J. M. (2010). *Gait Analysis: Normal and Pathological Function, 2nd Edn.* Thorofare, NJ: SLACK Incorporated.

Richards, C. L., and Olney, S. J. (1996). Hemiparetic gait following stroke. Part II: recovery and physical therapy. *Gait Posture* 4, 149–162. doi: 10.1016/0966-6362(96)01064-8

Routson, R. L., Kautz, S. A., and Neptune, R. R. (2014). Modular organization across changing task demands in healthy and poststroke gait. *Physiol. Rep.* 2:e12055. doi: 10.14814/phy2.12055

Saunders, J. B., Inman, V. T., and Eberhart, H. D. (1953). The major determinants in normal and pathological gait. *J. Bone Joint Surg. Am.* 35-A, 543–558. doi: 10.2106/00004623-195335030-00003

Stecco, A., Stecco, C., Raghavan, P. (2014). Peripheral mecahnisms contributing to spasticity and implications for treatment. *Curr. Phys. Med. Rehabil. Rep.* 2, 121–127. doi: 10.1007/s40141-014-0052-3

Tenniglo, M. J., Nederhand, M. J., Prinsen, E. C., Nene, A. V., Rietman, J. S., and Buurke, J. H. (2014). Effect of chemodenervation of the rectus femoris muscle in adults with a stiff knee gait due to spastic paresis: a systematic review with a meta-analysis in patients with stroke. *Arch. Phys. Med. Rehabil.* 95, 576–587. doi: 10.1016/j.apmr.2013.11.008

Ting, L. H., and McKay, J. L. (2007). Neuromechanics of muscle synergies for posture and movement. *Curr. Opin. Neurobiol.* 17, 622–628. doi: 10.1016/j.conb.2008.01.002

Verma, R., Arya, K. N., Sharma, P., and Garg, R. K. (2012). Understanding gait control in post-stroke: implications for management. *J. Bodyw. Mov. Ther.* 16, 14–21. doi: 10.1016/j.jbmt.2010.12.005

Winter, D. A. (1992). Foot trajectory in human gait: a precise and multifactorial motor control task. *Phys. Ther.* 72, 45–56. doi: 10.1093/ptj/72.1.45

Zorowitz, R. D., Gillard, P. J., and Brainin, M. (2013). Poststroke spasticity: sequelae and burden on stroke survivors and caregivers. *Neurology* 80, S45–S52. doi: 10.1212/WNL.0b013e3182764c86

7

Altered Neuromodulatory Drive may Contribute to Exaggerated Tonic Vibration Reflexes in Chronic Hemiparetic Stroke

*Jacob G. McPherson[1,2], Laura M. McPherson[1,2,3], Christopher K. Thompson[4,5], Michael D. Ellis[2], Charles J. Heckman[2,5] and Julius P. A. Dewald[2,6]**

[1] Department of Biomedical Engineering, Florida International University, Miami, FL, United States, [2] Department of Physical Therapy and Human Movement Sciences, Northwestern University Feinberg School of Medicine, Chicago, IL, United States, [3] Department of Physical Therapy, Florida International University, Miami, FL, United States, [4] Department of Physical Therapy, Temple University, Philadelphia, PA, United States, [5] Department of Physiology, Northwestern University Feinberg School of Medicine, Chicago, IL, United States, [6] Department of Biomedical Engineering, Northwestern University, Evanston, IL, United States

***Correspondence:**
Julius P. A. Dewald
j-dewald@northwestern.edu

Exaggerated stretch-sensitive reflexes are a common finding in elbow flexors of the contralesional arm in chronic hemiparetic stroke, particularly when muscles are not voluntarily activated prior to stretch. Previous investigations have suggested that this exaggeration could arise either from an abnormal tonic ionotropic drive to motoneuron pools innervating the paretic limbs, which could bring additional motor units near firing threshold, or from an increased influence of descending monoaminergic neuromodulatory pathways, which could depolarize motoneurons and amplify their responses to synaptic inputs. However, previous investigations have been unable to differentiate between these explanations, leaving the source(s) of this excitability increase unclear. Here, we used tonic vibration reflexes (TVRs) during voluntary muscle contractions of increasing magnitude to infer the sources of spinal motor excitability in individuals with chronic hemiparetic stroke. We show that when the paretic and non-paretic elbow flexors are preactivated to the same percentage of maximum prior to vibration, TVRs remain significantly elevated in the paretic arm. We also show that the rate of vibration-induced torque development increases as a function of increasing preactivation in the paretic limb, even though the amplitude of vibration-induced torque remains conspicuously unchanged as preactivation increases. It is highly unlikely that these findings could be explained by a source that is either purely ionotropic or purely neuromodulatory, because matching preactivation should control for the effects of a potential ionotropic drive (and lead to comparable tonic vibration reflex responses between limbs), while a purely monoaminergic mechanism would increase reflex magnitude as a function of preactivation. Thus, our results suggest that increased excitability of motor pools innervating the paretic limb post-stroke is likely to arise from both ionotropic and neuromodulatory mechanisms.

Keywords: stroke, motor control, stretch reflex, bulbospinal monoaminergic drive, motoneurons, sensorimotor integration

INTRODUCTION

Focal ischemic stroke causes changes in descending neural drive that alter spinal motor excitability (Stinear et al., 2007; Heckman et al., 2009; Bradnam et al., 2012; McMorland et al., 2015; McPherson et al., 2017, 2018; Owen et al., 2017). This can occur through direct effects on spinal neurons and/or by facilitating adaptive processes associated with shifts in the overall balance of spinal excitation and inhibition. In the chronic state post-stroke, spinal motor excitability generally increases in regions that control the paretic limbs; in regions innervating the non-paretic limbs, excitability remains at approximately pre-injury levels or is increased to a lesser degree (Lee et al., 1987; Powers et al., 1989; Thilmann et al., 1990, 1991; Ibrahim et al., 1993; McPherson et al., 2011, 2017; Hu et al., 2015). Increased spinal motor excitability could theoretically be related to alterations in ionotropic drive (i.e., signaling via ligand-gated channels that directly elicits excitatory or inhibitory post-synaptic potentials), neuromodulatory drive (i.e., signaling via metabotropic receptors to modify the intrinsic excitability of the cell), or both. However, it is currently unknown which of these options primarily underlies increased spinal motor excitability in paretic motor pools because the results of previous investigations could have plausibly been explained by either phenomenon alone (Powers et al., 1989; McPherson et al., 2008; Mottram et al., 2009, 2010).

Stretch-sensitive reflexes are a useful assay of spinal motor excitability. For example, exaggerated mechanical and electromyographical responses to imposed joint excursions in paretic limbs have proven to be both conspicuous and enduring findings in chronic hemiparetic stroke. These reflex exaggerations are known clinically as spasticity (Lance, 1980). Reflexive contractions developed during maintained muscle or tendon vibration can also be used to assess spinal motor excitability (Eklund and Hagbarth, 1966; Hagbarth and Eklund, 1966; Gillies et al., 1971; Matthews, 1984; McPherson et al., 2008). These contractions are known as tonic vibration reflexes (TVRs). We have previously shown that TVRs are dramatically amplified in resting muscles of the paretic arm compared to homologous muscles of the non-paretic arm, and robust muscle activation persists in the paretic arm long after removal of the vibration (McPherson et al., 2008). The finding of both amplification and prolongation of motor output in paretic muscles is important because it may point to an increased influence of descending monoaminergic neuromodulatory pathways. Indeed, a hallmark of monoaminergic actions on somatic motoneurons is the development of persistent inward currents (PICs) in motoneuron dendrites, which uniquely amplify and prolong motoneuron output in response to excitatory synaptic inputs (Schwindt and Crill, 1977; Powers and Binder, 2001; Heckman et al., 2003, 2009).

However, some signs of an increased neuromodulatory influence appear to diminish when muscles are volitionally preactivated. For example, we and others have demonstrated that stretch reflex amplitude equilibrates between paretic and non-paretic muscles when the muscles are preactivated to the same extent prior to stretch (Lee et al., 1987; Burne et al., 2005; Mottram et al., 2009, 2010; McPherson et al., 2017). Additionally, some estimates of PIC amplitude are indistinguishable between paretic and control muscles during volitional ramp contractions (Mottram et al., 2009, 2010). Although equivocal, these findings are usually taken as evidence that a tonic, low-level ionotropic drive mediates the resting excitability imbalance between arms rather than an increased neuromodulatory drive (Mottram et al., 2009, 2010). In this scenario, the tonic ionotropic drive provides a sub-threshold depolarization to the resting motoneuron pool. The pre-reflex volitional descending drive depolarizes the motoneuron pool above spiking threshold, eclipsing the tonic ionotropic drive and effectively washing out the resting excitability imbalance. As a result, reflex amplitude is comparable in both limbs and increases as a function of pre-reflex muscle activation.

Here, we characterize TVRs in elbow flexors of the paretic and non-paretic arms of individuals with chronic hemiparetic stroke at three levels of preactivation. In particular, we quantify TVR-evoked elbow flexion joint torque amplitude and rise time, metrics that can be used to infer the spinal neuromodulatory state (McPherson et al., 2008; Revill and Fuglevand, 2017). We predicted that TVR-evoked torque would equilibrate between paretic and non-paretic arms when muscles were preactivated to the same degree prior to vibration, based on parallels with torque responses to stretch reflexes elicited by imposed joint excursion. Contrary to our prediction, we found pronounced amplification of TVR responses in the paretic arm despite matching preactivation levels between limbs. Perhaps more conspicuously, however, the magnitude of TVR-evoked torque did not scale with preactivation level in either limb. This finding stands in contrast to the well-documented positive correlation between preactivation level and reflex amplitude in response to imposed joint excursion (Ibrahim et al., 1993; Burne et al., 2005; McPherson et al., 2017). We also found that the rise time of TVR-evoked torque was significantly more rapid with increasing preactivation in the paretic limb compared to the non-paretic limb. Given these surprising results, we then corroborated our findings in a proof-of-principle decerebrate cat preparation that also allowed visualization of individual motor unit firing characteristics. In this model, descending monoaminergic drive is elevated and invariant to synaptic input, and force output is *not* influenced by volition. Thus, force output in this model is due only to three factors: the sustained monoaminergic drive, Ia input (via vibration), and the resulting input-output function of the motoneurons. We interpret these results as evidence that both an ionotropic and monoaminergic neuromodulatory drive are likely to contribute to the apparent increased excitability of motor pools innervating paretic muscles post-stroke.

MATERIALS AND METHODS

Human-Subjects Experiments

Participant Characteristics and Ethics Statement

Ten individuals fulfilled all criteria for involvement in the study and subsequently completed the experimental protocol. The same individuals also participated in our original study of TVR responses post-stroke (McPherson et al., 2008). Each of these individuals (mean age: 59 ± 10 yrs) sustained a first-ever cortical or subcortical stroke at least 1 year prior to enrollment in the investigation (range: 40–124 months) and had lingering motor deficits on one side of the body. Fugl-Meyer motor assessment (FMA) scores ranged from 13 to 43 of a possible 66, representing severe to moderate impairment, and Ashworth scores (available for 6 of 10 participants) ranged from 2 to 4 (scoring: 0, 1, 2, 3, 4). Participant demographic and clinical data are summarized in **Table 1.**

For inclusion in the study, all participants were required to possess at least 90 degrees passive range of motion in shoulder flexion, shoulder abduction, and elbow flexion/extension. Participants were additionally required to exhibit some volitional control of elbow flexion/extension in order to obtain maximum voluntary torques (MVTs). The absence of inflammatory conditions at the shoulder, elbow, wrist and fingers was verified by overpressure at the end-range of motion. Potential participants were excluded from the study if the demonstrated minimal (50–66 on the FMA) or very severe (0–9 on the FMA) impairment, significant impairment of upper extremity tactile sensation or proprioception (O'Sullivan and Schmitz, 2001), or difficulties sitting for extended periods of time. All participants were required to have discontinued use of antispastic medications at least 6 months prior to enrollment; more recent or ongoing use was grounds for exclusion from the study.

All participants provided informed consent to participate in the investigation, which was approved by the Institutional Review Board of Northwestern University in accordance with the ethical standards stipulated by the 1964 Declaration of Helsinki for research involving human participants.

Experimental Setup

Participants were secured to a Biodex experimental chair (Biodex Medical Systems, Shirley, NY) by shoulder and lap belt restraints. The forearm, wrist and hand of each participant's paretic and non-paretic arms were fitted with custom fiberglass casts. The casted arm was coupled at the level of the wrist to a 6 degree-of-freedom load cell (Model 45E15A; JR3, Woodland, CA), and

TABLE 1 | Participant demographic and clinical data.

Participant	Age	Biological sex	Paretic arm	Fugl-meyer motor assessment	Ashworth score
1	68	M	R	18	2
2	40	M	L	40	2
3	53	F	R	13	2
4	59	M	R	14	4
5	61	M	L	43	2
6	50	F	R	21	2
7	65	M	L	18	NA
8	59	M	L	24	NA
9	77	M	R	30	NA
10	51	F	R	26	NA

Fugl-Meyer: 0–66; Ashworth: 0, 1, 2, 3, 4; NA, not available.

the limb was positioned such that it retained 75° of shoulder abduction, 40° of shoulder flexion, and 90° of elbow flexion. The test apparatus supported the weight of the limb throughout these experimental protocols.

Experimental Protocol

While interfaced with the isometric testing setup described above, participants were first required to generate MVTs in elbow flexion and extension. Visual feedback of performance was provided in real time for all trials. To obtain a reliable estimate of the true maximum torque capability in each direction, collection of MVTs continued until 3 trials were obtained within 10% of one another, without the last trial being the greatest.

For the TVR protocol, participants remained interfaced with the isometric setup used for testing MVTs, and a therapeutic massage vibrator (frequency: 112 Hz, model 91, Daito-Thrive, Showa-cho, Japan) was placed over the distal muscle belly of the biceps brachii. TVR trial onset and offset were indicated to the participant and experimentalist by auditory cues. TVR trials began after the experimentalist determined that the participant was fully relaxed (via real-time EMG and torque feedback). Upon trial onset, participants were first instructed to generate and maintain either 5 or 15% of their elbow flexion MVT, guided by visual feedback. Once the requisite torque was achieved, visual feedback was extinguished, and vibration commenced. The vibratory stimulus lasted for 5 s. Following each trial, participants were given at least a 15–30 s rest period to allow the limb to relax before beginning the next trial. First-pass trial acceptability was examined on-line by visual feedback provided to the experimentalist, and trials were excluded from further analysis if postural or unconstrained extremity movements occurred during the trial or if participants closed their eyes and appeared to fall asleep. Approximately 20 TVR response trials were collected at each of the 5 and 15% elbow flexion levels, and the protocol was performed on both the paretic and non-paretic limbs.

Data Analysis

Analyses of TVR-evoked elbow flexion torque were used as outcome measures in this study, computed using custom Matlab software (The MathWorks, Natick, MA). A Jacobian-based algorithm converted forces and moments recorded by the loadcell into elbow flexion/extension torques. The resulting torque curves were filtered with an eighth-order low-pass Butterworth filter with cutoff frequency of 50 Hz. Window averages of individual TVR trials were taken from 3.5 to 5.0 s after trial onset, corresponding to the preactivation phase, and from 9.5 to 10.0 s post-trial onset, corresponding to the last 500 ms of the vibration phase. We did not extract data during the post-vibration period because reflexive torque and EMG responses could not be reliably decoupled from volitional efforts to decrease elbow flexion torque. Preactivation windows and during-vibration windows were then ensemble-averaged for each participant and limb (paretic and non-paretic) for use in subsequent group analyses.

To quantify TVR-evoked torque amplitude, we computed the change in torque from preactivation to during-vibration for each participant's ensemble-averaged torque response. We computed this difference at each preactivation level (0, 5, 15%), and these values were subsequently used in group statistical analyses. Because of the likely difference in elbow flexion strength between paretic and non-paretic limbs, we calculated the TVR-evoked torque amplitude using both unnormalized torque (Nm) and normalized torque (% MVT). This dual approach ensured that between-limb results would not be inflated by normalization of paretic torque to lower MVT values.

We used two approaches to quantify the temporal profile of the rising phase of the TVR-evoked torque response. First, we computed the slope of a linear fit between each participant's preactivation torque and the time at which TVR-evoked torque reached 85% of the maximum stable response (Equation 1):

$$\textit{Rising slope of TVR evoked torque} = \frac{(torque_{85\%max} - torque_{preac})}{time_{85\%max} - time_{Vib.ON}} [\%MVT]/sec \quad (1)$$

Second, because TVR-evoked torque generally exhibits a non-linear temporal profile, we used non-linear least squares estimation to determine the optimal fit of each group mean ensemble-averaged torque response (i.e., paretic and non-paretic, each at 5 and 15% preactivation) to a function of the form:

$$\textit{Modeled TVR evoked torque} = a*(1 - e^{-t/b}) \quad (2)$$

In this equation, term a generally represents the amplitude of the TVR-evoked torque (add preactivation torque to a to approximate the final steady-state torque amplitude in the plots below), term b is the time constant describing the rate of rise of TVR-evoked torque, and t is elapsed time. The model was fit to experimental data from the time of vibration onset to the time of vibration offset; a and b are coefficients fit by the optimization routine and t is elapsed time. The parameters of this model are not intended to reflect specific biophysical features of motoneuron firing.

Statistical Analysis

For TVR-evoked torque amplitude, all statistical analyses were calculated on the normalized torque values. Unnormalized torque values are presented for comparison. A 2 × 3 repeated measures ANOVA was used to determine the main effects of limb (paretic, non-paretic) and preactivation level (0, 5, 15%), as well as the limb-by-preactivation level interaction, on normalized TVR-evoked torque amplitude. To reiterate, all participants included in this investigation were included in our original study of TVR responses post-stroke (McPherson et al., 2008), enabling data to be pooled across experiments to generate the new analyses presented here. Two sets of *post-hoc* t-tests were used. First, t-tests were used to determine differences between limbs at each preactivation level, with Bonferroni correction for multiple comparisons. Second, t-tests within each limb were used to evaluate differences between all combinations of preactivation levels, using Tukey correction for multiple comparisons within each limb.

For the slope of TVR-evoked torque, there were 60 total values (2 limbs × 3 preactivation levels × 10 participants). Several outliers were detected in both paretic and non-paretic values, which were excluded from further analysis. Outliers were defined as values exceeding 3 scaled median absolute deviations from the median. Given that a 2-way repeated measures ANOVA (which is most appropriate for this experimental design) requires no missing cases, the following method was used to account for the missing data and allow for a repeated measures ANOVA. First, if a participant had missing data for more than one preactivation level, all data for that participant was removed. This resulted in removing data from two participants for the non-paretic limb (with $N = 8$ remaining) and data from one participant in the paretic limb (with $N = 9$ remaining). Together, these removals reduced the total number of torque values from 60 to 51. There were two missing cases at one preactivation level for the non-paretic limb (for one participant at 0% and for another participant at 15%). Values for these cases were imputed by taking the average of values from the seven other participants. For the paretic limb, there was one missing case at the 0% condition, and the value was imputed by taking the average of the eight other participants for this condition. As a result, the number of total values that were imputed was 3 out of 51, or 5.9%. This method allowed for an ANOVA with a repeated factor of preactivation; however, because the number of participants for each limb was not the same, the factor of limb could not be repeated. Therefore, a mixed-model 2 × 3 ANOVA was used to determine the main effects of limb (paretic, non-paretic) and preactivation level (repeated measure; 0, 5, 15%) as well as the limb-by-preactivation level interaction on TVR-evoked slope magnitude. Between-limb *post-hoc* t-tests were used to determine differences in slope between paretic and non-paretic limbs at each preactivation level, with Bonferroni correction for multiple comparisons. Within-limb *post-hoc* t-tests were used to evaluate differences between all combinations of preactivation levels, using Tukey correction for multiple comparisons within each limb. Finally, a 2-way non-repeated measures ANOVA was also calculated without accounting for the missing data to ensure that the above analyses were not biased by methods used for accounting for missing data. Results from this ANOVA were virtually identical to those from the 2-way repeated measures ANOVA that is presented in the Results section below, with the same significant ANOVA effects and *post-hoc* test results.

To evaluate the goodness-of-fit of the non-linear model of TVR-evoked torque, we computed the variance accounted for (VAF) and sum-of-squared error (SSE) of the model. The effect of preactivation on the model parameters associated with the TVR-evoked portion of the torque profile was examined qualitatively for each limb.

Results of all analyses were considered significant at the $p < 0.05$ level, and p-values for the t-tests are presented in the results after application of corrections for multiple comparisons. All statistical analyses were performed in Prism (GraphPad software, Inc., version 7.0a).

Animal Experiments

As a first step toward providing additional mechanistic context for our human-subjects findings, we conducted a set of proof-of-principle TVR experiments in a decerebrate cat model. The primary goal of this model was to determine the impact of increasing preactivation level on the amplitude and rate of rise of TVR-evoked force. We chose the decerebrate cat preparation because it has a well-documented elevation of descending monoaminergic drive that does not scale with motor output (Crone et al., 1988) thus paralleling one potential mechanism underlying our chronic hemiparetic stroke findings. Further, we examined the motor unit firing patterns underlying the TVR-evoked forces to evaluate the effect of preactivation on motor unit rate modulation and recruitment during and after vibration.

Experimental Setting and Ethics Statement

Data were also collected in one adult cat sourced from a designated breeding establishment for scientific research. The animal was housed at Northwestern University's Center for Comparative Medicine, an AAALAC accredited animal research program. All procedures were approved by the Institutional Animal Care and Use Committee at Northwestern University and conform with accepted ethics standards (Grundy, 2015).

Surgical Procedure

Anesthesia was induced with 4% isoflurane and a 1:3 mixture of N_2O and O_2. Anesthetic depth was monitored via blood pressure, heart and respiratory rate, and withdrawal reflexes. Once surgically anesthetized, a tracheostomy was performed and a permanent tracheal tube was implanted. Isoflurane (0.5–2.5%) and gasses were delivered through the tube for the duration of the surgery. The animal was then transferred to a stereotaxic frame and immobilized by a head clamp, spinal clamp on the L2 dorsal vertebral process, and bilateral hip pins at the iliac crest. The left hindlimb was fixed with pins at the knee and clamps at the ankle, and the right hindlimb was secured using a clamp on the lower leg. The left soleus was dissected, isolated, and its distal tendon was attached to a load cell via a calcaneus bone chip in series with a linear variable differential transformer and customized voice coil. A distal, cutaneous branch of the right superficial peroneal nerve was dissected and a cuff electrode was secured around the nerve. The animal was then decerebrated at the precollicular level and anesthesia was discontinued (animals lack sentience after decerebration; Silverman et al., 2005). A thermistor was then placed in the esophagus and core temperature was maintained at 35–37°C. At the end of the experiment, the animal was euthanized using a 2 mM/kg solution of KCl in addition to a bilateral thoracotomy.

Data Collection

Referenced monopolar EMG activity was acquired using a custom 64-channel electrode array that covered the surface of the exposed soleus. The array consisted of 64 individual rigid silver pins, 7.5 mm in length and 0.7 mm in diameter, configured in a 5 × 13 matrix with an interelectrode distance of 2.54 mm. A ground electrode was place on the animal's back and a reference electrode was placed on the upper thigh. EMG data were bandpass filtered (100–900 Hz), amplified (0.5–2 k) and digitized (5,120 Hz) by a 12-bit A/D converter (EMG-USB 2, 256-channel EMG amplifier, OT Bioelettronica, Torino, Italy). Force data from the soleus muscle were simultaneously acquired.

With the animal's hindlimbs fixed, the soleus was activated by stimulating the contralateral superficial peroneal nerve through a cuff electrode (voltage-controlled stimulation; 50 Hz; 1 ms pulse width). This elicits the crossed-extension reflex and a maintained contraction. The magnitude of contraction is generally proportional to the applied voltage, and here, we used voltages ranging from 3.5 to 5 V. This evoked sub-maximal contractions up to ~25% of maximum force output, as confirmed by the appearance of force saturation with voltages at or above 6 V in this animal. After at least 2 s of stimulation (to acquire a stable baseline preactivation), 3–5 s of vibration of the soleus tendon commenced (~130 Hz; ~80 μm). This elicited a TVR. Electrical stimulation of the contralateral peroneal nerve continued for the duration of vibration, and we varied the applied voltage between trials to explore the impact of vibration at a range of preactivation levels.

Data and Statistical Analysis

Force data from the soleus was analyzed similarly to the elbow flexion torque data from the human subjects experiments. Preactivation force was calculated as the average of force values generated during the 0.5 s prior to vibration onset. TVR-evoked force amplitude was calculated as the change in force from the preactivation value to the average torque between 1 and 2 s post-vibration onset. The rising slope of the TVR-evoked force was calculated as with Eqn. 1 for the human data. The time to 85% max TVR-evoked force was calculated relative to vibration onset. Separate Pearson correlation calculations were used to determine if increasing preactivation level was associated with changes in TVR-evoked force amplitude, rising slope of the TVR-evoked force, or the time to 85% max TVR-evoked force.

To examine motor unit recruitment and rate modulation patterns underlying the TVR-evoked force due to different levels of preactivation, multi-channel EMG data from each trial were decomposed into individual motor unit spike trains using a blind source separation approach (Holobar et al., 2010, 2014; Negro et al., 2016). The instantaneous firing rate for each motor unit spike train was calculated as the reciprocal of the inter-spike interval.

RESULTS

TVR-Evoked Torque Amplitude

Across participants, maximum voluntary elbow flexion torque for the paretic limb averaged 34.85 Nm, whereas the non-paretic elbow flexion MVT averaged 62.29 Nm. Elicitation of the TVR in the paretic and non-paretic limbs in all cases resulted in an increase in net elbow flexion torque above the target preactivation level (**Figure 1**). Qualitatively, this torque developed rapidly upon vibration onset in the paretic limb and either monotonically increased during vibration or reached a stable plateau following the initial rising phase. The non-paretic limb demonstrated a more gradual increase in torque following vibration onset, which was also characterized by a monotonic rise or an initial increase followed by a plateau.

Table 2 shows the TVR-evoked torque amplitude (unnormalized and normalized; left and middle panels,

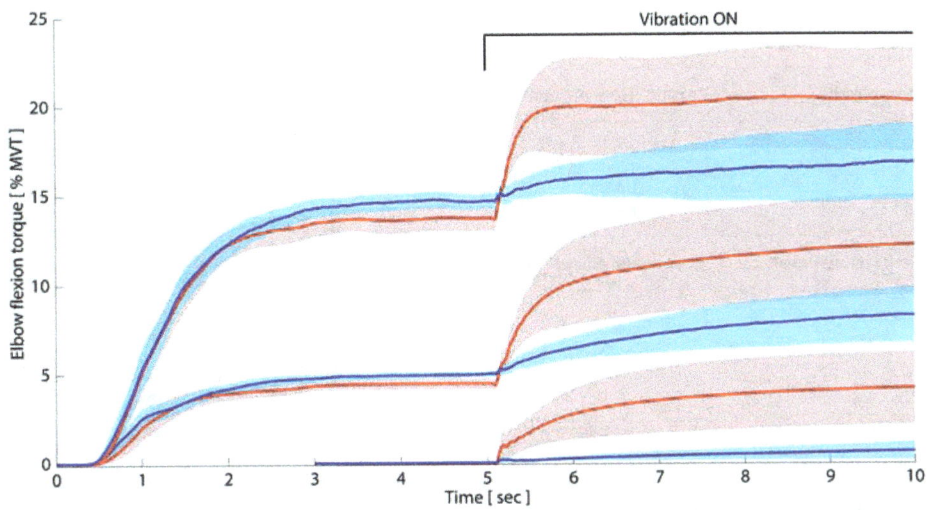

FIGURE 1 | Paretic limb tonic vibration reflexes remain exaggerated despite preactivation. Paretic and non-paretic elbow flexors were preactivated to 5 and 15% of MVT, respectively, before vibration began. Despite matching preactivation levels between limbs, group average ($N = 10$) paretic TVRs (pink) significantly exceeded non-paretic TVRs (blue). Bottom paretic and non-paretic traces are TVR responses in relaxed elbow flexors, with data adapted with permission from McPherson et al. (2018). Shaded region around each TVR curve represents ± 95% confidence interval. *Y-axis:* elbow flexion torque as percent of maximum; *x-axis:* time in seconds. Permission to adapt images from McPherson et al. (2008) is afforded by the American Physiological Society under original author rights.

TABLE 2 | TVR-evoked torque amplitude.

	TVR-evoked torque amplitude (Difference from preactivation to vibration-ON)						Torque amplitude during vibration (incl. preactivation torque) (% MVT)		
	Unnormalized Torque (Nm)			Normalized Torque (%MVT)					
Preactivation	**0%**	**5%**	**15%**	**0%**	**5%**	**15%**	**0%**	**5%**	**15%**
Paretic	1.20 ± 0.98	2.52 ± 1.32	2.25 ± 1.23%	3.75 ± 3.18%	7.79 ± 5.19%	7.41 ± 5.22%	4.48 ± 3.88%	12.02 ± 5.00%	21.00 ± 4.65%
Non-Paretic	0.35 ± 0.54	1.76 ± 1.27	0.88 ± 1.72	0.64 ± 0.94%	3.23 ± 2.55%	2.15 ± 3.52%	0.72 ± 1.03%	8.15 ± 2.59%	16.79 ± 3.65%

Data presented as mean ± standard deviation.

respectively) for both limbs at the three preactivation levels, as well as the normalized absolute torque values during vibration (i.e., those including preactivation torque; right panel). The data from the 0% MVT level is reproduced with permission from our previous work (McPherson et al., 2008). At the 5% MVT preactivation level in the paretic limb, vibration induced an increase in torque from 4.23% MVT during the preactivation period to 12.02% MVT during vibration (difference: 7.79% MVT, 2.52 Nm). In the non-paretic limb, preactivation to 5% MVT led to a TVR-evoked torque increase from 4.92 to 8.15% MVT (difference: 3.23% MVT, 1.76 Nm; **Table 2**). At the 15% MVT preactivation level, vibration induced an increase in torque from 13.39 to 21.00% MVT in the paretic limb (difference: 7.41% MVT, 2.25 Nm) and an increase in torque from 14.46 to 16.79% MVT in the non-paretic limb (difference: 2.15% MVT, 0.88 Nm).

The 2 × 3 repeated measures ANOVA revealed significant main effects of limb ($p = 0.004$) and preactivation level ($p = 0.0004$) on normalized TVR-evoked torque amplitude, and a non-significant limb-by-preactivation level interaction ($p = 0.16$). Examining the significant main effect of limb, paretic limb values were greater than non-paretic values, averaging 6.32% MVT across pre-activation levels vs. 2.00% MVT. The uniform increase in paretic vs. non-paretic TVR-evoked torque amplitude at all preactivation levels (i.e., significant main effect of limb and non-significant limb-by-preactivation interaction) was contrary to our prediction that the torque response would become similar across limbs with preactivation vs. the relaxed condition.

Results from within-limb *post-hoc t*-tests are summarized in **Table 3**, top panel. Paretic normalized TVR-evoked torque amplitude values from the 0% condition were significantly less than those from the 5 and 15% conditions ($p = 0.009$ and $p = 0.025$, respectively). Notably, however, there was no difference in TVR-evoked torque amplitude in the paretic limb between trials with torque preactivation of 5 and 15% MVT ($p = 0.84$). The same analysis in the non-paretic limb revealed a significant difference between the 0 and 5% conditions only ($p = 0.007$); comparisons of 0 vs. 15% ($p = 0.32$) and 5 vs. 15% ($p = 0.30$) were not statistically significant. Results from between-limb *post-hoc t*-tests are summarized in **Table 3**, bottom panel. As expected from the significant main effect of limb and non-significant

TABLE 3 | *Post-hoc* comparisons of TVR-evoked torque.

	TVR-evoked torque amplitude		Slope of torque rise	
Within-limb	**Paretic**	**Non-paretic**	**Paretic**	**Non-paretic**
0% vs. 5% MVT	**	**	*ns*	*ns*
0% vs. 15% MVT	*	*ns*	****	*ns*
5% vs. 15% MVT	*ns*	*ns*	****	*ns*
Between-limb	**Paretic vs. Non-Paretic**		**Paretic vs. Non-Paretic**	
0% MVT	**		*ns*	
5% MVT	****		*ns*	
15% MVT	****		****	

*Asterisks indicate significant differences at *p < 0.05, **p < 0.01, or ****p < 0.0001. ns indicates p > 0.05. Post-hoc comparisons computed from normalized torque.*

limb-by-preactivation interaction, paretic TVR-evoked torque amplitude values were higher than non-paretic values at all preactivation levels.

Slope of TVR-Evoked Torque

Qualitatively, the rate of rise of TVR-evoked torque in the paretic limb appears to increase with increasing preactivation. Further, the rate of rise in the paretic limb appears to be more rapid than that of the non-paretic limb at matched levels of preactivation (**Figure 1**). We evaluated these observations quantitatively by computing the slope of the rising TVR-evoked torque according to Equation (1), including a new analysis of TVR responses previously collected with 0% preactivation (adapted from McPherson et al., 2008; **Figure 2**). The 2×3 mixed-model ANOVA revealed significant main effects of limb ($p = 0.002$) and preactivation level ($p < 0.0001$) as well as a significant limb-by-preactivation level interaction ($p = 0.0002$). A 2-way non-repeated measures ANOVA, without imputation, likewise revealed significant main effects of limb ($p = 0.0003$) and preactivation level ($p = 0.0002$) and a significant limb-by-preactivation level interaction ($p = 0.0008$). The nature of the significant interaction can be appreciated from visual inspection of **Figure 2**. Slope values for the paretic limb increased with preactivation level, but slope values for the non-paretic limb remained constant. Paretic group mean slope of TVR-evoked torque averaged 1.0, 3.5, and 12.5% MVT/s (for 0, 5, and 15% MVT preactivation levels, respectively), and 0.2, 1.6, and 1.4% MVT/s in the non-paretic limb. As such, the significant main effect of preactivation level was driven by the paretic limb values.

Post-hoc t-tests comparing between-limb differences in the slope of TVR-evoked torque at each pre-activation level revealed a significant difference at the 15% condition ($p < 0.0001$) and not the 0 or 5% conditions ($p = 0.99$ and $p = 0.95$, respectively) (**Table 3**, bottom panel).

Post-hoc t-tests comparing within-limb differences in the slope of TVR-evoked torque between each combination of the three preactivation levels (**Table 3**, top panel) revealed that in the paretic limb, values for the 0 and 5% conditions were significantly less than those of the 15% condition ($p < 0.0001$ for both comparisons), but there was no significant difference

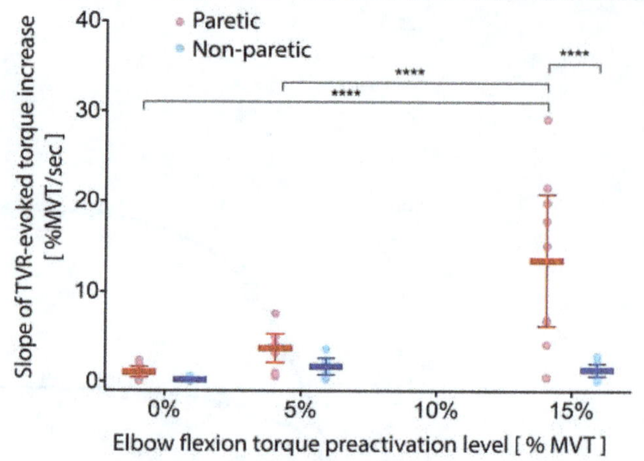

FIGURE 2 | Slope of TVR-evoked torque increases with preactivation only in paretic limb. As preactivation level increases, the slope of TVR-evoked torque increases in the paretic (pink/red) but not the non-paretic (light blue/royal blue) elbow flexors. Differences between limbs emerge at the 15% preactivation level. Individual circles represent single participant values; horizontal lines indicate group means, with error bars corresponding to 95% confidence intervals. *Y-axis*: slope of TVR-evoked torque (%MVT per second); *x-axis*: elbow flexion torque preactivation level expressed as percent of MVT. $^{****}p < 0.0001$.

between values for the 0 and 5% conditions ($p = 0.31$). The same analysis in the non-paretic limb revealed no significant differences in the slope of TVR-evoked torque among any preactivation level comparisons (p-values ranging from 0.72 to 0.98).

Modeled TVR-Evoked Torque Profile

Because the temporal profile of TVR-evoked torque is non-linear, particularly during the first ~1 s of vibration, we also modeled TVR-evoked torque as an exponential function according to Equation (2). All data were well-fit by this model, as can be appreciated visually in **Figure 3A** (black lines superimposed on data records). In **Table 4,** we present the optimal parameters for each group mean torque response at each preactivation level, as well as the SSE and VAF for each fit.

In **Figure 3B**, we plot parameters a and b from the model (left and right panels, respectively) for the paretic (pink) and non-paretic (blue) limbs as a function of preactivation level. These two parameters describe the shape of the during-vibration profile. Parameter a, most closely associated with the amplitude of TVR-evoked torque, tends to increase as a function of preactivation level for the paretic limb but not the non-paretic limb. Parameter b, reflective of the rate-of-rise of the TVR-evoked torque, is lower overall in the paretic limb—indicating more rapid torque development during vibration—and qualitatively appears to decrease as preactivation level increases.

Because parameters of modeled TVR-evoked torque data from the non-paretic limb had relatively less change across preactivation levels than those of the paretic limb, we also computed the VAF when applying the model fit *from* the 5% preactivation data *to* the 15% preactivation data (separately for the non-paretic and paretic limbs). This manipulation gives an estimate of similarity between TVR-evoked responses at increasing preactivation levels, particularly during the rising phase of the contraction. We found that the optimal parameters for describing the 5% preactivation response in the non-paretic limb also accounted for 98.25% of the variability in the 15% preactivation trials in the same limb (**Figure 4**; purple trace overlaid on raw data). Conversely, for the paretic limb only 75.41% of the variability in the 15% preactivation data could be explained by the optimal fit to the 5% preactivation torque responses (down from 96.33%; **Figure 4**; purple trace overlaid on raw data). This finding, too, is consistent both with the relative invariance of linear slope in the non-paretic limb to preactivation level and the strong dependency of paretic limb linear slope on preactivation.

TVR Responses in Decerebrate Cat Preparation

To examine mechanisms of why the TVR did not vary with preactivation level, we undertook studies of the TVR in a decerebrate cat preparation. We reasoned that if the same pre-activation invariance occurred in this preparation, it would reflect the basic input-output behavior of the motor pool in response to stable, sustained Ia input (in the presence of increased spinal monoamines) instead of some type of compensation by descending inputs.

We found that the pattern of TVR-evoked force in the decerebrate cat was strikingly similar to that of the paretic elbow flexors in individuals with chronic hemiparetic stroke (**Figure 5**). Specifically, we found that increasing preactivation force was *not* associated with a larger TVR-evoked force amplitude, with virtually no correlation between the two variables ($r = -0.10$; $p = 0.8$). In comparison, there was a higher correlation between preactivation force and the rising slope of the TVR-evoked force ($r = 0.48$) and time to 85% max TVR-evoked force ($r = -0.62$); however, neither of these correlations reached significance at the $p < 0.05$ level with the amount of data available ($p = 0.19$ and $p = 0.08$).

To further investigate how the TVR-evoked torque arose, we utilized motor unit spike trains to characterize motor unit recruitment and rate modulation. Motor unit spike trains for two TVR trials with different preactivation levels are represented in **Figure 6** by their instantaneous firing rates. Thirty-six motor units were decomposed from the trial with lower preactivation (left panel) and 39 motor units were decomposed from the trial with higher preactivation (right panel). Qualitatively, motor units followed expected trends of recruitment order and rate modulation during preactivation and vibration: increasing preactivation increased the number of motor units recruited before vibration, and vibration led both to recruitment of additional motor units and an increased firing rate in motor units previously recruited with preactivation (**Figure 6**). However, it can be seen that for both levels of preactivation, recruitment of additional motor units is the dominant contributor to the development of TVR-evoked force, with an increased firing rate of previously recruited motor units contributing to a lesser extent.

The decerebrate cat preparation also allowed us to examine potential post-vibration force production (given the lack of descending voluntary drive as a confounding factor), and, by extension, the ability of a purely spinal mechanism to account for any such effects. When vibration was discontinued, force

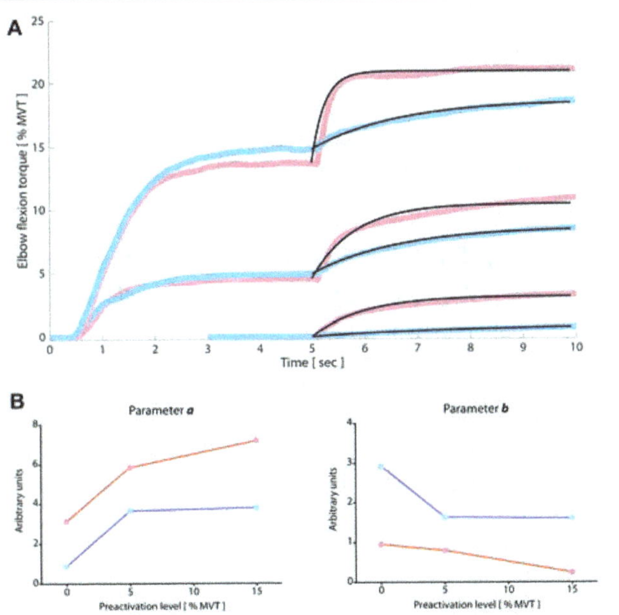

FIGURE 3 | TVR torque responses modeled by a composition of exponential functions. **(A)** Paretic and non-paretic TVR responses were well fit by exponential functions (black lines from 5 to 10 s), with Variances Accounted For of approximately >94% in all cases. Vibration commences at 5 s and continues for the duration of the plot. *Y-axis:* elbow flexion torque, expressed as a percentage of max; *x-axis:* time in seconds. Pink (paretic) and blue (non-paretic) traces are group averaged data ($N = 10$). **(B)**. Optimal parameters of exponential fit expressed as function of preactivation level. Pink/red: paretic limb; blue: non-paretic limb. Qualitatively, parameter *a* is greater in the paretic than the non-paretic limb; it trends toward an increased magnitude with increasing preactivation in the paretic limb but plateaus in the non-paretic limb. Parameter *b* is lower in the paretic limb than the non-paretic limb and decreases as a function of increasing preactivation. Permission to adapt images from McPherson et al. (2008) is afforded by the American Physiological Society under original author rights.

TABLE 4 | Modeled TVR-evoked torque.

	Preactivation level (% MVT)	a	b	SSE	VAF
Paretic	0%	3.14	0.96	97.3	97.14%
	5%	5.86	0.8	549.37	94.21%
	15%	7.21	0.25	247.17	96.33%
Non-paretic	0%	0.9	2.93	2.98	98.90%
	5%	3.66	1.64	31.84	99.44%
	15%	3.82	1.61	111.9	98.13%

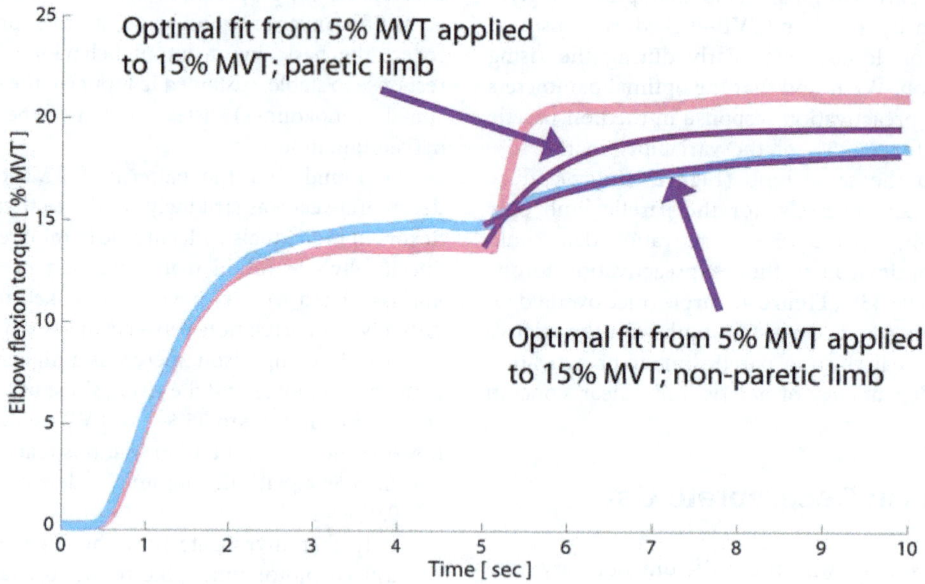

FIGURE 4 | Initial TVR-evoked torque development is invariant to preactivation magnitude in the non-paretic but not the paretic limb. Blue trace: non-paretic limb at 15% MVT preactivation; pink trace: paretic limb; black traces: optimal fits of an exponential composition to paretic and non-paretic data, respectively; purple traces: overlay of optimal fit of each limb's TVR-evoked torque at 5% MVT preactivation onto the 15% MVT preactivation records. In the non-paretic limb, the optimal fit at 5% MVT is able to explain ~98% of the variance in the torque response at 15% MVT preactivation. Conversely, the 5% MVT fit is only able to explain ~75% of the variance in torque response at 15% MVT in the paretic limb.

persisted at an elevated level until peroneal nerve stimulation was discontinued (**Figures 5, 6**; force produced after $t = \sim 3.5$–4.5 s). This persistent elevated force was accompanied by sustained firing of the vibration-recruited motor units despite removal of the vibration stimulus. Interestingly, we also observed differences between the two trials in the proportion of vibration-recruited motor units that demonstrated sustained firing. For the trial with lower preactivation, 32 of the 33 vibration-recruited motor units demonstrated sustained firing. For the trial with higher preactivation, however, only 12 of the 24 vibration-recruited motor units demonstrated sustained firing through the end of the trial.

DISCUSSION

We demonstrated that TVR-evoked torque amplitude in the paretic arm of individuals with chronic hemiparetic stroke significantly exceeds that of the non-paretic arm when muscles are preactivated to the same degree. Interestingly, within both the paretic and the non-paretic arm, TVR-evoked torque amplitude did not increase further when preactivation increased from 5 to 15% MVT. The rising *slope* of TVR-evoked torque did, however, increase with increasing preactivation in the paretic arm, whereas non-paretic values were not influenced by preactivation. Likewise, parameters extracted from the nonlinear model of TVR-evoked torque changed as a function of preactivation level only in the paretic arm. These findings contrast with the results of many classical stretch reflex paradigms, which suggest that reflex amplitude should equilibrate between paretic and non-paretic muscles when preactivation is matched (Lee et al., 1987; Burne et al., 2005; McPherson et al., 2017). Below, we discuss potential neural mechanisms that could underlie our findings.

Increased TVR-Evoked Torque Amplitude in the Paretic vs. Non-paretic Limb

One potential explanation for the increased amplitude of TVR-evoked torque in the paretic compared to the non-paretic arm (**Figure 1**) could be an increased monoaminergic drive to spinal motoneurons from the brainstem ponto-medullary reticular formation (PMRF). The PMRF has both a descending motor and a descending neuromodulatory component (Holstege and Kuypers, 1987), and recent evidence suggests that the motor component is progressively recruited post-stroke as volitional force production increases in the paretic arm (McPherson et al., 2018). The neuromodulatory component uses the monoamines serotonin and norepinephrine to regulate spinal excitability (Holstege and Kuypers, 1987; Hochman et al., 2001; Heckman et al., 2003), and is co-activated with the motor component (Veasey et al., 1995; Jacobs et al., 2002; Chan et al., 2006; Schwarz et al., 2008). Monoamines are uniquely excitatory to motoneurons, for example amplifying post-synaptic potentials 3–5-fold via PICs (Schwindt and Crill, 1977; Perrier and Hounsgaard, 2003; Heckman et al., 2009) while depolarizing the resting membrane potential and hyperpolarizing the spike threshold (Fedirchuk and Dai, 2004; Harvey et al., 2006). Thus, an increased descending monoaminergic drive could result in elevated TVR responses in paretic muscles through greater PIC-mediated amplification of motoneurons and/or by additional motor unit recruitment during vibration. It should be noted,

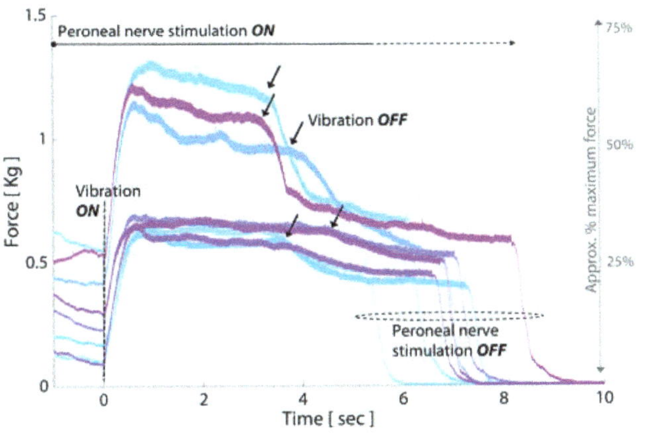

FIGURE 5 | TVR responses in decerebrate cat follow similar trends to paretic elbow flexors post-stroke as preactivation increases. Each colored line represents the force evoked in response to a single TVR trial at a given level of preactivation. Crossed extension reflex is initiated prior to vibration onset ($t = 0$ s) to achieve a stable preactivation force and is maintained throughout the duration of vibration. *Y-axis*: evoked force (Kg); *x-axis*: time (sec); black arrows: vibration offset. TVR-evoked force amplitude exhibits negligible change with increased preactivation, and involuntary force production is maintained after cessation of vibration (black arrows) and until peroneal nerve stimulation is stopped.

however, that previous investigations have yet to find changes in PIC amplitude in paretic muscles relative to non-paretic muscles post-stroke (Mottram et al., 2009, 2010), although methodological differences prevent a direct comparison to the findings presented here. Also, it should be noted for clarification that a *decrease* in monoaminergic drive may contribute to hyperreflexia after spinal cord injury (as opposed to the hypothetical increase described here post-stroke), because a lack of monoamines below the lesion appears to drive adaptive processes that result in constitutive activity of monoaminergic receptors on motoneurons (Murray et al., 2010).

Alternatively, it is possible that a tonic excitatory ionotropic drive to paretic motor pools could have contributed to the increased TVR amplitude we observed in the paretic arm. Such a drive could arise from ionotropic reticulospinal or vestibulospinal pathways following stroke-induced damage to primary motor resources (Mottram et al., 2009, 2010; Miller and Dewald, 2012; Miller D. M. et al., 2014; McMorland et al., 2015; McPherson et al., 2017), and would provide a maintained depolarizing input to motor pools innervating the paretic muscles. This would bring motoneurons closer to firing threshold, enabling vibration to more readily recruit them. It could also depolarize a small portion of the motor pool above firing threshold, leading to spontaneous motoneuron firing (Mottram et al., 2010)—a common finding post-stroke.

Our findings contrast with some aspects of the ionotropic drive hypothesis, particularly as they relate to other studies that cite this mechanism as possible explanation for exaggerated stretch-sensitive reflexes post-stroke. For example, when stretch reflexes are evoked by imposed joint excursions in the paretic and non-paretic arms at matched levels of preactivation, the difference in reflex response between arms is often extinguished (Lee et al., 1987; Burne et al., 2005; McPherson et al., 2017). Results from these studies suggest that the postulated tonic ionotropic drive is low enough that even small amounts of preactivation normalize the difference in resting excitability attributed to the tonic drive. Although a key assumption of the tonic ionotropic drive hypothesis is that preactivation is an effective means of balancing the excitability offset between limbs, it remains unknown if this is indeed the case. Nevertheless, if preactivation *does* abolish the resting excitability imbalance between limbs, then our results cannot be explained solely by a tonic ionotropic drive to motor pools innervating the paretic muscles. If that were the case, then TVR responses in paretic and non-paretic limbs would equilibrate with preactivation.

Changes in spinal circuits post-stroke could have also contributed to the increased TVR amplitude we observed in the paretic arm, although our experimental paradigm and analyses were not able to directly measure or clearly infer the potential contribution of such changes to our results. Nevertheless, there is evidence that the net effect of Group Ib afferent feedback transitions to from a combination of inhibition and excitation (Houk et al., 1970; Conway et al., 1987; Pearson and Collins, 1993; Prochazka et al., 1997) to preferential excitation in motor pools innervating the paretic muscles post-stroke (Delwaide and Oliver, 1988). While tendon vibration provides a strong volley of a Group Ia afferent feedback from muscle spindles, it also provides afferent information from Golgi tendon organs via Group Ib fibers. Given that Golgi tendon organs/Group Ib fibers are progressively activated by vibration as background muscle tension increases (Fallon and Macefield, 2007), a lateralized shift in Ib feedback toward excitation could explain a portion of our elevated paretic limb TVR responses. Further, if descending monoaminergic drive is indeed increased, interneuron responses to Group Ia and Ib feedback could be potentiated (Jankowska et al., 2000). And, while the effects of monoamines on Group II-evoked responses are both complex and incompletely characterized (Jankowska et al., 2000; Grey et al., 2001; Kurtzer et al., 2018), changes in this feedback mechanism would likely alter TVR responses as well. Likewise, a reduction of presynaptic inhibition, which is associated with spasticity following multiple sclerosis, spinal cord injury, and possibly stroke (Faist et al., 1994; Aymard et al., 2000; Morita et al., 2001; Nielsen et al., 2005; Lamy et al., 2009), could differentially alter reflex gain between arms and contribute to elevated TVR responses in the paretic arm.

Invariance of TVR-Evoked Torque Amplitude to Increasing Preactivation

It is unclear why the magnitude of TVR-evoked torque did not increase in either limb when preactivation increased from 5 to 15% MVT. Indeed, it is well accepted that the amplitude of stretch reflexes elicited by imposed joint excursions increases with increasing preactivation in paretic, non-paretic, and control limbs. Further, Henneman's size principle (Binder et al., 1983; Bawa et al., 1984; Henneman, 1985) suggests that, at low force levels, recruitment of progressively larger force motor units

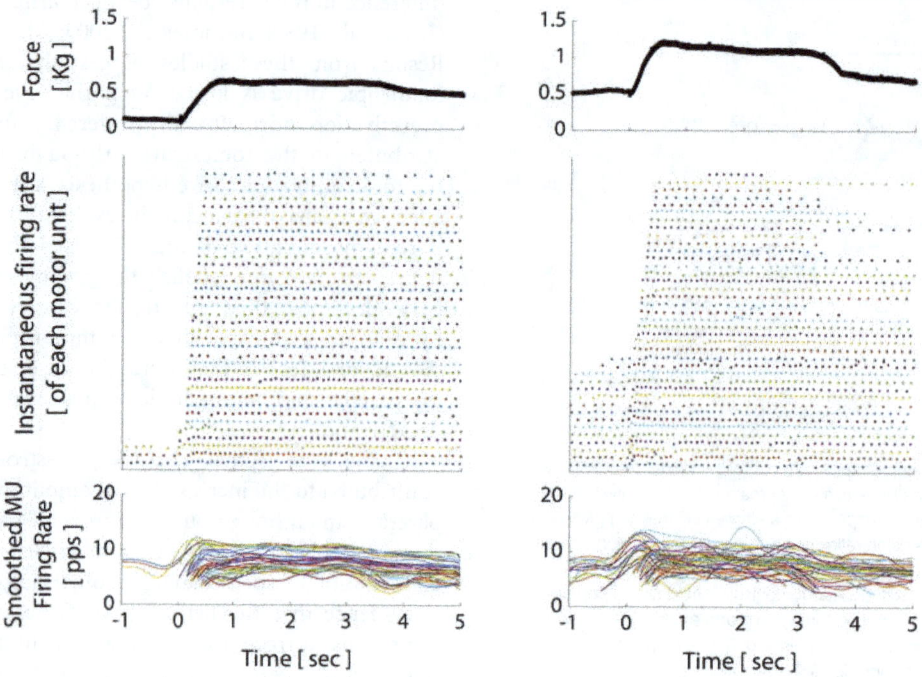

FIGURE 6 | Motor unit firing patterns in decerebrate cat during crossed extension reflex and TVR trials. Top panel: muscle force; middle panel: instantaneous firing rate individual motor units recruited during the corresponding force trace (each color/row represents a separate motor unit); bottom panel: smoothed motor unit firing rates during the corresponding force trace. X-axis for all panels: elapsed time, relative to onset of vibration. Increasing preactivation force (mediated by the crossed extension reflex) led to increasing motor unit recruitment, as seen in left and right middle panels from $t = -1$:0 s. Vibration onset was marked primarily by further increases in motor unit recruitment and less so by increases in firing rate of previously recruited units. After vibration stops (at $t = 3.5$ s), persistent motor unit firing is evident, particularly in low-threshold units; a hallmark of motoneuron PICs.

will impart an upwards curvature to the input-output function, regardless of the motoneuron input mixture (Heckman, 1994). This should cause TVR-evoked torque amplitude to increase with pre-activation level in both arms.

Two potential mechanisms could contribute to this unexpected finding. In the first, synaptic inhibition could simultaneously increase and decrease in direct proportion to preactivation level, a phenomenon known as "proportional," or "balanced," inhibition (Powers et al., 2012; Powers and Heckman, 2017). Because monoaminergic actions on motoneurons are exquisitely sensitive to synaptic inhibition (Johnson and Heckman, 2014), even small amounts of additional inhibition during contraction could prevent the predicted increase in TVR response amplitude. In the second scenario, monoaminergic drive to the paretic limb could be elevated yet relatively static post-stroke, contributing approximately the same net amount of excitation across the preactivation levels tested here. Because the non-paretic limb is presumably less reliant on monoaminergic drive for motoneuron activation than the paretic limb (due to an intact corticospinal tract), it is more likely to maintain an appropriate level of baseline inhibition, retain the capacity for presynaptic and reciprocal inhibition, and use a homeostatic "push-pull" method to regulate the excitation/inhibition balance during contraction (Powers et al., 2012; Powers and Heckman, 2017). These characteristics would enable more precise control of synaptic integration, potentially leading to similar levels of motoneuron recruitment during vibration for the relatively low submaximal contractions investigated here.

Corroboration With Animal Model

To further explore our finding that paretic limb TVR-evoked torque amplitude was not different between 5 and 15% preactivation levels post-stroke, we investigated the impact of increasing preactivation level on the amplitude and rate of rise of TVR-evoked force in a decerebrate cat model. This model has a strong descending monoaminergic drive, the magnitude of which is not modified by vibration or crossed-extension reflex inputs (Lee and Heckman, 1996; Hyngstrom et al., 2008). Thus, force output in this model is due only to three factors: the sustained monoaminergic drive, Ia input (via vibration), and the resulting input-output function of the motoneurons. Like our human-subjects findings, the magnitude of TVR-evoked force in the cat did not scale with preactivation level. Also similar to our human-subjects findings, there was a stronger correlation between preactivation level and rate of rising force; however, the correlation was not statistically significant in cat data. Also, because vibration is very selective for Ia inputs in the decerebrate cat model (Hyngstrom et al., 2008), the similarity of our cat and human-subjects results suggests that monosynaptic Ia feedback was the predominant driver of motoneuron activation in the human-subjects torque as well, with less influence from Ib or other sensory inputs.

Importantly, the decerebrate cat model also enabled us to investigate force production *after* vibration was discontinued, which was not possible in our human-subjects experiments. We found maintained, elevated force post-vibration rather than a return to preactivation level or the relaxed state. This behavior is characteristic of PICs in motoneurons (Heckman et al., 2008) and is consistent with post-vibration TVR responses seen in humans when no preactivation is present, as was detailed in our previous study (McPherson et al., 2008). The finding that sustained firing of vibration-recruited motor units accompanied the post-vibration force maintenance is highly consistent with activation of PICs, which characteristically enable a motoneuron to continue firing after removal of the excitatory stimulus that recruited it. Further, our observation that a greater percentage of motor units exhibited sustained firing in the trial with lower preactivation (32 of 33) compared to the trial with higher preactivation (12 of 24) is consistent with the greater impact that PICs have on sustained firing in low vs. higher threshold motor units (Heckman et al., 2008).

Together, these findings corroborate and extend key aspects of our overall unexpected human-subjects findings, and reinforce the notion that monoaminergic mechanisms are a potential component of the observed paretic arm TVR responses. However, it should be noted that in the decerebrate cat there is no natural analog to the non-paretic arm in humans, and it is unknown how the afferent drive provided by peripheral nerve stimulation in the cat compares to volitional preactivation in humans with regard to its inhibitory and excitatory content.

Slope of TVR-Evoked Torque and Modeled Torque Gain

We found that the slope of TVR-evoked torque amplitude and the gain of the modeled torque both increased with increasing preactivation in the paretic limb. These findings are consistent with an increased influence of monoamines in paretic motor pools, which could result in a combination of larger PICs in recruited motoneurons, more motoneurons recruited, and/or a reduced time to PIC activation as preactivation increases.

PIC activation time is proportional to the difference in membrane potential and PIC threshold potential (Heckman and Lee, 2001). Thus, as membrane potential depolarizes toward PIC threshold, the time required to activate the PIC by a given stimulus is reduced. Here, this phenomenon could occur when transitioning from the relaxed case to 5 and 15% MVT preactivation: as preactivation increases, an increasing amount of motoneurons are brought near to or above their PIC threshold. Assuming that monoaminergic drive would be elevated to paretic motoneurons compared to non-paretic motoneurons, PICs will be more rapidly activated in paretic motoneurons when vibration begins. The net effect of an increased PIC activation rate will be a faster rate of force production, and thus a higher TVR slope and gain. By comparison, the lower slope and modeled torque gain in the non-paretic limb could reflect a lack of robust neuromodulatory effects.

Comparison With Stretch Reflex Studies

Finally, an intriguing question raised by these results is why TVR responses continue to be elevated in the paretic limb compared to the non-paretic limb at matched levels of preactivation, yet stretch reflex responses equilibrate under analogous conditions. It is conceivable that this distinction is related to the potency of vibration as an input to motor pools compared to imposed joint excursions. Indeed, it has been suggested that vibration elicits more robust activation of Ia afferents than group Ib or II fibers, which may be activated more strongly by joint excursion (Matthews, 1984). More specifically, if vibration elicits a larger response in spinal motor pools than joint excursion, then lingering imbalances in motor pool excitability that were not well controlled by preactivation could "re-appear" through enhanced motor unit recruitment during vibration. Or, put another way, if joint excursion is a relatively modest stimulus, it may not recruit substantially more motor units over those already recruited via preactivation. This could mask persistent excitability imbalances.

This explanation seems unlikely, however, both because spindle-mediated feedback appears to be unchanged post-stroke (Hagbarth et al., 1973) and because our TVR paradigm actually appears to evoke a relatively small motor output compared to the joint excursions typically used to gauge motor excitability. Indeed, we found that when preactivated to 5% MVT, vibration only increased net elbow flexion torque output to ~13% MVT in the paretic limb. By comparison, a rapid joint excursion (270°/s) at 5% MVT preactivation can routinely drive reflex responses that exceed 20–25% MVT (McPherson et al., 2017), even though the stretch duration is only ~300 ms (compared to 5 s for vibration). Further, if our paretic limb TVR responses are compared to previously reported stretch reflex data post-stroke (McPherson et al., 2017), we find that they most closely match an approximately quasi-static imposed joint excursion (6°/s) in terms of rise time and amplitude. Thus, it remains an open question as to why the two stimuli modalities yield such differing responses.

Limitations

Our study has important limitations. First, we reiterate that because our human-subjects experiments used indirect probes of spinal neural excitability, our interpretation of the underlying mechanisms remains inferential. Additionally, we did not conduct TVR analyses in individuals without neurological injury. Although this choice was motivated by an attempt to limit variability, the ipsilesional arm is not truly unaffected post-stroke, and thus, future studies are warranted. We also did not acquire elbow flexion/extension torque after cessation of vibration in the human-subjects portion of the study. While this choice was made to avoid the confound of volitional activity in any persistent muscle activation post-TVR, it prevents our study from assessing the impact of preactivation on persistent motoneuron firing—an important component of PICs. And finally, regarding the decerebrate cat experiments: because the primary purpose of this preliminary cat model was to provide context for the mechanical response to vibration in a situation with known elevation of monoaminergic drive, we did not design the protocol with the specific goal of acquiring EMG data amenable to studying PICs. As a result, we are not able to make inferences about PICs from these data.

CONCLUSIONS

Our results suggest that a combination of both ionotropic and neuromodulatory mechanisms likely underlie the exaggerated TVR responses we observed in the paretic elbow flexors post-stroke, although the relative impact of each remains unclear. The finding that TVR-evoked torque amplitude did not change with preactivation level could imply a more pronounced role for synaptic inhibition in motor pools innervating the paretic muscles than previously thought. For example, an increase in inhibitory drive as volitional motor output increases (Powers and Heckman, 2017; Revill and Fuglevand, 2017) would reduce PIC-mediated effects on motoneuron firing dynamics, potentially stabilizing TVR-evoked torque output. Advanced yet available technologies such as high-density surface EMG grids and motor unit decomposition algorithms, which can be incorporated into both human experiments and animal preparations (Miller L. C. et al., 2014; McPherson et al., 2016; Johnson et al., 2017), will be essential for more fully characterizing these effects.

AUTHOR CONTRIBUTIONS

All authors contributed to the conception and design of the work; JM, LM, CT, ME contributed to the acquisition of data; JM, LM, CT contributed to analysis of data; all authors contributed to the interpretation of data and drafting, revising and approving the manuscript for publication. All authors are in agreement to be accountable for all aspects of the work.

FUNDING

This work was supported by NIH grants: R01NS054269, R01HD039343, and R01NS047567.

REFERENCES

Aymard, C., Katz, R., Lafitte, C., Lo, E., Penicaud, A., Pradat-Diehl, P., et al. (2000). Presynaptic inhibition and homosynaptic depression: a comparison between lower and upper limbs in normal human subjects and patients with hemiplegia. *Brain* 123 (Pt 8), 1688–1702. doi: 10.1093/brain/123.8.1688

Bawa, P., Binder, M. D., Ruenzel, P., and Henneman, E. (1984). Recruitment order of motoneurons in stretch reflexes is highly correlated with their axonal conduction velocity. *J. Neurophysiol.* 52, 410–420. doi: 10.1152/jn.1984.52.3.410

Binder, M. C., Bawa, P., Ruenzel, P., and Henneman, E. (1983). Does orderly recruitment of motoneurons depend on the existence of different types of motor units? *Neurosci. Lett.* 36, 55–58.

Bradnam, L. V., Stinear, C. M., Barber, P. A., and Byblow, W. D. (2012). Contralesional hemisphere control of the proximal paretic upper limb following stroke. *Cereb. Cortex* 22, 2662–2671. doi: 10.1093/cercor/bhr344

Burne, J. A., Carleton, V. L., and O'dwyer, N. J. (2005). The spasticity paradox: movement disorder or disorder of resting limbs? *J. Neurol. Neurosurg. Psychiatr.* 76, 47–54. doi: 10.1136/jnnp.2003.034785

Chan, E., Steenland, H. W., Liu, H., and Horner, R. L. (2006). Endogenous excitatory drive modulating respiratory muscle activity across sleep-wake states. *Am. J. Respir. Crit. Care Med.* 174, 1264–1273. doi: 10.1164/rccm.200605-597OC

Conway, B. A., Hultborn, H., and Kiehn, O. (1987). Proprioceptive input resets central locomotor rhythm in the spinal cat. *Exp. Brain Res.* 68, 643–656. doi: 10.1007/BF00249807

Crone, C., Hultborn, H., Kiehn, O., Mazieres, L., and Wigstrom, H. (1988). Maintained changes in motoneuronal excitability by short-lasting synaptic inputs in the decerebrate cat. *J. Physiol.* 405, 321–343. doi: 10.1113/jphysiol.1988.sp017335

Delwaide, P. J., and Oliver, E. (1988). Short-latency autogenic inhibition (IB inhibition) in human spasticity. *J. Neurol. Neurosurg. Psychiatr.* 51, 1546–1550. doi: 10.1136/jnnp.51.12.1546

Eklund, G., and Hagbarth, K. E. (1966). Normal variability of tonic vibration reflexes in man. *Exp. Neurol.* 16, 80–92. doi: 10.1016/0014-4886(66)90088-4

Faist, M., Mazevet, D., Dietz, V., and Pierrot-Deseilligny, E. (1994). A quantitative assessment of presynaptic inhibition of Ia afferents in spastics. Differences in hemiplegics and paraplegics. *Brain* 117 (Pt 6), 1449–1455.

Fallon, J. B., and Macefield, V. G. (2007). Vibration sensitivity of human muscle spindles and Golgi tendon organs. *Muscle* Nerve 36, 21–29. doi: 10.1002/mus.20796

Fedirchuk, B., and Dai, Y. (2004). Monoamines increase the excitability of spinal neurones in the neonatal rat by hyperpolarizing the threshold for action potential production. *J. Physiol.* 557, 355–361. doi: 10.1113/jphysiol.2004.064022

Gillies, J. D., Burke, D. J., and Lance, J. W. (1971). Supraspinal control of tonic vibration reflex. *J. Neurophysiol.* 34, 302–309. doi: 10.1152/jn.1971.34.2.302

Grey, M. J., Ladouceur, M., Andersen, J. B., Nielsen, J. B., and Sinkjaer, T. (2001). Group II muscle afferents probably contribute to the medium latency soleus stretch reflex during walking in humans. *J. Physiol.* 534, 925–933. doi: 10.1111/j.1469-7793.2001.00925.x

Grundy, D. (2015). Principles and standards for reporting animal experiments in The Journal of Physiology and Experimental Physiology. *J. Physiol.* 593, 2547–2549. doi: 10.1113/JP270818

Hagbarth, K. E., and Eklund, G. (1966). Tonic vibration reflexes (TVR) in spasticity. *Brain Res.* 2, 201–203. doi: 10.1016/0006-8993(66)90029-1

Hagbarth, K. E., Wallin, G., and Lofstedt, L. (1973). Muscle spindle responses to stretch in normal and spastic subjects. *Scand. J. Rehabil. Med.* 5, 156–159.

Harvey, P. J., Li, X., Li, Y., and Bennett, D. J. (2006). 5-HT2 receptor activation facilitates a persistent sodium current and repetitive firing in spinal motoneurons of rats with and without chronic spinal cord injury. *J. Neurophysiol.* 96, 1158–1170. doi: 10.1152/jn.01088.2005

Heckman, C. J. (1994). Computer simulations of the effects of different synaptic input systems on the steady-state input-output structure of the motoneuron pool. *J. Neurophysiol.* 71, 1727–1739. doi: 10.1152/jn.1994.71.5.1727

Heckman, C. J., Johnson, M., Mottram, C., and Schuster, J. (2008). Persistent inward currents in spinal motoneurons and their influence on human motoneuron firing patterns. *Neuroscientist* 14, 264–275. doi: 10.1177/1073858408314986

Heckman, C. J., and Lee, R. H. (2001). "Advances measuring active dendritic currents in spinal motoneurons *in vivo*," in *Motor Neurobiology of the Spinal Cord*, ed T. C. Cope (Boca Raton, FL: CRC Press), 89–106.

Heckman, C. J., Lee, R. H., and Brownstone, R. M. (2003). Hyperexcitable dendrites in motoneurons and their neuromodulatory control during motor behavior. *Trends Neurosci.* 26, 688–695. doi: 10.1016/j.tins.2003.10.002

Heckman, C. J., Mottram, C., Quinlan, K., Theiss, R., and Schuster, J. (2009). Motoneuron excitability: the importance of neuromodulatory inputs. *Clin. Neurophysiol.* 120, 2040–2054. doi: 10.1016/j.clinph.2009.08.009

Henneman, E. (1985). The size-principle: a deterministic output emerges from a set of probabilistic connections. *J. Exp. Biol.* 115, 105–112.

Hochman, S., Garraway, S., Machacek, D., and Shay, B. (2001). "5-HT receptors and the neuromodulatory control of spinal cord function," in *Motor*

Neurobiology of the Spinal Cord, ed T. C. Cope (Boca Raton, FL: CRC Press), 47–87.

Holobar, A., Minetto, M. A., Botter, A., Negro, F., and Farina, D. (2010). Experimental analysis of accuracy in the identification of motor unit spike trains from high-density surface EMG. *IEEE Trans. Neural Syst. Rehabil. Eng.* 18, 221–229. doi: 10.1109/TNSRE.2010.2041593

Holobar, A., Minetto, M. A., and Farina, D. (2014). Accurate identification of motor unit discharge patterns from high-density surface EMG and validation with a novel signal-based performance metric. *J. Neural Eng.* 11:016008. doi: 10.1088/1741-2560/11/1/016008

Holstege, J. C., and Kuypers, H. G. (1987). Brainstem projections to spinal motoneurons: an update. *Neuroscience* 23, 809–821. doi: 10.1016/0306-4522(87)90160-6

Houk, J. C., Singer, J. J., and Goldman, M. R. (1970). An evaluation of length and force feedback to soleus muscles of decerebrate cats. *J. Neurophysiol.* 33, 784–811. doi: 10.1152/jn.1970.33.6.784

Hu, X., Suresh, N. L., Chardon, M. K., and Rymer, W. Z. (2015). Contributions of motoneuron hyperexcitability to clinical spasticity in hemispheric stroke survivors. *Clin. Neurophysiol.* 126, 1599–1606. doi: 10.1016/j.clinph.2014.11.005

Hyngstrom, A. S., Johnson, M. D., and Heckman, C. J. (2008). Summation of excitatory and inhibitory synaptic inputs by motoneurons with highly active dendrites. *J. Neurophysiol.* 99, 1643–1652. doi: 10.1152/jn.01253.2007

Ibrahim, I. K., Berger, W., Trippel, M., and Dietz, V. (1993). Stretch-induced electromyographic activity and torque in spastic elbow muscles. Differential modulation of reflex activity in passive and active motor tasks. *Brain* 116 (Pt 4), 971–989. doi: 10.1093/brain/116.4.971

Jacobs, B. L., Martin-Cora, F. J., and Fornal, C. A. (2002). Activity of medullary serotonergic neurons in freely moving animals. *Brain Res. Brain Res. Rev.* 40, 45–52. doi: 10.1016/S0165-0173(02)00187-X

Jankowska, E., Hammar, I., Chojnicka, B., and Heden, C. H. (2000). Effects of monoamines on interneurons in four spinal reflex pathways from group I and/or group II muscle afferents. *Eur. J. Neurosci.* 12, 701–714. doi: 10.1046/j.1460-9568.2000.00955.x

Johnson, M. D., and Heckman, C. J. (2014). Gain control mechanisms in spinal motoneurons. *Front. Neural Circuits* 8:81. doi: 10.3389/fncir.2014.00081

Johnson, M. D., Thompson, C. K., Tysseling, V. M., Powers, R. K., and Heckman, C. J. (2017). The potential for understanding the synaptic organization of human motor commands via the firing patterns of motoneurons. *J. Neurophysiol.* 118, 520–531. doi: 10.1152/jn.00018.2017

Kurtzer, I., Bouyer, L. J., Bouffard, J., Jin, A., Christiansen, L., Nielsen, J. B., et al. (2018). Variable impact of tizanidine on the medium latency reflex of upper and lower limbs. *Exp. Brain Res.* 236, 665–677. doi: 10.1007/s00221-017-5162-6

Lamy, J. C., Wargon, I., Mazevet, D., Ghanim, Z., Pradat-Diehl, P., and Katz, R. (2009). Impaired efficacy of spinal presynaptic mechanisms in spastic stroke patients. *Brain* 132, 734–748. doi: 10.1093/brain/awn310

Lance, J. W. (1980). The control of muscle tone, reflexes, and movement: Robert Wartenberg Lecture. *Neurology* 30, 1303–1313. doi: 10.1212/WNL.30.12.1303

Lee, R. H., and Heckman, C. J. (1996). Influence of voltage-sensitive dendritic conductances on bistable firing and effective synaptic current in cat spinal motoneurons *in vivo*. *J. Neurophysiol.* 76, 2107–2110. doi: 10.1152/jn.1996.76.3.2107

Lee, W. A., Boughton, A., and Rymer, W. Z. (1987). Absence of stretch reflex gain enhancement in voluntarily activated spastic muscle. *Exp. Neurol.* 98, 317–335. doi: 10.1016/0014-4886(87)90245-7

Matthews, P. B. (1984). Observations on the time course of the electromyographic response reflexly elicited by muscle vibration in man. *J. Physiol.* 353, 447–461. doi: 10.1113/jphysiol.1984.sp015346

McMorland, A. J., Runnalls, K. D., and Byblow, W. D. (2015). A neuroanatomical framework for upper limb synergies after stroke. *Front. Hum. Neurosci.* 9:82. doi: 10.3389/fnhum.2015.00082

McPherson, J. G., Chen, A., Ellis, M. D., Yao, J., Heckman, C. J., and Dewald, J. P. A. (2018). Progressive recruitment of contralesional cortico-reticulospinal pathways drives motor impairment post stroke. *J. Physiol.* 596, 1211–1225. doi: 10.1113/JP274968

McPherson, J. G., Ellis, M. D., Heckman, C. J., and Dewald, J. P. (2008). Evidence for increased activation of persistent inward currents in individuals with chronic hemiparetic stroke. *J. Neurophysiol.* 100, 3236–3243. doi: 10.1152/jn.90563.2008

McPherson, J. G., Stienen, A. H. A., Drogos, J. M., and Dewald, J. P. A. (2017). Modification of spastic stretch reflexes at the elbow by flexion synergy expression in individuals with chronic hemiparetic stroke. *Arch. Phys. Med. Rehabil.* 99, 491–500. doi: 10.1016/j.apmr.2017.06.01

McPherson, J. G., Stienen, A. H., Drogos, J. M., and Dewald, J. P. (2011). The relationship between the flexion synergy and stretch reflexes in individuals with chronic hemiparetic stroke. *IEEE Int. Conf. Rehabil. Robot.* 2011:5975516. doi: 10.1109/ICORR.2011.5975516

McPherson, L. M., Negro, F., Thompson, C. K., Sanchez, L., Heckman, C. J., Dewald, J., et al. (2016). Properties of the motor unit action potential shape in proximal and distal muscles of the upper limb in healthy and post-stroke individuals. *Conf. Proc. IEEE Eng. Med. Biol. Soc.* 2016, 335–339. doi: 10.1109/EMBC.2016.7590708

Miller, D. M., Klein, C. S., Suresh, N. L., and Rymer, W. Z. (2014). Asymmetries in vestibular evoked myogenic potentials in chronic stroke survivors with spastic hypertonia: evidence for a vestibulospinal role. *Clin. Neurophysiol.* 125, 2070–2078. doi: 10.1016/j.clinph.2014.01.035

Miller, L. C., and Dewald, J. P. (2012). Involuntary paretic wrist/finger flexion forces and EMG increase with shoulder abduction load in individuals with chronic stroke. *Clin. Neurophysiol.* 123, 1216–1225. doi: 10.1016/j.clinph.2012.01.009

Miller, L. C., Thompson, C. K., Negro, F., Heckman, C. J., Farina, D., and Dewald, J. P. (2014). High-density surface EMG decomposition allows for recording of motor unit discharge from proximal and distal flexion synergy muscles simultaneously in individuals with stroke. *Conf. Proc. IEEE Eng. Med. Biol. Soc.* 2014, 5340–5344. doi: 10.1109/EMBC.2014.6944832

Morita, H., Crone, C., Christenhuis, D., Petersen, N. T., and Nielsen, J. B. (2001). Modulation of presynaptic inhibition and disynaptic reciprocal Ia inhibition during voluntary movement in spasticity. *Brain* 124, 826–837. doi: 10.1093/brain/124.4.826

Mottram, C. J., Suresh, N. L., Heckman, C. J., Gorassini, M. A., and Rymer, W. Z. (2009). Origins of abnormal excitability in biceps brachii motoneurons of spastic-paretic stroke survivors. *J. Neurophysiol.* 102, 2026–2038. doi: 10.1152/jn.00151.2009

Mottram, C. J., Wallace, C. L., Chikando, C. N., and Rymer, W. Z. (2010). Origins of spontaneous firing of motor units in the spastic-paretic biceps brachii muscle of stroke survivors. *J. Neurophysiol.* 104, 3168–3179. doi: 10.1152/jn.00463.2010

Murray, K. C., Nakae, A., Stephens, M. J., Rank, M., D'amico, J., Harvey, P. J., et al. (2010). Recovery of motoneuron and locomotor function after spinal cord injury depends on constitutive activity in 5-HT2C receptors. *Nat. Med.* 16, 694–700. doi: 10.1038/nm.2160

Negro, F., Muceli, S., Castronovo, A. M., Holobar, A., and Farina, D. (2016). Multi-channel intramuscular and surface EMG decomposition by convolutive blind source separation. *J. Neural Eng.* 13:026027. doi: 10.1088/1741-2560/13/2/026027

Nielsen, J. B., Petersen, N. T., Crone, C., and Sinkjaer, T. (2005). Stretch reflex regulation in healthy subjects and patients with spasticity. *Neuromodulation* 8, 49–57. doi: 10.1111/j.1094-7159.2005.05220.x

O'Sullivan, S. B., and Schmitz, T. J. (2001). *Physical Rehabilitation.* Philadelphia, PA: F.A. Davis Company.

Owen, M., Ingo, C., and Dewald, J. P. A. (2017). Upper extremity motor impairments and microstructural changes in bulbospinal pathways in chronic hemiparetic stroke. *Front. Neurol.* 8:257. doi: 10.3389/fneur.2017.00257

Pearson, K. G., and Collins, D. F. (1993). Reversal of the influence of group Ib afferents from plantaris on activity in medial gastrocnemius muscle during locomotor activity. *J. Neurophysiol.* 70, 1009–1017. doi: 10.1152/jn.1993.70.3.1009

Perrier, J. F., and Hounsgaard, J. (2003). 5-HT2 receptors promote plateau potentials in turtle spinal motoneurons by facilitating an L-type calcium current. *J. Neurophysiol.* 89, 954–959. doi: 10.1152/jn.00753.2002

Powers, R. K., and Binder, M. D. (2001). Input-output functions of mammalian motoneurons. *Rev. Physiol. Biochem. Pharmacol.* 143, 137–263. doi: 10.1007/BFb0115594

Powers, R. K., Campbell, D. L., and Rymer, W. Z. (1989). Stretch reflex dynamics in spastic elbow flexor muscles. *Ann. Neurol.* 25, 32–42. doi: 10.1002/ana.410250106

Powers, R. K., Elbasiouny, S. M., Rymer, W. Z., and Heckman, C. J. (2012). Contribution of intrinsic properties and synaptic inputs to motoneuron discharge patterns: a simulation study. *J. Neurophysiol.* 107, 808–823. doi: 10.1152/jn.00510.2011

Powers, R. K., and Heckman, C. J. (2017). Synaptic control of the shape of the motoneuron pool input-output function. *J. Neurophysiol.* 117, 1171–1184. doi: 10.1152/jn.00850.2016

Prochazka, A., Gillard, D., and Bennett, D. J. (1997). Implications of positive feedback in the control of movement. *J. Neurophysiol.* 77, 3237–3251. doi: 10.1152/jn.1997.77.6.3237

Revill, A. L., and Fuglevand, A. J. (2017). Inhibition linearizes firing rate responses in human motor units: implications for the role of persistent inward currents. *J. Physiol.* 595, 179–191. doi: 10.1113/JP272823

Schwarz, P. B., Yee, N., Mir, S., and Peever, J. H. (2008). Noradrenaline triggers muscle tone by amplifying glutamate-driven excitation of somatic motoneurones in anaesthetized rats. *J. Physiol.* 586, 5787–5802. doi: 10.1113/jphysiol.2008.159392

Schwindt, P., and Crill, W. E. (1977). A persistent negative resistance in cat lumbar motoneurons. *Brain Res.* 120, 173–178. doi: 10.1016/0006-8993(77)90510-8

Silverman, J., Garnett, N. L., Giszter, S. F., Heckman, C. J. II., Kulpa-Eddy, J. A., Lemay, M. A., et al. (2005). Decerebrate mammalian preparations: unalleviated or fully alleviated pain? A review and opinion. *Contemp. Top. Lab. Anim. Sci.* 44, 34–36.

Stinear, C. M., Barber, P. A., Smale, P. R., Coxon, J. P., Fleming, M. K., and Byblow, W. D. (2007). Functional potential in chronic stroke patients depends on corticospinal tract integrity. *Brain* 130, 170–180. doi: 10.1093/brain/awl333

Thilmann, A. F., Fellows, S. J., and Garms, E. (1990). Pathological stretch reflexes on the "good" side of hemiparetic patients. *J. Neurol. Neurosurg. Psychiatr.* 53, 208–214. doi: 10.1136/jnnp.53.3.208

Thilmann, A. F., Fellows, S. J., and Garms, E. (1991). The mechanism of spastic muscle hypertonus. Variation in reflex gain over the time course of spasticity. *Brain* 114 (Pt 1A), 233–244.

Veasey, S. C., Fornal, C. A., Metzler, C. W., and Jacobs, B. L. (1995). Response of serotonergic caudal raphe neurons in relation to specific motor activities in freely moving cats. *J. Neurosci.* 15, 5346–5359.

8

Differential Dopamine D1 and D3 Receptor Modulation and Expression in the Spinal Cord of Two Mouse Models of Restless Legs Syndrome

*Samantha Meneely[1], Mai-Lynne Dinkins[1], Miki Kassai[1], Shangru Lyu[2], Yuning Liu[2], Chien-Te Lin[1,3], Kori Brewer[4], Yuqing Li[2,5] and Stefan Clemens[1]**

[1] Department of Physiology, Brody School of Medicine, East Carolina University, Greenville, NC, United States, [2] Department of Neurology, College of Medicine, University of Florida, Gainesville, FL, United States, [3] East Carolina Diabetes and Obesity Institute, Brody School of Medicine, East Carolina University, Greenville, NC, United States, [4] Department of Emergency Medicine, Brody School of Medicine, East Carolina University, Greenville, NC, United States, [5] Wuxi Medical School, Jiangnan University, Wuxi, China

***Correspondence:**
Stefan Clemens
clemenss@ecu.edu

Restless Legs Syndrome (RLS) is often and successfully treated with dopamine receptor agonists that target the inhibitory D3 receptor subtype, however there is no clinical evidence of a D3 receptor dysfunction in RLS patients. In contrast, genome-wide association studies in RLS patients have established that a mutation of the *MEIS1* gene is associated with an increased risk in developing RLS, but the effect of *MEIS1* dysfunction on sensorimotor function remain unknown. Mouse models for a dysfunctional D3 receptor (D3KO) and Meis1 (Meis1KO) were developed independently, and each animal expresses some features associated with RLS in the clinic, but they have not been compared in their responsiveness to treatment options used in the clinic. We here confirm that D3KO and Meis1KO animals show increased locomotor activities, but that only D3KO show an increased sensory excitability to thermal stimuli. Next we compared the effects of dopaminergics and opioids in both animal models, and we assessed D1 and D3 dopamine receptor expression in the spinal cord, the gateway for sensorimotor processing. We found that Meis1KO share most of the tested behavioral properties with their wild type (WT) controls, including the modulation of the thermal pain withdrawal reflex by morphine, L-DOPA and D3 receptor (D3R) agonists and antagonists. However, Meis1KO and D3KO were behaviorally more similar to each other than to WT when tested with D1 receptor (D1R) agonists and antagonists. Subsequent Western blot analyses of D1R and D3R protein expression in the spinal cord revealed a significant increase in D1R but not D3R expression in Meis1KO and D3KO over WT controls. As the D3R is mostly present in the dorsal spinal cord where it has been shown to modulate sensory pathways, while activation of the D1Rs can activate motoneurons in the ventral spinal cord, we speculate that D3KO and Meis1KO represent two complementary animal models for RLS, in which the mechanisms of sensory (D3R-mediated) and motor (D1R-mediated) dysfunctions can be differentially explored.

Keywords: RLS animal models, dopamine, D1 receptor, D3 receptor, Meis1, sensorimotor function, spinal cord

INTRODUCTION

Background on RLS

Restless Legs Syndrome (RLS) is a highly prevalent (5–10% of the population, Ghorayeb and Tison, 2010; Earley et al., 2011), but also underappreciated aging-associated neurological sensorimotor disorder that severely disrupts sleep and affects quality of life. First described in 1685 (Willis, 1685) and clinically confirmed in the mid-twentieth century (Ekbom, 1944, 1945, 1960), RLS is a clinical disorder in which overlapping genetic risk factors may play a role in the emergence of the symptoms (Trenkwalder et al., 2016). Genome-wide association studies in RLS patients have established several chromosome loci associated with RLS, notably *MEIS1* and *BTBD9* (Stefansson et al., 2007; Winkelmann et al., 2007), of which a point mutation in the *MEIS1* gene has the highest odd ratios with RLS (Winkelmann, 2008; Schormair et al., 2011, 2017; Winkelmann et al., 2011). Meis1 plays a role in the early development of the nervous system (Spieler et al., 2014; Marcos et al., 2015), and is essential to specify cell fates and differentiation patterns along the proximodistal axis of the limbs (Mercader et al., 1999, 2009). Intriguingly, a dysfunction of the *MEIS1* homolog in *C. elegans* is associated with an altered projection phenotype of dopamine neurons (M. Aschner, Albert Einstein College of Medicine, personal communication), suggesting a possible interaction between *MEIS1* and dopamine (DA) function.

RLS is often and successfully treated with DA receptor agonists that target the inhibitory D2-like receptor subtype, in particular D3 (Stiasny et al., 2000; Ferri et al., 2010; Manconi et al., 2011a; Garcia-Borreguero et al., 2016), and it has been suggested that a dysfunction of the descending A11 DA system in the hypothalamus may be involved in RLS by predominantly affecting the D3R system (Clemens et al., 2006; Lanza et al., 2017). There exist three DA receptors that mediate inhibitory actions via *Gi*-coupled pathways (D2, D3, and D4), and the D3R subtype has a very high affinity to DA (Robinson et al., 1994; Cote and Kuzhikandathil, 2014). Yet despite the efficacy of the D3R compounds in treating RLS symptoms, there is no clinical evidence of A11 dysfunction in patients (Earley et al., 2009). However, a dysfunction of the DA system has been linked to altered iron homeostasis or iron-deficient diet (Dowling et al., 2011; Klinker et al., 2011; Dauvilliers and Winkelmann, 2013; Earley et al., 2014).

Animal Models of RLS

Mouse models for a dysfunctional D3 receptor (D3KO) and Meis1 (Meis1KO) were developed independently (Accili et al., 1996), and each animal expresses some features associated with RLS in the clinic. Both D3KO and Meis1KO express increased locomotor activity (Accili et al., 1996; Salminen et al., 2017), but only D3KO show an increased sensory excitability both in the isolated spinal cord (Clemens and Hochman, 2004) and *in vivo* (Keeler et al., 2012). The thermal pain withdrawal reflex depends on spinal cord circuits that can be recruited experimentally to assess compromised function of the underlying neural networks, both with the spinal cord and extending into the periphery. The previously reported increased excitability of the D3KO mouse to thermal stimuli suggests a possible role of C-fiber mediated pathways that convey altered sensations from deep within the muscle tissue (Clemens et al., 2006; Keeler et al., 2012). Further, as recent data suggest that the inhibitory D3 receptor can form functional heteromeric dimers with the excitatory D1 receptor (Marcellino et al., 2008), it is conceivable that the increased excitability observed in D3KO may be the result of an increased expression of the excitatory dopamine D1 receptor (D1R) (Brewer et al., 2014).

We here compared the effects of dopaminergic treatment on spinal reflexes as a tool to assess sensorimotor function (Eccles and Lundberg, 1959; Nielsen, 2004; Barriere et al., 2005) in Meis1KO and D3KO animal models, and we assessed D1R and D3R expressions the spinal cord, the gateway for sensorimotor processing. We found that Meis1KO share most of the tested behavioral properties with their wild type (WT) controls, including the modulation of the thermal pain withdrawal reflex by morphine, L-DOPA and D3 receptor (D3R) agonists and antagonists. However, Meis1KO and D3KO also shared behavioral similarities when tested with D1 receptor (D1R) agonists and antagonists, while the matching WTs were unresponsive to these drugs. Subsequent Western blot analyses of D1R and D3R protein expression in the spinal cord revealed a significant increase in D1R expression in Meis1KO and D3KO over the WT controls, while D3R expression was not significantly different across all 3 groups. Our data show that changes in spinal D1R expression and behavioral responses to D1R compounds are similar between Meis1KO and D3KO, while the increased sensitivity at baseline is present only in D3KO. We provide a model that separates D3KO and Meis1KO into two complimentary models of RLS that represent sensory and motor dysfunctions, respectively.

METHODS

Animals

All experimental procedures were approved by the Institutional Animal Care and Use Committees at East Carolina University and University of Florida, and were fully compliant with the National Institutes of Health guide for the care and use of Laboratory animals (NIH Publications No. 80-23). All efforts were made to minimize the number of animals used, and a total of 55 male mice (age range ∼9–12 months) were tested in this study. Behavioral testing was performed on *Meis1* heterozygous knockout mice (*Meis1*+/Δ, Meis1KO, $n = 15$) and their appropriate wild-type (WT) controls (C57BL/6J, $n = 12$), dopamine D3 receptor knockout mice (D3KO; strain B6.129S4-Drd3^{tm1dac}/J (stock # 002958, Jackson Laboratory, Bar Harbor, ME), $n = 13$) and their appropriate WT controls (C57BL/6J, $n = 15$) (Clemens and Hochman, 2004; Brewer et al., 2014). *Meis1 loxP mice* were from Drs. Copeland and Sadek (Kocabas et al., 2012), and Meis1+/Δ were generated by crossing *Meis1 loxP* with Emx1-cre mice (Guo et al., 2000). *Emx1* expresses in testis germ cells, so that when germ cells contain both *Emx1*-cre and *Meis1 loxP*, cre-mediated recombination occurs and leads to a deletion of the *loxP*-flanked sequence. Male mice heterozygous for both *Meis1 loxP* and *Emx1*-cre were then bred with WT female mice. The deletion of *Meis1* gene occurred during the development and *Meis1*+/Δ mice were derived. Finally, *Meis1*+/Δ mice were crossed with WT mice to generate experimental mice. Animals were housed with free access to food, water, and enrichments under a 12-h light/dark cycle at room temperature.

Behavioral Assessments–Hargreaves

Behavioral testing procedures have been described in detail recently (Keeler et al., 2012; Brewer et al., 2014). Thermal withdrawal latencies (Hargreaves' method) were obtained in each cohort by using the IITC plantar analgesia meter (IITC Series 8, IITC Inc., Woodland Hills, CA). Experiments were performed between 9 am and 1 pm, to minimize the circadian variation. The week before testing started, animals were acclimated on 3–4 days to the experimental room and the Hargreave's system, by placing them individually into the Plexiglas cubicles for an average of 2 h. In week 1 of the testing period, we tested the effects of vehicle injections (0.9% NaCl, i.p., ~90–120 μl per animal). Animals were tested 5 times per session, with resting periods for each individual animal between tests of 5–10 min. Stimulation cut-off for each test was set to 30 s test duration, to prevent the possibility of a heat-induced injury. Once initiated, recording sessions for all 5 trials lasted no longer than 60–90 min for all animals tested that day. After vehicle assessments, we subsequently compared all drug effects (i.p. injections, injection volumes matching the vehicle volumes) against the data obtained after the respective vehicle injections in each animal cohort. We started the tests 1 h after vehicle or drug injections. Each drug test was separated from the next drug treatment by an at least 3-day recovery period, to minimize any potential drug interactions possibly skewing the latency measurements. After ~5–6 weeks, we again tested the responses to vehicle injections in two cohorts and found no significant differences from the values obtained at baseline (data not shown).

Behavioral Assessments–Locomotor Activity

Spontaneous locomotor activities were recorded for Meis1KO and their WT controls with a VersaMax Legacy open field apparatus connected to a computerized Digiscan System (Accuscan Instruments, Inc. OH), and for D3KO and their controls with a TSE LabMaster System (TSE Systems, Chesterfield, MO). Infrared sensors were used to record ambulatory activity in the X-Y plane). Counts across all these axes were summed to give total ambulatory activity. Meis1KO and their WT controls were monitored for 7 days. Only the data from the last 4 days were pooled and analyzed. For D3KO and their controls, after 2 days of acclimation, data were collected for 2 consecutive days to calculate locomotor activity.

Compounds Tested

We tested the effects of levodopa (L-DOPA, 10 mg/kg, Acros Organics, Geel, Belgium), the D3 receptor agonist, pramipexole (0.5 mg/kg, ApexBio Technology LLC, Houston, TX), the D3 receptor antagonist, SB277011-A (10 mg/kg, Abcam Cambridge, MA), the D1 agonist, SKF 38393 (10 mg/kg, Tocris, Ellisville, MO), the D1 receptor antagonist, SCH 39166 (5 mg/kg, Tocris, Ellisville, MO), and morphine (morphine sulfate salt pentahydrate, 2 mg/kg, Sigma-Aldrich St. Louis, MO). Drug concentrations were chosen based on previous publications by others and us (Acquas and Di Chiara, 1999; Williams et al., 2006; Brewer et al., 2014; Solís et al., 2015; Dinkins et al., 2017)

Tissue Harvesting and Protein Isolation

Mice were deeply anesthetized with isoflurane and decapitated before spinal cords were dissected out, immediately placed in RNAlater (Thermo Fisher Scientific, Waltham, MA), and stored at −20°C until use. Spinal cords were homogenized in 1 ml of RIPA buffer with protease and phosphatase inhibitors (0.12 ml/ml RIPA buffer, Sigma-Aldrich #P2714 and 0.012 ml/ml of RIPA buffer, Sigma-Aldrich #P5726 St. Louis, MO, respectively). The homogenized spinal cords were centrifuged (13,000 rpm, 4°C, 15 min), and supernatants were aliquoted and stored individually at −80°C. Following homogenization, standard protein concentrations were established with a Bradford protein assay (Quickstart Bradford reagent, Bio-Rad #500205), and plates were read on an Epoch Microplate Spectrophotometer (BioTek, Winooski, VT) at 595 nm using the Gen5.1 software package (BioTek, Winooski, VT).

Western Blot

For Western blots, 30 μg of each lumbar spinal cord protein samples were denatured using 2x Laemmli buffer containing 5% β-mercaptoethanol and 1% SDS at 95°C for 10 min and loaded onto a 12% Criterion™ TGX Stain-Free™ Protein Gel (#5678045, Bio-Rad, Hercules, CA) and run ~45 min at 200 V. The proteins were transferred to a low fluorescent PVDF membrane using Trans-Blot® Turbo™ RTA Midi LF PVDF Transfer Kit (#170-4275, Bio-Rad, Hercules, CA). Membranes were probed with the primary antibodies and with secondary antibodies (LI-COR, Lincoln, NE) by the iBind™ Flex Western Device (SLF2000, Thermo Fisher, Waltham, MA) based on sequential Lateral Flow (SLF) technology using iBind™ Flex Fluorescent Detection (FD) Solution Kit (SLF 2019, Thermo Fisher, Waltham, MA). Membranes were imaged with an Odyssey imaging system (Odyssey Clx, LI-COR, Lincoln, NE).

Antibodies

The primary antibodies used for Western blot to detect receptor-specific protein expression were: anti-dopamine receptor D1 (Abcam 78021, 1:500 Cambridge, MA) and anti-dopamine receptor D3 (Abcam 42114, 1:1,000 Cambridge, MA). The secondary antibodies used were goat anti-rabbit 680RD (925-68071, 1:4,000, LI-COR Biosciences, Lincoln, NE) and goat anti-mouse 680RD (925-68070, 1:4,000, LI-COR Biosciences, Lincoln, NE).

Statistical Analysis

Following the experiments, behavioral data were transferred and stored in Excel format, then analyzed and plotted offline with SigmaPlot (Version 11, SPSS Science, San Jose, California). For statistical comparisons, we employed parametric or non-parametric comparisons as appropriate when comparing multiple groups (One-Way ANOVA, RM ANOVA, or ANOVA on Ranks) with appropriate *post-hoc* comparisons (Holms-Sidak, Dunn's); *t*-tests or paired *t*-tests were used for comparison between two sets of data (treatment against respective control vehicle treatment only). Significance levels were set at $p < 0.05$. For Western blot analysis, images were analyzed with ImageStudio and ImageJ (1.50i National Institutes of Health, USA) and statistical analyses were performed with SigmaPlot 11.0.

RESULTS

Thermal Pain Withdrawal Latencies Under Baseline Conditions

We first tested and compared pain withdrawal latency responses in Meis1KO and D3KO lines under baseline conditions (after sham injection, i.p., 0.9% NaCl, 100 μl/30 g), and compared them to their respective controls. Meis1KO and their respective controls were tested as two independent cohorts. In cohort 1 the average WT latency was 10.2 ± 1.1 s, while Meis1KO latencies were 10.2 ± 0.5 s ($p = 0.97$, $n = 7$ each, power: 0.05). In cohort 2 (tested about 1 year later) the average WT latency was 6.6 ± 0.4 s, while Meis1KO latencies were 6.7 ± 0.9 s ($p = 0.92$, $n = 6$ [WT] and $n = 7$ [Meis1KO], power: 0.05). Thus despite the difference between the two Meis1KO cohorts and their WT controls, there was no effect within each cohort between WT and knockout. In contrast, individual withdrawal latencies in D3KO ranged per trial from 4.8 to 11.1 s, (average: 8.5 ± 0.24 s, $n = 7$) while the latencies of their respective WTs (WT_{D3KO}) ranged from 5.9 to 13.7 s (average: 6.5 ± 0.33 s, $n = 7$). A *t*-test comparison revealed that the difference between WT_{D3KO} and D3KO was significant ($p < 0.001$, power: 0.99).

To illustrate the effect of the genotype alone on thermal pain withdrawal reflex latencies, we normalized the WT_{meis1} response to 100% and compared them with the effects in the genetically modified animals (**Figure 1**). We found that pain withdrawal latencies of Meis1KO and their respective controls (WT_{meis1}) were not significantly different from each other (WT_{meis1}: 99.9 ± 6.1% S.E. $n = 13$, Meis1KO: 101 ± 6.7 % S.E., $n = 14$, $p = 0.97$, *t*-test, power: 0.5), while those of D3KO were significantly reduced over their respective WTs (WT_{D3KO}: 99.99 ± 2.8%; D3KO: 77.3 ± 3.9%, S.E., $p < 0.001$, *t*-test, both: $n = 7$, power: 0.99).

Morphine Modulation of Withdrawal Latencies

While opioids are commonly used for treating chronic neuropathic pain, they have also become a treatment of choice in dopamine agonist-refractory RLS (Trenkwalder et al., 2015; Gemignani et al., 2016). As we have previously shown that the D3KO mouse expresses a morphine-tolerant phenotype if treated with low doses of morphine (Brewer et al., 2014), we next addressed the question if the Meis1KO mouse follows the WT or the D3KO phenotype when challenged with morphine (**Figure 2**). In Meis1KO cohort 1, WT withdrawal latencies increased from 6.8 ± 0.45 s to 9.1 ± 1.2 s ($n = 6$), while responses of Meis1KO increased from 6.3 ± 1.2 s to 10.1 ± 1.1 s ($n = 7$). Similarly, in cohort 2, WT withdrawal latencies increased from 6.5 ± 1.2 s to 9.3 ± 1.9 s ($n = 5$), while responses of Meis1KO increased from 6.3 ± 0.6 s to 7.9 ± 1.9 s ($n = 7$). After normalization to each WT_{meis1} control, the data are as follows: WT_{meis1}; Ctrl: 99.3 ± 7.1%; after treatment: 132.5 ± 14.8%, $p = 0.08$, paired *t*-test, $n = 11$, power: 0.83, **Figure 2A1**; Meis1KO; Ctrl: 99.2 ± 5.7%; after treatment: 143 ± 16.6%, $p = 0.024$, paired *t*-test, $n = 14$, power: 0.59, **Figure 2A2**. For WT_{D3KO} the raw data were as follows; Ctrl: 8.3 ± 0.3 s; after treatment: 11.4 ± 0.6 s ($n = 7$), while D3KO were not responsive to 2 mg/kg morphine (Ctrl: 6.6 ± 0.4 s; after treatment: 6.1 ± 0.4 s, $n = 7$). After normalization to the pre-treatment control, the data for WT_{D3KO} are: 99.8 ± 2.8%; after treatment: 137.1 ± 7%, $p = 0.002$, paired *t*-test, power: 0.99; **Figure 2B1**. In contrast, normalized the data for the D3KO are: Ctrl 100.6 ± 5%; after treatment: 95.1 ± 6.6%, $p = 0.62$, paired *t*-test, power: 0.05, **Figure 2B2**). Together, these data suggest that WT_{meis1}, WT_{D3KO}, and Meis1KO animals respond similar to morphine, while D3KO are not affected.

Dopaminergic Modulation of Withdrawal Latencies

Dopaminergics are the first line of therapy in the treatment of RLS symptoms, and they can cover a range from L-DOPA to highly specific D3 receptor agonists. We therefore sought to first test the effects of L-DOPA on thermal withdrawal latencies in the different animal strains before testing the effects of the more selective receptor agonists and antagonists. We found that treatment with 10 mg/kg L-DOPA did not significantly alter withdrawal latencies in WT controls, Meis1KO or D3KO (data not shown).

We next tested the effects of the D3-receptor preferring agonist, pramipexole (PPX, **Figures 3**, **4**). In WT_{meis1}, treatment with PPX (0.5 mg/kg) increased withdrawal latencies from 100.2 ± 6.6% to 144.4 ± 13.7%, ($p = 0.008$, paired *t*-test, $n = 11$, power: 0.81, **Figure 3A1**; raw data for WT_{meis1} cohort 1: Ctrl 6.1 ± 0.7 s, PPX 9.6 ± 1.3 s, $n = 6$; cohort 2: Ctrl 7.2 ± 0.5 s; PPX: 8.6 ± 0.9 s, $n = 5$). In Meis1KO, the PPX treatment also led to a significant increase in withdrawal latencies from 100.1 ± 8.9% to 131.3 ± 12.3% ($p = 0.017$, paired *t*-test, $n = 14$, power: 0.65, **Figure 3A2**; raw data for Meis1KO cohort 1: Ctrl 6.7 ± 0.9 s, PPX 9.1 ± 1.2 s, $n = 7$; cohort 2: Ctrl 7.2 ± 0.9 s; PPX: 7.8 ± 1 s, $n = 7$). The effect of PPX was similar in the WT of the D3KO mice (WT_{D3KO}) to the effect observed in WT_{meis1} and Meis1KO, but it did not alter the responses in the D3KO. In WT_{D3KO}, withdrawal latencies rose significantly from 100 ± 6.3% (Ctrl) to 204.8 ± 9% (PPX, $p < 0.001$, paired *t*-test, $n = 8$, power: 1.0, **Figure 3B1**). In contrast, PPX did not have any significant effect in D3KO (Ctrl: 100 ± 5.6%, PPX: 108.4 ± 5.6%, $p = 0.47$, *t*-test, $n = 6$, power: 0.5, **Figure 3B2**). The raw data were as follows: WT_{D3KO}; Ctrl 6.6 ± 0.5 s, PPX 12.9 ± 1.8 s, $n = 8$; D3KO; Ctrl 9.3 ± 0.6 s; PPX: 10.1 ± 0.8 s, $n = 9$.

Additionally, treatment with the D3 receptor antagonist, SB 277011, significantly decreased withdrawal latencies in Meis1KO

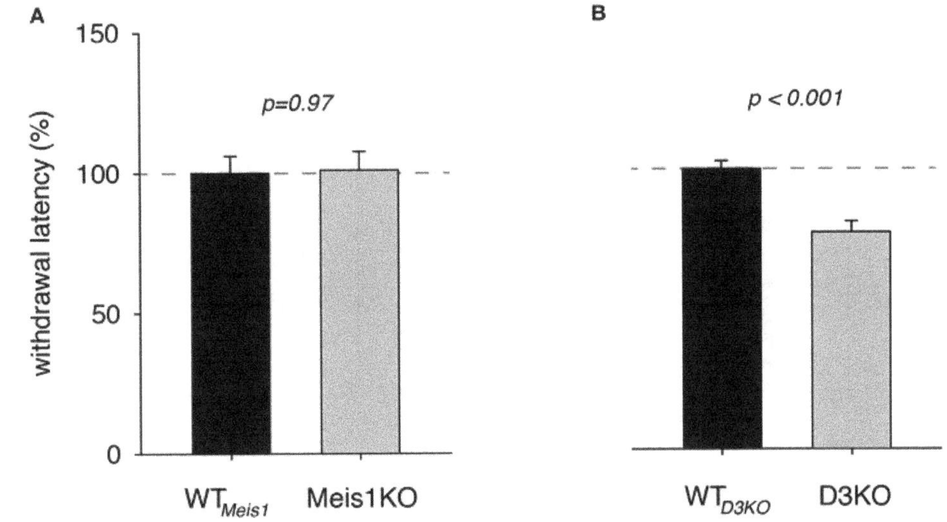

FIGURE 1 | Thermal pain withdrawal latencies under vehicle (control) conditions. **(A)** Normalized representation of data from Meis1KO mice and their respective WT controls (WT_{meis1}). WT $_{meis1}$ latencies (black bar) were similar to those of Meis1KO (gray bar). **(B)** Normalized representation of data from D3KO animals and respective WT controls (WT $_{D3KO}$). WT $_{D3KO}$ latencies (black bar) were significantly higher than those of the D3KO (gray bar).

but not D3KO (**Figure 4**). In MeislKO, withdrawal latencies dropped from 99.5 ± 6.3% (Ctrl) to 78.5 ± 4.4% (SB277, $p = 0.004$, $n = 7$, paired t-test, power: 0.96, **Figure 4A**). However, we did not observe any significant effect in D3KO mice (Ctrl: 99.9 ± 5.3%, SB277: 92.8 ± 3.6%, $p = 0.28$, $n = 6$, paired t-test, power: 0.09, **Figure 4B**). The raw data were as follows: MeislKO; Ctrl 7.2 ± 0.6 s, SB277 5.2 ± 0.2 s, $n = 7$; D3KO; Ctrl 7.9 ± 0.3 s; SB277: 7.8 ± 0.2 s, $n = 6$. Overall, treatment with the D3 receptor modulators led to similar effects in WT and MeislKO and contrasted those in D3KO.

As recent findings from our lab point to a possible involvement of the D1 receptor in the face of D3 dysfunction (Brewer et al., 2014) or prolonged D3R agonist exposure (Dinkins et al., 2017), we next tested the effects of the D1 receptor agonist, SKF 38393 (SKF, **Figure 5**). We found that treatment with SKF had no significant effect in WT_{meis1} animals (Ctrl: 99.9 ± 8.2%; SKF: 92 ± 6.4%, $p = 0.77$, paired t-test, $n = 5$, power: 0.05, **Figure 5A1**), while the same treatment led to significant decrease of withdrawal latencies in MeislKO (Ctrl: 99.9 ± 8.2%; SKF: 82.4 ± 5.7%, $p = 0.001$, paired t-test, $N = 7$, power: 0.98, **Figure 5A2**). The raw data were as follows: WT_{Meis1}; Ctrl 6.6 ± 0.3 s, SKF 6.2 ± 0.5 s; MeislKO; Ctrl 6.9 ± 0.5 s; SKF: 5.4 ± 0.3 s.

In WT_{D3KO} animals, SKF effects were similar to WT_{meis1} (Ctrl: 100.1 ± 6.6%, SKF: 92.2 ± 5.9%, $p = 0.37$, $n = 5$, power: 0.051, **Figure 5B1**), while the responses in D3KO were similar to those in MeislKO (Ctrl: 99.8 ± 3.9%, SKF: 71.6 ± 3.6%, $p < 0.001$, $n = 6$, power: 1.0, **Figure 5B2**). The raw data were as follows: WT_{D3KO}; Ctrl 16.8 ± 1.9 s, SKF 14 ± 1.2 s; D3KO; Ctrl 8.4 ± 0.9 s; SKF: 5.9 ± 0.8 s. In contrast to the D1 receptor agonist SKF 38393, the D1 receptor antagonist, SCH 39166, displayed no differential effects in WT controls, MeislKO or D3KO animals (WT_{Meis1} animals: Ctrl: 100.3 ± 7.2%, SCH: 102.3 ± 12%, $p = 0.89$, paired t-test, $n = 5$, power: 0.05, MeislKO: Ctrl: 100.3 ± 6.9%, SCH: 110.6 ± 11%, $p = 0.4$, paired t-test, $n = 7$, power: 0.05; D3KO: Ctrl: 99.7 ± 5.5%, SCH: 111.6 ± 8.8%, $p = 0.3$, paired t-test, $n = 6$, power: 0.07). Taken together, the results of these dopaminergic modulators suggest that D3 receptor-mediated actions affect WT and MeislKO similarly, while activation of D1 receptor signaling pathways exert similar effects in MeislKO and D3KO but not WTs.

D1R and D3R Protein Expression in the Lumbar Spinal Cord of WT, Meis1KO, and D3KO Animals

As treatments with D3- and D1 receptor-preferring agonists and antagonists respectively led to different outcomes, we next tested if the expression of these dopamine receptor subtypes was differentially regulated in MeislKO and D3KO over WT (**Figures 6, 7**). We found that D3 receptor protein expression did not significantly differ between WT_{Meis1}, MeislKO, and D3KO (WT: 99.1 ± 3.5%; MeislKO: 128.7 ± 8.5%; D3KO: 126.5 ± 11.5%, $p = 0.16$, One-Way ANOVA; **Figure 6**). Note that the D3KO expresses a dysfunctional D3 receptor that is not embedded into the membrane (Clemens et al., 2005). In contrast to the D3 receptor, when we probed for D1 receptor expression in the spinal cord, we found significantly increased D1 receptor protein levels in both MeislKO and D3KO over WT controls (WT: 99.9 ± 8.4%; MeislKO: 158.4 ± 13.5%; D3KO: 162 ± 12%, $p = 0.003$, One-Way ANOVA, **Figure 7**).

Increased Locomotor Activity in Meis1KO And D3KO Animals

As the pharmacological and Western blot data suggested a role of the D1 receptor system in the control of spinal cord function, and as D1 receptor activation can recruit spinal cord networks

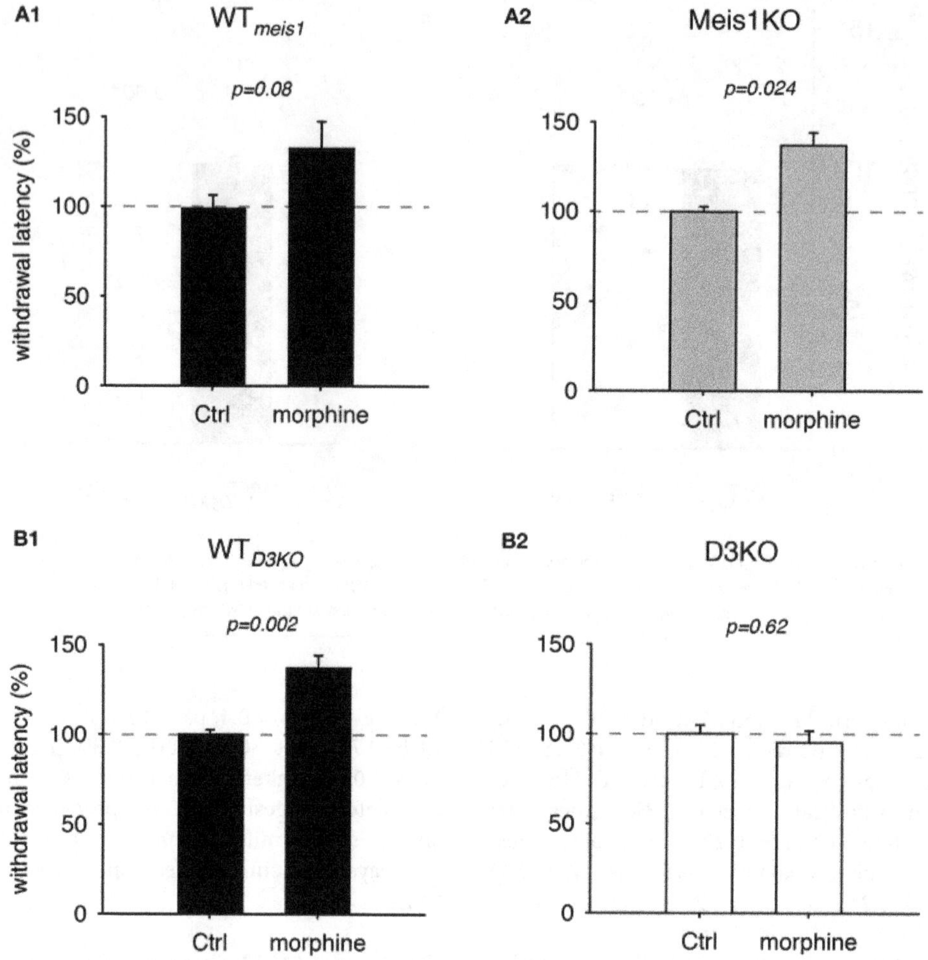

FIGURE 2 | Thermal pain withdrawal latencies of WT, Meis1KO, and D3KO under sham (Ctrl) and morphine conditions. **(A1)** Normalized representation of data from WT_{meis1} animals. Morphine significantly increased withdrawal latencies. **(A2)** Normalized representation of data from the pooled Meis1KO animals. As in WT_{meis1}, morphine significantly increased withdrawal latencies. **(B1)** Normalized representation of data from WT_{D3KO} animals. Morphine significantly increased withdrawal latencies. **(B2)** Normalized representation of data from D3KO animals. Unlike in both WT lines and Meis1KO, morphine had no effect on withdrawal latencies in D3KO.

to generate locomotor-like activities, we next tested if Meis1KO and D3KO show altered locomotor activities over their respective WT controls (**Figure 8**). We found that Meis1KO exhibited significantly increased locomotor activities compared to their WT (WT_{meis1}: 86.1 ± 13.7 m/day, $n = 7$; Meis1KO: 399.7 ± 35.5 m/day, $n = 8$, $p < 0.001$, t-test, power: 1.0), and that D3KO showed a similar significant increase over their WT controls (WT_{D3KO}: 343.2. ± 41.3 m/day, $n = 16$; D3KO: 587 ± 120 m/day, $n = 8$, $p = 0.035$, t-test, power: 0.48).

DISCUSSION

Here we compared thermal pain withdrawal latencies in two animal models of RLS, D3KO, and Meis1KO mice against wild type (WT) controls under different drug treatment conditions. We found that, under baseline conditions (sham), withdrawal latencies of WT and Meis1KO were similar, while those of D3KO were decreased, suggesting heightened excitability in these animals to a thermal stimulus and confirming earlier *in vivo* and *in vitro* studies (Keeler et al., 2012). DA acts via both excitatory (D1 and D5 receptor) and inhibitory (D2, D3, and D4 receptor) receptor subtypes, and D3KO animals express increased locomotor and rearing activities, indicating an inhibitory role of the D3 receptor in the control of these motor behaviors (Accili et al., 1996). Moreover, while present in all laminae of the spinal cord (Zhu et al., 2007), the D3 receptor is most densely expressed in the dorsal horn (Levant, 1998), suggesting a strong modulatory effect of D3 receptor-mediated pathways in this sensory area of the cord. Further, the lack of function of the inhibitory D3 receptor in the isolated spinal cord *in vitro* was sufficient to increase the number or large-reflex spinal reflex amplitudes when compared to WT controls (Clemens and Hochman, 2004). Similar to D3KO, Meis1KO show a pattern of hyperactivity but contrary to D3KO, express no significant nociceptive differences in a hotplate test (Salminen et al., 2017). This is consistent with our findings under baseline

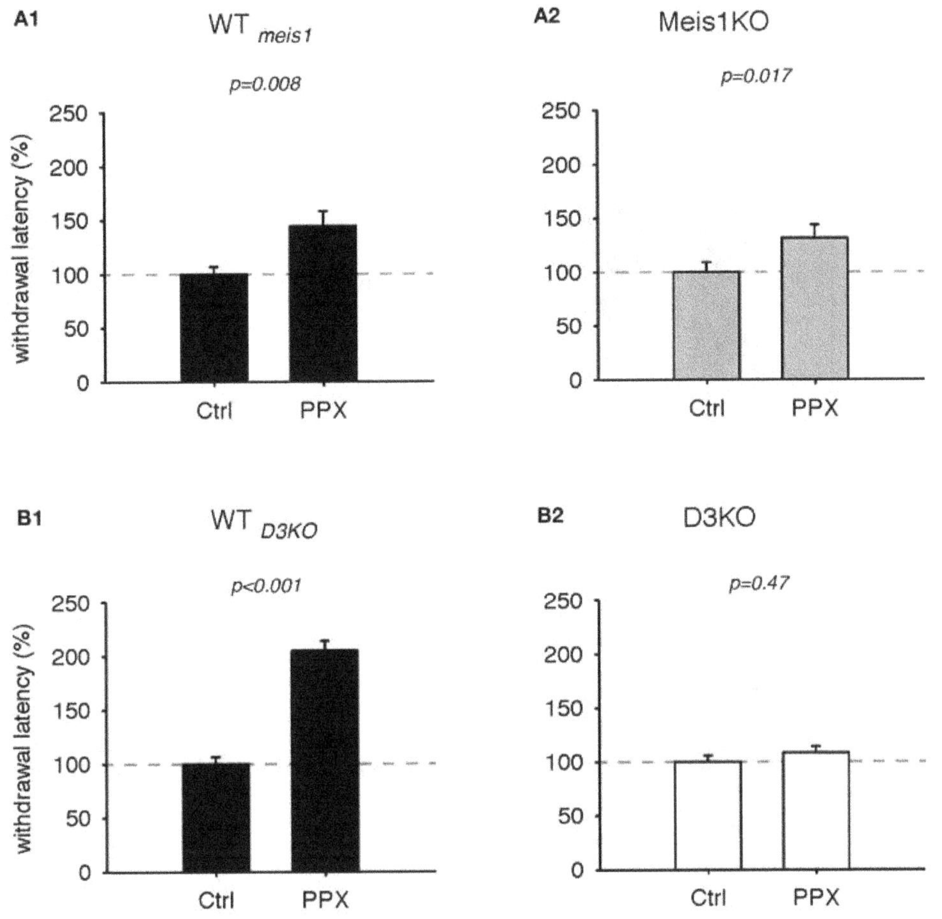

FIGURE 3 | Thermal pain withdrawal latencies of WT, Meis1KO, and D3KO before and after D3 receptor agonist (PPX) treatment. **(A1)** Normalized representation of data from WT_{meis1} animals. PPX significantly increased withdrawal latencies. **(A2)** Normalized representation of data from the Meis1KO animals. As in WT_{meis1}, PPX significantly increased withdrawal latencies. **(B1)** Normalized representation of data from WT_{D3KO} animals. PPX significantly increased withdrawal latencies. **(B2)** Normalized representation of data from D3KO animals. Unlike in both WT lines and Meis1KO, the D3 receptoer agonist PPX had no effect on withdrawal latencies in D3KO.

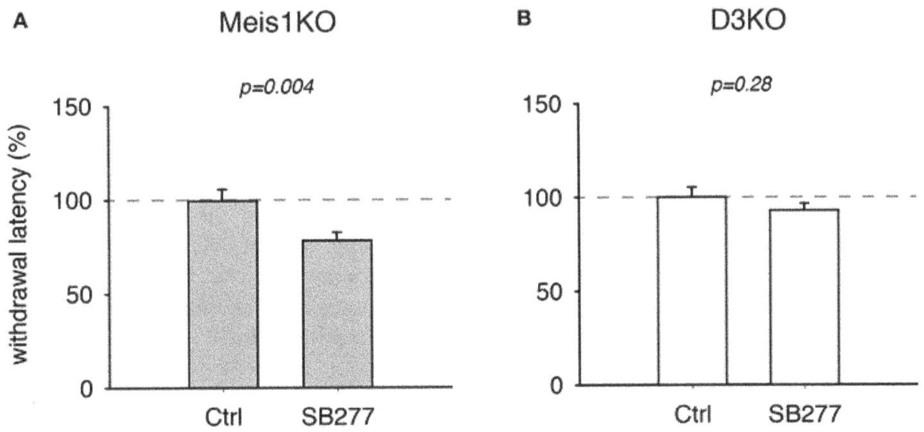

FIGURE 4 | Thermal pain withdrawal latencies of Meis1KO and D3KO before and after treatment with the D3R antagonist SB 277011. **(A)** In Meis1KO, SB277 significantly decreased withdrawal latencies. **(B)** In D3KO, treatment with SB277 did not lead to any significant changes in withdrawal latencies.

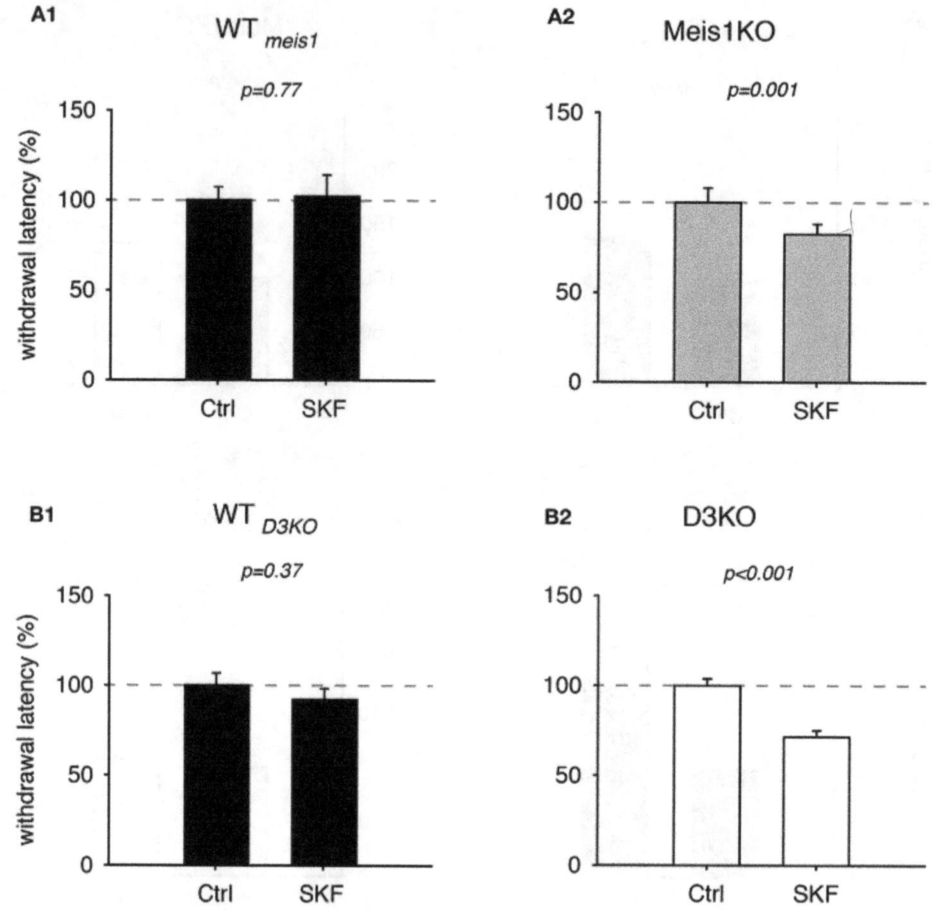

FIGURE 5 | Thermal pain withdrawal latencies of WT, Meis1KO, and D3KO before and after D1 receptor agonist (SKF) treatment. **(A1)** Normalized representation of data from WT_{meis1} animals. SKF did not have a significant effect on withdrawal latencies. **(A2)** Normalized representation of data from the Meis1KO animals. SKF significantly increased withdrawal latencies. **(B1)** Normalized representation of data from WT_{D3KO} animals. SKF did not significantly alter withdrawal latencies in WT_{D3KO}. **(B2)**. Normalized representation of data from D3KO animals. As in Meis1KO, the D1 receptor agonist significantly decreased withdrawal latencies in D3KO.

conditions where Meis1KO and WT express similar withdrawal thermal pain latencies, whereas reflex latencies are decreased in D3KO (**Figure 1**).

Effects of Morphine

Opioids are powerful modulators of nociceptive pathways, and we have shown previously that low morphine exposure (at 2 mg/kg, i.p.) was unsuccessful in modulating thermal pain withdrawal reflexes in D3KO and that this effect could be mimicked by acutely blocking D3 receptors in the isolated WT spinal cord preparation (Brewer et al., 2014). There, we also reported that the lack of a morphine effect in the D3KO animal was associated with an increased expression of the D1 receptor subtype in the spinal cord. While we did not perform other behavioral tests on pain (i.e. von Frey testing for mechanical pain), we confirmed the earlier D3KO findings here. We also found that Meis1KO and WT respond to morphine similarly (**Figure 2**). These data suggest that their opioid receptor pathways are alike, and preliminary Western blots indicate that the protein expression of the phosphorylated MOR is similar between WT and Meis1KO, but significantly increased in D3KO (data not shown). We are currently assessing if those receptor changes are found systemwide in the CNS or whether they are confined to specific (dorsal or ventral) areas of the spinal cord.

Effects of L-Dopa

We used L-DOPA (levodopa) as the immediate precursor of DA, to test the effects of raised DA levels on sensorimotor function in the three animal lines but observed no clear effect in either animal line. While L-DOPA plays an important modulatory role in controlling, at least temporarily, RLS symptoms (Akpinar, 1982; Paulus and Schomburg, 2006; Stiasny-Kolster et al., 2013), it can exert differential effects on monosynaptic and oligo- or polysynaptic nociceptive and non-nociceptive reflexes, where it depresses monosynaptic reflexes of flexors but not extensors, but also depresses transmission in nociceptive flexor reflex pathways (Schomburg and Steffens, 1998). There are several not mutually exclusive scenarios that may explain lack of any significant effect in our experiments: i) we only tested L-DOPA at a single dose of 10 mg/kg thus it is possible that lower or higher doses

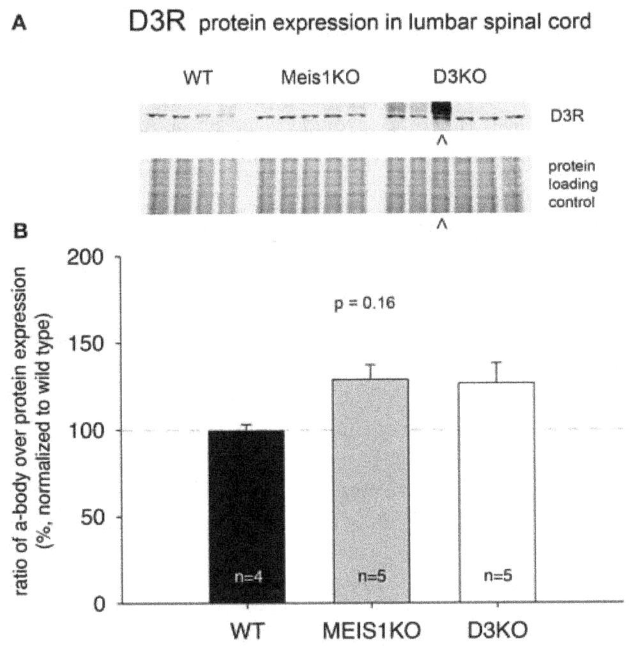

FIGURE 6 | D3R expression in the lumbar spinal cord. **(A)**. Western blot of D3R protein expression in the spinal cord. Top: D3R protein band; bottom: protein loading control. **(B)**. Quantification of D3R protein expression in the spinal cord, normalized to protein loading control / lane. D3R expression was not significantly altered in Meis1KO and D3KO animals. ^: D3KO lanes that were excluded from the subsequent analysis.

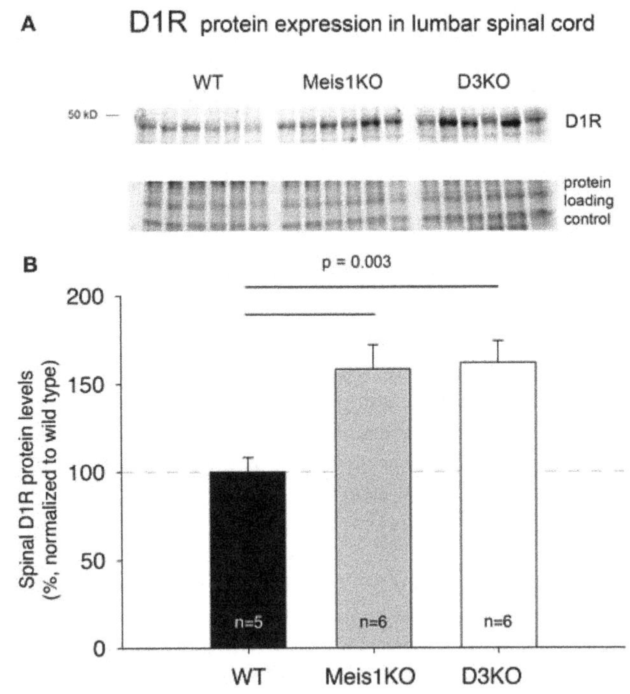

FIGURE 7 | D1R expression in the lumbar spinal cord. **(A)** Western blot of D1R protein expression in the spinal cord. Top: D1R protein band; bottom: protein loading control. **(B)** Quantification of D1R protein expression in the spinal cord, normalized to protein loading control / lane. D1R expression was significantly increased in Meis1KO and D3KO over WT animals.

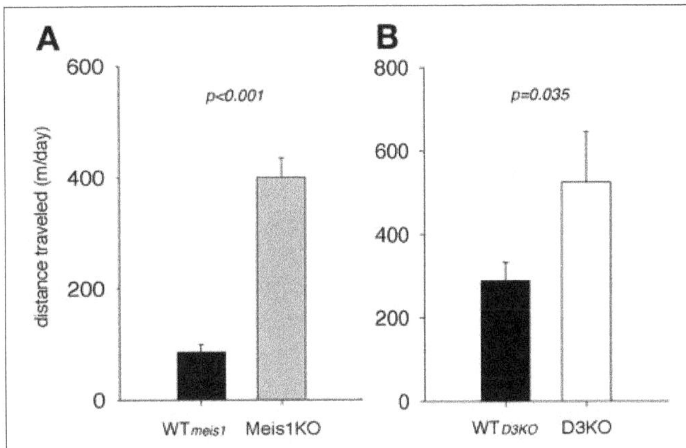

FIGURE 8 | Spontaneous locomotor activities of Meis1KO and D3KO and their respective controls. **(A)** Meis1KO. Meis1KO displayed significantly increased locomotor activities per 24 h over their WT controls (WT_{Meis1}). **(B)** Similar to Meis1KO, D3KO animals ran significantly longer distances per day over their controls (WT_{D3KO}).

would have yielded different results. However, doses of less than 10 mg/kg have been sufficient to provide behavioral effects and induce L-DOPA-induced dyskinesia in 6-hydroxydopamine lesioned mice (Lundblad et al., 2004). ii) Increasing dopamine levels with L-DOPA does not necessarily target the different DA receptor subtypes similarly. It is conceivable that high-affinity D3 receptor-activated inhibitory pathways compete with low-affinity D1 receptor-activated excitatory pathways, resulting in a net zero effect of this drug. iii), L-DOPA may act on the different components of sensory pain pathways differently; for example, in high spinal cats the onset of reflex facilitation induced by noxious radiant heat and mediated by A∂ fibers is delayed after injection of L-DOPA, while the late component persisted (Schomburg et al., 2011).

Effects of D3R and D1R Agonists and Antagonists

While the conversion of L-DOPA to DA can lead to an activation of both inhibitory and excitatory receptor subtypes, we hypothesize that our findings reflect a strong influence of the D3 receptor in mediating the behavioral responses tested. The D3 receptor has a very high affinity to DA (Cote and Kuzhikandathil, 2014), thus an initial DA increase will primarily (but not exclusively) mediate an inhibitory response that should be missing in the D3KO. Both D3 and D1 receptors are expressed in the lumbar spinal cord (Zhu et al., 2007), and DA can up- or downregulate cellular and network functions in a dose-dependent manner (Missale et al., 1998; Thirumalai and Cline, 2008; Clemens et al., 2012). Current DA-based RLS treatment options center around D3 receptor agonists (Ferini-Strambi et al., 2016; Ferré et al., 2017), but their effect is reduced over time and can cause a worsening of the symptoms (augmentation)

(Allen et al., 2011; García-Borreguero and Williams, 2011; Earley et al., 2017; Trenkwalder et al., 2017). While we have previously shown that D3 receptor agonists and antagonists can oppositely regulate spinal reflex amplitudes (SRAs) of WT *in vitro* while they do not alter SRAs in D3KO (Clemens and Hochman, 2004), we here wanted to test how these neuromodulators act *in vivo*, and how their effects compare with the Meis1KO animals (**Figure 4**). Treatment with both D3 receptor modulators (agonist pramipexole; PPX, and antagonist SB277011-A; SB277) led to nearly identical outcomes in WT and Meis1KO respectively, and had, as expected, no effect in the D3KO. In WT and Meis1KO, PPX had a strong analgesic effect that was counteracted by SB277, suggesting a similar role for the D3 receptor in modulating the thermal nociceptive pathway in these two animal strains. As the D3 receptor in the spinal cord is most prominently expressed in the sensory neurons of the dorsal horn (Levant, 1998), it is tempting to speculate that reduced DA levels at this sensory interface in the evening or at night (Carlsson et al., 1980; Sowers and Vlachakis, 1984) might reduce descending inhibitory control and thus contribute to the emergence of the circadian symptoms in RLS ("urge to move"). Of particular note is that such a reduced functional state of the D3 receptor in the dorsal horn could also arise independent of circadian DA levels, either by Meis1-dependent compromised projections of descending DA fibers from the A11 nucleus (M. Aschner, personal communication) or with the normal aging-related gradual decline of DA levels (Haycock et al., 2003) and a subsequent reduction in the expression levels of inhibitory *Gi*-coupled DA receptors (Mesco et al., 1991; Valerio et al., 1994). As with the circadian DA fluctuations, low DA levels would first affect the D3R and thus reduce overall DA-mediated inhibition. The D3KO animal then could serve as a model to specifically assess the mechanisms that follow a D3 receptor dysfunction in the sensory part of the spinal cord.

In contrast to D3 receptor modulators, the effects of the D1 receptor agonist was similar between Meis1KO and D3KO, but had no effect in WT. We suspect that the increase in spinal D1R protein expression (discussed below) may be the component that drives this behavioral outcome. We here confirmed that both Meis1KO and D3KO animals express increased locomotor activities (Accili et al., 1996; Salminen et al., 2017), and there is ample evidence that, in the isolated spinal cord preparation, D1R agonists can activate the central pattern generator (CPG) for locomotion (Kiehn and Kjaerulff, 1996) (Starr and Starr, 1993; Lapointe and Guertin, 2008; Urs et al., 2011; Sharples et al., 2015). As the locomotor CPG is contained to the ventral aspect of the thoraco-lumbar spinal cord (Kjaerulff and Kiehn, 1996; Kiehn, 2006, 2016) and the D1 receptor is more strongly expressed in ventral than sensory areas of the spinal cord (Zhu et al., 2007), D1 receptor-mediated actions may predominantly target motor-related over sensory functions in the spinal cord. Intriguingly, periodic limb movements during sleep (PLMS) are often associated with RLS (Wetter and Pollmächer, 1997; Moore et al., 2014; Li et al., 2016), and PLMS scores are regularly used to quantify RLS severity (Happe et al., 2001; Manconi et al., 2011b; Winkelmann et al., 2017). The similar responsiveness of Meis1KO and the D3KO to the D1 receptor modulators and their heightened motor activity suggest that the excitability of the spinal CPG may be upregulated in these animals, possibly via a D1 receptor-dependent beta-arrestin 2/phospho-ERK signaling complex that selectively mediates the locomotor CPG (Urs et al., 2011), which then could provide a target to understand the development of PLMS in future mechanistic studies.

D3R and D1R Protein Expression in the Spinal Cord

All DA receptor-mRNAs are expressed in the neurons of the rodent spinal cord (Zhu et al., 2007), although it is unclear if this translates also to proteins similarly, and if it is also the case in primates and man. For example, in non-human primates the D1 receptor is missing in the cord (Barraud et al., 2010), however its functions may be compensated for by the D5 receptor subtype, which also activates adenylyl cyclase (Missale et al., 1998). Using standard Western blot techniques, we tested for D3 receptor and D1 receptor protein expression in the lumbar spinal cord of the three animal models tested behaviorally. While we found no significant difference in D3 receptor expression across WT, Meis1KO and D3KO (**Figure 6**), we observed a significant upregulation of D1 receptor protein expression in Meis1KO and D3KO over WT (**Figure 7**). While present at relatively low levels in the spinal cord (Zhu et al., 2007), quantitative autoradiography has revealed that the D3 receptor is predominantly expressed in the dorsal horn (Levant, 1998), where it is in a prime position to modulate sensory pathways. In contrast, D1 receptor activation is regularly used to induce fictive locomotion in the isolated spinal cord preparation (Lapointe and Guertin, 2008; Han and Whelan, 2009; Sharples et al., 2015), suggesting a strong influence of the D1 receptor system to activate these more ventrally located circuits. Thus an increase in the availability or activation of D1 receptors in D3KO animals could explain an increase in an overall increase in the overall excitability and activity, similar to that observed with normal aging (Keeler et al., 2016).

The presence of a D3 receptor protein in the D3KO may appear unexpected, but the D3KO mouse used in our studies is not a genetic knockout of the D3 receptor; rather it is a targeted mutation of the D3 receptor gene in the second intracellular loop of the predicted protein sequence that prevents the incorporation of the D3R into the membrane (Accili et al., 1996). While this mutation does not preclude the transcription and translation of the D3 receptor, it prevents its insertion into the cell membrane (Zhu et al., 2008), rendering it functionally inactive (Clemens and Hochman, 2004). The lack of a difference between WT and Meis1KO supports the behavioral effects of the D3 receptor compounds and underlines the similarities between these two models with regard to the modulation of their sensory circuits.

In contrast to the D3 receptor data, the results of the D1 receptor protein expression point to a similarity of Meis1KO and D3KO, but not with either of them and the WT. We have shown previously that D3KO express not only decreased thermal pain withdrawal latencies but also an increased spinal D1 receptor protein expression (Brewer et al., 2014), and it is possible that in these animals a lack of synergistic D1-D3 receptor intra-membrane receptor-receptor interactions may account for the underlying mechanism that is responsible for this behavioral outcome (Marcellino et al., 2008). However, our data do not completely answer the question if there is a spatial component to the differences in D3 receptor and D1 receptor protein expression in the cord between the two genetically-modified animals and their WT controls. While we performed our Western blot experiments on lumbar spinal segments only, we did not anticipate the outcome that point to potential differential changes in sensory and motor circuits, and hence did not further dissect out and differentiate the outcomes between ventral versus dorsal aspects within those segments.

The Caveat of Using Dopaminergics *in vivo* to Test Sensorimotor Circuits in the Spinal Cord

Descending DA projections to and the presence of DA receptors in the spinal cord are well established (Holstege et al., 1996; van Dijken et al., 1996; Levant, 1998; Zhu et al., 2007), yet we cannot exclude the possibility that any of the drugs tested may have triggered changes in descending pathways, which in turn altered spinal reflex circuit excitabilities. Possible alternate approaches to test whether the DA effects are systemwide or truly spinal, which was beyond the scope of this study, would be to test the modulatory effects of these compounds in acutely anesthetized and spinalized animals, or by employing intrathecal drug delivery or conditional knockout approaches. In fact, data from a preliminary study, in which a D3 receptor-specific blocker was applied intrathecally, indicate that such an intrathecal approach alone can alter locomotor patterns and spinal D1 receptor expression (Jensen et al., 2014).

D3KO and Meis1KO–Complementary Models of RLS?

Figure 9 presents a comparative model, in which we summarize baseline properties, behavioral responses to the drugs tested, and D1 and D3 receptor protein expression data between WT, Meis1KO, and D3KO. WT and Meis1KO are similar with regard to sensory excitability at baseline (sham), their behavioral responses to morphine and D3 receptor modulators, and the expression levels of the spinal D3 receptor. Importantly, WT are different from D3KO with regard to baseline, opioid response, D1 receptor modulators, and D1 receptor expression. While Meis1KO and D3KO differ from each other in baseline and opioid response, they react similarly to D1 receptor modulators, and they express similarly increased D1 receptor protein expression levels in the lumbar spinal cord. As Meis1KO show at baseline only an increased locomotor activity, but normal sensory excitability, and as locomotor circuits are located in the ventral

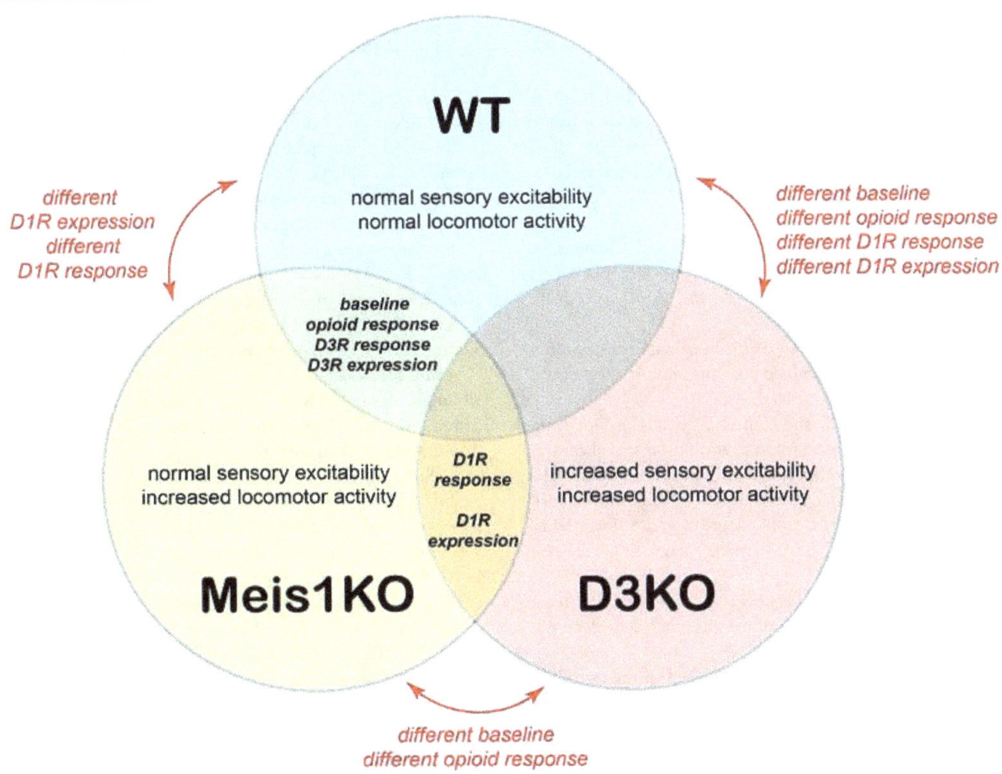

FIGURE 9 | Model of relationships between WT, Meis1KO, and D3KO animals. WT and Meis1KO share a similar baseline under control conditions, respond similarly to opioids, and have a similar D3R expression in the spinal cord. However, they differ in their responses to D1R modulators. WT and D3KO have different baselines under control conditions and respond differently to opioids, D3R, and D1R modulators. Meis1KO and D3KO have different baselines under control conditions, but respond similarly to D1R modulators, and have similar D1R expression levels in the spinal cord.

horn of the spinal cord, we posit that the Meis1KO mouse may serve as a model to specifically explore the mechanisms affiliated with the motor-related aspects of RLS (i.e. PLMS). In contrast, the increased sensory excitability and locomotor activity in D3KO suggest that both sensory and motor circuits are functionally upregulated in the spinal cord of this mouse, and that this model may be used to examine the impact of both sensory and motor pathways affiliated with RLS.

AUTHOR CONTRIBUTIONS

SM, M-LD, SL, YunL, C-TL, and MK performed the experiments. SM, M-LD, MK, C-TL, and SC analyzed the data. SC and YuqL designed the experiments. SM, KB, YuqL, and SC wrote the manuscript. SM, M-LD, MK, SL, YunL, YuqL, C-TL, KB, YL, and SC approved of the manuscript.

ACKNOWLEDGMENTS

Funding support for this study was provided in part by a National Institute of Health grant (R01NS082244), the Office of Research and Graduate Studies at East Carolina University, the Restless Legs Syndrome Foundation, and the Department of Physiology at the Brody School of Medicine. We thank B. and M. Neuhaus for their help with designing the model diagram, Drs. Neal G. Copeland and Hesham A. Sadek for providing the Meis1 loxP mice, and Kelly Dexter for breeding and genotyping the Meis1KO mice.

REFERENCES

Accili, D., Fishburn, C. S., Drago, J., Steiner, H., Lachowicz, J. E., Park, B. H., et al. (1996). A targeted mutation of the D3 dopamine receptor gene is associated with hyperactivity in mice. *Proc. Natl. Acad. Sci. U. S. A.* 93, 1945–1949. doi: 10.1073/pnas.93.5.1945

Acquas, E., and Di Chiara, G. (1999). Local application of SCH 39166 reversibly and dose-dependently decreases acetylcholine release in the rat striatum. *Eur. J. Pharmacol.* 383, 275–279. doi: 10.1016/S0014-2999(99)00660-3

Akpinar, S. (1982). Treatment of restless legs syndrome with levodopa plus benserazide. *Arch Neurol.* 39:739. doi: 10.1001/archneur.1982.00510230065027

Allen, R. P., Ondo, W. G., Ball, E., Calloway, M. O., Manjunath, R., Higbie, R. L., et al. (2011). Restless legs syndrome (RLS) augmentation associated with dopamine agonist and levodopa usage in a community sample. *Sleep Med.* 12, 431–439. doi: 10.1016/j.sleep.2011.03.003

Barraud, Q., Obeid, I., Aubert, I., Barriere, G., Contamin, H., McGuire, S., et al. (2010). Neuroanatomical study of the A11 diencephalospinal pathway in the non-human primate. *PLoS ONE* 5:e13306. doi: 10.1371/journal.pone.0013306

Barriere, G., Cazalets, J. R., Bioulac, B., Tison, F., and Ghorayeb, I. (2005). The restless legs syndrome. *Prog Neurobiol.* 77, 139–165. doi: 10.1016/j.pneurobio.2005.10.007

Brewer, K. L., Baran, C. A., Whitfield, B. R., Jensen, A. M., and Clemens, S. (2014). Dopamine D3 receptor dysfunction prevents anti-nociceptive effects of morphine in the spinal cord. *Front. Neural Circuits.* 8, 62-01 62–10. doi: 10.3389/fncir.2014.00062

Carlsson, A., Svennerholm, L., and Winblad, B. (1980). Seasonal and circadian monoamine variations in human brains examined post mortem. *Acta Psychiatr. Scand. Suppl.* 280, 75–85. doi: 10.1111/acps.1980.61.s280.75

Clemens, S., Belin-Rauscent, A., Simmers, J., and Combes, D. (2012). Opposing modulatory effects of D1- and D2-like receptor activation on a spinal central pattern generator. *J. Neurophysiol.* 107, 2250–2259. doi: 10.1152/jn.00366.2011

Clemens, S., and Hochman, S. (2004). Conversion of the modulatory actions of dopamine on spinal reflexes from depression to facilitation in D3 receptor knock-out mice. *J. Neurosci.* 24, 11337–11345. doi: 10.1523/JNEUROSCI.3698-04.2004

Clemens, S., Rye, D., and Hochman, S. (2006). Restless legs syndrome: revisiting the dopamine hypothesis from the spinal cord perspective. *Neurology* 67, 125–130. doi: 10.1212/01.wnl.0000223316.53428.c9

Clemens, S., Sawchuk, M. A., and Hochman, S. (2005). Reversal of the circadian expression of tyrosine-hydroxylase but not nitric oxide synthase levels in the spinal cord of dopamine D3 receptor knockout mice. *Neuroscience* 133, 353–357. doi: 10.1016/j.neuroscience.2005.03.002

Cote, S. R., and Kuzhikandathil, E. V. (2014). *In vitro* and *in vivo* characterization of the agonist-dependent D3 dopamine receptor tolerance property. *Neuropharmacology* 79, 359–367. doi: 10.1016/j.neuropharm.2013.11.023

Dauvilliers, Y., and Winkelmann, J. (2013). Restless legs syndrome: update on pathogenesis. *Curr. Opin. Pulm. Med.* 19, 594–600. doi: 10.1097/MCP.0b013e328365ab07

Dinkins, M.-L., Lallemand, P., and Clemens, S. (2017). Long-term treatment with dopamine D3 receptor agonists induces a behavioral switch that can be rescued by blocking the dopamine D1 receptor. *Sleep Med.* 40, 47–52. doi: 10.1016/j.sleep.2017.10.001

Dowling, P., Klinker, F., Stadelmann, C., Hasan, K., Paulus, W., and Liebetanz, D. (2011). Dopamine D3 receptor specifically modulates motor and sensory symptoms in iron-deficient mice. *J. Neurosci.* 31, 70–77. doi: 10.1523/JNEUROSCI.0959-10.2011

Earley, C. J., Allen, R. P., Connor, J. R., Ferrucci, L., and Troncoso, J. (2009). The dopaminergic neurons of the A11 system in RLS autopsy brains appear normal. *Sleep Med.* 10, 1155–1157. doi: 10.1016/j.sleep.2009.01.006

Earley, C. J., Allen, R. P., and Hening, W. (2011). Restless legs syndrome and periodic leg movements in sleep. *Handb. Clin. Neurol.* 99, 913–948. doi: 10.1016/B978-0-444-52007-4.00015-1

Earley, C. J., Connor, J., Garcia-Borreguero, D., Jenner, P., Winkelman, J., Zee, P. C., et al. (2014). Altered Brain iron homeostasis and dopaminergic function in Restless Legs Syndrome (Willis-Ekbom Disease). *Sleep Med.* 15, 1288–1301. doi: 10.1016/j.sleep.2014.05.009

Earley, C. J., Uhl, G. R., Clemens, S., and Ferre, S. (2017). Connectome and molecular pharmacological differences in the dopaminergic system in restless legs syndrome (RLS): plastic changes and neuroadaptations that may contribute to augmentation. *Sleep Med.* 31, 71–77. doi: 10.1016/j.sleep.2016.06.003

Eccles, R. M., and Lundberg, A. (1959). Supraspinal control of interneurones mediating spinal reflexes. *J. Physiol.* 147, 565–584. doi: 10.1113/jphysiol.1959.sp006262

Ekbom, K. A. (1944). Asthenia crurum pasasthetica (irritable legs). *Acta Med. Scand.* 118, 197–209. doi: 10.1111/j.0954-6820.1944.tb17800.x

Ekbom, K. A. (1945). Restless legs syndrome. *Acta Med. Scand.* 158, 4–122.

Ekbom, K. A. (1960). Restless legs syndrome. *Neurology* 10, 868–873. doi: 10.1212/WNL.10.9.868

Ferini-Strambi, L., Marelli, S., and Galbiati, A. (2016). Clinical pharmacology and efficacy of rotigotine (Neupro(R) patch) in the treatment of restless leg syndrome. *Expert Opin. Drug Metab. Toxicol.* 12, 967–975. doi: 10.1080/17425255.2016.1194393

Ferré, S., Earley, C., Gulyani, S., and Garcia-Borreguero, D. (2017). In search of alternatives to dopaminergic ligands for the treatment of restless legs syndrome: iron, glutamate, and adenosine. *Sleep Med.* 31, 86–92. doi: 10.1016/j.sleep.2016.08.019

Ferri, R., Manconi, M., Arico, D., Sagrada, C., Zucconi, M., Bruni, O., et al. (2010). Acute dopamine-agonist treatment in restless legs syndrome: effects on sleep architecture and NREM sleep instability. *Sleep* 33, 793–800. doi: 10.1093/sleep/33.6.793

Garcia-Borreguero, D., Silber, M., Winkelman, J. W., B. H., and Bainbridge, J., Buchfuhrer, M. J., et al. (2016). Guidelines for the first-line treatment of restless legs syndrome/Willis–Ekbom disease, prevention and treatment of dopaminergic augmentation: a combined task force of the IRLSSG, EURLSSG, and the RLS-foundation. *Sleep Med.* 211, 1–11. doi: 10.1016/j.sleep.2016.01.017

García-Borreguero, D., and Williams, A. M. (2011). Dopaminergic augmentation of restless legs syndrome: the scope of the problem. *Sleep Med.* 12, 425–426. doi: 10.1016/j.sleep.2011.03.004

Gemignani, F., Melpignano, A., Milioli, G., Riccardi, S., and Parrino, L. (2016). Restless legs syndrome: a new entity of neuropathic pain? Treatment with prolonged release oxycodone/naloxone combination. *J. Parkinson. Restless Legs Syndrome.* 6, 23–27. doi: 10.2147/JPRLS.S77560

Ghorayeb, I., and Tison, F. (2010). Restless legs syndrome epidemiology. *Presse Med.* 39, 564–570. doi: 10.1016/j.lpm.2009.08.006

Guo, H., Hong, S., Jin, X. L., Chen, R. S., Avasthi, P. P., Tu, Y. T., et al. (2000). Specificity and efficiency of Cre-mediated recombination in Emx1-Cre knock-in mice. *Biochem. Biophys. Res. Commun.* 273, 661–665. doi: 10.1006/bbrc.2000.2870

Han, P., and Whelan, P. J. (2009). Modulation of AMPA currents by D(1)-like but not D(2)-like receptors in spinal motoneurons. *Neuroscience* 158, 1699–1707. doi: 10.1016/j.neuroscience.2008.11.040

Happe, S., Klösch, G., Saletu, B., and Zeitlhofer, J. (2001). Treatment of idiopathic restless legs syndrome (RLS) with gabapentin. *Neurology* 57, 1717–1719. doi: 10.1212/WNL.57.9.1717

Haycock, J. W., Becker, L., Ang, L., Furukawa, Y., Hornykiewicz, O., and Kish, S. J. (2003). Marked disparity between age-related changes in dopamine and other presynaptic dopaminergic markers in human striatum. *J. Neurochem.* 87, 574–585. doi: 10.1046/j.1471-4159.2003.0 2017.x

Holstege, J. C., Van Dijken, H., Buijs, R. M., Goedknegt, H., Gosens, T., and Bongers, C. M. (1996). Distribution of dopamine immunoreactivity in the rat, cat and monkey spinal cord. *J. Comp. Neurol.* 376, 631–652. doi: 10.1002/(SICI)1096-9861(19961223)376:4<631::AID-CNE10>3.0.CO;2-P

Jensen, A. M., Salvad,è, A., Samir, S., Morales, G., Manconi, M., and Clemens, S. (2014). *Block of Dopamine D3 Receptors Induces Hind Limb Movements During Sleep and is Accompanied by an Increase in Spinal D1 Receptor Protein Expression.* Program No 14822. Washington, DC: Society for Neuroscience, Online.

Keeler, B. E., Baran, C. A., Brewer, K. L., and Clemens, S. (2012). Increased excitability of spinal pain reflexes and altered frequency-dependent modulation in the dopamine D3-receptor knockout mouse. *Exp. Neurol.* 238, 273–283. doi: 10.1016/j.expneurol.2012.09.002

Keeler, B. E., Patel, M. M., Lallemand, P., de Castro Brás, L. E., and Clemens, S. (2016). Opposing aging-related shift of excitatory dopamine D1and inhibitory D3 receptor protein expression in striatum and spinal cord. *J. Neurophysiol.* 115, 363–369. doi: 10.1152/jn.00390.2015

Kiehn, O. (2006). Locomotor circuits in the mammalian spinal cord. *Annu. Rev. Neurosci.* 29, 279–306. doi: 10.1146/annurev.neuro.29.051605.112910

Kiehn, O. (2016). Decoding the organization of spinal circuits that control locomotion. *Nat. Rev. Neurosci.* 17, 224–238. doi: 10.1038/nrn.2016.9

Kiehn, O., and Kjaerulff, O. (1996). Spatiotemporal characteristics of 5-HT and dopamine-induced rhythmic hindlimb activity in the *in vitro* neonatal rat. *J. Neurophysiol.* 75, 1472–1482. doi: 10.1152/jn.1996.75.4.1472

Kjaerulff, O., and Kiehn, O. (1996). Distribution of networks generating and coordinating locomotor activity in the neonatal rat spinal cord *in vitro*: a lesion study. *J. Neurosci.* 16, 5777–5794. doi: 10.1523/JNEUROSCI.16-18-057 77.1996

Klinker, F., Hasan, K., Dowling, P., Paulus, W., and Liebetanz, D. (2011). Dopamine D(3) receptor deficiency sensitizes mice to iron deficiency-related deficits in motor learning. *Behav. Brain Res.* 220, 358–361. doi: 10.1016/j.bbr.2011.02.022

Kocabas, F., Zheng, J., Thet, S., Copeland, N. G., Jenkins, N. A., DeBerardinis, R. J., et al. (2012). Meis1 regulates the metabolic phenotype and oxidant defense of hematopoietic stem cells. *Blood* 120, 4963–4972. doi: 10.1182/blood-2012-05-432260

Lanza, G., Bachmann, C. G., Ghorayeb, I., Wang, Y., Ferri, R., and Paulus, W. (2017). Central and peripheral nervous system excitability in restless legs syndrome. *Sleep Med.* 31, 49–60. doi: 10.1016/j.sleep.2016. 05.010

Lapointe, N. P., and Guertin, P. A. (2008). Synergistic effects of D1/5 and 5-HT1A/7 receptor agonists on locomotor movement induction in complete spinal cord-transected mice. *J. Neurophysiol.* 100, 160–168. doi: 10.1152/jn.90339.2008

Levant, B. (1998). Differential distribution of D3 dopamine receptors in the brains of several mammalian species. *Brain Res.* 800, 269–274. doi: 10.1016/S0006-8993(98)00529-0

Li, X., Allen, R. P., Earley, C. J., Liu, H., Cruz, T. E., Edden, R. A., et al. (2016). Brain iron deficiency in idiopathic restless legs syndrome measured by quantitative magnetic susceptibility at 7 tesla. *Sleep Med.* 22, 75–82. doi: 10.1016/j.sleep.2016.05.001

Lundblad, M., Picconi, B., Lindgren, H., and Cenci, M. A. (2004). A model of L-DOPA-induced dyskinesia in 6-hydroxydopamine lesioned mice: relation to motor and cellular parameters of nigrostriatal function. *Neurobiol. Dis.* 16, 110–123. doi: 10.1016/j.nbd.2004.01.007

Manconi, M., Ferri, R., Zucconi, M., Clemens, S., Giarolli, L., Bottasini, V., et al. (2011b). Preferential D2 or preferential D3 dopamine agonists in restless legs syndrome. *Neurology* 77, 110–117. doi: 10.1212/WNL.0b013e3182242d91

Manconi, M., Ferri, R., Zucconi, M., Clemens, S., Rundo, F., Oldani, A., et al. (2011a). Effects of acute dopamine-agonist treatment in restless legs syndrome on heart rate variability during sleep. *Sleep Med.* 12, 47–55. doi: 10.1016/j.sleep.2010.03.019

Marcellino, D., Ferré, S., Casado, V., Cortes, A., Le Foll, B., Mazzola, C., et al. (2008). Identification of dopamine D1-D3 receptor heteromers. Indications for a role of synergistic D1-D3 receptor interactions in the striatum. *J. Biol. Chem.* 283, 26016–26025. doi: 10.1074/jbc.M710349200

Marcos, S., González-Lázaro, M., Beccari, L., Carramolino, L., Martin-Bermejo, M. J., Amarie, O., et al. (2015). Meis1 coordinates a network of genes implicated in eye development and microphthalmia. *Development* 142, 3009–3020. doi: 10.1242/dev.122176

Mercader, N., Leonardo, E., Azpiazu, N., Serrano, A., Morata, G., Martinez, C., et al. (1999). Conserved regulation of proximodistal limb axis development by Meis1/Hth. *Nature* 402, 425–429. doi: 10.1038/46580

Mercader, N., Selleri, L., Criado, L. M., Pallares, P., Parras, C., Cleary, M. L., et al. (2009). Ectopic Meis1 expression in the mouse limb bud alters P-D patterning in a Pbx1-independent manner. *Int. J. Dev. Biol.* 53, 1483–1494. doi: 10.1387/ijdb.072430nm

Mesco, E. R., Joseph, J. A., Blake, M. J., and Roth, G. S. (1991). Loss of D2 receptors during aging is partially due to decreased levels of mRNA. *Brain Res.* 545, 355–357. doi: 10.1016/0006-8993(91)91314-Q

Missale, C., Nash, S. R., Robinson, S. W., Jaber, M., and Caron, M. G. (1998). Dopamine receptors, from structure to function. *Physiol. Rev.* 78, 189–225. doi: 10.1152/physrev.1998.78.1.189

Moore, H.t, Winkelmann, J., Lin, L., Finn, L., Peppard, P., and Mignot, E. (2014). Periodic leg movements during sleep are associated with polymorphisms in BTBD9, TOX3/BC034767, MEIS1, MAP2K5/SKOR1, and PTPRD. *Sleep* 37, 1535–1542. doi: 10.5665/sleep.4006

Nielsen, J. B. (2004). Sensorimotor integration at spinal level as a basis for muscle coordination during voluntary movement in humans. *J. Appl. Physiol.* 96, 1961–1967. doi: 10.1152/japplphysiol.01073.2003

Paulus, W., and Schomburg, E. D. (2006). Dopamine and the spinal cord in restless legs syndrome: does spinal cord physiology reveal a basis for augmentation? *Sleep Med Rev.* 10, 185–196. doi: 10.1016/j.smrv.2006.01.004

Robinson, S. W., Jarvie, K. R., and Caron, M. G. (1994). High affinity agonist binding to the dopamine D3 receptor: chimeric receptors delineate a role for intracellular domains. *Mol. Pharmacol.* 46, 352–356.

Salminen, A. V., Garrett, L., Schormair, B., Rozman, J., Giesert, F., Niedermeier, K. M., et al. (2017). Meis1: effects on motor phenotypes and the sensorimotor system in mice. *Dis. Model. Mech.* 10, 981–991. doi: 10.1242/dmm.030080

Schomburg, E. D., Dibaj, P., and Steffens, H. (2011). Role of L-DOPA in spinal nociceptive reflex activity: higher sensitivity of Adelta versus C fibre-evoked nociceptive reflexes to L-DOPA. *Physiol Res.* 60, 701–703. Available online at: http://www.biomed.cas.cz/physiolres/pdf/60/60_701.pdf

Schomburg, E. D., and Steffens, H. (1998). Comparative analysis of L-DOPA actions on nociceptive and non-nociceptive spinal reflex pathways in the cat. *Neurosci. Res.* 31, 307–316. doi: 10.1016/S0168-0102(98)00058-3

Schormair, B., Plag, J., Kaffe, M., Gross, N., Czamara, D., Samtleben, W., et al. (2011). MEIS1 and BTBD9: genetic association with restless leg syndrome in end stage renal disease. *J. Med. Genet.* 48, 462–466. doi: 10.1136/jmg.2010.087858

Schormair, B., Zhao, C., Bell, S., Tilch, E., Salminen, A. V., Putz, B., et al. (2017). Identification of novel risk loci for restless legs syndrome in genome-wide association studies in individuals of European ancestry: a meta-analysis. *Lancet Neurol.* 16, 898–907. doi: 10.1016/S1474-4422(17)30327-7

Sharples, S. A., Humphreys, J. M., Jensen, A. M., Dhoopar, S., Delaloye, N., Clemens, S., et al. (2015). Dopaminergic modulation of locomotor network activity in the neonatal mouse spinal cord. *J. Neurophysiol.* 113, 2500–2510. doi: 10.1152/jn.00849.2014

Solís, O., Garcia-Montes, J. R., Gonzalez-Granillo, A., Xu, M., and Moratalla, R. (2015). Dopamine D3 Receptor Modulates l-DOPA-Induced Dyskinesia by Targeting D1 Receptor-Mediated Striatal Signaling. *Cereb. Cortex.* 27, 435–446. doi: 10.1093/cercor/bhv231

Sowers, J. R., and Vlachakis, N. (1984). Circadian variation in plasma dopamine levels in man. *J. Endocrinol. Invest.* 7, 341–345. doi: 10.1007/BF03351014

Spieler, D., Kaffe, M., Knauf, F., Bessa, J., Tena, J. J., Giesert, F., et al. (2014). Restless legs syndrome-associated intronic common variant in Meis1 alters enhancer function in the developing telencephalon. *Genome Res.* 24, 592–603. doi: 10.1101/gr.166751.113

Starr, M. S., and Starr, B. S. (1993). Facilitation of dopamine D1 receptor-but not dopamine D1/D2 receptor-dependent locomotion by glutamate antagonists in the reserpine-treated mouse. *Eur. J. Pharmacol.* 250, 239–246. doi: 10.1016/0014-2999(93)90387-W

Stefansson, H., Rye, D. B., Hicks, A., Petursson, H., Ingason, A., Thorgeirsson, T. E., et al. (2007). A genetic risk factor for periodic limb movements in sleep. *N. Engl. J. Med.* 357, 639–647. doi: 10.1056/NEJMoa072743

Stiasny, K., Wetter, T. C., Trenkwalder, C., and Oertel, W. H. (2000). Restless legs syndrome and its treatment by dopamine agonists. *Parkinsonism Relat. Disord.* 7, 21–25. doi: 10.1016/S1353-8020(00)00041-9

Stiasny-Kolster, K., Pfau, D. B., Oertel, W. H., Treede, R. D., and Magerl, W. (2013). Hyperalgesia and functional sensory loss in restless legs syndrome. *Pain* 154, 1457–1463. doi: 10.1016/j.pain.2013.05.007

Thirumalai, V., and Cline, H. T. (2008). Endogenous dopamine suppresses initiation of swimming in prefeeding zebrafish larvae. *J. Neurophysiol.* 100, 1635–1648. doi: 10.1152/jn.90568.2008

Trenkwalder, C., Allen, R., Hogl, B., Paulus, W., and Winkelmann, J. (2016). Restless legs syndrome associated with major diseases: a systematic review and new concept. *Neurology* 86, 1336–1343. doi: 10.1212/WNL.0000000000002542

Trenkwalder, C., Canelo, M., Lang, M., Schroeder, H., Kelling, D., Berkels, R., et al. (2017). Management of augmentation of restless legs syndrome with rotigotine: a 1-year observational study. *Sleep Med.* 30, 257–265. doi: 10.1016/j.sleep.2015.10.006

Trenkwalder, C., Winkelmann, J., Inoue, Y., and Paulus, W. (2015). Restless legs syndrome-current therapies and management of augmentation. *Nat. Rev. Neurol.* 11, 434–445. doi: 10.1038/nrneurol.2015.122

Urs, N. M., Daigle, T. L., and Caron, M. G. (2011). A dopamine D1 receptor-dependent beta-arrestin signaling complex potentially regulates morphine-induced psychomotor activation but not reward in mice. *Neuropsychopharmacology* 36, 551–558. doi: 10.1038/npp.2010.186

Valerio, A., Belloni, M., Gorno, M. L., Tinti, C., Memo, M., and Spano, P. (1994). Dopamine D2, D3, and D4 receptor mRNA levels in rat brain and pituitary during aging. *Neurobiol. Aging.* 15, 713–719. doi: 10.1016/0197-4580(94)90053-1

van Dijken, H., Dijk, J., Voom, P., and Holstege, J. C. (1996). Localization of dopamine D2 receptor in rat spinal cord identified with immunocytochemistry and *in situ* hybridization. *Eur. J. Neurosci.* 8, 621–628. doi: 10.1111/j.1460-9568.1996.tb01247.x

Wetter, T. C., and Pollmächer, T. (1997). Restless legs and periodic leg movements in sleep syndromes. *J. Neurol.* 244, S37–45. doi: 10.1007/BF03160570

Williams, S., Mmbaga, N., and Chirwa, S. (2006). Dopaminergic D1 receptor agonist SKF 38393 induces GAP-43 expression and long-term potentiation in hippocampus *in vivo*. *Neurosci. Lett.* 402, 46–50. doi: 10.1016/j.neulet.2006.03.075

Willis, T. (1685). *Of the Diseases of the Brain and the Genus Nervosum.* London, UK: The London Practice of Physick. Bassett and Crooke.

Winkelmann, J. (2008). Genetics of restless legs syndrome. *Curr. Neurol. Neurosci. Rep.* 8, 211–216. doi: 10.1007/s11910-008-0033-y

Winkelmann, J., Czamara, D., Schormair, B., Knauf, F., Schulte, E. C., Trenkwalder, C., et al. (2011). Genome-wide association study identifies novel restless legs syndrome susceptibility loci on 2p14 and 16q12.1. *PLoS Genet.* 7:e1002171. doi: 10.1371/journal.pgen.1002171

Winkelmann, J., Schormair, B., Lichtner, P., Ripke, S., Xiong, L., Jalilzadeh, S., et al. (2007). Genome-wide association study of restless legs syndrome identifies common variants in three genomic regions. *Nat. Genet.* 39, 1000–1006. doi: 10.1038/ng2099

Winkelmann, J., Schormair, B., Xiong, L., Dion, P. A., Rye, D. B., and Rouleau, G. A. (2017). Genetics of restless legs syndrome. *Sleep Med.* 31, 18–22. doi: 10.1016/j.sleep.2016.10.012

Zhu, H., Clemens, S., Sawchuk, M., and Hochman, S. (2007). Expression and distribution of all dopamine receptor subtypes (D1 - D5) in the mouse lumbar spinal cord: a real-time polymerase chain reaction and non-autoradiographic *in situ* hybridization study. *Neuroscience* 149, 885–897. doi: 10.1016/j.neuroscience.2007.07.052

Zhu, H., Clemens, S., Sawchuk, M., and Hochman, S. (2008). Unaltered D1, D2, D4, and D5 dopamine receptor mRNA expression and distribution in the spinal cord of the D3 receptor knockout mouse. *J. Comp. Physiol. A Neuroethol. Sens. Neural Behav. Physiol.* 194, 957–962. doi: 10.1007/s00359-008-0368-5

9

Electroacupuncture Inhibits Visceral Nociception via Somatovisceral Interaction at Subnucleus Reticularis Dorsalis Neurons in the Rat Medulla

Lingling Yu[1,2], Liang Li[2], Qingguang Qin[2], Yutian Yu[2], Xiang Cui[2], Peijing Rong[2] and Bing Zhu[2]**

[1] *Department of Neurology, Tongji Hospital, Tongji Medical College, Huazhong University of Science and Technology, Wuhan, China,*
[2] *Institute of Acupuncture and Moxibustion, China Academy of Chinese Medical Sciences, Beijing, China*

Correspondence:
Peijing Rong
drrongpj@163.com
Bing Zhu
zhubing@mail.cintcm.ac.cn

Electroacupuncture (EA) is an efficacious treatment for alleviating visceral pain, but the underlining mechanisms are not fully understood. This study investigated the role of medullary subnucleus reticularis dorsalis (SRD) neurons in the effects of EA on visceral pain. We recorded the discharges of SRD neurons extracellularly by glass micropipettes on anesthetized rats. The responses characteristics of SRD neurons to different intensities of EA (0.5, 1, 2, 4, 6, and 8 mA, 0.5 ms, and 2 Hz) on acupoints "Zusanli" (ST 36) and "Shangjuxu" (ST 37) before and during noxious colorectal distension (CRD) were analyzed. Our results indicated that SRD neurons responded to either a noxious EA stimulation ranging from 2 to 8 mA or to noxious CRD at 30 and 60 mmHg by increasing their discharge frequency at an intensity-dependent manner. However, during the stimulation of both CRD and EA, the increasing discharges of SRD neurons induced by CRD were significantly inhibited by 2–8 mA of EA. Furthermore, SRD neurons can encode the strength of EA, where a positive correlation between current intensity and the magnitude of neuronal responses to EA was observed within 2–6 mA. Yet, the responses of SRD neurons to EA stimulation reached a plateau when EA exceeded 6 mA. In addition, 0.5–1 mA of EA had no effect on CRD-induced nociceptive responses of SRD neurons. In conclusion, EA produced an inhibiting effect on visceral nociception in an intensity-dependent manner, which probably is due to the somatovisceral interaction at SRD neurons.

Keywords: electroacupuncture, visceral pain, colorectal distension, subnucleus reticularis dorsalis, analgesia

INTRODUCTION

Visceral pain is one of the most common symptoms in patients with gastrointestinal disorders (Sach et al., 2002). It is usually associated with impaired health-related quality of life and a significant health care burden (Chang, 2004; Spiegel et al., 2004). Electroacupuncture (EA) therapy is an effective analgesic by delivering of electrical current to acupoints via acupuncture needles connected to an electrical stimulator (Zhao, 2008). Many behavioral studies have confirmed that EA stimulation exerts good effects on rats with acute or chronic visceral hyperalgesia (Qi and Li, 2012; Wang et al., 2012). In addition, EA therapy has been proven to be effective in treating visceral pain in long-term follow-up clinical trials (MacPherson et al., 2017). It is generally accepted that EA analgesia is an integrative process of afferent impulses between pain regions and acupoints at convergence neurons and this process involves different levels of central structures, such as spinal dorsal horn (Rong et al., 2005), nucleus tractus solitarius (Liu et al., 2014) and periaqueductal gray (Wang et al., 2014). However, the involvement of other convergence neurons in EA analgesia is still unknown.

Accumulating evidence suggests that subnucleus reticularis dorsalis (SRD), the caudal-most aspect of the medulla, plays an important role in the transmission and modulation of nociceptive information (Villanueva et al., 1996). Neurons within SRD are not only activated exclusively by somatic noxious stimuli (mechanical, thermal, or chemical noxious stimuli) applied to widespread areas of the body (Villanueva et al., 1988, 1990), but also respond to noxious visceral stimuli (Roy et al., 1992). Owing to the widespread nociceptive convergence, SRD neurons might contribute to the processing of visceral nociception. In fact, SRD has been verified as a critical region in the pain-inhibiting effect of diffuse noxious inhibitory controls (DNIC) (Bouhassira et al., 1992; Villanueva and Le Bars, 1995). In order to explore the role of SRD neurons in the effects of EA on visceral nociception, the response characteristics of SRD neurons to different intensities of EA before and during noxious CRD was observed and investigated in the present study.

MATERIALS AND METHODS

Animals Preparations

Thirty eight male Sprague-Dawley rats, weighing 220–280 g, were purchased from the Laboratory Animal Center of China Academy of Military Medical Sciences [License number: SCXK-(Military)-2016-0024]. This study was carried out in accordance with the recommendations of the Guideline on the Humane Care and Use of Laboratory Animals issued by the Ministry of Science and Technology of the People's Republic of China in 2006. The protocol was approved by the CACMS Animal Ethics Committee (No. 20160218). Rats were housed in standard laboratory conditions under artificial 12 h light/dark cycle and at an ambient temperature of 22 ± 0.5. Food and water were available *ad libitum*. After an overnight fast of 12 h, rats were deeply anesthetized with 10% urethane (1.0–1.2 g/kg) and artificially ventilated through a tracheal cannula. Body temperature was maintained at 37 ± 0.5 by means of a feedback controlled homoeothermic heating blanket system.

Colorectal Distension

Visceral nociceptive stimulus was generated by noxious CRD. Briefly, A 6 cm balloon was gently inserted into descending colon at 4 cm depth through the anus. During the recording sessions, the balloon in the colon was consecutively inflated with air to produce pressure and the intracolonic pressure was monitored with a pressure transducer. The pressure of CRD stimulation applied to rats was 30 and 60 mmHg. In order to prevent possible sensitization triggered by overstimulation of the colorectum, the interval between two CRD stimulations was at least 10 min.

Recordings

Rats were mounted in a stereotaxic frame with the head fixed in a ventroflexed position by means of a metallic bar cemented to the skull. The caudal medulla was exposed by removing the overlying musculature, atlantooccipital membrane, and dura mater.

Unitary extracellular recordings were made with glass micropipettes (8–12 MΩ) filled with a mixture of 2% pontamine sky blue dye and 0.1 M of natrium aceticum. Micropipettes were inserted on the right side of the medulla, 1.0–2.0 mm caudal to the obex, and 0.5–1.5 mm lateral to the midline.

Single unit activities were fed into a window discriminator and displayed on an oscilloscope screen. The output of the window discriminator and amplifier were fed into a data acquisition system developed by ADInstrument (Power Lab) through a personal computer and Chart 5.0 was used to compile histograms and waveform files for further analysis.

Electroacupuncture

The rats were treated with EA via a pair of non-insulated acupuncture needles. The needles were inserted into the skin 3 mm apart at the right side of the acupoints "Zusanli" (ST36) and "Shangjuxu" (ST37), which is located in the ipsilateral side of the inserted location of micropipettes. The needles were then connected to an electrical stimulator (88–102G, Nihon Kohden). During a 30 s EA session, intensities of 0.5, 1, 2, 4, 6, and 8 mA were applied in random order. The duration and frequency of electrical stimulation were set at 0.5 ms and 2 Hz.

Experimental Procedure

(1) After locating a neuron with stable discharges, noxious (pinch) and innocuous (brush) skin stimuli were used to identify the targeted neurons. Since SRD neurons were excited by noxious stimulation to widespread areas of the body including foot, tail and finger, but did not response to innocuous stimuli, we first observed neuronal response to pinch and brush stimulation to foot, tail and finger to identify SRD neurons. Only the neurons that can be excited by pinch stimulation to widespread areas of the body characterized as SRD neurons and were used for further study.

(2) Second, responses of SRD neurons to different intensities of single EA stimulation were compared. The baseline activity was recorded for 5 s, then followed by 10 s EA stimulation, then another 5 s recovery of neuronal discharge was recorded after EA stimulation had stopped.

(3) Third, responses of SRD neurons to graded intensities of CRD stimulation were observed. The baseline activity was recorded for 10 s, followed by 10 s CRD stimulation, then another 10 s of recovery of neuronal discharge was recorded after CRD had stopped.

(4) Fourth, the responses of SRD neurons to different intensities of EA during CRD were observed. A standard conditioned recording procedure was administered for 60 s. Recording of 5 s baseline activities and 5 s recovery neuronal activities were acquired before and after 50 s CRD recording

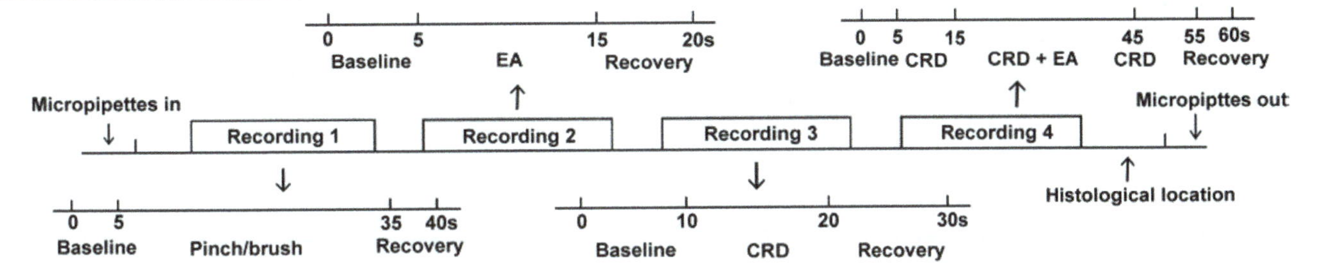

FIGURE 1 | Timeline of experimental prodedure.

procedure. During the CRD recording procedure, an initial 10 s response of neuron activities to CRD were recorded, 30 s of EA stimulation was administrated and the response of neurons to both EA and CRD was recorded, followed by recording of 10 s of responses to CRD.

The interval between any two stimulations was at least 10 min. The timeline of recording protocol was presented in **Figure 1**.

Histological Location

After single unit recordings, the recording sites were marked by electrophoretic deposition of pontamine sky blue and checked by HE coloration. Locations of the recording sites were then determined with reference to the rat brain atlas.

Data Collection and Statistical Analysis

Neuronal discharges per second (identified as $\bar{X} \pm SE\%$) were calculated with PowerLab, Chart 5.0, and SPSS13.0. One way ANOVA and linear regression analyses were used for statistical purposes. $P < 0.05$ was deemed statistically significant.

RESULTS

General Characteristics of SRD Neurons on Medulla

A total of 68 units were recorded within medulla, among which 82.35%(56/68) were characterized as SRD neurons with a "whole body receptive field." Other neuronal types, such as spinal nucleus of trigeminal, were not considered in this paper. Examination of the rat brain slices verified that the recording sites (n = 12) were located in the dorsomedial part of the SRD (**Figure 2**).

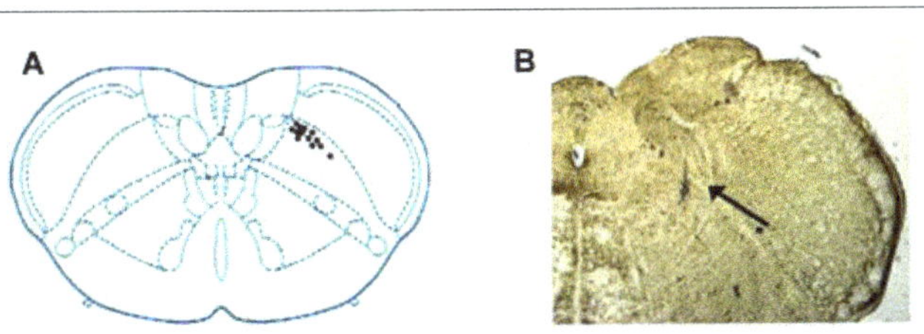

FIGURE 2 | Location of SRD neurons in the medulla. **(A)** Locations of recording sites were marked according to the brain atlas of the rat. **(B)** An individual example showing the location of an SRD neuron marked by pontamine sky blue. Blue dye represents the sites, as indicated by an arrow.

SRD neurons could be characterized by their response to mechanical and electrical stimuli, our initial approach is to identify these neurons by their responses to pinch and brush stimuli at various part of the rat's body, which was defined as conditional noxious and innocuous mechanical stimuli. As presented in **Figure 3**, SRD neurons that were recorded responded to noxious pinch stimulation of the foot, tail and finger with increasing neuronal discharges (**Figures 3A–C**), but did not respond to innocuous burshing stimulation of the foot, tail and finger (**Figures 3D–F**).

Effects of EA With Different Intensities on SRD Neurons Before CRD

The neuronal response to graded EA stimulation at acupoints ST 36 and ST 37 was observed on 7 SRD neurons. An individual example of neuronal discharges evoked by graded intensity of

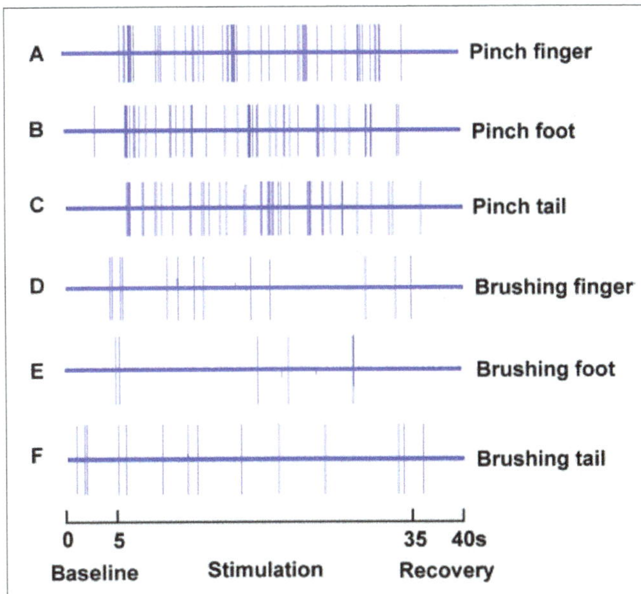

FIGURE 3 | Response characteristics of SRD neurons to innocuous and noxious stimuli. SRD neurons increased neuronal discharges to noxious pinch stimuli of the finger **(A)**, foot **(B)**, and tail **(C)**, but they did not response to innocuous brush stimuli of the finger **(D)**, foot **(E)**, and tail **(F)**.

EA stimulation is presented in **Figure 4**. We found that SRD neurons did not respond to low intensity of EA stimulation (0.5–1 mA), but were significantly activated by high intensity of EA stimulation (2–8 mA). After EA stimulation, the average discharge frequency of SRD neurons was significantly increased from 0.08 ± 0.06 spikes/s at baseline to 1.78 ± 0.42 spikes/s (2 mA), 5.47 ± 0.65 spikes/s (4 mA), 8.89 ± 0.65 spikes/s (6 mA) and 9.03 ± 0.92 spikes/s (8 mA) ($P < 0.05$). There is also a

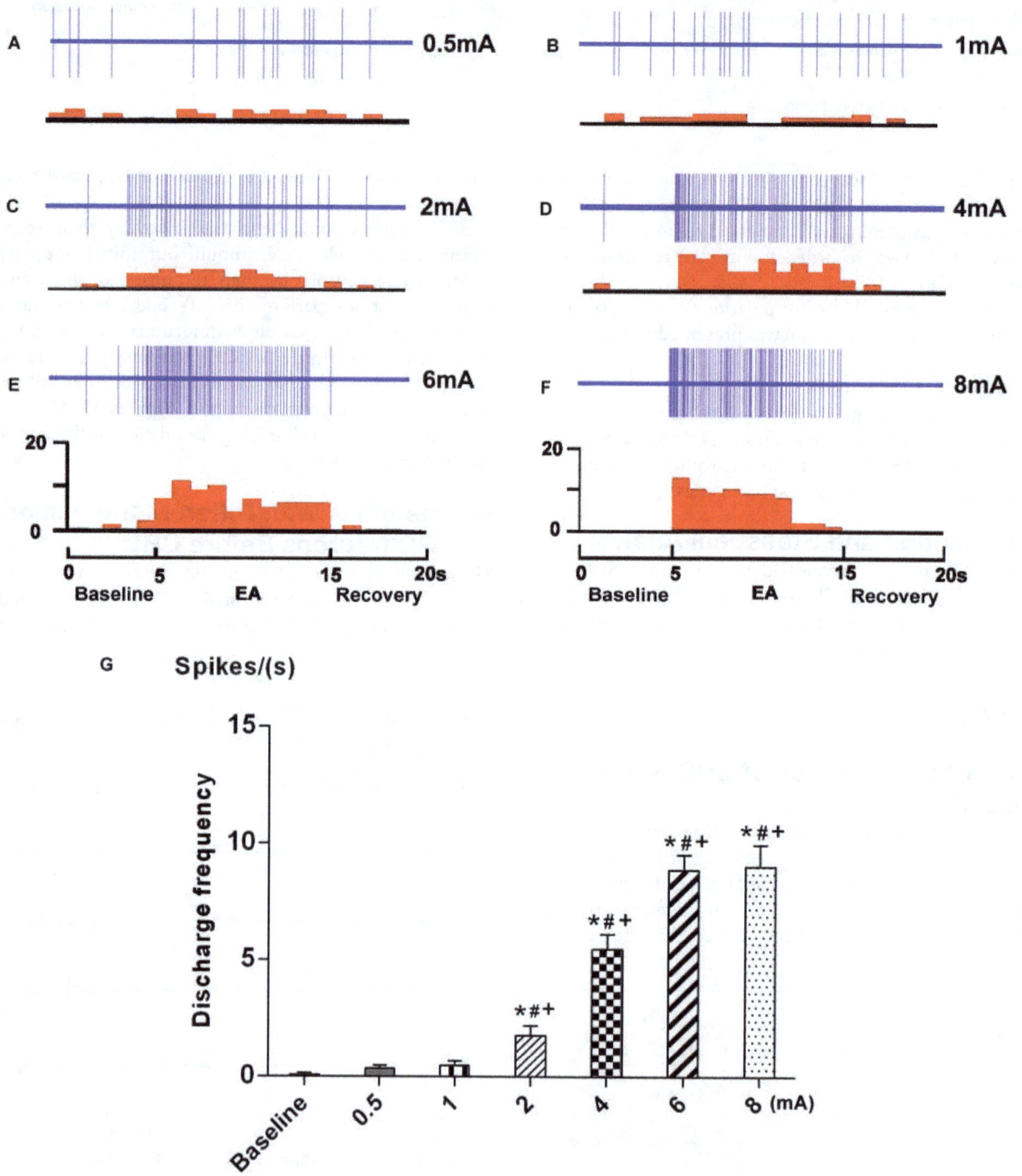

FIGURE 4 | Response characteristics of SRD neurons to graded EA. **(A–F)** Representative examples showing the responses of SRD neuron to graded EA stimulation. The upper rows show the unit discharges at different stimulations and the lower rows show these discharges in histogram. EA (Electroacupuncture) **(G)** A histogram showing the dicharges of SRD neurons (n = 7) were significantly activated by EA at 2–8 mA. $^{*}p < 0.05$ compared with baseline; $^{\#}p < 0.05$ compared with 0.5 mA EA; $^{+}p < 0.05$ compared with 1 mA EA.

significant difference between the effects of high intensity of EA (2–8 mA) and low intensity of EA (0.5–1 mA) ($P < 0.05$).

Furthermore, SRD neurons increased their discharges linearly when the intensity of current was raised from 2 to 6 mA; Further increased the current beyond 6 mA resulted in a plateau effect on neuronal responses. These observations indicated that SRD neurons responsed to noxious EA stimuli, and could encode the intensity of EA stimuli within a specific range.

Effects of EA With Different Intensities on the Discharges of SRD Neurons During CRD

In this experiment, we examined 7 SRD neurons on their reactions to CRD stimulation. As showed in **Figure 5**, SRD neurons responsed to 30–60 mmHg CRD with increasing discharge rates. After the stimulation of 30 mmHg CRD, the average discharges of SRD neurons were significantly increased from 0.96 ± 0.32 spikes/s at baseline to 2.97 ± 0.32 spikes/s ($P < 0.001$); when CRD was set at 60 mmHg, the average discharges of SRD neurons were increased to 11.87 ± 0.79 spikes/s($P < 0.001$). This indicates that noxious CRD stimulation could activate the activity of SRD neurons and of significant dose–effect relation.

During the stimulation of 60 mmHg CRD, the response of SRD neurons to different intensities of EA was observed. As illustrated in **Figure 6**, the increased discharges of SRD neurons induced by CRD could be inhibited by EA at 2–8 mA. However, low intensity of EA (0.5–1 mA) had no significant inhibitory effect on CRD induced noxious discharges of SRD neurons.

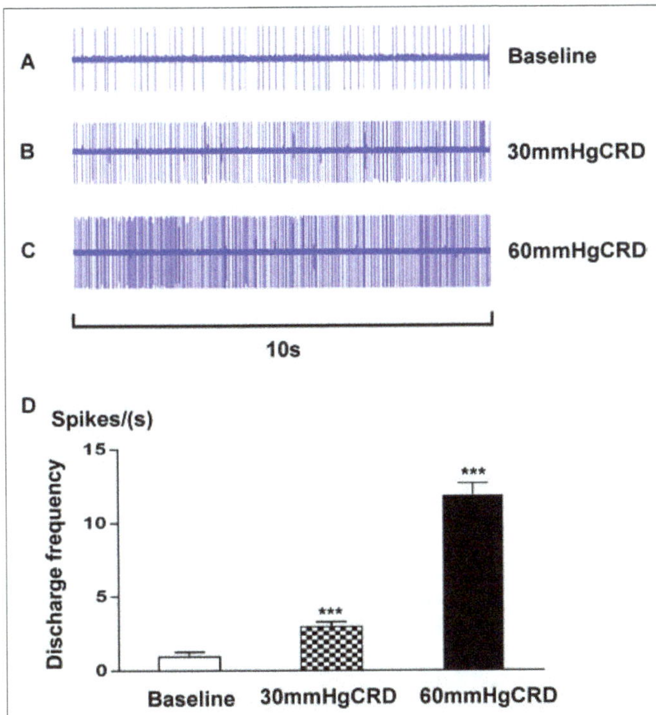

FIGURE 5 | Response characteristics of SRD neurons to graded CRD. **(A–C)** Representative examples showing the responses of SRD neuron to 30–60 mmHg CRD stimulation. **(D)** Cumulative results showing the discharges of SRD neurons ($n = 7$) were significantly activated by 30–60 mmHg CRD stimulation. ***$p < 0.001$ compared with baseline.

When the intensity of the current was set at 2 mA, EA produced a slight, but significant inhibition on the discharges of SRD neurons. The average discharges decreased from 13.02 ± 1.15 spikes/s of CRD to 9.51 ± 0.98 spikes/s, with an inhibiting percentage of 29.91 ± 6.24% ($P < 0.05$, $n = 7$). There is also a significantly difference between the effects of 2 mA EA and 0.5 mA EA ($P < 0.05$), as well as 2 mA EA and 1 mA EA ($P < 0.05$).

When the intensity of the current was set at 4 mA, EA produced a moderate inhibition, the average discharges of SRD neurons decreased from 12.63 ± 1.02 spikes/s of CRD to 5.84 ± 0.74 spikes/s, with an inhibiting percentage of 57.59 ± 4.25 % ($P < 0.05$, $n = 7$). There is also a significantly difference between the effects of 4 mA EA and 0.5 mA EA ($P < 0.05$), as well as 4 mA EA and 1 mA EA ($P < 0.05$).

When the intensity of the current was set at 6 mA, EA produced a stronger inhibition, the average discharges of SRD neurons decreased from 13.15 ± 1.08 spikes/s of CRD to 2.30 ± 0.88 spikes/s, with an inhibiting percentage of 83.36 ± 6.31 % ($P < 0.05$, $n = 7$). There is also a significantly difference between the effects of 6 mA EA and 0.5 mA EA ($P < 0.05$), as well as 6 mA EA and 1 mA EA ($P < 0.05$).

When the intensity of EA was set at 8 mA, EA still produced a strong inhibition, yet this inhibitory effects of EA on the noxious responses of SRD neurons had reached a plateau. After EA, the average discharges of SRD neurons decreased from 13.39 ± 1.02 spikes/s of CRD to 3.65 ± 1.13 spikes/s, with a inhibiting percentage of 73.00 ± 8.14 % ($P < 0.05$, $n = 7$). Although there is also a significantly difference between the effects of 8 mA EA and 0.5 mA EA ($P < 0.05$), as well as 8 mA EA and 1 mA EA ($P < 0.05$). There is no significantly difference between the effects of 8 mA EA and 6 mA EA.

These results indicated that the noxious responses of SRD neurons to CRD could be inhibited by EA in an intensity dependent manner, but such an inhibiting effect of EA reached a plateau when the current exceeded 6 mA.

DISCUSSION

Although EA has been practiced in China since the early 1950s and is widely used for analgesia in clinic, the mechanisms of EA analgesia on visceral pain are not fully understood. In this study, we explored the role of SRD in EA analgesia on visceral pain. Our results demonstrated that the activities of SRD neurons were activated by either a single noxious CRD or 2–8 mA of EA stimulation by increasing their spontaneous discharges. However, the increased discharges of SRD neurons resulted from the stimulation of noxious CRD could be inhibited by 2–8 mA of EA stimulation. These results suggest that visceral nociception could be inhibited by EA via somatovisceral interaction onto SRD neurons.

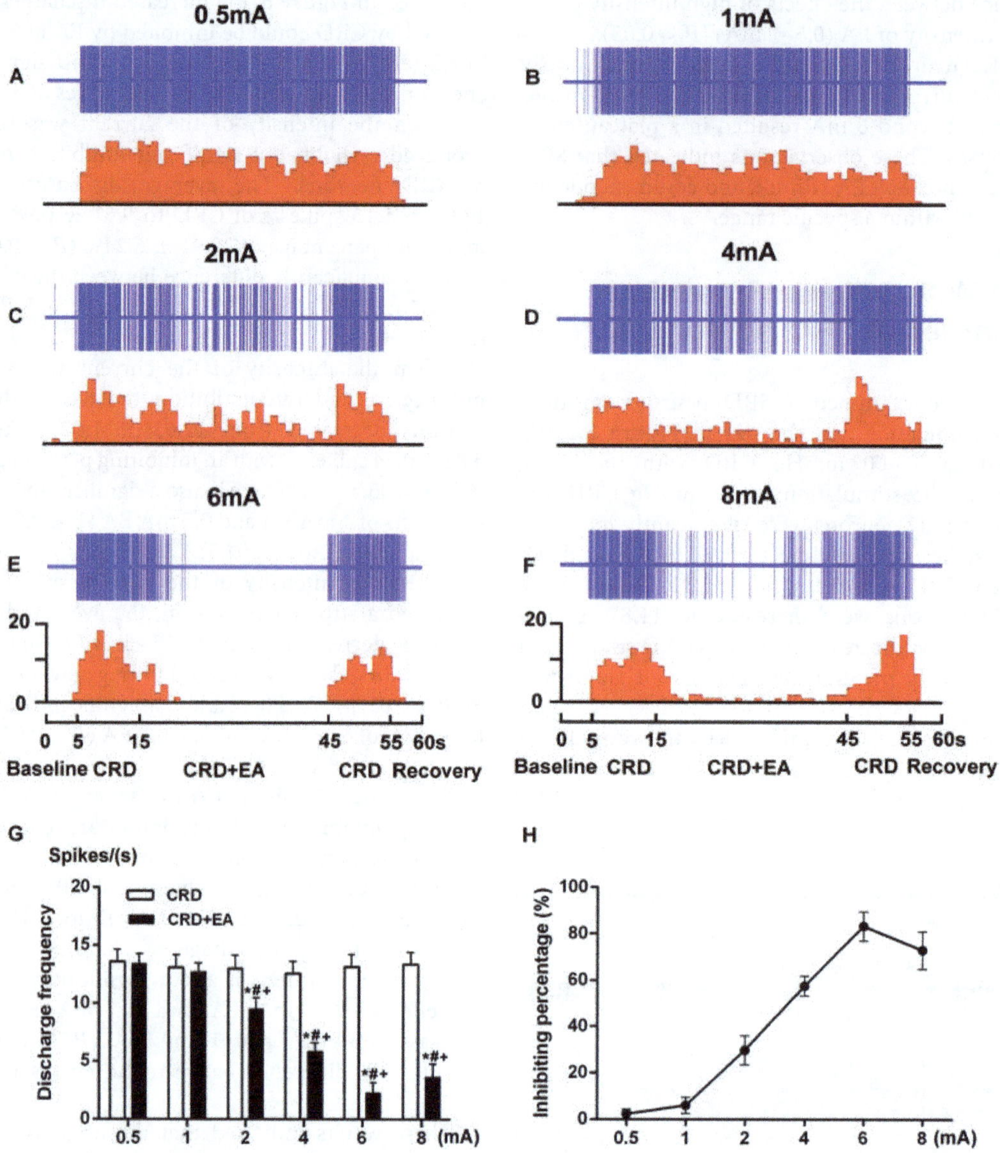

FIGURE 6 | Response characteristics of SRD neurons to different intensities of EA during CRD. **(A–F)** Representative examples showing a decrease in discharges of SRD neurons during the CRD + EA sequence was elicited by EA at 2–8 mA. The upper rows show the unit discharges at different stimulations and the lower rows show these discharges in histogram. Note: CRD (Colorectal distention), CRD + EA (CRD plus EA). **(G)** This histogram shows that CRD induced discharges of SRD neurons were inhibited by EA at 2–8 mA. Data consists of the average spikes per second (mean ± SEM). $^{*}p < 0.05$ compared with CRD; $^{\#}p < 0.05$ compared with 0.5 mA EA; $^{+}p < 0.05$ compared with 1 mA EA. **(H)** This stimulus–response curve shows the percentage of inhibition induced by EA. A positive linear relationship between intensity and inhibition percentage of inhibition was observed within 2–6 mA ($Y = 10.79 \log X + 3.387$, $P < 0.001$). Further increased the intensity to 8 mA induced a significant decrease in inhibition percentage.

The antinociceptive effects of EA on visceral nociception were observed on acupoints ST 36 and ST 37. According to traditional acupuncture theory, the two acupoints are lower confluent acupoint of the meridians of stomach and large intestine, and are used for the treatment of gastrointestinal disease. It has been confirmed by animal experiments that EA and acupuncture stimulation applied at acupoints ST 36 and ST 37 exerts good effects on rats with acute visceral hyperalgesia induced by acetic acid (Qi et al., 2016, 2018) and CRD (Rong et al., 2005). In addition, ST 36 has a specific effect on CRD-induced changes in blood pressure, abnormal electrogastrogram and gastric tension (Chen et al., 2011). In the present study, we observed that noxious EA stimulation of ST 36 and ST 37 is effective in inhibiting visceral nociception at SRD level. Together with previous studies, these findings provide evidence for the efficacy of ST 36 and ST 37 in treating visceral gastrointestinal pain.

SRD could play a specific role in processing nociceptive information. It was a well delimited area within the caudal most aspect of the medulla. Previous electrophysiological studies had clearly demonstrated the response properties of neurons within SRD to somatic and visceral inputs. The great majority of neurons within SRD did not exhibit spontaneous activity, but these neurons were activated exclusively by thermal, mechanical, and electrical noxious stimulation on any part of the body surface, thus exhibiting a "whole body" receptive field (Villanueva et al., 1988, 1990). In addition, SRD neurons also responded to noxious visceral stimulation (Li et al., 2013; Yu et al., 2014). Similarly, the present study observed the activation responses of SRD neurons evoked by noxious pinch stimulation applied to the foot, tail and finger, and also by noxious CRD stimulation and high intensity of EA stimulation within 2–8 mA. However, SRD neurons did not response to innocuous brush stimulation nor to low intensity of EA stimuli within 0.5–1 mA. Interestingly, the threshold of the intensity for Aδ–and C–fiber activation evoked by EA stimulation was approximately 1.68 ± 0.53 mA and 4.78 ± 0.45 mA, respectively (Zhu et al., 2004). Therefore, EA with the intensity of 2–8 mA could be identified as noxious stimulation. This indicated that SRD neurons have similar characteristics of responses to EA stimulation as to other somatic stimulation, receive solely noxious information.

EA achieves analgesic effects on visceral pain via somatovisceral interactions between pain regions and acupoints at different level of central nervous system. The inhibition of visceral nociception induced by acupuncture has been observed at spinal wide dynamic range neurons in our previous study (Rong et al., 2005). However, the inhibition was abolished by blockade of the central descending pathway, indicating that the effects of EA on visceral nociception may not only modulate by spinal level, but many others in supraspinal center. Accumulating evidences showed that the occurrence of a reciprocal connection between dorsal reticular structure and spinal neurons (Villanueva et al., 1991; Almeida et al., 1993). SRD is an important structure in spino-reticulo-spinal loop, which implicated in the modulating of ascending noxious information (Almeida et al., 1993). In this study, we clearly demonstrated that the nociceptive response of SRD neurons induced by noxious CRD stimulation could be inhibited by EA stimulation within the intensity of 2–8 mA. Because SRD neurons receive only noxious inputs, the nociceptive responses of SRD neurons were not affected by EA stimulation within the intensity of 0.5–1 mA. Our findings provide evidence for the interaction of visceral and EA inputs onto SRD neurons. Together with previous electrophysiological studies (Bing et al., 1991), we reasoned that SRD may be involved in EA analgesia on visceral pain by means of spino-reticulo-spinal feed-back mechanism.

The mechanisms underlying EA induced segmental and extrasegmental analgesia are differ. Electrophysiological studies on somatic pain have shown that segmental analgesia of homotopic EA stimulation can be elicited by the activation of Aβ- and part of Aδ - fibers, whereas extrasegmental analgesia of heterotopic EA stimulation is only effective with intensities strong enough to excite Aδ–or C–fibers (Xu et al., 2003; Zhu et al., 2004; Xin et al., 2016). It is very likely that SRD neurons are involved in the mechanism of the widespread extrasegmental antinociceptive effects of EA.

When the intensity of EA increased to noxious range, EA stimulation produced apparent inhibition of the nociceptive responses in the SRD neurons. The widespread extrasegmental analgesia induced by noxious EA stimuli can also be illustrated by DNIC that was proposed by Le Bars et al. (1979a). DNIC refer to the phenomena that noxious response of convergent neurons of the dorsal horn and/or medullary dorsal horn was inhibited by heterotopic noxious stimuli (Cadden et al., 1983; Cadden and Morrison, 1991). SRD has been verified as an important supraspinal relay in DNIC. Similar to the response properties of SRD neurons, DNIC is triggered only by A δ–and C–fibers (Le Bars et al., 1979b). The arrival of nociceptive inputs to medulla can activate SRD neurons and trigger DNIC function, and then trigger a negative feedback to nociceptive signals (Le Bars, 2002). Actually, 2 Hz EA exert analgesic effect on chronic pain by improve DNIC function (Yuan et al., 2018).

We also found that there is a positive relationship between current intensity and the magnitude of neuronal responses to EA within 2–6 mA, while the responses of SRD neurons to EA reached a plateau beyond 6 mA. The encoding property of SRD neurons to EA closely resembles the encoding property of SRD neurons to electrical stimuli (Villanueva et al., 1989). SRD neurons can encode the intensity of electrical stimuli, especially within the noxious range (Villanueva et al., 1989, Gall et al., 2000), For instance, they responded to the graded intensity of electrical stimuli in the range of 1.5–6.0 mA (Villanueva et al., 1989). However, we must point out that if the electrical current is strong enough to excite C–fibers, EA treatment will inevitably cause unbearable pain in clinical practice. As such, if the intensity of EA exceeds a certain range, this treatment is not suitable for analgesia in patients. The present results show that 6 mA may be sufficient to elicit the optimal analgesic effects on visceral pain rats.

CONCLUSION

The present study emphasizes the important role of SRD neurons in EA analgesia on visceral pain. In normal state, the spontaneous activity of SRD neurons could be activated by EA within 2–8 mA. However, during CRD, the nociceptive responses of SRD neurons could be inhibited by EA within 2–8 mA. In summary, we speculated that the transmission of visceral nociceptive could be inhibited by EA via somatovisceral interaction at SRD neurons.

AUTHOR CONTRIBUTIONS

LY, LL, and QQ performed the experiments. BZ designed the experiments. LY and YY analyzed the data and drafted the manuscript. All the authors discussed the results, reviewed the final manuscript, and approved it for the publication.

FUNDING

This work was funded by National Natural Science Foundation of China (No. 81403475) and the Fundamental Research Funds for the Central Public Welfare Research Institutes (Nos. ZZZD16001 and ZZ10-006).

REFERENCES

Almeida, A., Tavares, I., Lima, D., and Coimbra, A. (1993). Descending projections from the medullary dorsal reticular nucleus make synaptic contacts with spinal cord lamina I cells projecting to that nucleus: an electron microscopic tracer study in the rat. *Neuroscience* 55, 1093–1106. doi: 10.1016/0306-4522(93)90323-8

Bing, Z., Villanueva, L., and Le Bars, D. (1991). Acupuncture-evoked responses of subnucleus reticularis dorsalis neurons in the rat medulla. *Neuroscience* 44, 693–703. doi: 10.1016/0306-4522(91)90088-6

Bouhassira, D., Villanueva, L., Bing, Z., and le Bars, D. (1992). Involvement of the subnucleus reticularis dorsalis in diffuse noxious inhibitory controls in the rat. *Brain Res.* 595, 353–357. doi: 10.1016/0006-8993(92)91071-L

Cadden, S. W., and Morrison, J. F. (1991). Effects of visceral distension on the activities of neurones receiving cutaneous inputs in the rat lumbar dorsal horn; comparison with effects of remote noxious somatic stimuli. *Brain Res.* 558, 63–74. doi: 10.1016/0006-8993(91)90714-7

Cadden, S. W., Villanueva, L., Chitour, D., and Le Bars, D. (1983). Depression of activities of dorsal horn convergent neurones by propriospinal mechanisms triggered by noxious inputs; comparison with diffuse noxious inhibitory controls (DNIC). *Brain Res.* 275, 1–11. doi: 10.1016/0006-8993(83)90412-2

Chang, L. (2004). Review article: epidemiology and quality of life in functional gastrointestinal disorders. *Aliment. Pharmacol. Ther.* 20(Suppl. 7), 31–39. doi: 10.1111/j.1365-2036.2004.02183.x

Chen, S. P., Gao, Y. H., Wang, J. Y., and Liu, J. L. (2011). Effects of electroacupuncture at different points on colorectal distention-induced changes in blood pressure, electrogastrogram, gastric tension and gastric blood flow. *J. Tradit. Chin. Med.* 31, 360–366. doi: 10.1016/S0254-6272(12)60019-3

Gall, O., Villanueva, L., Bouhassira, D., and Le Bars, D. (2000). Spatial encoding properties of subnucleus reticularis dorsalis neurons in the rat medulla. *Brain Res.* 873, 131–134. doi: 10.1016/S0006-8993(00)02524-5

Le Bars, D. (2002). The whole body receptive field of dorsal horn multireceptive neurones. *Brain Res. Brain Res. Rev.* 40, 29–44. doi: 10.1016/S0165-0173(02)00186-8

Le Bars, D., Dickenson, A. H., and Besson, J. M. (1979a). Diffuse noxious inhibitory controls (DNIC). I. Effects on dorsal horn convergent neurones in the rat. *Pain* 6, 283–304. doi: 10.1016/0304-3959(79)90049-6

Le Bars, D., Dickenson, A. H., and Besson, J. M. (1979b). Diffuse noxious inhibitory controls (DNIC). II. Lack of effect on non-convergent neurones, supraspinal involvement and theoretical implications. *Pain* 6, 305–327.

Li, L., Yu, L., Rong, P., Ben, H., Li, X., Zhu, B., et al. (2013). Visceral nociceptive afferent facilitates reaction of subnucleus reticularis dorsalis to acupoint stimulation in rats. *Evid. Based Complement. Alternat. Med.* 2013:931283. doi: 10.1155/2013/931283

Liu, K., Gao, X. Y., Li, L., Ben, H., Qin, Q. G., Zhao, Y. X., et al. (2014). Neurons in the nucleus tractus solitarius mediate the acupuncture analgesia in visceral pain rats. *Auton. Neurosci.* 186, 91–94. doi: 10.1016/j.autneu.2014.08.004

MacPherson, H., Tilbrook, H., Agbedjro, D., Buckley, H., Hewitt, C., and Frost, C. (2017). Acupuncture for irritable bowel syndrome: 2-year follow-up of a randomised controlled trial. *Acupunct. Med.* 35, 17–23. doi: 10.1136/acupmed-2015-010854

Qi, D., Wu, S., Zhang, Y., and Li, W. (2016). Electroacupuncture analgesia with different frequencies is mediated via different opioid pathways in acute visceral hyperalgesia rats. *Life Sci.* 160, 64–71. doi: 10.1016/j.lfs.2016.06.025

Qi, D. B., and Li, W. M. (2012). Effects of electroacupuncture on expression of c-fos protein and N-methyl-D-aspartate receptor 1 in the rostral ventromedial medulla of rats with chronic visceral hyperalgesia. *Zhong Xi Yi Jie He Xue Bao* 10, 416–423. doi: 10.3736/jcim20120410

Qi, D. B., Zhang, S. H., Zhang, Y. H., Wu, S. Q., and Li, W. M. (2018). A rat model for studying electroacupuncture analgesia on acute visceral hyperalgesia. *Exp. Anim.* 67, 51–61. doi: 10.1538/expanim.17-0063

Rong, P. J., Zhu, B., Huang, Q. F., Gao, X. Y., Ben, H., and Li, Y. H. (2005). Acupuncture inhibition on neuronal activity of spinal dorsal horn induced by noxious colorectal distention in rat. *World J. Gastroenterol.* 11, 1011–1017. doi: 10.3748/wjg.v11.i7.1011

Roy, J. C., Bing, Z., Villanueva, L., and Le Bars, D. (1992). Convergence of visceral and somatic inputs onto subnucleus reticularis dorsalis neurones in the rat medulla. *J. Physiol.* 458, 235–246. doi: 10.1113/jphysiol.1992.sp019415

Sach, J., Bolus, R., Fitzgerald, L., Naliboff, B. D., Chang, L., and Mayer, E. A. (2002). Is there a difference between abdominal pain and discomfort in moderate to severe IBS patients? *Am. J. Gastroenterol.* 97, 3131–3138. doi: 10.1111/j.1572-0241.2002.07110.x

Spiegel, B. M., Gralnek, I. M., Bolus, R., Chang, L., Dulai, G. S., Mayer, E. A., et al. (2004). Clinical determinants of health-related quality of life in patients with irritable bowel syndrome. *Arch. Intern. Med.* 164, 1773–1780. doi: 10.1001/archinte.164.16.1773

Villanueva, L., Bing, Z., Bouhassira, D., and Le Bars, D. (1989). Encoding of electrical, thermal, and mechanical noxious stimuli by subnucleus reticularis dorsalis neurons in the rat medulla. *J. Neurophysiol.* 61, 391–402. doi: 10.1152/jn.1989.61.2.391

Villanueva, L., Bouhassira, D., Bing, Z., and Le Bars, D. (1988). Convergence of heterotopic nociceptive information onto subnucleus reticularis dorsalis neurons in the rat medulla. *J. Neurophysiol.* 60, 980–1009. doi: 10.1152/jn.1988.60.3.980

Villanueva, L., Bouhassira, D., and Le Bars, D. (1996). The medullary subnucleus reticularis dorsalis (SRD) as a key link in both the transmission and modulation of pain signals. *Pain* 67, 231–240. doi: 10.1016/0304-3959(96)03121-1

Villanueva, L., Cliffer, K. D., Sorkin, L. S., Le Bars, D., and Willis, W. D. Jr. (1990). Convergence of heterotopic nociceptive information onto neurons of caudal medullary reticular formation in monkey (Macaca fascicularis). *J. Neurophysiol.* 63, 1118–1127. doi: 10.1152/jn.1990.63.5.1118

Villanueva, L., de Pommery, J., Menetrey, D., and Le Bars, D. (1991). Spinal afferent projections to subnucleus reticularis dorsalis in the rat. *Neurosci. Lett.* 134, 98–102. doi: 10.1016/0304-3940(91)90517-W

Villanueva, L., and Le Bars, D. (1995). The activation of bulbo-spinal controls by peripheral nociceptive inputs: diffuse noxious inhibitory controls. *Biol. Res.* 28, 113–125.

Wang, K., Xiang, X. H., Qiao, N., Qi, J. Y., Lin, L. B., Zhang, R., et al. (2014). Genomewide analysis of rat periaqueductal gray-dorsal horn reveals time-, region- and frequency-specific mRNA expression changes in response to electroacupuncture stimulation. *Sci. Rep.* 4:6713. doi: 10.1038/srep06713

Wang, S. J., Yang, H. Y., and Xu, G. S. (2012). Acupuncture alleviates colorectal hypersensitivity and correlates with the regulatory mechanism of TrpV1 and p-ERK. *Evid. Based Complement. Alternat. Med.* 2012:483123. doi: 10.1155/2012/483123

Xin, J., Su, Y., Yang, Z., He, W., Shi, H., Wang, X., et al. (2016). Distinct roles of ASIC3 and TRPV1 receptors in electroacupuncture-induced segmental and systemic analgesia. *Front. Med.* 10:465–472. doi: 10.1007/s11684-016-0482-7

Xu, W. D., Zhu, B., Rong, P. J., Bei, H., Gao, X. Y., and Li, Y. Q. (2003). The pain-relieving effects induced by electroacupuncture with different intensities at homotopic and heterotopic acupoints in humans. *Am. J. Chin. Med.* 31, 791–802. doi: 10.1142/s0192415x03001478

Yu, L. L., Li, L., Rong, P. J., Zhu, B., Qin, Q. G., Ben, H., et al. (2014). Changes in responses of neurons in spinal and medullary subnucleus reticularis dorsalis to acupoint stimulation in rats with visceral hyperalgesia. *Evid. Based Complement. Alternat. Med.* 2014:768634. doi: 10.1155/2014/768634

Yuan, X.-C., Zhu, B., Jing, X.-H., Xiong, L.-Z., Wu, C.-H., Gao, F., et al. (2018). Electroacupuncture potentiates cannabinoid receptor-mediated descending inhibitory control in a mouse model of knee osteoarthritis. *Front. Mol. Neurosci.* 11:112. doi: 10.3389/fnmol.2018.00112

Zhao, Z. Q. (2008). Neural mechanism underlying acupuncture analgesia. *Prog. Neurobiol.* 85, 355–375. doi: 10.1016/j.pneurobio.2008.05.004

Zhu, B., Xu, W. D., Rong, P. J., Ben, H., and Gao, X. Y. (2004). A C-fiber reflex inhibition induced by electroacupuncture with different intensities applied at homotopic and heterotopic acupoints in rats selectively destructive effects on myelinated and unmyelinated afferent fibers. *Brain Res.* 1011, 228–237. doi: 10.1016/j.brainres.2004.03.034

10

Adjustment of Synchronization Stability of Dynamic Brain-Networks Based on Feature Fusion

Haifang Li, Rong Yao, Xiaoluan Xia, Guimei Yin, Hongxia Deng and Pengfei Yang*

College of Information and Computer, Taiyuan University of Technology, Taiyuan, China

***Correspondence:**
Haifang Li
lihaifang@tyut.edu.cn

When the brain is active, the neural activities of different regions are integrated on various spatial and temporal scales; this is termed the synchronization phenomenon in neurobiological theory. This synchronicity is also the main underlying mechanism for information integration and processing in the brain. Clinical medicine has found that some of the neurological diseases that are difficult to cure have deficiencies or abnormalities in the whole or local integration processes of the brain. By studying the synchronization capabilities of the brain-network, we can intensively describe and characterize both the state of the interactions between brain regions and their differences between people with a mental illness and a set of controls by measuring the rapid changes in brain activity in patients with psychiatric disorders and the strength and integrity of their entire brain network. This is significant for the study of mental illness. Because static brain network connection methods are unable to assess the dynamic interactions within the brain, we introduced the concepts of dynamics and variability in a constructed EEG brain functional network based on dynamic connections, and used it to analyze the variability in the time characteristics of the EEG functional network. We used the spectral features of the brain network to extract its synchronization features and used the synchronization features to describe the process of change and the differences in the brain network's synchronization ability between a group of patients and healthy controls during a working memory task. We propose a method based on the fusion of traditional features and spectral features to achieve an adjustment of the patient's brain network synchronization ability, so that its synchronization ability becomes consistent with that of healthy controls, theoretically achieving the purpose of the treatment of the diseases. Studying the stability of brain network synchronization can provide new insights into the pathogenic mechanism and cure of mental diseases and has a wide range of potential applications.

Keywords: EEG, working memory, EEG dynamic brain network, brain network synchronization stability, brain network synchronization adjustment and control

INTRODUCTION

The brain is a complex system that exhibits various subsystems on different spatial and temporal scales. These subsystems are recurrent networks, that is, very large clusters of neurons that repeatedly interact with each other. Individual neurons are microscopic and change at a different time rate than macroscopic neural populations. After Babloyantz et al. (1986) first used nonlinear dynamics theory to study EEG signals in 1985, research on EEG signals rapidly entered the era of nonlinear dynamics. Various theories and methods of nonlinear dynamics have opened up new possibilities for analyzing EEG data. Eliasmith et al. (2012) presented a 2.5 million neuron model of the brain (called "Spaun") that bridged this gap by exhibiting many different behaviors. The model is presented by only visual image sequences, and it draws all its responses with a physically modeled arm. Although simplified, the model captures many aspects of neuroanatomy, neurophysiology, and psychological behavior.

Hutt (2010) studied the main characteristics of a single neuron and its interactions by establishing a standard mathematical model and applied the model to explain experimental results from the delayed feedback system of weak electric fish and from electroencephalography (EEG). Liley et al. (2002) used nonlinear differential equations based on the human brain's physiological structure and medical anatomy to define a mathematical model of brain neuron clusters in states of both excitement and inhibition. With the establishment of neuron models, neuroscientists have conducted extensive and in-depth studies on neural network dynamics using various neuronal models to try to reveal the hidden secrets of the brain (Stam et al., 2007; Liu et al., 2008, 2014; De Han et al., 2009; Sun et al., 2009; Bartolomei et al., 2010; Skidmore et al., 2011).

Currently, many studies (Zhao et al., 2008; Qun, 2009; Gao et al., 2014b; Ruizhen et al., 2017) have shown that when the brain is active, the neural activities of different regions are integrated on a variety of spatial and temporal scales; this is known as the synchronization phenomenon in neurobiological theory. Synchronization is the basic mechanism for information integration and processing. Clinical medicine studies have shown that some of the neurological diseases that are difficult to cure have deficiencies or abnormalities in the whole or local integration process of the brain. Scientists have discovered a variety of synchronous behaviors in the neuronal system. The results of these studies show that the synchronization behavior of neuronal firing not only affects daily learning, brain memory, calculation, and motor control but can also be used to explain some neurological diseases such as epilepsy and Parkinson's disease.

The human brain is a complex network. Synchronization capability is an important indicator of complex networks. Therefore, brain network synchronization research has gradually attracted the attention of brain scientists and has made great advances. For example, Ma et al. (2014) and Hongli et al. (2013) found that the synchronization of the brain network of Alzheimer's patients was lower than that of a control group. Hou et al. (Dong et al., 2014; Feng-Zhen et al., 2014) analyzed the brain network of epilepsy patients using the network connectivity index to understand whether the brain network of patients with epilepsy is different from a normal brain network, and also investigated the brain electrical signal synchronization of patients with cerebral infarction. Rosário et al. (2015) proposed a new brain network edge association method that involves motif synchronization, primarily by calculating the number of occurrences of certain patterns between any two time-series to provide information about the degree and direction of synchronization between two nodes in the network. Sakkalis et al. (2013) used amplitude square coherence, phase synchronization estimation, and robust nonlinear state space generalized synchronization assessment methods to calculate the synchrony between all the pairs of channels in alcohol addiction patients. The experimental results showed that, during a rehearsal procedure, the alcohol addiction patients showed a loss of synchrony and an impaired lateralization of the brain activity.

Although previous studies have used synchrony to study neurodegenerative diseases, most of the current studies about the differences in brain function between patients with mental disorders and normal subjects investigated traditional features of brain network properties (node degree, mean-clustering-coefficient, global-efficiency, small-world attributes, etc.) (Micheloyannis et al., 2006; Zhang et al., 2013a,b, 2015; Müller et al., 2018). Researching these traditional features can clearly aid in understanding the topological characteristics of the brain network, but these features do not fully reflect the structure of the brain network. As a result, clinicians cannot find a unique and effective index for determining the specific diagnosis that a subject should receive. The spectral properties of complex networks (Li and Zhang, 1997; Xiao, 2012; Sato and Iwai, 2014; Liu and Shen, 2017) can provide a comprehensive measure of the global structure of the network. Any change in a local attribute feature is reflected in changes in the spectrum.

Therefore, to find more significant indicators of the differences between mental patients and healthy controls, we built a brain network based on complex network theory, used the spectral features of the brain network to identify the synchronization characteristics, and used the synchronous features to characterize the patients and the healthy controls. Thus, we studied the process by which the brain's synchronization ability changed during the working memory process and its difference between the two groups. We also proposed a method based on fusing traditional features and spectral features to adjust the synchronization ability of the brain networks of patients so that their synchronization ability will be consistent with those of healthy controls. Theoretically we can achieve the goal of treating diseases. Studying brain network synchronization can help to more clearly explain the dynamic process of the collective behavior of a large number of nodes in a complex brain network and may be able to prevent the harm that comes from some types of synchronizations. Thus, this research may provide a new direction for studying the pathological mechanisms of brain diseases. The brain network mechanisms of healthy controls and patients have very important practical significance and academic value.

The paper is organized as follows: Section EEG Dataset Description and Preprocessing briefly describes the dataset of EEG signals employed in our research. Section Methods presents information about the methods used in this study, including constructing the brain-network, extracting synchronization features, and synchronizing optimization algorithms. Section Experimental Results and Analysis provides the experiments undertaken in the framework of the study, the experimental procedures used, and the experimental results obtained. Finally, section Limitations describes the conclusions derived from the study and some thoughts, with regard to future work.

EEG DATASET DESCRIPTION AND PREPROCESSING

EEG Dataset Description

The dataset used in this work was task state EEG data. The experimental paradigm used the modified Sternberg's SMST (Manoach et al., 1999) (short-term memory scanning task) paradigm (see **Figure 1**) The dataset included 34 psychiatric (in this study we used schizophrenic) patients and 34 healthy people (controls), none of whom had any record of drug abuse or diagnosis of neuropsychiatric disease in the past 6 months. The age range of the patient group was 20–51 years old, and the average age was (40.1 ± 11.1) years old; the healthy control group age range was 21–58 years old, and the average age was (37.1 ± 13.8) years old. Age, sex, and education level did not differ significantly between the two groups. All the members of both groups had normal vision or corrected visual acuity, had no color disturbance, and were right-handed (Zhao et al., 2011).

Data Preprocessing

Data collection was completed at a hospital psychiatry research center on a NeuroScan 64-lead EEG acquisition device. The sampling frequency was 500 Hz, the impedance was kept below 5 kΩ, the ground electrode was AFz, and the reference electrode was physically connected to the left and right mastoids. The vertical electro-oculogram recording was from electrodes placed above and below the left eye, and the horizontal electro-oculogram recording was from electrodes placed on the right eyelid margin (Stam et al., 2007).

The preprocessing was performed on the EEGLab (https://sccn.ucsd.edu/eeglab/download.php) platform on Matlab, which converted the reference data of the original data, removing the electrooculogram, filtering, segmenting, and removing artifacts to yield noiseless and clean EEG data. An average reference electrode was selected as the reference electrode, and the low-pass and high-pass noise were removed by filtering in the range of 0.5–50 Hz. The ocular electrical artifacts in the data were removed using the negative entropy-based FastICA method (Joyce et al., 2010; Jiaqing et al., 2018). Compared with the traditional blind source separation algorithm, this method does not require the ocular electrical signal as the reference electrode, avoiding the mixing of new noise during the EE signal acquisition process and reducing the collection workload. In addition, volume conduction can affect the output of synchronization measures when using EEG signals, because EEG is bipolar by nature. This means that EEG signals are composed of a difference between an electrode of interest and a reference (Guevara et al., 2005; Peraza et al., 2012). We used surface Laplacian transform methods (Matlab toolbox CSD) (Kayser and Tenke, 2006a,b) to eliminate the mixing effect of volume conduction. During the data acquisition process the data were labeled as S1–S10, in which S1–S5 represented the encoding phases, S6–S8 represented the maintenance phases, and S9–S10 represented the retrieval phases (see **Figure 2**). The data were filtered and retained by θ (4–7 Hz), α (7–14 Hz), β1 (14–20 Hz), β2 (for 20–30 Hz), and γ (30–40 Hz) signals in five frequency bands. From these data, 20 segments were selected from the different frequency bands in the different stages, and each was spliced. Duration of the EEG trajectory in the encoding, maintenance, and retrieval phases were 100 s, 60 s, and 50 s, respectively.

METHODS

Unweighted Complex Dynamic Brain-Networks Construction

In the experiment, 60 scalp electrode channels were selected as the nodes of the brain network. The phase-locking value (PLV) coherence function was chosen for the edges of the network. This function was used to calculate the correlation between two electrode channels to form a 60 × 60 PLV correlation matrix. PLV can separate phase and amplitude components. Because EEG data can be affected by transient amplitude changes such as eye movements, PLV is quite suitable for this data. This paper uses a wavelet transform to extract phase information. The short time Fourier transform (STFT) method uses a sliding window to intercept the signal and performs a Fourier transform on the signal in the window to obtain the spectrum formula of the signal at any time (1), where STFT of $f(t)$: computed for each window centered at $t = t'$; t' is the time parameter; μ is the frequency parameter; $f(t)$ is the signal to be analyzed; $W(t - t')$ is the windowing function.

$$STFT(t', \mu) = \int f(t)\, W(t - t')e^{-j2\pi\mu t}dt \tag{1}$$

Specifically, the PLV definition (Xu et al., 2014) is Equation (2), where N represents the number of brain network nodes (In

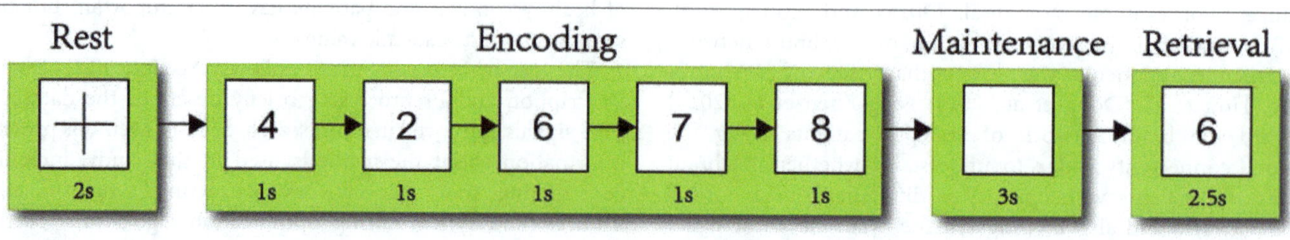

FIGURE 1 | Short-term memory scanning task (SMTS) paradigm. Subjects needed to remember the numbers appearing on the screen during the encoding stage and recall these during the maintenance stage. Finally, in the retrieval stage, the subjects were required to determine whether the number had appeared by searching their memory.

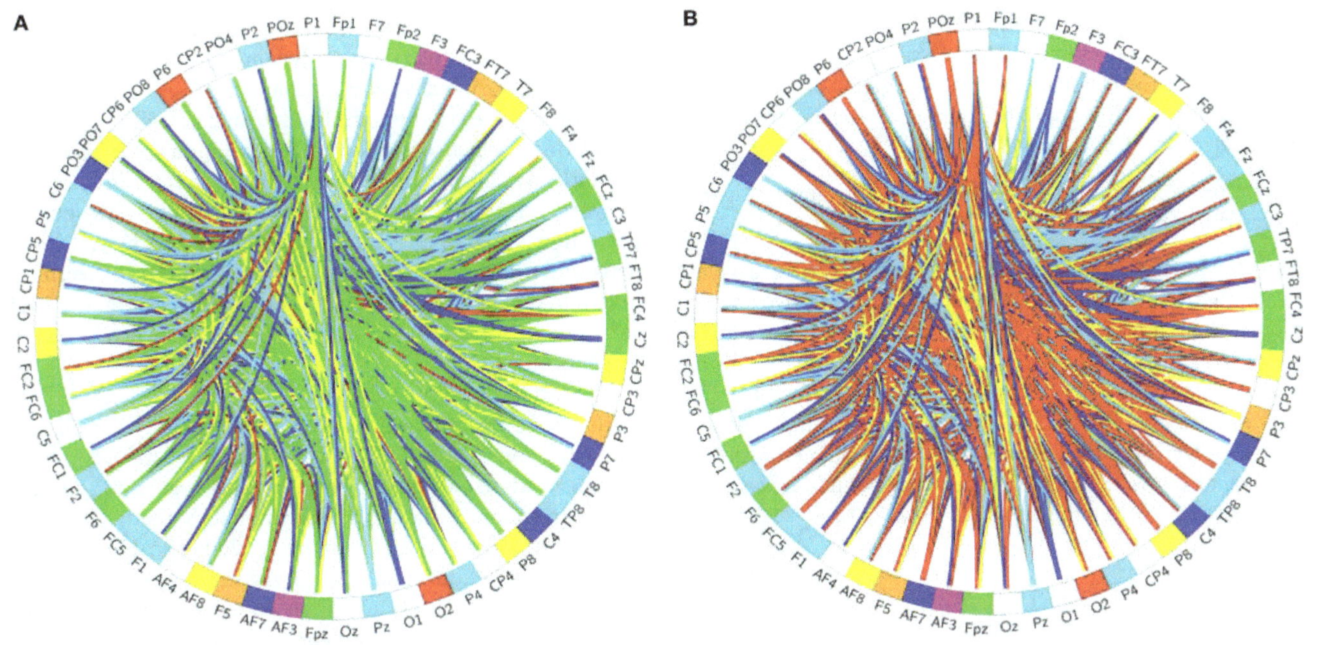

FIGURE 2 | Brain-network. **(A)** Represents the healthy controls, **(B)** represents the patients.

this paper $N = 60$); $\Delta\ \varphi_n(t) = \varphi_x(t) - \varphi_y(t)$ represents the phase difference between the two channel time-frequency points t; and PLV ϵ [0,1].

$$PLV\ (t) = \frac{1}{N}\left|\sum_{n=1}^{N} exp(j(\triangle\Phi_n(t)))\right| \tag{2}$$

The study of dynamic functional networks or time-varying brain function networks is an emerging field in brain function connection research. Its purpose is to study the dynamic nature or variability of functional connections over time. It has been applied to the analysis and diagnosis of brain diseases in fMRI and has in EEG signal analysis. Common methods for studying time-varying functional connections include important transfer point detection, time-frequency decomposition methods, and time window methods (Rosário et al., 2015). Of these, the sliding time window method is currently the most widely used. Existing research found that the brain network clearly shows time-variability and dynamics even over a short period of time and that the size of the time window is related to changes in the topological properties of the brain network (Sakkalis et al., 2013). The time window selected for the PLV cannot be too large. If it is too large, the signal may not be reasonably stable during this time period. Therefore, referring to existing research in a PLV phase synchronicity measurement study (Yi et al., 2014) and existing related research (Gysels and Celka, 2004; Gao et al., 2014a; Bola et al., 2015), we selected a sliding time window (step size of 0.04 s) in the range of 0.04–0.48 s. To determine the size of the PLV sliding time window, the classification accuracy of the network attributes was calculated within a given range of 0.04–0.48 s. The classification accuracy between the groups was determined. The final time window was determined to be 0.12 s.

The experiment was related to previous research on the small-world characteristics of the human brain (Guo et al., 2013). The sparsity range chosen was 30 to 40% with a step size of 2%; the network was constructed separately for each of the 20 trials. The networks for the 34 patients and 34 healthy controls were constructed separately for the encoding, maintenance, and retrieval stages and for the alpha and theta bands. A total of 48,960 brain networks were constructed.

Brain-Network Feature Extraction

The traditional features of brain networks are usually attributes of the network and include global attributes and local attributes (Guo et al., 2013). Our experiment calculated four local attributes, which were degree, inference, clustering coefficient, and local efficiency, and six global attributes, which were global efficiency, modularity index, positive and negative matching degree, feature path length, average clustering coefficient, and average local efficiency. The feature extraction in this research included two stages: The first stage extracted the distinctive features from the traditional features; the second stage extracted the features of the brain network spectrum; and spectral feature calculations provided the synchronization features.

The first stage:

A. Extraction of significant differences from global features

We compared the global attribute values between the patient group and the healthy controls in the same frequency band and at the same sparsity in the same stage. We used the Kolmogorov-Smirnov (KS) test ($P < 0.05$) to indicate that the node difference between the patients' brain networks and those of the healthy controls was significant. A significant difference attribute was put into a support vector machine (SVM) classifier as a feature. Based on an analysis of the classification result, a global attribute with a significant difference at a specific stage and a specific frequency band was selected.

B. Extraction of significant differences and nodes from local attributes

To characterize the overall level of a property Y over a given sparsity range (Guo et al., 2013; Hao, 2013), these two papers from our research group used the area under the curve (AUC) to characterize the value of the entire sparsity range Y^{AUC} in the selected sparsity range. Its definition is shown in formula (3), where ΔS represents the space between the sparse upper bound Sn and the lower bound S1 span, which is the step size for the change in sparseness. In this study, the upper bound Sn was 40%, the next S1 was 30%, and the step size ΔS was 2%.

$$Y^{AUC} = \sum_{k=1}^{n-1} [Y(S_k) + Y(S_{k-1})] \times \Delta S/2 \tag{3}$$

In our current experiment, the sparsity range was fused by calculating the AUC. Throughout the entire sparsity range, we identified the nodes that had significant differences between the patients and the healthy controls. We tested the AUC value of each subject's local attribute value in the sparsity range at a certain stage and a certain frequency band. Then, we selected the local attribute AUC value splicing of the significant difference node as a feature to classify, and obtained locally significant attributes and significant nodes that differed significantly between the patients and healthy controls.

The second stage extracted the brain network spectrum characteristics and calculated the brain network synchronization characteristics according to section Synchronization Criteria. The spectral features of a network generally refer to the set of all the eigenvalues of the Laplacian matrix.

Synchronization Criteria

Network synchronization is a very common and important nonlinear phenomenon. There are many different types of network synchronization, such as common constant synchronization, phase synchronization, generalized synchronization, etc. Identical synchronization is defined as:

Definition 1:

Let $x_i(t, X_0)$ be a solution of the complex dynamic network

$$\dot{x} = f(x_i) + g_i(x_1, x_2, x_3, \ldots x_N), \quad i = 1, 2, \ldots, N \tag{4}$$

where $X_0 = \left((x_1^0)^T, (x_2^0)^T, \ldots, (x_N^0)^T, \right)^T \in R^{N^*N}, f: D \to R^n$ and $g_i: D \times D \to R^n (\ i = 1, 2, \ldots, N)$ are all continuously differentiable , $D \subseteq R^n$,and meet $g(x_1, x_2, \ldots, x_n) = 0$. There is any non-empty open set $C \subseteq F$ in the domain, which can make any $x_i(t, X_0) \in F$ and

$$\lim_{t\to\infty} \|x_i(t, X_0) - s_i(t, X_0)\| = 0 \, i = 1, 2, \ldots, N$$

for any $x_i^0 \in C, i = 1, 2, \ldots, N$ and $t \geq 0, i = 1, 2, \ldots, N$, where $s_i(t, X_0)$ is an effective solution space of equation $\dot{x} = f(x)$, and $X_0 \in F$, then the complex dynamics network can reach the identity synchronous steady state, and $C \times \ldots \times C$ is called the synchronous area of the complex dynamic network.

Identical synchronization is a common phenomenon of network synchronization, which shows that all nodes in the network are in the same state at a particular time point. In Definition 1, $s(t, X_0)$ is the synchronous steady state of the network, and $x_1 = x_2 = \ldots = x_N$ is the synchronization manifold of the network state space; that is, each physical oscillator tends to be in a described state when a network is synchronized.

Definition 2:

In 1998, Pecora and Carroll (Pecora and Carroll, 1990; Kashtan and Alon, 2005) studied the stability of the synchronization of linear coupled networks and developed the main stability function discrimination method. In 2002, Wang and Chen (Lü and Guanrong, 2005; Jin-Hu, 2010; Gao et al., 2014b; Zhou et al., 2014) studied the problem of the synchronization stability of coupled oscillators in a continuous system and proposed a dynamic network consisting of N identical vibrators whose dynamic equation is:

$$\dot{\boldsymbol{x}}_i = \boldsymbol{f}(\boldsymbol{x}_i) - \boldsymbol{c} \sum_{j=1}^{N} \mathbf{l}_{ij} \boldsymbol{H}(\boldsymbol{x}_j) \quad , \boldsymbol{i} = \mathbf{1}, \mathbf{2}, \ldots\ldots \boldsymbol{N} \tag{5}$$

where $x_i = (x_{i1}, x_{i2}, \ldots, x_{in})^T \in R^N$ are the node's state variable; $\mathbf{x_i} = \mathbf{f(x_i)}$ describes the state of a single node when there is no coupling; c is the strength of the brain network coupling that has been constructed; H is a node state variable indicating which variables are passed between the coupled nodes; **L** is the Laplacian matrix of the brain network; $\mathbf{l_{ij}}$ is the matrix element of L and contains the information of the network topology.

When the coupling matrix is a Laplacian matrix:If L is a positive semidefinite symmetric matrix and the row sum is 0, then the eigenvalue of L satisfies the following when the network remains connected:

①matrix L has only one eigenvalue with a multiplicity of 1 and its corresponding eigenvector is

$(1,1,1 \ldots \ldots 1)^T$

②The remaining N-1 eigenvalues of the matrix L are positive real numbers, that is: $0 = \lambda1 < \lambda2 \leq \lambda3 \leq \lambda4 \leq \ldots\ldots \leq \lambda N$。

Definition 3:

When the coupling matrix L satisfies Definition 2, the synchronization ability of the network can be expressed by the spectral features of the coupling matrix L. According to the different situations of the synchronization area, a dynamic network (Definition 2) can be divided into two categories. One (type 1) is that the synchronization field of the network is semi-unbounded, and its synchronization ability passes through the minimum non-zero spectral feature λ2 of the corresponding Laplacian matrix L. The larger the value of λ2, the stronger the synchronization ability. The other type (type 2) is that the synchronization domain of the network is bounded, and its synchronization capability can be characterized by the ratio R of the maximum non-zero spectral characteristics of the corresponding Laplacian matrix L to the smallest non-zero spectral features. The smaller the value of R, the stronger the synchronization capability.

Note:

$$R = \lambda N/\lambda 2 \tag{6}$$

Proof:

Construct a brain network of experimental datasets and compute the spectral features of the L-matrix. The experimental results shown in **Figure 3** show that the spectral features of the brain network were all positive. The data verification used in this paper satisfies the synchronization criterion condition type 2. That is, the synchronization ability of the network can be measured by calculating the parameter R.

Defining the Coupling Formula L*

Currently, the adjustment of the synchronization capability of complex network power systems (Wigand et al., 2015; Hongyue et al., 2017; Ruizhen et al., 2017) is mainly based on the network topology, adaptive synchronization control of dynamic equations, and network coupling methods. Considering the particularity of a brain network in the practical application process, that is, that the brain network structure is not easy to change and that the dynamic system is more complex and difficult to control, we here propose a method based on the fusion of traditional features and spectral features to achieve the ability of brain network synchronization for patients. In theory, adjusting a disease brain network so that it is synchronized with that of normal people could be a way to treat the disease.

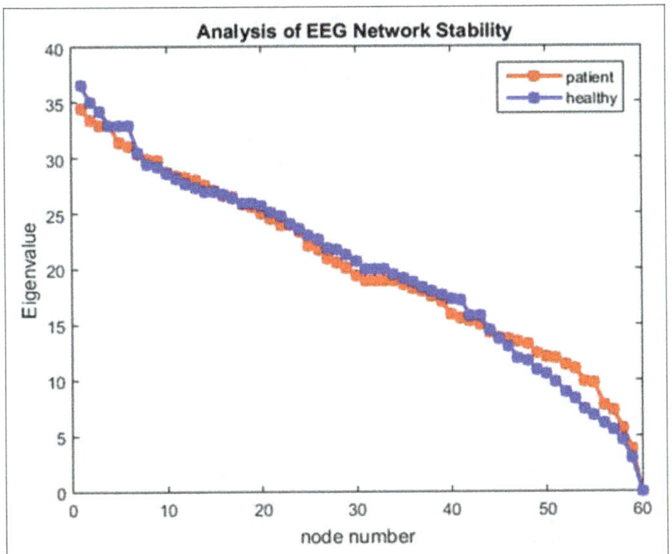

FIGURE 3 | EEG Working memory data Laplacian eigenvalue spectrum (descending order) diagram.

The definition of the T&S(Traditional and Spectral)coupling matrix $\mathbf{L}^*$equationis:

$$L^* = L{*}G \tag{7}$$

where matrix L is the original Laplacian matrix of the complex network dynamics equation, which represents the network spectrum characteristics. Matrix G is the distinctive feature of the extracted brain network.

Formula (7) can be written as formula (8):

$$l^*_{ij} = l^*_{ij} g_i^{\ aa} * g_j^{\ bb} \tag{8}$$

Where ∀ aa, bb∈ R, we can adjust the parameters aa, bb to enhance or weaken the synchronization ability of the network. The combinations of parameters aa, bb are: ① parameters aa, bb are both positive; ② parameters aa, bb are one positive and one negative; ③ parameters aa, bb are both negative.

Define the T&S coupling matrix $\mathbf{L}^*$ [Equation (7)], If the T&S coupling matrix $\mathbf{L}^*$ satisfies definition 3 of section Synchronization Criteria,

which is:

$\mathbf{L}^*$ is a positive semidefinite symmetric matrix;

$\mathbf{L}^*$ line sum is 0;

Then the synchronization capability of the brain network is the ratio R of the spectral features of the T&S coupling matrix $\mathbf{L}^*$.

Mathematical proof:

① If the matrix $\mathbf{L}^*$ is a real symmetric matrix know all eigenvalues of $\mathbf{L}^*$ are real numbers;

② If the matrix $\mathbf{L}^*$ is a positive semi-definite matrix know all eigenvalues of $\mathbf{L}^*$ are positive or 0;

③The following only proves that the matrix $\mathbf{L}^*$ satisfies the row sum to 0;

Proof:

Write formula (7) as a matrix:

$$L^* = L{*}G^{aa}{*}G^{bb} \tag{9}$$

Where

$G = diag\ \{k_1, k_2 \ldots\ldots k_N\}$ is a diagonal matrix composed of a distinctive feature of the brain network.

TABLE 1 | Extracted nodes that showed differences in encoding/alpha/sparsity 34%.

ELECTRODE NUMBER—ELECTRODE NAME		
59-POZ	3-FP2	51-PO3
58-P2	60-P1	29-Pz
36-AF4	57-PO4	31-FPz
16-Cz	22-TP8	17-CPz
15-FC4	27-O2	28-O1
35-AF8	43-FC6	5-FC3
9-F4	10-Fz	11-FCz
13-TP7	14-FT8	32-AF3

TABLE 2 | The average Pearson correlation coefficient for the 10 healthy controls.

Normal/Encoding/Alpha	NO.1	NO.2	NO.3	NO.4	NO.5	NO.6	NO.7	NO.8	NO.9	NO.10	AVE
Assortativity	0.59	0.20	0.57	0.237	0.571	0.059	0.602	0.326	0.549	0.152	0.385
Mean-Clustering-Coef	**0.79**	**0.531**	**0.567**	**0.259**	**0.697**	**0.834**	**0.824**	**0.595**	**0.718**	**0.588**	**0.6105**
Transitivity	**0.82**	**0.546**	**0.566**	**0.595**	**0.701**	**0.703**	**0.653**	**0.666**	**0.544**	**0.795**	**0.6588**
Global-Efficiency	**−0.769**	**−0.430**	**−0.554**	**−0.708**	**−0.718**	**−0.787**	**−0.787**	**−0.572**	**−0.892**	**−0.852**	**−0.7069**
Modularity	−0.234	0.163	−0.378	−0.337	0.369	0.063	0.549	−0.405	0.114	−0.484	−0.0579
Mean-Path-Length	**0.774**	**0.530**	**0.754**	**0.717**	**0.709**	**0.797**	**0.789**	**0.633**	**0.899**	**0.906**	**0.774**

Bold indicates that the conclusion is drawn from the bold part.

The sum of all elements in the i-th row of matrix L^* is:

$$L_J{}^* = \sum_{i=1,j\neq i}^{N} L_{ij} g_i^{aa} * g_j^{bb} = \left(\sum_{i=1,j\neq i}^{N} L_{ij} g_i^{aa}\right) * g_j^{bb}$$
$$= \left(\sum_{i=1,j\neq i}^{N} L_{ij} g_i^{aa} - \left(\sum_{i=1,i\neq j}^{N} L_{ij} g_j^{-aa} g_i^{aa} g_j^{aa}\right)\right) * g_j^{bb}$$
$$= \sum_{i=1,i\neq j}^{N} L_{ij} g_i^{aa} g_j^{bb} - \sum_{i=1,i\neq j}^{N} L_{ij} g_i^{aa} g_j^{bb} = 0 \quad (10)$$

Through mathematics and experiments (**Figure 3**) prove: When the network remains connected, the spectral features of L^*satisfy: (1) The matrix L^*has only one eigenvalue with a multiplier of 1 and its corresponding eigenvector (1,1,1,1, … … $1)^T$; (2) The remaining N-1 eigenvalues of the matrix $L^*$are positive real numbers, that is: $0 = \lambda 1 < \lambda 2 \leq \lambda 3 \leq \lambda 4 \leq \ldots\ldots \leq \lambda N$.

EXPERIMENTAL RESULTS AND ANALYSIS

Experiment 1:Brain-Network Significant Difference Features and Node Extraction

Experiment 1 investigated the encoding stage.

①Using the method of feature extraction described in section Brain-Network Feature Extraction, the distinctive features obtained in the first stage extraction included: assortativity (depending on the trend of nodes in the network, it can be divided into an assortative or disassortative network. Assortative means that a node tends to be connected to its similar node; otherwise, the network is said to be disassortative), mean-clustering-coefficient, transitivity (transitivity is the ratio of "triangles to triplets" in the network), global efficiency, modulus, and mean path length (in the current study, we reanalyzed EEG data from our previous publications Liting et al., 2017; Yuchi et al., 2017).

②We calculated the Pearson correlation coefficient of the features extracted from the first stage and the second stage and identified the features that were strongly correlated. We randomly selected 10 normal subjects and 10 patients with 7 significant differences in characteristics and used their network spectral characteristics (R) to calculate the Pearson correlation coefficients (**Tables 2, 3**). **Table 1** shows the nodes that differed significantly between the patient and healthy controls, as identified using the KS test.

Tables 2, 3 show that there was a strong positive correlation between the synchronization of the brain network and the mean-clustering-coefficient, transitivity, mean path length, and node degree and that there was a strong negative correlation with global efficiency.

The criteria for evaluating the Pearson correlation coefficient are: (1) 0.8–1.0 means that the two are highly correlated; (2) 0.6–0.8 means that the two are significantly correlated; (3) 0.4–0.6 means that the two are mildly correlated (4) 0.2–0.4 means that the two are weakly related; (5) 0.0–0.2 means that the two are very weakly related.

Experiment 2:Brain-Network Synchronization Stability Analysis

Differences in Synchronous Processing

In this process, 20 brain networks were constructed for each subject's 20 trial EEG signals and were used to extract the synchronization features (R) of the brain network's spectral features. The patients and healthy controls could be represented by their synchronization features and by the time required to reach the initial synchronization. The process by which brain synchronization occurs during memory processing differs between healthy subjects and patients. **Table 4** is the range of changes in the mean values of the synchronization characteristics for the 34 patients and 34 healthy controls in the encoding, maintenance, and retrieval stages; **Figure 4** is the initial synchronization of the time chart for the 10 patients and 10 healthy controls who were randomly selected during the encoding, maintenance, and retrieval stages; **Table 5** shows the mean and variance at the initial synchronization in **Figure 4**.

Table 4 shows that there was a significant difference in the synchronization between the patients and the healthy controls in the encoding phase and that the patient's synchronization ability was stronger than that of the normal subjects. This may be because patients have cognitive impairments in memory and their thinking and speech are often confused. Therefore, they showed considerable differences from the healthy controls in the encoding phase of working memory. An analysis of **Table 5** shows that the normal subjects achieved synchronization earlier than the patients.

Determining Significant Differences in the Synchronization Stability of Area S

A. Discovering-significant-differences-in-area-s

The PLV binary matrix corresponding to 48,960 brain networks constructed using data from the patients and the healthy controls is shown in **Figures 5A–C** shows the difference significant area, S, a mathematical representation of the difference between

TABLE 3 | The average Pearson correlation coefficient for the 10 patients' group.

Patient/Encoding/Alpha	NO.1	NO.2	NO.3	NO.4	NO.5	NO.6	NO.7	NO.8	NO.9	NO.10	AVE
Assortativity	0.25	0.32	0.29	0.275	0.683	0.847	0.314	0.383	0.545	0.604	0.4522
Mean-Clustering-Coef	**0.59**	**0.814**	**0.683**	**0.745**	**0.773**	**0.818**	**0.844**	**0.819**	**0.545**	**0.668**	**0.730**
Transitivity	**0.57**	**0.667**	**0.581**	**0.551**	**0.774**	**0.804**	**0.851**	**0.823**	**0.716**	**0.703**	**0.65883**
Global-Efficiency	**−0.735**	**−0.801**	**−0.530**	**−0.582**	**−0.804**	**−0.898**	**−0.841**	**−0.830**	**−0.885**	**−0.829**	**−0.7736**
Modularity	−0.285	0.092	−0.379	−0.119	−0.154	−0.062	−0.551	0.486	−0.150	−0.174	−0.1295
Mean-Path-Length	**0.667**	**0.802**	**0.635**	**0.709**	**0.804**	**0.797**	**0.848**	**0.839**	**0.902**	**0.826**	**0.667**

Bold indicates that the conclusion is drawn from the bold part.

TABLE 4 | Comparison of synchronization differences between healthy controls and patients.

NORMAL GROUP AND PATIENT GROUP R-MEAN		
	Normal	Patient
Encoding	**5–19**	**5–8**
Maintenance	5–13	5–8
Retrieval	5–8	5–8

Bold indicates that the conclusion is drawn from the bold part.

5a and 5b; **Figure 5D** is a brain electrode position diagram corresponding to a 5c S region in the brain map.

Comparing the differences (**Figures 5A,B**) we found that the significant differences in the brain network between normal subjects and patients were located in the S region (**Figure 5C**). The specific manifestations were as follows: The normal controls' S-area connections were tightly organized and the patients' S-area connections were sparsely disordered. This is likely because psychiatric (specifically schizophrenic in this study) patients have cognitive impairments in memory, and their thinking and speech are often confused. Therefore, in memory processing, the connections between the brain regions of the brains of the psychiatric patients were disorganized, but the brain connections of the normal controls showed obvious signs of organization.

From the above analysis, we concluded that the area that was significantly different between the patients and the healthy controls was region S, so the corresponding brain area was primarily located in the occipital lobe.

B. Regional-s-synchronization-stability-analysis

Using the information about the significant difference node (**Table 1**) extracted in Experiment1: Brain-Network Significant Difference Features and Node Extraction the coupling between a certain node in the brain network and the other nodes was removed, and the synchronous characteristics R of brain networks that were randomly selected from the patients and healthy controls (if the other subject conditions were kept constant) were the same. The subjects were compared based on the order of magnitude (**Figure 6**). In **Figure 6**, the abscissa represents the decoupling node number (the electrode corresponding to the node number in **Table 6**), and the ordinate represents the synchronization eigenvalue of the brain network after decoupling.

Figure 6 shows that, in the encoding stage, when node numbers 59, 3, 51, 58, 60, ..., 9, 10, 11 were successively removed, the trends of the patients and the healthy controls in the **Figure 6A** were similar to those in **Figure 6B**. Particularly when the node numbers 16, 22, 17, 15, 27, 28 were sequentially removed, the synchronicity between the patient and the normal person increased. In addition, the node numbers 16, 22, 17, 15, 27, 28 all belong to the red area S, and the ability to remove these nodes one at a time was enhanced. The data shown in **Figure 6** also indicate that, as the density of the red zone S edge decreased, the synchronization ability was stronger, and as the edge density increased, the worse the synchronization ability became (**Figures 5A,B** as healthy controls).

Without changing the coupling relationship of the red region S (**Figure 5C**), the effect of the influence on the synchronization ability of the brain network was observed by enhancing the edge strength of the red region S. **Figures 7A,B** show the changes in the synchronization ability of the red region S edge strengths of the 20 brain networks of a specific patient and a specific individual from the healthy controls from 1, 1.5...3.5 times (In the encoding phase, we chose a period of consecutive 100 s for each participant, constructing a brain network every 5 s).

It can be seen from **Figure 7** that for the same edge strength, the change in the synchronization ability between the patients and the healthy controls exhibited opposite trends and tended to be uniform; the strength of the internal bridging of S is more obvious. However, if the edge strength was too great, it simultaneously reduced the ability of the healthy subjects' network and the patients' network to synchronize.

Experiment 3: Synchronization Stability and Brain-Network Adjustment

From the analysis of the differences in the synchronization ability of the brain network between the patients and healthy controls in section Experiment 2:Brain-Network synchronization stability analysis, we found that the two groups differed considerably in their brains' synchronization ability and that these differences are concentrated in the local area S. That is, the smaller the S edge density, the stronger the synchronization ability. To achieve the goal of curing disease, this section primarily discusses the theory of complex network synchronization control to explore ways in which a patient's brain network could be given a certain "treatment" that would make the patient's synchronization ability consistent with the synchronization ability of normal people.

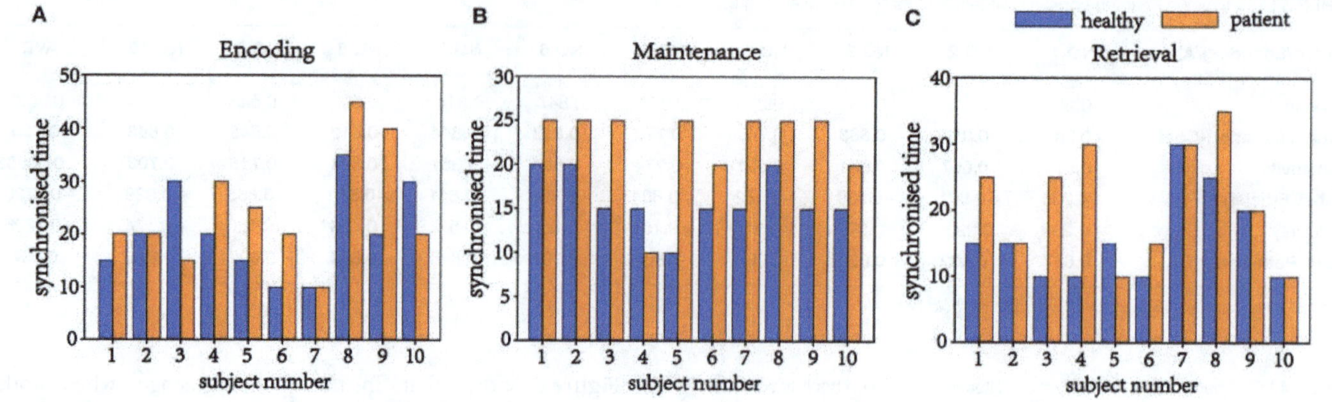

FIGURE 4 | Time of initial synchronization in the healthy controls and the patients. **(A)** is the encoding stage, **(B)** is the maintenance stage, and **(C)** is the retrieval stage.

TABLE 5 | Time to initial synchronization in patients and healthy controls.

Subject	Stage/band (alpha)	Average value (ms)	Standard deviation (ms)
Patients	Encoding	27	9.798
	Maintenance	26.5	10.259
	Retrieval	22	7.810
Normal	Encoding	18	6.782
	Maintenance	21	5.385
	Retrieval	15.5	6.874

This section proposes a method based on the fusion of traditional features and spectral features to achieve the adjustment of the patient's brain network synchronization ability, so that its synchronization ability would be consistent with normal subjects, theoretically achieving the purpose of treatment of diseases. Applying the T&S coupling formula defined in section Defining the Coupling Formula **L***, the patient's brain network synchronization ability could be adjusted by selecting appropriate values of the T&S coupling matrix **L*** parameters aa or bb. The feasibility and validity of the method were verified by specific data.

Coupling Matrix L^*Parameter Selection

The experiment investigated the patients' brain networks. Based on the results of the Pearson correlation coefficient calculation in section Experiment1:Brain-Network Significant Difference Features and Node Extraction, the clustering coefficient of the matrix G and the mean path length were used to adjust the brain's synchronization ability. **Figure 8** shows the change in the synchronization ability of the patient's brain network when the matrix G takes the clustering coefficient; **Figure 9** shows the synchronization stability of the brain network when the matrix G takes the path length. The abscissa indicates the value of the parameter bb, and the ordinate indicates the corresponding brain network synchronization feature value. The parameters chosen in the experiment were arbitrary and have no practical meaning. Other values could also be selected.

Adjustment-A

Figure 8A shows the result when the parameters aa and bb are both positive; 8b shows the result when parameter aa is negative and bb is positive; 8c shows the result when the parameters aa and bb are both negative.

In **Figure 8A**, when the parameters aa and bb are positive numbers, the results are as follows: When parameter bb is fixed, the network synchronization capability is proportional to the value of parameter aa; when parameter aa is constant, the synchronization capability of the network has an anti-proportional relationship to the value of parameter bb.

In **Figure 8B**, when parameter aa is negative and bb is positive, the network synchronization capability changes are more complex. When parameter aa < -1.5, the trend of the network synchronization capability is exactly the same as that in graph c. When the parameter aa> -1.5, the synchronization trend of the network is exactly the same as that in graph a.

In **Figure 8C**, when the parameters aa and bb are both negative numbers, the results are as follows: When parameter bb is fixed, the network synchronization ability is inversely proportional to the value of parameter aa. When parameter aa is constant, the network synchronization ability increases with parameter bb and then decreases, and the network synchronization ability gradually changes to become consistent with the original synchronization capabilities.

Adjustment-B

Figure 9A shows the results when the parameters aa and bb are both positive; 9b shows the results when parameter aa is negative and bb is positive; 9c shows the results when parameters aa and bb are both negative.

In **Figure 9A**, when the parameters aa and bb are both positive, the results are as follows: When parameter bb is fixed, the network synchronization capability is directly proportional to the value of parameter aa; when parameter aa is fixed, the synchronization capability of the network is directly proportional

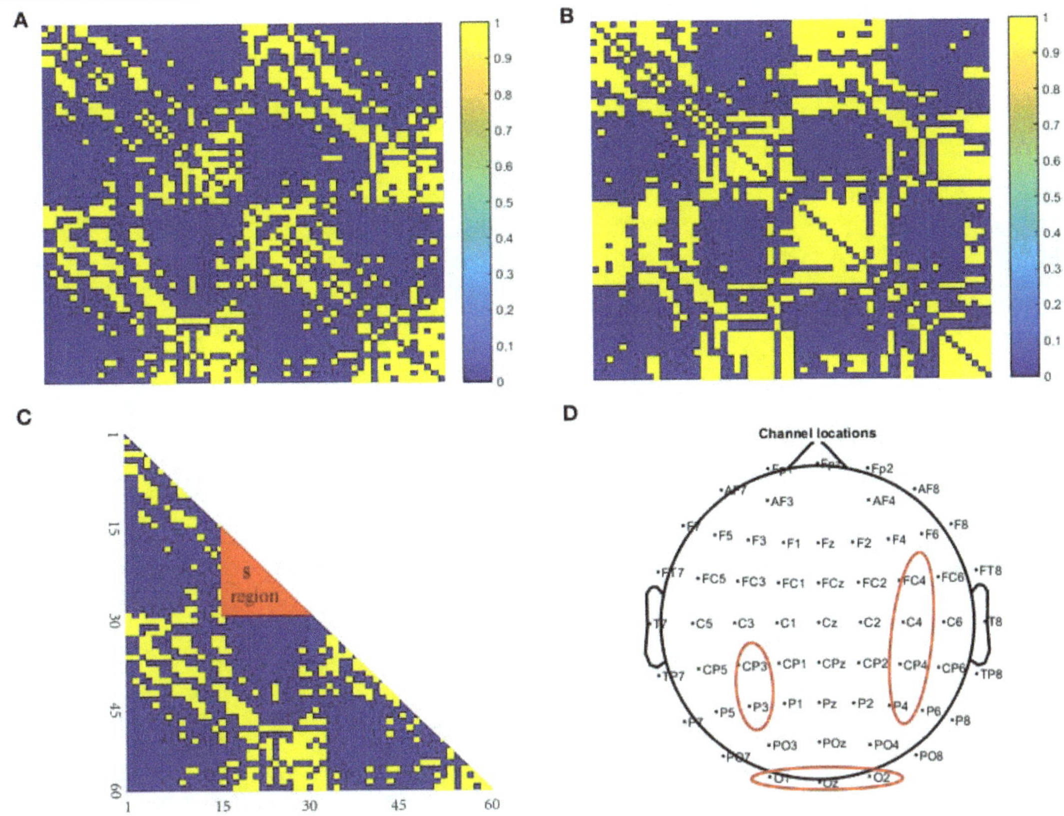

FIGURE 5 | Brain network structure. **(A)** is a binary matrix constructed using the healthy controls; **(B)** is a binary matrix constructed using the patient subjects; **(C)** is the difference significant area S, a mathematical representation of **(A,B,D)** is a brain electrode position diagram corresponding to a **(C)** S region in the brain map.

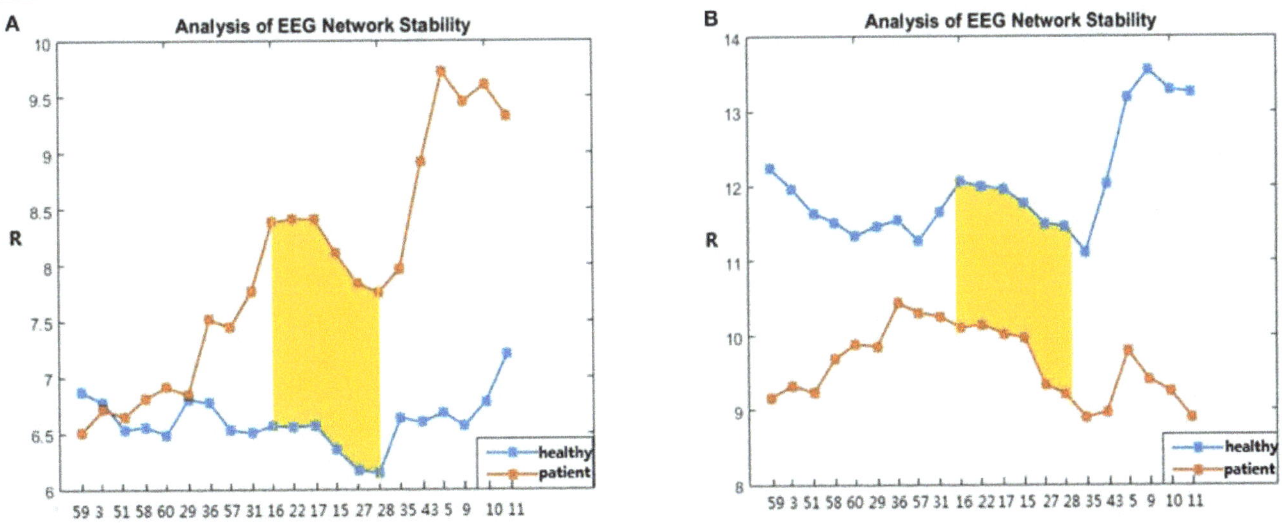

FIGURE 6 | R-value changes with the coupling of the S area in patients and healthy controls. The patient subject graphed here was #6 and the healthy control subject was #4 in **(A)**, and the patient subject graphed in **(B)** was #4 and the healthy control subject was #6.

to the value of parameter bb. This shows that, when the coupling matrix selects the path length as the "weighted" mode, the network synchronization capability is proportional to the values of the parameters aa and bb.

In **Figure 9B**, when parameter aa is negative and bb is positive, the results are as follows: When parameter bb is fixed, the network synchronization capability is directly proportional to the value of parameter aa; when parameter aa is fixed,

TABLE 6 | EEG signal 64 electrode name numbering table.

Ele-No.	EN	Ele-No.	EN	Ele-No.	EN	Ele-No.	EN	Ele-No.	EN
1	Fp1	14	FT8	27	O2	40	F2	53	CP6
2	F7	15	FC4	28	O1	41	FC1	54	PO8
3	Fp2	16	Cz	29	Pz	42	C5	55	P6
4	F3	17	CPz	30	Oz	43	FC6	56	CP2
5	FC3	18	CP3	31	Fpz	44	FC2	57	PO4
6	FT7	19	P3	32	AF3	45	C2	58	P2
7	T7	20	P7	33	AF7	46	C1	59	POz
8	F8	21	T8	34	F5	47	CP1	60	P1
9	F4	22	TP8	35	AF8	48	CP5	61	VEOU
10	Fz	23	C4	36	AF4	49	P5	62	VEOL
11	FCz	24	P8	37	F1	50	C6	63	HEOL
12	C3	25	CP4	38	FC5	51	PO3	64	HEOR
13	TP7	26	P4	39	F6	52	PO7		

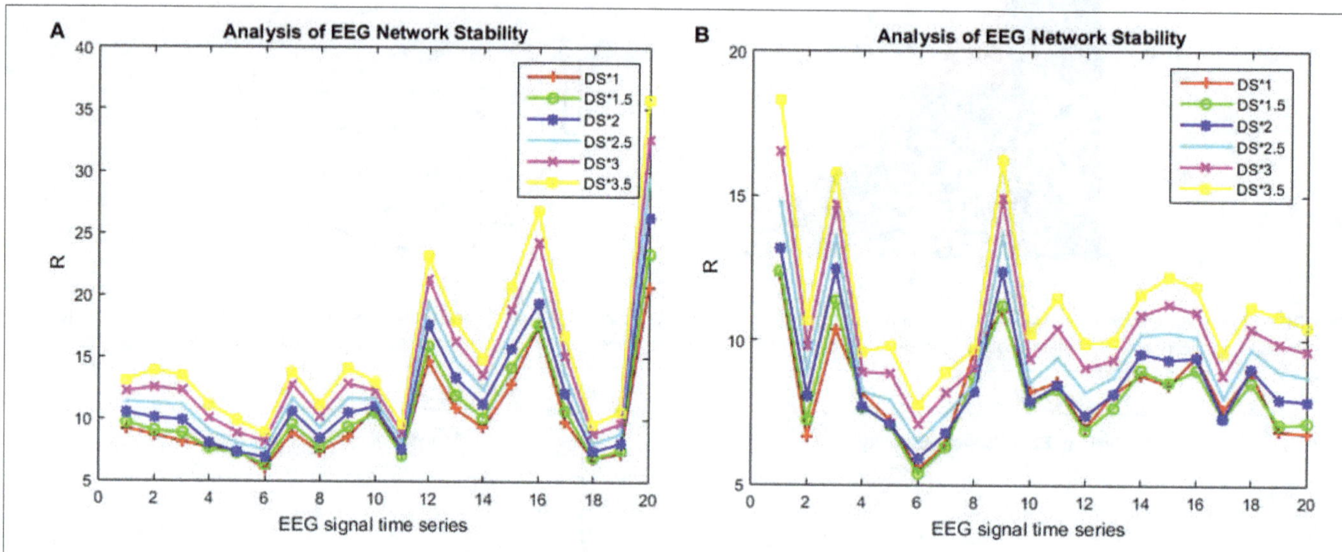

FIGURE 7 | *R*-value changes with the strength of the S area in patients and healthy controls. The patient subject graphed here was #6 in **(A)** and the healthy control subject was #4 in **(B)**.

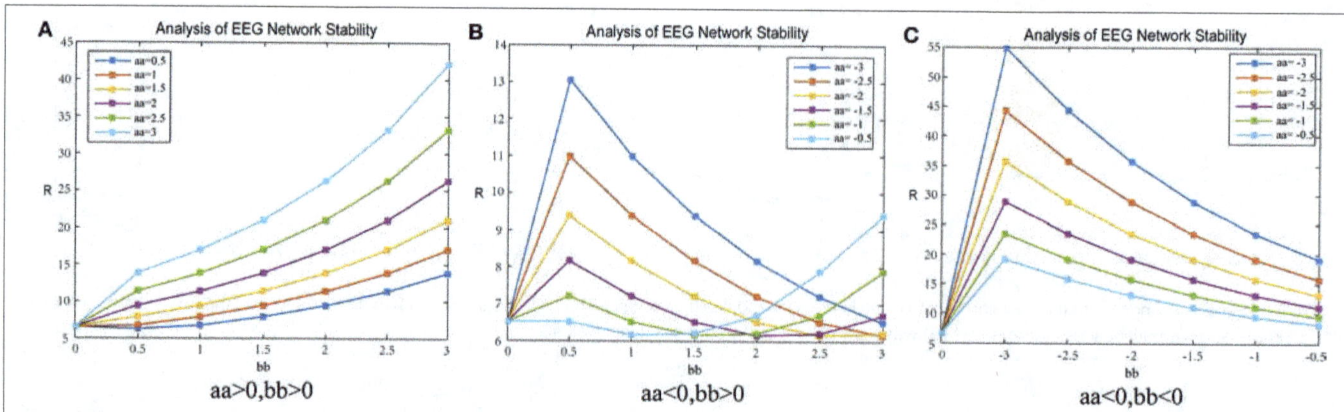

FIGURE 8 | *R*-value changes in a patient subject. Matrix G represents mean-clustering-coef and the data are from patient #6. **(A)** shows the parameters aa, bb are positive. **(B)** shows the parameter aa is negative, bb is positive. **(C)** shows the parameter aa, bb are negative.

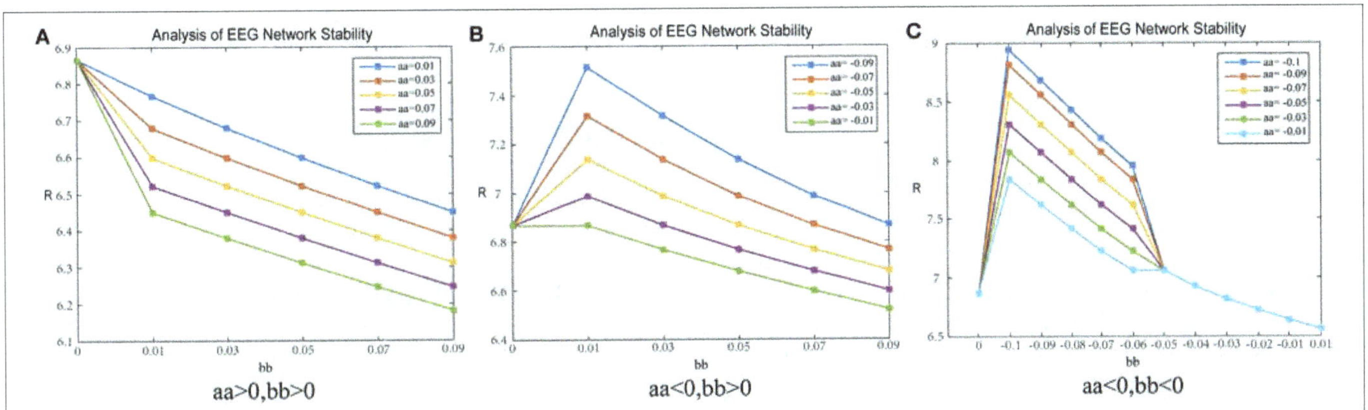

FIGURE 9 | *R*-value changes in a healthy subject. Matrix G represents mean-path-length and the data are from patient #6. **(A)** shows the parameters aa, bb are positive. **(B)** shows the parameter aa is negative, bb is positive. **(C)** shows the parameter aa, bb are negative.

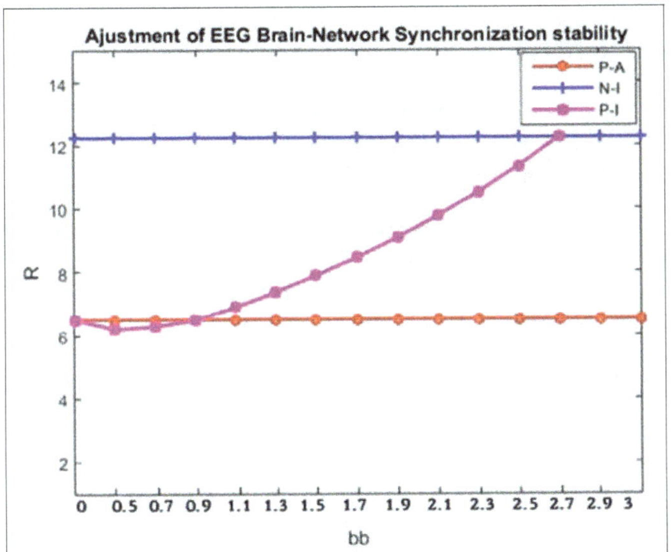

FIGURE 10 | Adjustment of patient's brain- network synchronization ability. The data are from patient #6 and healthy control subject number #4. The abscissa is the value of parameter bb, and the ordinate is the corresponding brain network synchronization feature value. P-A indicates the synchronization ability of the patient after the brain network adjustment; P-I indicates the synchronization ability of the patient before the brain network adjustment; N-I indicates normal synchronization ability.

the relationship between the synchronization capability of the network and the value of the parameter bb is first weakened and then enhanced to match the initial synchronization ability. After weakening, the enhancement tends to be consistent with the original synchronization ability.

In **Figure 9C**, when parameters aa and bb are negative, the network synchronization capability changes are more complex. When parameter bb is fixed and bb < -0.05, the synchronization capability of the network is proportional to the value of parameter aa; when parameter bb is fixed and bb > -0.05, the network synchronization capability is enhanced and does not change with parameter aa; when parameter aa is constant, the synchronization capability of the network decreases with an increase in parameter bb, and then the enhancement gradually changes to become stronger than the original synchronization capability.

Adjusting the Patient Synchronization Stability

Based on the conclusions in Coupling Matrix L ^* Parameter Selection, the best values of parameters aa and bb could be selected to be applied to the patient, so that the synchronization ability of the brain network of a patient and the brain synchronization ability of a normal person would tend to be consistent. Next, the clinician would refer to the equivalent of **Figure 8A** to identify the parameter transformation and would select aa $= 0.5$. The patient's brain network synchronization ability would finally be adjusted using parameter bb (**Figure 10**). In **Figure 10**, it can be seen that when aa $= 0.5$ and bb $= 2.5$, the patient's synchronization ability should be consistent with that of a normal person. In this way, the goal of curing disease can theoretically be achieved.

LIMITATIONS

The current study involved several limitations that should be considered. First, the effect of offline processing of EEG traces on brain network dynamics synchronization was not considered, so it is unclear how the synchronization differences obtained in an offline analysis of the EEG can pave a way for the treatment of unspecified neuropsychiatric diseases. In addition, EEG signals recorded from the scalp surface are generally highly correlated. Each channel is a linear mixture of concurrently active brain and non-brain electrical sources, whose activities are volume conducted to the scalp electrodes with broadly overlapping patterns (Nunez et al., 1997). Therefore, we used surface Laplacian transform methods to eliminate the mixed effect of volume conduction (Makeig et al., 1996; Jung et al., 2001; Delorme et al., 2012). Also, our study did not provide specific values for the parameters aa and bb, so the values of aa and bb were arbitrarily chosen. The purpose was only to verify the validity of the T&S coupling formula proposed in this study. As for its application in clinical trials, it may be necessary to correlate the aa and bb parameters with certain biological characteristics of the human body (such as blood flow). Consequently, we should pay more attention to these aspects and add related experiments in future research.

CONCLUSION

In this study, a brain network was constructed based on complex network theory. The synchronization characteristics of the brain network were calculated using the spectral features of the brain network. The synchronization process characterizes the differences and changes in the brain network synchronization ability between a patient and healthy subjects during the process of making memories. Our experiments showed that the synchronization of aa differed significantly between the patients and the healthy controls and that this synchronization is concentrated in the S region. In addition, these experiments further indicated that the effect of S on the synchronization ability in this S region was that the density of the S region was smaller, and the synchronization ability was stronger. To achieve the purpose of treating patients, we proposed a method based on the fusion of traditional features and spectral features to achieve the adjustment of a patient's brain network synchronization ability. The KS test, SVM classification, and other methods were used to extract traditional features and nodes that showed significant differences; we designed a T&S coupling method that fuses traditional features with spectral features and selects the appropriate parameter values aa or bb to adjust the patient's brain network synchronization capabilities. The data validated the feasibility of the method and theoretically achieved the purpose of treating disease. This study has only theoretically explored the treatment of disease through algorithms and has not been clinically applied. In the future, we will try to explore animal (rat) susceptibility factors, clinical manifestations, skull characteristics, and prognosis in depth, and we hope to find feasible measures (such as physical therapy) that can adjust these features.

ETHICS STATEMENT

All subjects were given written informed consent in accordance with the Declaration of Helsinki.

AUTHOR CONTRIBUTIONS

RY performed the experiment and completed the manuscript. XX, GY, HD, and PY provided suggestions for this study. HL provided the guidance throughout the study. HL had full access to all of the data in the study and takes responsibility for its integrity and the accuracy of the data analysis. All the authors have read through the manuscript, approved it for publication, and declared no conflict of interest.

FUNDING

This study Natural Science Foundation of China (61472270, 61873178, and 61876124) and the Natural Science Foundation of Shanxi (201801D121135). The sponsors had no role in the design or execution of the study, the collection, management, analysis, and interpretation of the data, or the preparation, review, and approval of the manuscript. This manuscript has not been published or presented elsewhere in part or in entirety and is not under consideration by any another journal.

ACKNOWLEDGMENTS

The authors also thank Rhoda E. Perozzi Ph.D. for linguistic assistance during the preparation of this manuscript and thank the reviewers for helpful comments.

REFERENCES

Babloyantz, A., Salazar, J. M., and Nicolis, C. (1986). Evidence of chaotic dynamics of brain activity during the sleep cycle. *Phys. Lett. A.* 111, 152–156. doi: 10.1016/0375-9601(85)90444-X

Bartolomei, F., Bosma, I., Klein, M., Baayen, J. C., Reijneveld, J. C., Postma, T. J., et al. (2010). How do brain tumors alter functional connectivity? A magnetoencephalography study. *Digest World Core Med. J.* 59, 128–138. doi: 10.1002/ana.20710

Bola, M., Gall, C., and Sabel, B. A., (2015). Disturbed temporal dynamics of brain synchronization in vision loss. *Cortex* 67, 134–146. doi: 10.1016/j.cortex.2015.03.020

De Han, W., Pijnenburg, Y. A., and Strijers, R. L. (2009). Functional neural network analysis in fronto temporal dementia and Alzheimer's disease using EEG and graph theory. *BMC Neuro sci.* 10:101. doi: 10.1186/1471-2202-10-101

Delorme, A., Palmer, J., Onton, J., Oostenveld, R., and Makeig, S., (2012). Independent EEG sources are dipolar. *PLoS ONE* 7:e30135. doi: 10.1371/ journal.pone.0030

Dong, Z. Q., Hou, F. Z., Dai, J. F., and Liu, X. F. (2014). An improved synchronous algorithm based on Kendall for analyzing epileptic brain network. *Acta Phys. Sinica. Chin. Ed.* 63, 208705–208705. doi: 10.7498/aps.63.208705

Eliasmith, C., Stewart, T. C., Choo, X., Bekolay, T., DeWolf, T., Tang, Y., et al. (2012). A large-scale model of the functioning brain. *Science* 338, 1202–1205. doi: 10.1126/science.1225266

Feng-Zhen, H., Jia-Fei, D., Xin-Feng, L., and Xiao-Lin, H. (2014). Phase synchrony in the cerebral infarction electroencephalogram based on the degree of network-links. *Acta Phys. Sinica.* 63, 257–264. doi: 10.7498/aps.63.040506

Gao, X., Cao, H., Ming, D., Qi, H., Wang, X., Wang, X., et al. (2014a). Analysis of EEG activity in response to binaural beats with different frequencies. *Int. J. Psychophysiol.* 94, 399–406. doi: 10.1016/j.ijpsycho.2014.10.010

Gao, X., Huang, J., Liu, S., Li, Y., Li, H., Li, L. et al. (2014b). Research on mechanisms of low temperature for blocking excessive synchronization discharge *in vitro* epilepsy model. *Chongqing Med.* 43, 2319–2322. doi: 10.3969/j.issn.1671-8348.2014.18.020

Guevara, R., Velazquez, J. L., Nenadovic, V., Wennberg, R., Senjanovic, G., and Dominguez, L. G. (2005). Phase synchronization measurements using electroencephalographic recordings: what can we really say about neuronal synchrony?[J]. *Neuroinformatics* 3, 301–313. doi: 10.1385/NI:3:4:301

Guo, H., Cao, X., and Liu, Z. (2013). Machine learning classifier using abnormal brain network topological metrics in major depressive disorder. *Neuroreport* 24, 51–51. doi: 10.1097/WNR.0b013e32835ca23a

Gysels, E., and Celka, P. (2004). Phase synchronization for the recognition of mental tasks in a brain-computer interface. *IEEE Trans. Neural Syst. Rehabil. Eng. A Public. IEEE Eng. Med. Biol. Soc.* 12:406. doi: 10.1109/TNSRE.2004.838443

Hao, G. (2013). *Analysis and Classification of Abnormal Topological Properties of Resting Brain Function Network in Depression.* Taiyuan University of Technology, Taiyuan, Shanxi.

Hongli, L. I., Jiang, W., Bin, D., and Xile, W. (2013). Analysis of mutual information and synchronism for epileptic EEG signals. *J. Comput. Eng. Appl.* 49, 19–192. doi: 10.3778/j.issn.1002-8331.1205-0234

Hongyue, Z., Suogang, W., and Shuping, T. (2017). Study on functional brain network of schizophrenia p50 sensory gating based on granger causality. *Space Med. Med. Eng.* 30, 203–207. doi: 10.16289/j.cnki.1002-0837.2017.03.009

Hutt, A. (2010). Oscillatory activity in excitable neural systems. *Contemp. Phys.* 51, 3–16. doi: 10.1080/00107510903293710

Jiaqing, L. I., Haifang, L. I., Yifan, B., Guimei, Y., and Liting, S. (2018). Research on recognizing and removing ocular artifact automatically from EEG signals. *Comput. Eng. Appl.* 54, 148–152. doi: 10.3778/j.issn.1002-8331.1702-0267

Jin-Hu, L. (2010). Synchronization of complex networks and consensus of complex multi-agent systems. *Complex Syst. Complex. Sci.* 57, 50–52. doi: 10.3969/j.issn.1672-3813.2010.02.013

Joyce, C. A., Gorodnitsky, I. F., and Kutas, M. (2010). Automatic removal of eye movement and blink artifacts from EEG data using blind component separation. *Psychophysiology* 41, 313–325. doi: 10.1111/j.1469-8986.2003.00141.x

Jung, T. P., Makeig, S., McKeown, M. J., Bell, A. J., Lee, T. W., and Sejnowski, T. J., (2001). Imaging brain dynamics using independent component analysis. *Proc. IEEE* 89, 1107–1122. doi: 10.1109/5.939827

Kashtan, N., and Alon, U. (2005). Spontaneous evolution of modularity and network motifs. *Proc. Natl. Acad. Sci. U.S.A.* 102, 13773–13778. doi: 10.1073/pnas.0503610102

Kayser, J., and Tenke, C. E. (2006a). Principal components analysis of Laplacian waveforms as a generic method for identifying ERP generator patterns: I. Evaluation with auditory oddball tasks. *Clin. Neurophysiol.* 117, 348–368. doi: 10.1016/j.clinph.2005.08.034

Kayser, J., and Tenke, C. E. (2006b). Principal components analysis of Laplacian waveforms as a generic method for identifying ERP generator patterns: II. Adequacy of low-density estimates. *Clin. Neurophysiol.* 117, 369–380. doi: 10.1016/j.clinph.2005.08.033

Li, J. S., and Zhang, X. D. (1997). A new upper bound for eigenvalues of the Laplacian matrix of a graph[J]. *Linear Algebr. Appl.* 265, 93–100. doi: 10.1016/S0024-3795(96)00592-7

Liley, D. T., Cadusch, P. J., and Dafilis, M. P. (2002). A spatially continuous mean field theory of electrocortical activity. *Network* 13, 67–113. doi: 10.1080/net.13.1.67.113

Liting, S., Guimei, Y., Shuping, T., Yanli, Z., Jinguo, Z., Dong, L., et al. (2017). Properties analysis of working memory EEG functional network in schizophrenia. *Comput. Eng. Appl.* 53, 25–30. doi: 10.3778/j.issn.1002-8331.1703-0114

Liu, Y., Liang, M., Zhou, Y., He, Y., Hao, Y., Song, M., et al. (2008). Disrupted small-world networks in schizophrenia. *Brain* 131, 945–961. doi: 10.1093/brain/awn018

Liu, Y., and Shen, J. (2017). Some results on the sum of the normalized Laplacian eigenvalues of graphs. *Adv. Math.* 46, 848–856. doi: 10.3969/j.issn.1000-5641.2010.01.003

Liu, Y., Yu, C., Zhang, X., Liu, J., Duan, Y., Alexander-Bloch, A. F., et al. (2014). Impaired long distance functional connectivity and weighted network architecture in Alzheimer's disease. *Cerebral Cortex.* 24, 1422–1435. doi: 10.1093/cercor/bhs410

Lü, J., and Guanrong, C. (2005). A time-varying complex dynamical network model and its controlled synchronization criteria. *IEEE Trans. Autom. Control* 50, 841–846. doi: 10.1109/TAC.2005.849233

Ma, C. C., Liu, A. J., Liu, A. H., Zhou, X. Y., and Zhou, S. N. (2014). Electroencephalogram global field synchronization analysis: a new method for assessing the progress of cognitive decline in Alzheimer's disease. *Clin. Eeg. Neurosci.* 45, 98–103. doi: 10.1177/1550059413489669

Makeig, S., Bell, A. J., Jung, T.-P., and Sejnowski, T. J. (1996). Independent component analysis of electroencephalographic data. Adv. *Neural Inform. Process. Syst.* 8, 145–151

Manoach, D. S., Press, D. Z., Thangaraj, V., Searl, M. M., Goff, D. C., Halpern, E., et al. (1999). Schizophrenic subjects activate dorsolateral prefrontal cortex during a working memory task, as measured by fMRI. *Biol. Psychiatry* 45:1128–1137. doi: 10.1016/S0006-3223(98)00318-7

Micheloyannis, S., Pachou, E., Stam, C. J., Vourkas, M., Erimaki, S., and Tsirka, V. (2006). Using graph theoretical analysis of multi channel EEG to evaluate the neural efficiency hypothesis. *Neurosci. Lett.* 402, 273–277. doi: 10.1016/j.neulet.2006.04.006

Müller, V., Sänger, J., and Lindenberger, U. (2018). Hyperbrain network properties of guitarists playing in quartet. *Ann. N. Y. Acad. Sci.* 1423, 198–210. doi: 10.1111/nyas.13656

Nunez, P. L., Srinivasan, R., Westdorp, A. F., Wijesinghe, R. S., Tucker, D. M., Silberstein, R. B., et al. (1997). EEG coherency: I: statistics, reference electrode, volumeconduction,Laplacians,corticalimaging,andinterpretationatmultiple scales. *Electroencephalogr. Clin. Neurophysiol.* 103, 499–515. doi: 10.1016/S0013-4694(97)00066-7

Pecora, L. M., and Carroll, T. L. (1990). Synchronization in chaotic systems. *Phys. Rev. Lett.* 64, 821–824. doi: 10.1103/PhysRevLett.64.821

Peraza, L. R., Asghar, A. U., Green, G., and Halliday, D. M. (2012). Volume conduction effects in brain network inference from electroencephalographic recordings using phase lag index[J]. *J. Neurosci. Methods* 207, 189–199. doi: 10.1016/j.jneumeth.2012.04.007

Qun, Z. (2009). On the study methods of electroencephalograph synchronization. *J. Biomed. Eng.* 26, 1353–1357. doi: 10.3321/j.issn:1001-5515.2009.06.040

Rosário, R. S., Cardoso, P. T., Muñoz, M. A., Montoya, P., and Miranda, J. G. V. (2015). Motif-Synchronization: A new method for analysis of dynamic brain networks with EEG. *Phys. A Stat. Mech. Appl.* 439, 7–19. doi: 10.1016/j.physa.2015.07.018

Ruizhen, Z., Yinan, T., Yuhan, S., Huanhuan, Z., and Mengya, W. (2017). Apparent receptor dynamics analysis of hippocampal excitatory synaptic transmission in rats and its application. *J. Gannan Med. College* 36, 103–106. doi: 10.3969/j.issn.1002-0217.2017.02.001

Sakkalis, V., Oikonomou, T., and Tsiaras, V. (2013). Graph-theoretic indices of evaluating brain network synchronization: application in an alcoholism paradigm. *Neuromethods* 91, 159–169. doi: 10.1007/7657_2013_62

Sato, H., and Iwai, T. (2014). Optimization algorithms on the Grassmann manifold with application to matrix eigenvalue problems. *Jpn. J. Ind. Appl. Math.* 31, 355–400. doi: 10.1007/s13160-014-0141-9

Skidmore, F., Korenkevych, D., Liu, Y., He, G., Bullmore, E., and Pardalos, P. M. (2011). Connectivity brain networks based on wavelet correlation analysis in Parkinson fMRI data. *Neurosci. Lett.* 499, 47–51 doi: 10.1016/j.neulet.2011.05.030

Stam, C. J., Jones, B. F., Nolte, G., Breakspear, M., and Scheltens, P. (2007). Small-world networks and functional connectivity in Alzheimer's disease. *Cerebral Cortex.* 17, 92–99. doi: 10.1093/cercor/bhj127

Sun, Y., Dai, Z., Li, J., Collinson, S. L., and Sim, K. (2009). Connectome alterations in schizophrenia. *Neuroimage* 47, S157–S157. doi: 10.1016/S1053-8119(09)71653-2

Wigand, M., Kubicki, M., Clemm von Hohenberg, C., Leicht, G., Karch, S., Eckbo, R., et al.. (2015). Auditory verbal hallucinations and the interhemispheric auditory pathway in chronic schizophrenia. *World J. Biol. Psychiatry* 16, 31–44. doi: 10.3109/15622975.2014.948063

Xiao, C. (2012). *Research on Quasi-Laplace Matrix Eigenvalues of Graphs.* University of Electronic Science and Technology, Chengdu, Sichuan.

Xu, B., Fu, Y., Shi, G., Yin, X., Wang, Z., Li, H., et al. (2014). Enhanced performance by time-frequency-phase feature for EEG-based BCI systems. *Sci. World J.* 2014:420561. doi: 10.1155/2014/420561

Yi, W., Qiu, S., Wang, K., Qi, H., Zhang, L., Zhou, P., et al. (2014). Evaluation of EEG Oscillatory patterns and cognitive process during simple and compound limb motor imagery. *PLoS ONE* 9:e114853. doi: 10.1371/journal.pone.0114853

Yuchi, L. I., Haifang, L. I., Dan, J., Guimei, Y., and Keyou, H. (2017). Phase synchronization analysis of emotional EEG based on complex network theory. *Comput. Eng. Appl.* 53, 230–235. doi: 10.3778/j.issn.1002-8331.1604-0007

Zhang, Y., Guo, D., Cheng, K., Yao, D., and Xu, P. (2015). The graph theoretical analysis of the ssvep harmonic response networks. *Cogn. Neurodyn.* 9, 305–315. doi: 10.1007/s11571-015-9327-3

Zhang, Y., Xu, P., Guo, D., and Yao, D. (2013b). Prediction of ssvep-based bci performance by the resting-state eeg network. *J. Neural Eng.* 10:066017. doi: 10.1088/1741-2560/10/6/066017

Zhang, Y., Xu, P., Huang, Y., Cheng, K., and Yao, D. (2013a). Ssvep response is related to functional brain network topology entrained by the flickering stimulus. *PLoS ONE* 8:e72654. doi: 10.1371/journal.pone.0072654

Zhao, L., Wang, B., and Yao, D. (2008). Research on analytical methods of phase synchronization in EEG. *Sheng Wu Yi Xue Gong Cheng Xue Za Zhi.* 25, 250–254. doi: 10.3321/j.issn:1001-5515.2008.02.005

Zhao, Y. L., Tan, S. P., Yang, F. D., Wang, L. L., Feng, W. F., Chan, R. C., et al. (2011). Dysfunction in different phases of working memory in schizophrenia: evidence from ERP recordings. *Schizophrenia Res.* 133, 112–119. doi: 10.1016/j.schres.2011.09.017

Zhou, T., Zhang, Z.-K., Chen, G.-R., Wang, X.-F., Shi, D.-H., Di, Z.-R., et al. (2014). The opportunities and challenges of complex networks research. *J. Univ. Electron. Sci. Technol. China.* 43, 1–5. doi: 10.3969/j.issn.1001-0548.2014.01.001

11

Age-Related Changes in Neuromodulatory Control of Bladder Micturition Contractions Originating in the Skin

Harumi Hotta, Harue Suzuki, Kaori Iimura and Nobuhiro Watanabe*

Department of Autonomic Neuroscience, Tokyo Metropolitan Institute of Gerontology, Tokyo, Japan

***Correspondence:**
Harumi Hotta
hhotta@tmig.or.jp

The brainstem is essential for producing micturition contractions of the urinary bladder. Afferent input from perineal skin evoked by gentle mechanical stimulation inhibits micturition contractions by decreasing both ascending and descending transmissions between the brainstem and spinal cord. Dysfunction of this inhibitory mechanism may be one cause of the increase in the prevalence of overactive bladder in old age. The aim of this study was to examine effect of aging on function of skin afferent fibers that inhibit bladder micturition contractions in rats. We used anesthetized male rats in three different age groups: young adult (4–5 months old), middle aged (6–9 months old), and aged (27–30 months old). The bladder was expanded to produce isovolumetric rhythmic micturition contractions. Skin afferent fibers were activated for 1 min either by electrical stimulation (0.5 ms, 0.2–10 V, 0.1–10 Hz) of the cutaneous branch of the pudendal nerve (CBPN) or by gentle mechanical skin stimulation with an elastomer roller. When skin afferent nerves were activated electrically, micturition contractions were inhibited in a similar manner in all age groups, with long latency inhibition induced by excitation of Aβ fibers and short latency inhibition by additional Aδ and C fiber excitation (at 1–10 Hz). On the contrary, when skin afferent nerves were activated mechanically by rolling, latency of inhibition following rolling stimulation was prolonged in aged rats. Single unitary afferent nerve activity of low-threshold mechanoreceptors (LTMs) from the cutaneous nerve was recorded. The discharge rate during rolling was not significantly reduced in Aβ units but was much lower in Aδ and C units in aged rats (0.4 and 0.5 Hz, respectively) than in young adult rats (3 and 7 Hz). These results suggest that the neural mechanism that inhibits bladder micturition contractions by skin afferent input is well maintained in old age, but the early inhibition by gentle skin stimulation is decreased because of reduced responses of Aδ- and C-LTMs.

Keywords: electrical stimulation, myelinated nerve fibers, unmyelinated nerve fibers, reflexes, urinary bladder, skin, mechanoreceptors, perineum

INTRODUCTION

The prevalence of lower urinary tract symptoms such as nocturia, urinary incontinence, and overactive bladder increases with older age (Homma et al., 2006; Irwin et al., 2006; Bosch and Weiss, 2010). Various age-related changes in bladder activity have been reported in humans and other animals. For example, a combination of detrusor overactivity with impaired contraction is seen in bladders in the elderly. In human bladder tissue, cholinergic bladder contractions decrease, while purinergic contractions increase with age (Yoshida et al., 2001). In rats, an increase in bladder volume, a reduced sensitivity of pelvic nerve afferents to bladder volume, and a reduced ability to raise bladder pressure in response to pelvic nerve efferent stimulation are associated with aging (Hotta et al., 1995). Pelvic nerve unmyelinated fibers with smaller diameters decrease in number in aged rats (Nakayama et al., 1998), and pelvic arterial insufficiency has been suggested to play an important role in the development of bladder dysfunctions in humans and other animals (Andersson et al., 2017). However, in addition to such peripheral factors, age-related changes in complex neuronal networks, including the spinal cord and brainstem, regulating bladder function might also be important. The micturition reflex is induced by positive feedback between the bladder and the pontine micturition center (PMC) in the brainstem and is facilitated or inhibited by various sensory inputs. Reduction in the inhibitory mechanism of the micturition reflex may contribute to susceptibility to overactive bladder due to aging. However, the age-related changes in the inhibitory mechanism of the micturition reflex remain to be determined.

In anesthetized adult animals, micturition contractions induced by bladder filling are inhibited by exciting somatic afferent nerves, either by electrical stimulation (Sato et al., 1980; Boggs et al., 2006; Tai et al., 2012; Ferroni et al., 2015) or with natural stimuli (Sato et al., 1975, 1977, 1992; Morrison et al., 1995; Budgell et al., 1998; Hotta et al., 2012). This is because the burst discharges of the pelvic nerve inducing bladder contractions are inhibited by somatosensory input (Sato et al., 1977, 1992, 1997; Hotta et al., 2012). We have recently reported the properties of somatic afferent nerves in the cutaneous branch of the pudendal nerve (CBPN) involved in the inhibition of bladder contraction. The excitation of Aβ fibers at 0.1–10 Hz for 1 min causes late inhibition, emerging several minutes after the end of stimulation, excitation of Aδ fibers at 1–10 Hz produced early inhibition, emerging immediately after stimulus onset, and excitation of C fibers at 1–10 Hz promoted both early and late inhibition (Onda et al., 2016). Similarly, gentle mechanical stimulation of the perineal skin surface with a roller that excites Aβ, Aδ, and C low-threshold mechanoreceptor (LTM) units to discharge at a rate of 2–8 Hz strongly inhibits micturition contraction (Hotta et al., 2012). Perineal rolling inhibits bladder contraction induced by electrical stimulation of the PMC or of the descending tract from the PMC and also inhibits afferent (ascending) transmission from the bladder to the PMC. Therefore, perineal rolling was suggested to shut down the positive feedback between the bladder and the PMC, resulting in inhibition of the micturition reflex (Hotta and Watanabe, 2015). It was shown by randomized clinical trial that perineal rolling reduces the nocturia associated with overactive bladder (Iimura et al., 2016). Such light stimulation to the skin may be applied spontaneously in daily life, and if this inhibitory mechanism is attenuated with age, it may be related to the cause of overactive bladder in the elderly.

The purpose of this study was to examine the effect of aging on the bladder micturition contraction inhibiting function of skin afferent nerve fibers. We employed anesthetized rats of three different age groups and compared the effect of perineal skin stimulation (gentle stimulation with a roller) on micturition contraction. We hypothesized that the inhibitory effect of mechanical skin stimulation is attenuated with age. For comparison, the effects of electrical stimulation of Aβ, Aδ, and C afferent nerve fibers in the skin were also examined. In the present study, age-related changes were observed following only mechanical skin stimulation, so we further examined the possibility of reduced responses of single unitary afferent Aβ-, Aδ-, and C-LTM fibers in the skin of the aged rats.

MATERIALS AND METHODS

The experiments were performed on 38 male Wistar or Fischer rats. There were no significant differences in their responses, so we combined all data from different strains. The animals were divided into three groups according to their different ages: (1) young adult (4–5 months old, $n = 15$, body weight 260–380 g), (2) middle aged (6–9 months old, $n = 10$, 360–410 g), and (3) aged (27–30 months old, $n = 13$, 330–435 g). The animals were bred at the Tokyo Metropolitan Institute of Gerontology (TMIG) and kept in a specific pathogen-free environment with free access to a commercial pelleted diet and filtered tap water with 2 ppm of chloride. This study was conducted in accordance with the Guidelines for Proper Conduct of Animal Experiments (established by the Science Council of Japan in 2006) and was approved by the animal care and use committee of TMIG. Basic preparation including anesthesia and artificial respiration, recordings of intravesical pressure of micturition contraction, skin stimulation with a roller, electrical stimulation and recordings of unit activity of cutaneous afferents were essentially the same as in our previous studies (Hotta et al., 2012; Onda et al., 2016).

General Surgery

The animals were anesthetized with urethane, after initial inhalation of 3% halothane or 3–4% isoflurane for 2–3 min. During the surgery, 0.3–1.0% halothane or isoflurane was additionally provided as required. An initial dose of urethane was given at 0.9–1.1 g/kg, subcutaneously (s.c.). Additional doses of 0.1–0.2 g/kg were administered intravenously (i.v.), if necessary, to maintain anesthesia at a relatively constant level as judged by the recorded blood pressure. The animals were artificially ventilated via a tracheal cannula to maintain the end-tidal CO_2 at 3.0–4.0%. Rectal temperature was maintained at 37–38°C by means of an automatically regulated heating pad and lamp (ATB-1100, Nihon Kohden, Tokyo). A jugular vein was catheterized for i.v. administration of supplemental anesthetics and other drugs. A common carotid artery was catheterized to record arterial blood pressure. Rats were euthanized by injecting an overdose of pentobarbital at the end of each experiment.

Recording of Intravesical Pressure

A laparotomy was performed, and a catheter was inserted into the bladder via the anterior urethra. The catheter was secured to the urethra by a thread, closing the urethral cavity. To measure intravesical pressure, the urethral catheter was connected to a transducer (TP-200T, Nihon Kohden, Tokyo) via a T-shaped connector. The other end of the T-shaped connector was connected to a syringe pump to manipulate bladder volume. The bladder was filled with saline at a speed of 0.1 ml/min by means of a syringe pump (EP-70, EICOM, Kyoto) connected to the bladder cannula. The saline infusion was stopped when micturition contractions (two or three consecutive contractions) were produced. Then, the micturition contractions continued rhythmically because the urethra had been closed to keep the bladder volume at a suitable range for the micturition reflex (Sato et al., 1992). The frequency of contractions was summarized as a time histogram of contractions counted every 2 min and expressed as contractions per min. Each contraction was counted as one contraction only when its amplitude was above one third of the prestimulus control size.

Cutaneous Stimulation

Gentle mechanical stimulation was applied to the skin of the perineum using a roller with a smooth, soft surface made of elastic polymer (Somaplane, Toyoresin Co., Shizuoka; 17 mm in diameter, 15 mm in length, weighing 4 g), as described previously (Hotta et al., 2012). The hair of the skin area to be stimulated was trimmed with a conventional clipper. The stimulus was applied to a skin area of about 3 cm^2 for a period of 1 min with a rolling speed of approximately 3 mm/s and a frequency of 10 strokes/min. Rolling was performed manually with a force (roller weight) of 4 g and was paced with an auditory cue.

Electrical Stimulation of Cutaneous Afferent Nerve

After cutting the skin of the lower back on the left side when in the prone position, the CBPN was separated and cut at greater than 20 mm caudal to the sacral plexus. The cavity was kept open by pulling back the edge of the cut skin with threads, and the cavity was filled with warm paraffin oil. The central cut segments of the nerve were placed on bipolar platinum-iridium wire stimulation electrodes, and repetitive rectangular pulses (0.5 ms) were delivered to the nerve. The evoked compound action potential of the CBPN was recorded 17–25 mm proximal from the stimulating site in some cases. During data collection, gallamine triethiodide (20 mg/kg, i.v.) was administered to avoid interference by skeletal muscle activity.

Recording of Unitary Afferent Nerve Activity from Perineal Skin

Single unitary afferent nerve activity was recorded from CBPN in five young adult rats and four aged rats. The CBPN was separated either in the prone position or the supine position and cut close to the sacral plexus. The peripheral cut segments of the nerve were placed on bipolar platinum-iridium wire recording electrodes. Action potentials of single units were amplified (MEG-2100, Nihon Kohden), audibly monitored through connection to a speaker, visually displayed on an oscilloscope (TS-8500, IWATSU, Tokyo), and digitized (Micro1401, Cambridge Electronic Design, UK) for later processing (Spike 2 software, Cambridge Electronic Design, UK). Receptive fields and mechanical thresholds of each unit were determined using 0.08–4.0 mN von Frey hairs (Touch-test sensory filaments, US Neurologicals). The conduction velocity of each single unit was measured to classify nerve fibers which had conduction velocities >15.6 m/s as Aβ fibers, fibers with conduction velocities between 2 and 15.6 m/s as Aδ fibers, and fibers with conduction velocities <2 m/s as C fibers, as described previously (Hotta et al., 2012).

Data Acquisition and Analysis

All analog signals obtained (including intravesical pressure and neuronal potentials) were digitized (Micro1401, Cambridge Electronic Design, UK) for display on a computer monitor and for on-line and off-line analysis using Spike 2 software (Cambridge Electronic Design). Statistical analysis was performed using Prism6 software (GraphPad Software Inc., La Jolla, CA, USA). Values were expressed as mean ± standard error (S.E.). One-way factorial analysis of variance (ANOVA) followed by the Fisher's least significant difference test was used for comparison of values among the three different age groups. The time course of changes in rhythmic micturition contractions induced by somatic stimulation was assessed using repeated measures two-way ANOVA (time and different age groups), followed by Dunnett's multiple comparison test. The properties of single afferent units in aged rats were compared with corresponding data from young adult rats using Student's *t*-test (unpaired). Statistical significance was set at the 5% level.

RESULTS

Baseline Bladder Conditions

Body weight and the basal state of bladder micturition contractions before application of any somatic stimuli were compared between the young adult, middle aged, and aged rat groups (**Table 1**). Body weight was significantly heavier in middle aged (391 ± 5 g; $p = 0.0002$) and aged (388 ± 11 g, $p = 0.0004$) groups than in the young adult group (332 ± 12 g). However, the bladder volume required to induce micturition contraction was significantly larger in the aged group (1.72 ± 0.30 ml; range 0.6–3.7 ml) than in the young adult (0.96 ± 0.13 ml; range 0.4–1.6 ml, $p = 0.0083$) and middle aged (1.12 ± 0.11 ml; range 0.5–1.6 ml, $p = 0.0342$) groups. Basal pressure, maximum pressure, amplitude, and frequency of micturition contractions did not differ significantly between the three groups. Systolic blood pressure, recorded simultaneously, ranged from 100 to 150 mmHg and did not significantly differ between the three groups.

TABLE 1 | Summary of body weight and baseline conditions of the bladders in young adult, middle-aged, and aged rats.

	Young adult (4–5 months old) $n = 11$	Middle aged (6–9 months old) $n = 10$	Aged (27–30 months old) $n = 9$
Body weight (g)	332 ± 12	391 ± 5**	388 ± 11**
Bladder volume (ml)	0.96 ± 0.13	1.12 ± 0.11	1.72 ± 0.30**,#
Basal pressure (mmH$_2$O)	116 ± 7	131 ± 14	137 ± 16
Maximum pressure (mmH$_2$O)	526 ± 47	475 ± 56	476 ± 25
Amplitude of contraction (mmH$_2$O)	410 ± 45	344 ± 50	339 ± 25
Frequency of contraction (times/min)	1.27 ± 0.18	0.85 ± 0.11	0.83 ± 0.08

*Values are mean ± SE; **p < 0.01 vs. young adult, #p < 0.05 vs. middle-aged rats, determined by Fisher's least significant difference tests.*

Inhibition of Micturition Contractions by Electrical Stimulation of Skin Afferent Nerves

By recording the strength–response curve of compound action potentials in the CBPN, we confirmed in young adult, middle aged, and aged rats that 0.2 V was suprathreshold for Aβ fibers but subthreshold for Aδ and C fibers, 1.0 V was suprathreshold for Aβ and Aδ fibers but subthreshold for C fibers, and 10 V was suprathreshold for all fibers. Electrical stimulation (pulse duration: 0.5 ms) was applied to the CBPN with these voltages at three different frequencies of 0.1, 1, and 10 Hz for 1 min, and changes in micturition contractions were examined in young adult (n = 5), middle aged (n = 4), and aged (n = 5) rats. The order of nine different stimulus parameters was randomized.

Figure 1 shows sample recordings in rats of different ages after application of 10-Hz electrical stimulation to CBPN afferents for 1 min with 1 V (**Figure 1A**) or 10 V (**Figure 1B**). With 1 V, micturition contractions completely stopped for 6–8 min and then recovered. With 10 V, micturition contractions completely stopped for >15 min. These responses were similar in all age groups. The time course of the effect of electrical stimulation of CBPN at three different voltage intensities (0.2, 1, and 10 V) and three different frequencies (0.1, 1, and 10 Hz) are summarized in **Figure 2**.

In all nine different stimulus parameters, effects of CBPN stimulation on contraction frequency were similar among different age groups (**Figure 2**). Two-way ANOVA revealed that the main effect of age was not statistically significant ($p > 0.19$) for all nine stimulus parameters. Interaction was also not significant ($p > 0.068$). However, there were significant time-dependent effects ($p < 0.019$) for eight of the stimulus parameters but not for stimulation at 0.1 Hz with 10-V intensity. Therefore, *post-hoc* tests were performed for the eight parameters on pooled data in all age groups of rats. With 0.2-V intensity at 0.1–10 Hz, the frequency of micturition contractions significantly decreased 7–11 min after the stimulus onset (late inhibition). With 1-V intensity at 1 Hz, the frequency of micturition contractions significantly decreased at 1–5 min (early inhibition) and throughout 1–11 min at 10 Hz (both early and late inhibition). With 10-V intensity at 1–10 Hz, contractions significantly decreased throughout 1–11 min; especially at 10 Hz, contractions were stopped completely in all except one case. Contractions recommenced 14–47 min later in all rat age groups.

Inhibition of Micturition Contractions by Gentle Mechanical Skin Stimulation

Figure 3 shows sample recordings from three rats in the different age groups, in which gentle mechanical stimulation was applied to the perineal skin with a roller for 1 min. Following stimulation, the frequency of micturition contractions decreased in all age groups. However, there was a difference in the time course of inhibition. The onset of inhibition following rolling stimulation of the skin was gradually delayed with age. In a typical case of a young adult rat (upper part of **Figure 3**), contractions stopped immediately during perineal stimulation and then recovered within 15 min. In a typical case of a middle-aged rat (**Figure 3** middle), the contractions continued for several min after stimulation ended and then stopped. In a typical example of an aged rat, the intercontraction interval was gradually increased after stimulation (lower part of **Figure 3**).

The time course of the effects of rolling stimulation is summarized from six rats for each group in **Figure 4**, as time histograms of contraction. A significant interaction ($p = 0.022$) was observed when the frequency of micturition contractions was compared between the three groups with two-way ANOVA. The main effect of time was also significant ($p < 0.0001$). However, the main effect of age was not significant ($p = 0.90$). Therefore, *post-hoc* multiple comparison tests of the effect of time were performed for each age group. The *post-hoc* analysis revealed that the time course differed in each group; the decrease in micturition contractions was significant from 1 to 7 and 11 min after stimulation in the young adult group and from 7 to 11 min in the middle-aged group but only at 11 min in the aged group (**Figure 4**).

The magnitude of the decrease of micturition contractions at 1 min (early inhibition) and 11 min (late inhibition) was expressed as a percentage of the prestimulus control level and compared among the three age groups (**Figure 5**). The magnitudes of early inhibition were −92% ± 8%, −42% ± 20%, and −8% ± 30% in the young adult, middle-aged, and aged rats, respectively (**Figure 5A**), gradually reducing with age ($p = 0.045$). The value in the aged rats was significantly lower than that in the young adult rats ($p = 0.015$). The value for the middle-aged rats was not significantly different between the other groups. In contrast, late inhibition (−79 ± 13%, −86 ± 9%, and −83 ± 11% in young adult, middle-aged, and aged rats, respectively) was not significantly different ($p = 0.90$) between the three age groups (**Figure 5B**). The responses in the aged

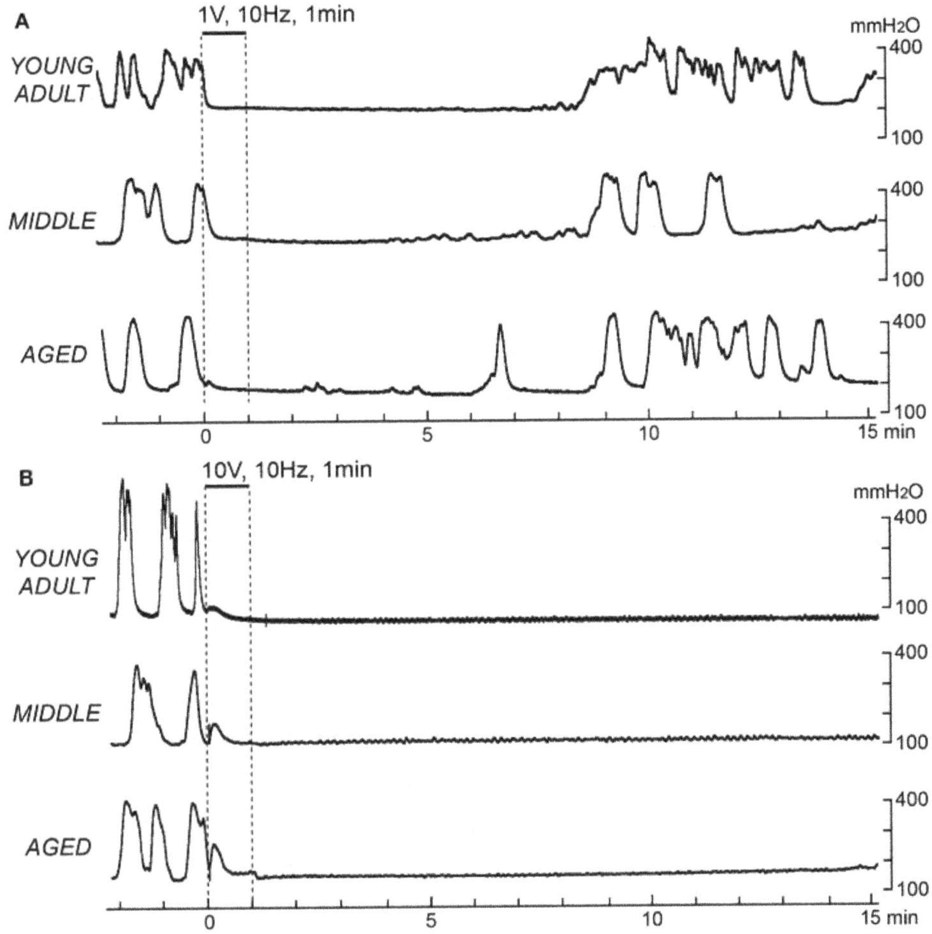

FIGURE 1 | Effects of electrical stimulation of cutaneous branch of the pudendal nerve afferents on rhythmic micturition contractions. Sample recordings in a young adult (upper), a middle-aged (middle), and an aged rat (lower) are shown. Stimulation for 1 min at 10 Hz with 1 V **(A)** and 10 V **(B)** is indicated by the upper horizontal bar and the vertical dashed lines, respectively.

group, in which late inhibition was predominant, were similar to those induced by selective excitation of Aβ afferents with 0.2-V electrical stimulation.

Response of Single Unitary Activity of Skin Afferent LTM Fibers

The above results showed that contraction inhibition by skin stimulation was delayed by aging although inhibition by electrical stimulation of CBPN afferents was well maintained. This suggests that the cause of the age-related changes in response to skin stimulation may be due to changes in the function of skin mechanoreceptors. Therefore, firing activity of skin afferent Aβ-, Aδ-, and C-LTM units in response to perineal rolling stimulation was examined in aged rats and compared with the results of young adult rats.

Figure 6 shows an example recording of single unitary afferent nerve activities of Aβ-, Aδ-, and C-LTM units in aged rats responsive to the perineal rolling stimulus. The conduction velocity of each unit was 16.1, 7.3, and 0.94 m/s, respectively. In each of these units, periodic activities synchronized with the movement of the rollers on the receptive field were observed. The average discharge frequency of Aβ, Aδ, and C fiber action potentials during stimulation for 60 s was 2.4, 1.5, and 0.5 Hz, respectively.

A total of 26 and 23 units were recorded in young adult and aged rats, including 12 and 9 units classified as Aβ fibers, 9 and 9 units classified as Aδ fibers, and 5 and 5 units classified as C fibers, respectively. In young adult and aged rats, the conduction velocities of Aβ fibers were 27.4 ± 1.6 m/s (with a range of 19.0–37.9 m/s) and 23.6 ± 1.6 m/s (16.1–30.0 m/s), Aδ fibers were 9.6 ± 1.1 m/s (5.5–15.3 m/s) and 8.6 ± 0.8 m/s (4.2–12.4 m/s), and C fibers were 0.90 ± 0.12 m/s (0.6–1.3 m/s) and 0.87 ± 0.17 m/s (0.43–1.35 m/s), respectively. All values in aged rats were equivalent to those in young adult rats.

The von Frey thresholds measured in 21 units from aged rats were within the range of 0.08–4 mN, which was the same as those in 24 units from young adult rats. However, in young adult rats, variations of the threshold in Aβ-, Aδ-, and C-LTM units were equal, whereas in the aged group, all C-LTM units responded to the lowest level of 0.08 mN stimulation.

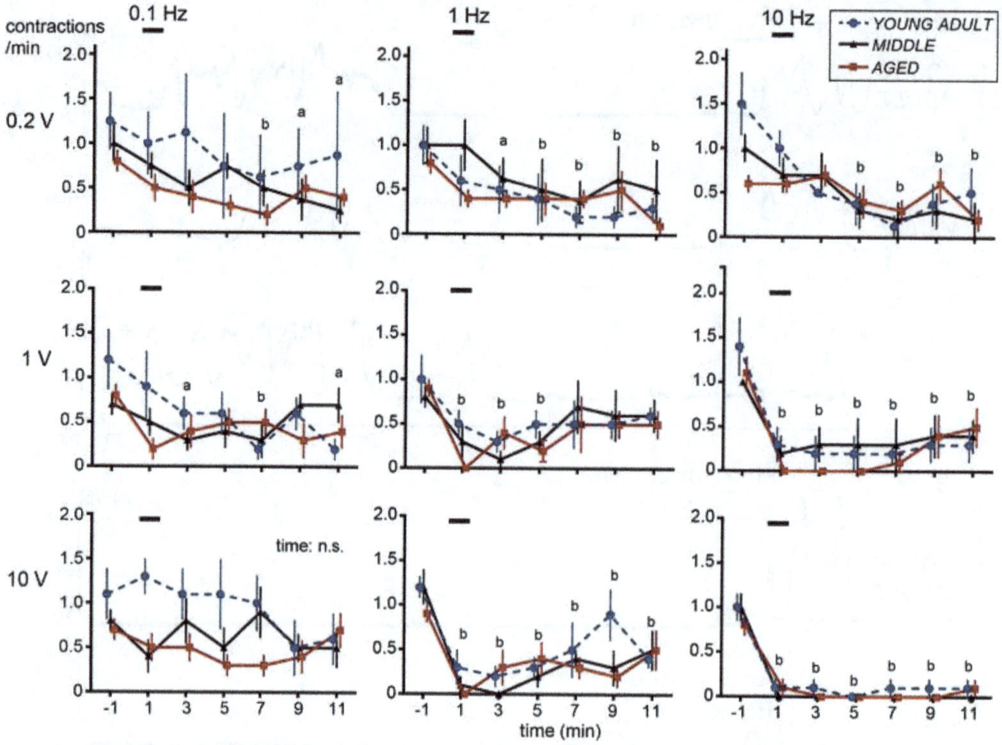

FIGURE 2 | Time histograms of micturition contractions after electrical stimulation of cutaneous branch of the pudendal nerve afferents compiled from five young adult rats (blue circles and dashed lines), four middle-aged rats (triangles and solid lines), and five aged rats (red squares and solid lines). Each rat was subjected to 1–2 trials. Each point represents mean ± SE (4–5 trials from 4–5 rats) for the number of contractions counted every 2 min, expressed as contractions per minute. Onset of stimulation was set as time zero; $^{a}p < 0.05$, $^{b}p < 0.01$, significant differences from prestimulus control values determined by Dunnett's multiple comparison test in pooled data from all three groups.

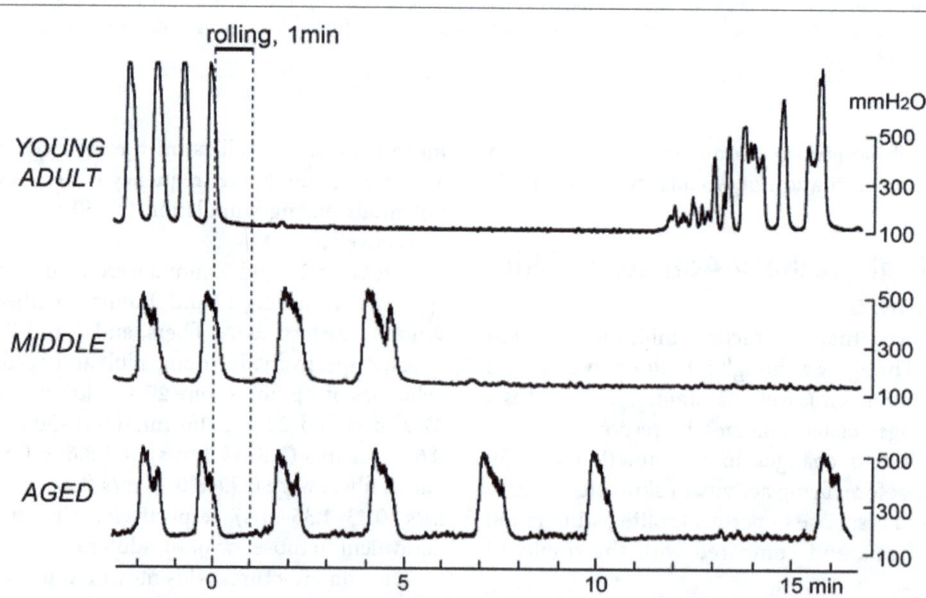

FIGURE 3 | Effects of gentle perineal skin stimulation by a roller on rhythmic micturition contractions. Sample recordings in a young adult **(upper)**, a middle-aged **(middle)**, and an aged **(lower)** rat are shown. Stimulation by perineal rolling for 1 min is indicated by the upper horizontal bar and vertical dashed lines.

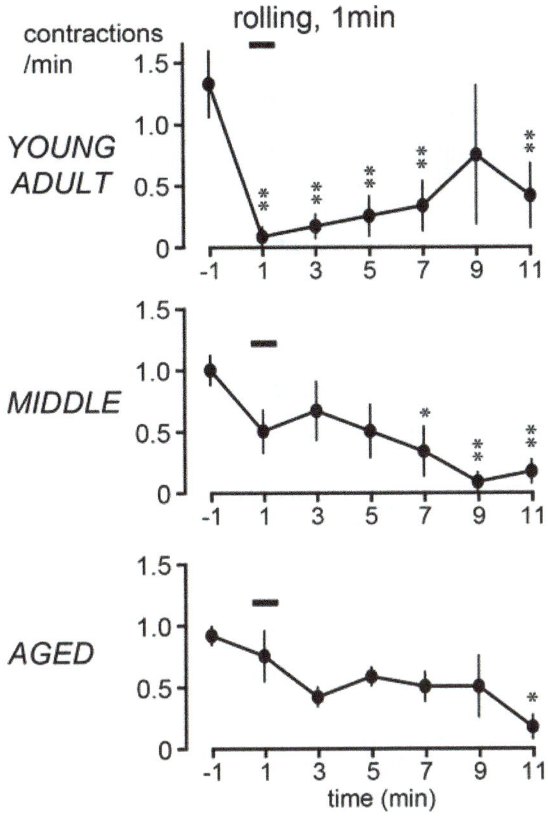

FIGURE 4 | Peristimulus time histograms of micturition contractions after perineal rolling stimulation, compiled from six rats each in young adult (upper), middle-aged (middle), and aged (lower) rats. Details of histogram are same as in **Figure 2**; *$p < 0.05$, **$p < 0.01$, significant differences from prestimulus control values determined by Dunnett's multiple comparison test.

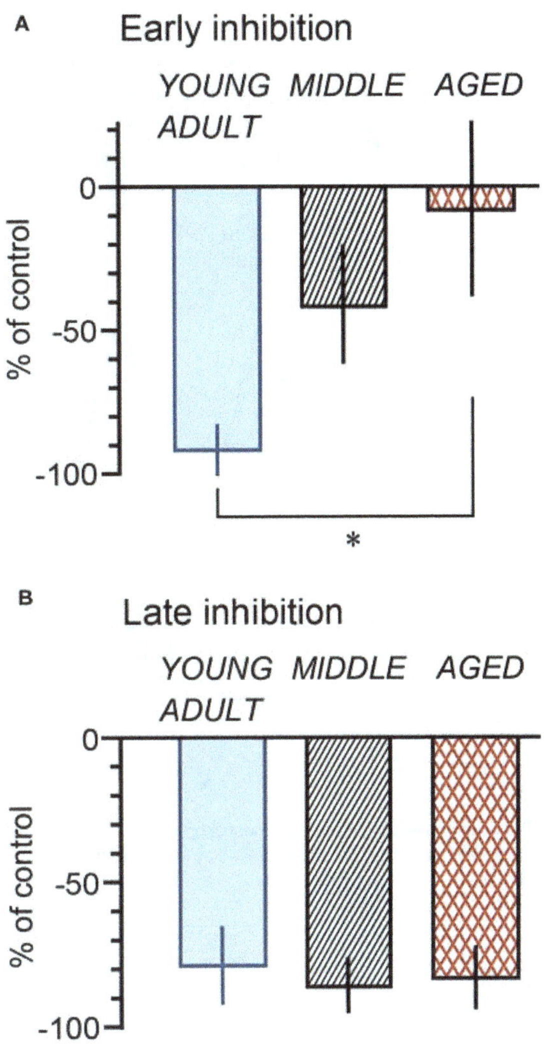

FIGURE 5 | Summary of magnitude of early (**A**: at 1 min) and late (**B**: at 11 min) inhibition by perineal rolling in young adult, middle-aged, and aged rats. Each column and vertical bar indicates the mean ± SE; *$p < 0.05$, significant differences determined by Fisher's least significant difference test.

In the young adult and aged rats, the mean discharge rates during cutaneous stimulation of the Aβ fibers were in the range of 0.03–11.2 (2.4 ± 0.9) Hz and 0.08–2.8 (1.1 ± 0.4) Hz, respectively (**Figure 7**), a slight but not significant ($p = 0.24$) reduction for the aged rats. However, the mean discharge rates during cutaneous stimulation of the Aδ fibers were 0.1–7.3 (2.9 ± 0.8) Hz and 0.02–1.5 (0.4 ± 0.2) Hz in the young adult and aged rats, respectively, showing significant reduction ($p = 0.0078$) in aged rats. Further, the mean discharge rates during cutaneous stimulation of the C fibers were 3.3–11.1 (7.3 ± 1.3) Hz in young adult rats, the highest among three fiber groups, but were much reduced to 0.1–1.1 (0.5 ± 0.2) Hz in aged rats ($p = 0.0007$; **Figure 7**).

DISCUSSION

In the present study, the inhibition of micturition contractions in response to gentle mechanical cutaneous stimulation delayed with age. The weaker bladder inhibition may be due to changes in the peripheral or central nervous system, bladder, or skin mechanoreceptors. However, inhibition in response to electrical stimulation of the skin afferent nerve was well maintained in aged rats and was similar to that in adult rats. Therefore, age-related functional changes in the peripheral or central nervous system or bladder do not appear to be involved in the changes in contraction inhibition. Moreover, the discharge rate of skin Aδ- and C-LTM afferent fibers during gentle mechanical stimulation was markedly reduced in aged rats compared to that in adult rats. These results suggest that age-related functional changes in skin mechanoreceptors, specifically in Aδ and C fibers that trigger early inhibition, are responsible for the delay of contraction inhibition.

Basal Condition of the Aged Bladder

The basal pressure, maximum pressure, amplitude, and frequency of micturition contractions were not significantly different between the young adult, middle-aged, and aged groups.

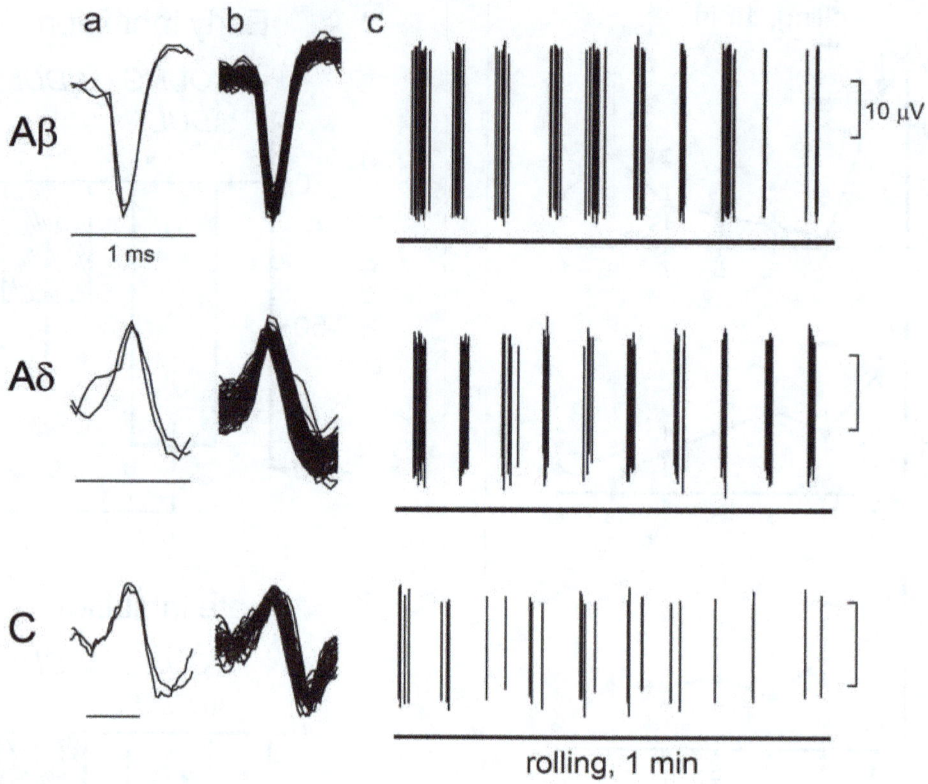

FIGURE 6 | Response of low-threshold mechanoreceptor (LTM) afferent nerve units during rolling. Examples of unitary afferent fiber recordings of Aβ-, Aδ- and C-LTM units in aged rats. **(a)** Action potentials evoked by electrical stimulation of the receptive field. **(b)** Superimposed action potentials recorded during manual rolling stimulation. **(c)** Responses of each unitary afferent fiber to rolling stimulation of the receptive field skin by a roller. A horizontal line indicates the period of rolling stimulation.

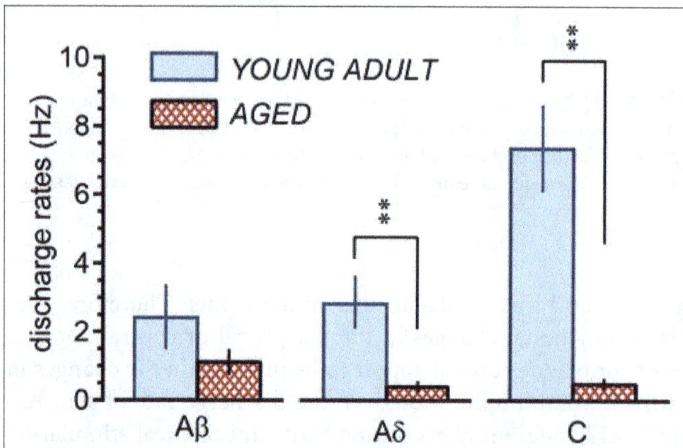

FIGURE 7 | Summary of discharge rates of low-threshold mechanoreceptor afferent nerve fibers during perineal rolling (1 min) in young adult and aged rats. Each column and vertical bar indicates the mean ± SE; $^{**}p < 0.01$, significant differences determined by Student's *t*-test.

However, the bladder volume inducing micturition contractions was about 70% larger in aged (27–30 months old) than in young adult (4–5 months old) and middle-aged (6–9 months old) rats. The results showing the increase in bladder capacity in aged rats are consistent with previous results comparing cystometrograms of young adult rats of 2–3 months old with aged rats of 26–29 months old. In that study, the volume at an intravesical pressure of 200 mmH_2O was 1.75 ± 0.26 ml in aged rats vs. 0.33 ± 0.05 ml in young-adult rats, and the cystometrograms were significantly shifted to the right in the aged rats (Hotta et al., 1995). Zhao et al. also reported that conscious, freely moving, old (28–30 months old) rats had increased bladder capacity, post-void residual volume, baseline, and intermicturition pressure but decreased micturition pressure compared with young (4–6 months old) rats. These changes were associated with decreased muscle mass and increased collagen deposition in the old bladder (Zhao et al., 2010). Recently, age-related increases in the collagen-smooth muscle ratio were also reported in old (85-week-old) mice using *ex vivo* two-photon laser scanning microscopy (Schueth et al., 2016).

Inhibition by Electrical Stimulation of Perineal Skin Afferents

The stimulation intensity and frequency dependence of inhibition of micturition contractions due to electrical stimulation in aged rats was essentially maintained as in younger adult rats. This result suggests that both the peripheral and central neural mechanisms involved in the somato-vesical inhibitory reflex are maintained in aged rats. Late inhibition was induced by activation of only Aβ fibers over a wide range of 0.1–10 Hz, but excitation of Aδ or C fibers at 1–10 Hz was required to induce early inhibition. These features are in accord with a previous study in adult rats (Onda et al., 2016). Complete inhibition by 10 V, 10-Hz stimulation was shown not to be affected by blocking capsaicin-sensitive C fibers in adult rats (Onda et al., 2016). The present results indicate that the mechanisms for late inhibition by excitation of Aβ fibers, early inhibition by additional excitation of Aδ fibers, and early and late inhibition by further excitation of C fibers, are all well-maintained during aging. Treatment of overactive bladder by electrical stimulation is used clinically, and many of the patients are elderly (Guo et al., 2014). The influence of age on the inhibition of micturition contractions induced by electrical stimulation has not previously been reported. Our results suggest that electrical stimulation therapy may be effective for the elderly, as for younger adults.

Inhibition by Gentle Stimulation of Perineal Skin

In contrast to the well-maintained inhibition of micturition contractions by electrical stimulation, inhibition by gentle mechanical skin stimulation changed with age. Although the inhibitory effect itself was maintained, the latency of inhibition was prolonged with age. The inhibition of micturition contractions following cutaneous rolling in the aged group was similar to that following electrical stimulation of only Aβ fibers. By recording the LTM unitary activity, the response of Aβ-LTM units during rolling was maintained in the aged group, but Aδ- and C-LTM unitary activity during rolling in aged rats was much lower than in adult rats. Mean discharge rates of Aδ- and C-LTM units in young adult rats were 3–7 Hz, whereas those in aged rats were 0.4–0.5 Hz. Therefore, considering that electrical stimulation of Aδ and C fibers at frequencies of 1–10 Hz was necessary for inducing early inhibition, lack of the early inhibition by skin stimulation in aged rats appears to be due to reduced responses of Aδ- and C-LTMs, and the late inhibition observed in aged rats appears to be caused by activity of Aβ-LTMs.

It has been shown in adult rats that rolling of the skin inhibits PMC neuronal activity induced by bladder distension and also inhibits bladder contraction by PMC stimulation (Hotta and Watanabe, 2015). The inhibitory effect on PMC activity may be delayed in aged rats, resulting in a delay of inhibition of micturition contractions. In humans, rolling stimulation, self-applied before bedtime for 1 min, has been shown to alleviate nocturia caused by overactive bladder in the elderly (Iimura et al., 2016). As a clinical effect of the rolling on nocturia, late inhibition rather than early inhibition would be important. However, the lack of rapid inhibition by gentle skin stimulation may be related to urge incontinence, which increases with age.

Age-Related Changes in Skin Mechanoreceptors

Tactile sensations involving Aβ fibers, such as sensing vibration, and the density of Pacinian corpuscles and Meissner bodies connecting to Aβ fibers decreases with age (reviews of Wickremaratchi and Llewelyn, 2006; Decorps et al., 2014). Although only one report has examined the function of single afferent Aβ units, there were no differences in the receptive field sizes and von Frey thresholds in the planter nerve of 6- and 24- to 27-month-old rats (Reinke and Dinse, 1996). Their result on hairless skin is consistent with our result on hairy skin. However, there have been no reports investigating age-related changes in single unitary activities of small diameter LTM fibers from the skin. Our study showed for the first time that the responses of Aδ- and C-LTM units are selectively decreased with age.

Aδ-LTMs and C-LTMs are abundantly present in the hairy skin of humans and animals (Adriaensen et al., 1983; Djouhri, 2016) and suggested to project to the limbic cortices (Olausson et al., 2002; Watanabe et al., 2013) but do not contribute to tactile sensation. This contrasts with Aβ fibers, which project to the neocortical primary somatosensory cortex and contribute to tactile sensation. Inhibition of the somato-cardiac sympathetic C-reflex by gentle touch (Hotta et al., 2010; Watanabe et al., 2012), mainly caused by activity of Aδ- and C-LTMs (Watanabe et al., 2015), was attenuated in aged rats (Watanabe et al., 2011). On the contrary, inhibition of adrenal sympathetic nerve activity by brushing, mainly caused by activity of Aβ- and Aδ-LTMs (Isa et al., 1985), was well maintained in the aged rats (Kurosawa et al., 1987). These different cutaneous effects of aging may be explained by our results showing the attenuated responses of Aδ- and C-LTMs and the well-maintained responses of Aβ-LTMs.

The frequency of discharges to mechanical stimuli and the size of the receptive fields of LTMs, including unmyelinated tactile afferents, generally depend on the strength of the indentation (Wessberg et al., 2003), and if the mechanical threshold is higher, the frequency of discharge in response to the same 4-g roller stimulus would lower. However, it is of note that for Aδ- and C-LTM units in aged rats, the von Frey threshold was not higher, but the response frequency during rolling was much lower than that in younger adult rats. This may be due to receptor-specific changes that evoke afferent volleys in Aδ- and C-LTMs, such as a decrease in the number and/or changes in the properties of fine Zigzag hairs in which Aδ- and C-LTMs are selectively distributed (Abraira and Ginty, 2013). It will be important to clarify the mechanisms of age-related changes in responses of Aδ- and C-LTMs in future studies.

CONCLUSION

In summary, we reported three important age-related results in response to gentle mechanical cutaneous and electrical stimulation: (1) inhibition of micturition contractions induced by gentle mechanical stimulation had a delayed onset, (2) discharge rate of Aδ and C-LTM skin afferent fibers was markedly reduced, and (3) inhibition of micturition contractions induced by electrical stimulation was well maintained during aging. Electrical stimulation can maintain the firing rate of the cutaneous afferent, which is different from mechanical rolling stimulation (**Table 2**). Therefore, we can conclude that the reduced firing rate in skin mechanoreceptors during mechanical stimulation is the cause of weak inhibition observed in aged rats study.

TABLE 2 | Summary of the present results.

Skin afferent fiber type	Electrical stimulation		Gentle mechanical stimulation	
	Afferent activity (Hz)	**Effect on bladder**	**Afferent activity (Hz)**	**Effect on bladder**
(A) YOUNG ADULT				
Aβ fiber	0.1–10	Late inhibition	2	Early and Late inhibition
Aδ fiber	1–10	Early inhibition	3	
C fiber	1–10	Early and Late inhibition	7	
(B) AGED				
Aβ fiber	0.1–10	Late inhibition	1	Late inhibition
Aδ fiber	1–10	Early inhibition	0.4	
C fiber	1–10	Early and Late inhibition	0.5	

The autonomic nerve itself is relatively resistant to aging (Hotta and Uchida, 2010), but the aging processes affecting tactile function begin from an early age (Verrillo, 1980; Giuseppe et al., 1994; Stevens and Patterson, 1995). This study showed for the first time the possibility that age-related changes in skin function may affect brainstem functions regulating visceral activities.

AUTHOR CONTRIBUTIONS

HH contributed to study design, data acquisition, data analysis, data interpretation and manuscript writing. HS contributed to data analysis, data interpretation and manuscript writing. KI contributed to data acquisition, data analysis and manuscript revising. NW contributed to study design, data interpretation and manuscript writing. All authors approved the final version of the manuscript and agreed to be accountable for all aspects of the work in ensuring that questions related to the accuracy or integrity of any part of the work are appropriately investigated and resolved.

FUNDING

The present study was supported by JPSP KAKENHI Grant Number JP17K01550.

REFERENCES

Abraira, V. E., and Ginty, D. D. (2013). The sensory neurons of touch. *Neuron* 79, 618–639. doi: 10.1016/j.neuron.2013.07.051

Adriaensen, H., Gybels, J., Handwerker, H. O., and Van Hees, J. (1983). Response properties of thin myelinated (A-delta) fibers in human skin nerves. *J. Neurophysiol.* 49, 111–122. doi: 10.1152/jn.1983.49.1.111

Andersson, K. E., Boedtkjer, D. B., and Forman, A. (2017). The link between vascular dysfunction, bladder ischemia, and aging bladder dysfunction. *Ther. Adv. Urol.* 9, 11–27. doi: 10.1177/1756287216675778

Boggs, J. W., Wenzel, B. J., Gustafson, K. J., and Grill, W. M. (2006). Frequency-dependent selection of reflexes by pudendal afferents in the cat. *J. Physiol.* 577, 115–126. doi: 10.1113/jphysiol.2006.111815

Bosch, J. L., and Weiss, J. P. (2010). The prevalence and causes of nocturia. *J. Urol.* 184, 440–446. doi: 10.1016/j.juro.2010.04.011

Budgell, B. S., Hotta, H., and Sato, A. (1998). Reflex responses of bladder motility after stimulation of interspinous tissues in the anesthetized rat. *J. Manipulative Physiol. Ther.* 21, 593–599.

Decorps, J., Saumet, J. L., Sommer, P., Sigaudo-Roussel, D., and Fromy, B. (2014). Effect of ageing on tactile transduction processes. *Ageing Res. Rev.* 13, 90–99. doi: 10.1016/j.arr.2013.12.003

Djouhri, L. (2016). Aδ-fiber low threshold mechanoreceptors innervating mammalian hairy skin: a review of their receptive, electrophysiological and cytochemical properties in relation to Aδ-fiber high threshold mechanoreceptors. *Neurosci. Biobehav. Rev.* 61, 225–238. doi: 10.1016/j.neubiorev.2015.12.009

Ferroni, M. C., Slater, R. C., Shen, B., Xiao, Z., Wang, J., Lee, A., et al. (2015). Role of the brain stem in tibial inhibition of the micturition reflex in cats. *Am. J. Physiol. Renal Physiol.* 309, F242–F250. doi: 10.1152/ajprenal.0013 5.2015

Giuseppe, R., Santo, D. S., Donato, F., Mariano, M., and Luciano, M. (1994). Comparison of tactile sensitivity in a group of elderly and young adults and children using a new instrument called a 'Tangoceptometer'. *Arch. Gerontol. Geriatr.* 18, 207–214. doi: 10.1016/0167-4943(94)90014-0

Guo, Z. F., Liu, Y., Hu, G. H., Liu, H., and Xu, Y. F. (2014). Transcutaneous electrical nerve stimulation in the treatment of patients with poststroke urinary incontinence. *Clin. Interv. Aging* 9, 851–856. doi: 10.2147/CIA.S61084

Homma, Y., Yamaguchi, O., Hayashi, K., and Neurogenic Bladder Society Committee (2006). Epidemiologic survey of lower urinary tract symptoms in Japan. *Urology* 68, 560–564. doi: 10.1016/j.urology.2006.03.035

Hotta, H., Masunaga, K., Miyazaki, S., Watanabe, N., and Kasuya, Y. (2012). A gentle mechanical skin stimulation technique for inhibition of micturition contractions of the urinary bladder. *Auton. Neurosci.* 167, 12–20. doi: 10.1016/j.autneu.2011.11.002

Hotta, H., Morrison, J. F., Sato, A., and Uchida, S. (1995). The effects of aging on the rat bladder and its innervation. *Jpn. J. Physiol.* 45, 823–836. doi: 10.2170/jjphysiol.45.823

Hotta, H., Schmidt, R. F., Uchida, S., and Watanabe, N. (2010). Gentle mechanical skin stimulation inhibits the somatocardiac sympathetic C-reflex elicited by excitation of unmyelinated C-afferent fibers. *Eur. J. Pain* 14, 806–813. doi: 10.1016/j.ejpain.2010.02.009

Hotta, H., and Uchida, S. (2010). Aging of the autonomic nervous system and possible improvements in autonomic activity using somatic afferent stimulation. *Geriatr. Gerontol. Int.* 10(Suppl. 1), S127–S136. doi: 10.1111/j.1447-0594.2010.00592.x

Hotta, H., and Watanabe, N. (2015). Gentle mechanical skin stimulation inhibits micturition contractions via the spinal opioidergic system and by decreasing both ascending and descending transmissions of the micturition reflex in the spinal cord. *PLoS ONE* 10:e0135185. doi: 10.1371/journal.pone.0135185

Iimura, K., Watanabe, N., Masunaga, K., Miyazaki, S., Hotta, H., Kim, H., et al. (2016). Effects of a gentle, self-administered stimulation of perineal skin for nocturia in elderly women: a randomized, placebo-controlled, double-blind crossover trial. *PLoS ONE* 11:e0151726. doi: 10.1371/journal.pone.0151726

Irwin, D. E., Milsom, I., Hunskaar, S., Reilly, K., Kopp, Z., Herschorn, S., et al. (2006). Population-based survey of urinary incontinence, overactive bladder, and other lower urinary tract symptoms in five countries: results of the EPIC study. *Eur. Urol.* 50, 1306–1315. doi: 10.1016/j.eururo.2006.09.019

Isa, T., Kurosawa, M., Sato, A., and Swenson, R. S. (1985). Reflex responses evoked in the adrenal sympathetic nerve to electrical stimulation of somatic afferent nerves in the rat. *Neurosci. Res.* 3, 130–144. doi: 10.1016/0168-0102(85)90026-4

Kurosawa, M., Sato, A., Sato, Y., and Suzuki, H. (1987). Undiminished reflex responses of adrenal sympathetic nerve activity to stimulation of baroreceptors and cutaneous mechanoreceptors in aged rats. *Neurosci. Lett.* 77, 193–198. doi: 10.1016/0304-3940(87)90585-4

Morrison, J. F., Sato, A., Sato, Y., and Yamanishi, T. (1995). The influence of afferent inputs from skin and viscera on the activity of the bladder and the skeletal muscle surrounding the urethra in the rat. *Neurosci. Res.* 23, 195–205. doi: 10.1016/0168-0102(95)00942-M

Nakayama, H., Noda, K., Hotta, H., Ohsawa, H., and Hosoya, Y. (1998). Effects of aging on numbers, sizes and conduction velocities of myelinated and unmyelinated fibers of the pelvic nerve in rats. *J. Auton. Nerv. Syst.* 69, 148–155. doi: 10.1016/S0165-1838(98)00013-7

Olausson, H., Lamarre, Y., Backlund, H., Morin, C., Wallin, B. G., Starck, G., et al. (2002). Unmyelinated tactile afferents signal touch and project to insular cortex. *Nat. Neurosci.* 5, 900–904. doi: 10.1038/nn896

Onda, A., Uchida, S., Suzuki, H., and Hotta, H. (2016). Stimulus frequency-dependent inhibition of micturition contractions of the urinary bladder by electrical stimulation of afferent Aβ, Aδ, and C fibers in cutaneous branches of the pudendal nerve. *J. Physiol. Sci.* 66, 491–496. doi: 10.1007/s12576-016-0468-x

Reinke, H., and Dinse, H. R. (1996). Functional characterization of cutaneous mechanoreceptor properties in aged rats. *Neurosci. Lett.* 216, 171–174. doi: 10.1016/0304-3940(96)13039-1

Sato, A., Sato, Y., and Schmidt, R. F. (1980). Reflex bladder activity induced by electrical stimulation of hind limb somatic afferents in the cat. *J. Auton. Nerv. Syst.* 1, 229–241. doi: 10.1016/0165-1838(80)90019-3

Sato, A., Sato, Y., and Schmidt, R. F. (1997). The impact of somatosensory input on autonomic functions. *Rev. Physiol. Biochem. Pharmacol.* 130, 1–328. doi: 10.1007/BFb0046598

Sato, A., Sato, Y., Shimada, F., and Torigata, Y. (1975). Changes in vesical function produced by cutaneous stimulation in rats. *Brain Res.* 94, 465–474. doi: 10.1016/0006-8993(75)90229-2

Sato, A., Sato, Y., Sugimoto, H., and Terui, N. (1977). Reflex changes in the urinary bladder after mechanical and thermal stimulation of the skin at various segmental levels in cats. *Neuroscience* 2, 111–117. doi: 10.1016/0306-4522(77)90072-0

Sato, A., Sato, Y., and Suzuki, A. (1992). Mechanism of the reflex inhibition of micturition contractions of the urinary bladder elicited by acupuncture-like stimulation in anesthetized rats. *Neurosci. Res.* 15, 189–198. doi: 10.1016/0168-0102(92)90004-V

Schueth,. A., Spronck, B., van Zandvoort, M. A., and van Koeveringe, G. A. (2016). Age-related changes in murine bladder structure and sensory innervation: a multiphoton microscopy quantitative analysis. *Age* 38:17. doi: 10.1007/s11357-016-9878-1

Stevens, J. C., and Patterson, M. Q. (1995). Dimensions of spatial acuity in the touch sense: changes over the life span. *Somatosens. Mot. Res.* 12, 29–47. doi: 10.3109/08990229509063140

Tai, C., Shen, B., Mally, A. D., Zhang, F., Zhao, S., Wang, J., et al. (2012). Inhibition of micturition reflex by activation of somatic afferents in posterior femoral cutaneous nerve. *J. Physiol.* 590, 4945–4955. doi: 10.1113/jphysiol.2012.239475

Verrillo, R. T. (1980). Age related changes in the sensitivity to vibration. *J. Gerontol.* 35, 185–193. doi: 10.1093/geronj/35.2.185

Watanabe, N., Ishii, K., Hotta, H., Oda, K., Sakata, M., Toyohara, J., et al. (2013). Differential human brain activity induced by two perceptually indistinguishable gentle cutaneous stimuli. *Neuroreport* 24, 425–430. doi: 10.1097/WNR.0b013e32836164d4

Watanabe, N., Miyazaki, S., Mukaino, Y., and Hotta, H. (2012). Effect of gentle cutaneous stimulation on heat-induced autonomic response and subjective pain intensity in healthy humans. *J. Physiol. Sci.* 62, 343–350. doi: 10.1007/s12576-012-0210-2

Watanabe, N., Piché, M., and Hotta, H. (2015). Types of skin afferent fibers and spinal opioid receptors that contribute to touch-induced inhibition of heart rate changes evoked by noxious cutaneous heat stimulation. *Mol. Pain* 11:4. doi: 10.1186/s12990-015-0001-x

Watanabe, N., Uchida, S., and Hotta, H. (2011). Age-related change in the effect of gentle mechanical cutaneous stimulation on the somato-cardiac sympathetic C-reflex. *J. Physiol. Sci.* 61, 287–291. doi: 10.1007/s12576-011-0146-y

Wessberg, J., Olausson, H., Fernström, K. W., and Vallbo, Å. B. (2003). Receptive field properties of unmyelinated tactile afferents in the human skin. *J. Neurophysiol.* 89, 1567–1575. doi: 10.1152/jn.00256.2002

Wickremaratchi, M. M., and Llewelyn, J. G. (2006). Effects of ageing on touch. *Postgrad. Med. J.* 82, 301–304. doi: 10.1136/pgmj.2005.039651

Yoshida, M., Homma, Y., Inadome, A., Yono, M., Seshita, H., Miyamoto, Y., et al. (2001). Age-related changes in cholinergic and purinergic neurotransmission in human isolated bladder smooth muscles. *Exp. Gerontol.* 36, 99–109. doi: 10.1016/S0531-5565(00)00175-3

Zhao, W., Aboushwareb, T., Turner, C., Mathis, C., Bennett, C., Sonntag, W. E., et al. (2010). Impaired bladder function in aging male rats. *J. Urol.* 184, 378–385. doi: 10.1016/j.juro.2010.03.004

12

Upregulation of AT_1 Receptor Mediates a Pressor Effect Through ROS-SAPK/JNK Signaling in Glutamatergic Neurons of Rostral Ventrolateral Medulla in Rats with Stress-Induced Hypertension

Liping Jiang[1†], Xuan Zhou[1†], Hongyu Yang[1], Ruijuan Guan[1], Yanlei Xin[1], Jijiang Wang[1], Linlin Shen[1], Danian Zhu[1], Shulan Ma[2] and Jin Wang[1*]*

[1] *Department of Physiology and Pathophysiology, School of Basic Medical Sciences, Fudan University, Shanghai, China,*
[2] *Training Center of Medical Experiments, School of Basic Medical Sciences, Fudan University, Shanghai, China*

***Correspondence:**
Shulan Ma
slma@fudan.edu.cn
Jin Wang
wangjin@shmu.edu.cn*

† These authors have contributed equally to this work

The present study examined whether angiotensin II (Ang II) mediates the pressor effect through nicotinamide adenine dinucleotide phosphate (NADPH) oxidase-derived reactive oxygen species (ROS)-mitogen-activated protein kinase (MAPK) signaling in the glutamatergic neurons of the rostral ventrolateral medulla (RVLM) in stress-induced hypertensive rats (SIHR). The SIHR model was established using electric foot-shocks combined with noises for 15 days. We observed that Ang II type 1 receptor (AT_1R) and the glutamatergic neurons co-localized in the RVLM of SIHR. Furthermore, glutamate levels in the intermediolateral column of the spinal cord were higher in SIHR than in controls. Microinjection of Ang II into the RVLM of SIHR activated stress-activated protein kinase/Jun N-terminal kinase (SAPK/JNK), extracellular signal-regulated protein kinase (ERK) 1/2, and p38MAPK. Compared with controls, the activation of SAPK/JNK, ERK1/2, p38MAPK, and ROS in the RVLM were higher in SIHR, an effect that was blocked by an NADPH oxidase inhibitor (apocynin) and an AT_1R antagonist (candesartan). RVLM microinjection of apocynin or a SAPK/JNK inhibitor (SP600125), but not an ERK1/2 inhibitor (U0126) or a p38MAPK inhibitor (SB203580), decreased AT_1R mRNA and mean arterial blood pressure (MABP) in SIHR. The increase of AT_1R protein expression and MABP was inhibited by intracerebroventricular infusion (ICV), for 14 days, of SP600125, but not U0126 or SB203580 in SIHR. We conclude that Ang II modulates the pressor effect through AT_1R-dependent ROS-SAPK/JNK signaling in glutamatergic neurons in the RVLM of SIHR.

Keywords: angiotensin II type 1 receptor, stress-induced hypertension, glutamatergic neurons, rostral ventrolateral medulla, NAPDH oxidase-ROS-SAPK/JNK signaling

---

Abbreviations: aCSF, artificial cerebrospinal fluid; Ang II, angiotensin II; AP-1, activator protein-1; APO, apocynin; AT_1R, angiotensin II type 1 receptors; BP, blood pressure; CAN, candesartan; FISH, fluorescence *in situ* hybridization; Glu, glutamate; HR, heart rate; ICV, intracerebroventricular; IML, intermediolateral column; MABP, mean arterial blood pressure; ROS, reactive oxygen species; RVLM, rostral ventrolateral medulla; SBP, systolic blood pressure; SHR, spontaneously hypertensive rats; SIH, stress-induced hypertension; SIHR, stress-induced hypertensive rats.

INTRODUCTION

Hypertension is a silent killer worldwide and an outcome of a convoluted interaction between genetic and environmental factors. The psychosocial stress caused by the fast-paced lifestyle of modern society, is an important risk factor for hypertension. Chronic stress leads to the generation of stress-induced hypertension (SIH) (Xia et al., 2008; Xiao et al., 2013; Zhang et al., 2013). Angiotensin II (Ang II) has important effects on the central modulation of cardiovascular activities. Ang II modulates sympathetic functions acting on a diverse range of receptors such as Ang II type 1 receptor (AT_1R) and type 2 receptor (AT_2R); the pressor effect of Ang II mainly results from the activation of AT_1R (Reja et al., 2006).

Oxidative stress is caused by the imbalance between free radicals and antioxidants—an essential factor in hypertension. It has been indicated that nicotinamide adenine dinucleotide phosphate (NADPH) oxidase-derived reactive oxygen species (ROS), particularly superoxide anions ($O_2^{\cdot -}$), are crucial intracellular messengers within Ang II signaling pathways (Hanna et al., 2002; Ushio-Fukai and Alexander, 2004). Ang II can upregulate mRNA and protein expression of NADPH oxidase subunits and augment production of ROS (Hausding et al., 2013; Wakui et al., 2013; Ding et al., 2015; Minas et al., 2015). In addition, ROS have been reported to participate in the modulation of sympathetic activities (Wang et al., 2002; Gao et al., 2004; Campese et al., 2005). NADPH oxidase-derived ROS act as essential intracellular messengers to activate downstream signaling molecules, including mitogen-activated protein kinase (MAPK) and transcriptional factors (Zhang et al., 2007; Bae et al., 2011; Lassegue et al., 2012). It is reported that Ang II activates stress-activated protein kinase/Jun N-terminal kinase (SAPK/JNK), extracellular signal-regulated protein kinase 1/2 (ERK1/2), and p38MAPK, which are critical protein kinases for gene expression and cell growth (Omura et al., 2005). A previous study demonstrated that chronic Ang II infusion elevated NADPH oxidase subunit protein expression, ROS production, as well as p38MAPK activation, leading to hypertension in Sprague Dawley rats (Bao et al., 2007).

The rostral ventrolateral medulla (RVLM) has an important impact on the maintenance of sympathetic activities. It is widely accepted that the neurons in the RVLM provide downward impulses to the sympathetic preganglionic neurons in the intermediolateral column (IML) of the spinal cord, which projects the sympathetic nerves that dominate the heart and blood vessels (Xiang et al., 2014). Our previous studies suggested that Ang II might activate glutamatergic neurons in the RVLM, resulting in the enhancement of blood pressure (BP) in Wistar and spontaneously hypertensive rats (SHR) (Hu et al., 2002). Moreover, AT1R, an angiotensin converting enzyme, mRNA and protein expression were significantly higher in the RVLM in stress-induced hypertensive rats (SIHR) compared with control rats (Du et al., 2013). It has been shown that the elevated glutamatergic inputs to the RVLM contribute to increased BP and sympathetic activities in Goldblatt hypertension (Carvalho et al., 2003) and spontaneous hypertension (Zha et al., 2013). However, the cellular and molecular mechanisms underlying the central roles of Ang II in SIHR remain to be identified. Therefore, this study evaluated the hypothesis that Ang II mediates pressor response through AT1R-dependent NADPH oxidase derived-ROS-MAPK signaling pathways in the glutamatergic neurons of the RVLM of SIHR.

MATERIALS AND METHODS

Animals

Adult male Sprague-Dawley rats (200–220 g) were randomly housed (5 per cage) at room temperature (22–27°C), on a 12/12 h light/dark schedule, and allowed free access to food and water. All experimental procedures were approved by the Animal Use and Care Committee of Shanghai Medical College, Fudan University and were performed in strict accordance with the guidelines of the National Institutes Health Guide for the Care and Use of Laboratory Animals.

Stress-Induced Hypertension Model

Rats were randomly allocated into normotension (control) and stressed-induced hypertension (SIH) groups. The SIH model was created as described in our previous studies (Xia et al., 2008; Xiao et al., 2013; Zhang et al., 2013). Briefly, the rats of SIH group were placed in a cage with a grid floor and received 2-h random electric foot-shocks paired with interval noise stimulation, twice daily, for 15 days. The control rats received the same treatment excluding the stressful stimuli. Systolic blood pressure (SBP) in conscious rats was measured using the tail-cuff method at 2 h after stress and obtaining the average of three measurements. The criterion for hypertension in this experiment was determined as an SBP greater than 140 mmHg. After the 15-day stimulation period, the rats in the SIH group with an SBP less than 140 mmHg were removed from the follow-up experiments.

MABP Measurements

After endotracheal intubation, the right carotid artery of each rat was cannulated to monitor BP continuously using a polygraph (Model SMUP-A, Department of Physiology and Pathophysiology, Shanghai Medical College of Fudan University, Shanghai, China). The heart rate (HR) was derived automatically from the BP phasic wave. During the experiment, the rectal temperature of rats was kept at 37 ± 0.5°C using a thermostat.

RVLM Microinjections

Similar to the procedures reported previously (Xiao et al., 2013), the rats were anesthetized with urethane/α-chloralose (urethane 0.75 g/kg; α-chloralose 70 mg/kg) intraperitoneally, and the bilaterally microinjection of test agents to the RVLM was performed with a micropipette (40–70 μm internal diameter) attached to a 0.5 μl microsyringe (Hamilton). The RVLM was located 0.8 mm from the first anterior branch of the hypoglossal nerve, 1.9 mm lateral, and 0.7 mm deeper toward the ventral surface. As a routine, a total volume of 50 nl was delivered to each side of the RVLM over 30 s to allow for complete diffusion of the test agents. The RVLM injection was verified by the presence of a transient pressor response (MABP greater than 15 mmHg) to an L-glutamate (2 nmol/50 nl) microinjection (Ross et al., 1984). Ang II, AT_1R antagonist candesartan, and NADPH oxidase inhibitor apocynin, were purchased from Sigma-Aldrich (St. Louis, MO, United States). The SAPK inhibitor SP600125, ERK1/2 inhibitor U0126, and p38MAPK inhibitor SB203580 were obtained from Sigma-Aldrich (St. Louis, MO, United States). Artificial cerebrospinal fluid (aCSF) or 1% dimethyl sulphoxide (the solvent of SP600125, U0126, or SB203580) was used as a vehicle control. To avoid the confounding effects of drug interactions, each animal received only one pharmacological treatment. After the experiments, 50 nl of pontamine sky blue was injected through the micropipette to confirm the position (rostroventrolateral reticular nucleus, lateral paragigantocellular nucleus).

Fluorescence *in situ* Hybridization (FISH)

The staining procedure was performed with an enhanced sensitive FISH detection kit (Servicebio, China). Six-micron cryosections were prepared ahead of time. We applied proteinase K (20 μg/ml) on the slice for 5 min to expose the nucleic acid and then washed the slides three times with 0.5M PBS. Following incubation with hybridization buffer at 37°C for 2 h, the slides were incubated with 50 μl of 8 ng/ul 5′,3′ double CY3-labeled RNA (VGLUT2 mRNA) detection probe and 5′,3′ double FAM-labeled RNA (AT_1R mRNA) detection probe (TSINGKE, China) in the same buffer at 37°C overnight. After the samples were washed with different concentrations of SSC buffers. After three 5 min washes in PBS for the last time, the slides were detected under a Nikon Ni-U microscope (Nikon, Japan) and pictures were collected.

Intracerebroventricular (ICV) Infusion

Anesthetized rats were fixed in a stereotaxic apparatus (NeruoStar, United States). After the bregma was identified, an ICV cannula was implanted for the infusion of the inhibitors, as described previously (Dange et al., 2014). Once the anterior fontanel was identified, an ICV cannula was implanted into the right lateral cerebral ventricle 0.8 mm caudal to bregma, 1.5 mm lateral to the bregma, and 3.8 mm ventral to the zero level (Pan et al., 2007). The cannula was fixed to the cranium using dental acrylic and two stainless steel screws. The pump body was implanted subcutaneously. The rats underwent a 14-day ICV infusion of the SAPK/JNK inhibitor (SP600125), ERK1/2 inhibitor (U0126), p38MAPK inhibitor (SB203580) (0.5 μl/hr, 0.6 mmol/L), NADPH oxidase inhibitor APO (0.5 μl/hr, 0.45 mmol/L) (Fang et al., 2013), or aCSF via osmotic micro-pumps (Alzet, Cupertino, CA, United States). The position of the cannula in the lateral cerebral ventricle was confirmed by the staining of all four ventricles after injection of 5 μl of evans blue dye at the end of the experiments.

Intermediolateral Column (IML) Microdialysis

After making an incision in the back to expose the T8 level of the thoracic segment and then removing the bone and meningeal membrane to expose the spinal cord surface, the microdialysis probe was inserted into the T8 spinal cord 0.45 mm lateral to the midline and 0.9 mm below the dorsal surface. The tip of the probe was in the IML. The probe was perfused (2 μl/min) with aCSF using a microdialysis pump (BASi, United States). Each dialysate sample was harvested for 10 min at a volume of 20 μl.

High-Performance Liquid Chromatography (HPLC)

Amino acids of dialysate samples were separated using reverse-phase HPLC (Waters 1525, United States) and fluorescence detection (Waters 2475, United States) with a reverse-phase column (C18, ultrasphere octadecyl silane). The derivatized reagent consisted of 5 ml of absolute ethanol, 5 ml of 0.1 mol/L sodium tetraborate, 27 mg of orthophthaldialdehyde (Sigma-Aldrich, St. Louis, MO, United States), and 40 μl of β-mercaptoethanol (Sigma-Aldrich, St. Louis, MO, United States). The sample (20 μl) was mixed with the derivatized reagent (10 μl) for 90 s and then injected into the HPLC system. The mobile phase, which contained 63% 0.1 mol/L KH_2PO4, 35% methanol, and 2% tetrahydrofuran, flowed through the system with a flow rate of 1.0 ml/min. The temperature of the column was 35°C. The excitation and emission wave lengths were 330 and 450 nm, respectively. For each sample, the analysis time was not more than 10 min.

Collection of Tissue Samples From the RVLM

On the 15th day, or after microinjections, rats were euthanized and their brains were removed and frozen on dry ice. Both sides of the ventrolateral medulla covering the RVLM (0.5–2.5 mm rostral to the obex and 1.4–2.4 mm lateral to the midline and medial to the spinal trigeminal tract) were dissected using a stainless steel micropunch (1 mm internal diameter) (Chan et al., 2007). Medullary tissues were stored at −80°C prior to protein analysis.

Western Blot Analysis

The samples of brain tissues were homogenized in RIPA lysis buffer with protease or phosphatase inhibitor (Roche, Basel, Switzerland) and then centrifuged (12000 rpm, 15 min, 4°C) to obtain supernatants. The total protein concentration of the supernatants was determined using the BCA assay kit (Pierce). Samples were loaded and separated on the SDS–PAGE gel (40 μg per well). The protein was transferred to the PVDF membrane (Millipore, MA, United States), which was incubated overnight with primary antibodies at 4°C and then probed with the corresponding secondary antibody. The primary antibodies were as follows: rabbit anti-AT_1R antibody (1:800 dilution, Abcam, MA, United States) (Czikora et al., 2015; Wang et al., 2018), rabbit anti-SAPK/JNK antibody, mouse anti-phospho-SAPK/JNK antibody, mouse anti-ERK1/2 antibody, rabbit anti-phospho-ERK1/2 antibody, rabbit anti-p38MAPK antibody, rabbit anti-phospho-p38MAPK antibody and rabbit anti-β-tublin antibody (1:1000 dilution, Cell Signaling Technology, Danvers, MA, United States). The membranes were detected by an ECL-Plus detection kit (Tiangen, Beijing, China), and scanned using Image Quant LAS 4000 (GE Healthcare Life Sciences, CT, United States). The images were quantified using the ImageJ densitometry system.

Measurement of ROS in the RVLM

The lucigenin-enhanced chemiluminescence assay was adopted to detect the ROS production in the RVLM (Chan et al., 2005). RVLM was homogenized in PBS (20 mM, pH 7.4) containing EDTA (0.01 mM). The homogenate was centrifuged at $1200 \times g$ for 10 min at 4°C and the supernatant was collected for ROS assay. Background chemiluminescence in a 2-ml buffer mixed with lucigenin (5 μmol/L) was detected for 5 min. Adding 100 μl supernatant, the chemiluminescence was detected for 30 min at room temperature. The production of ROS was determined and expressed as average light units per minute per milligram of protein.

Immunohistochemistry

The procedure for immunohistochemistry was described previously (Peng et al., 2009). One section from every six serial sections was picked up, with a total of five sections in each animal. Tissue sections were deparaffinized, rehydrated by graded ethanol series, pre-incubated with 5% BSA for an hour, and then incubated with mouse anti-phospho-SAPK/JNK antibody (1:50 dilution, Cell Signaling Technology, Danvers, MA, United States), rabbit anti-phospho-ERK1/2 antibody (1:200 dilution, Cell Signaling Technology, Danvers, MA, United States), or rabbit anti-phospho-p38MAPK antibody (1:400 dilution, Cell Signaling Technology, Danvers, MA, United States) at 4°C overnight. The sections were washed three times with PBS and then incubated with corresponding secondary antibodies. The color reaction was carried out with HRP-linked polymer detection system.

Quantitative Real-Time PCR

The total RNA was extracted from lung tissues using TRIzol Reagent (Invitrogen Corporation, CA, United States). First-strand cDNA was synthesized and amplified from 0.5 μg of total RNA using the ReverTra Ace qPCR RT Kit (Toyobo, Tokyo, Japan). Then the mRNA levels of AT_1R were measured by quantitative real-time PCR (iCyler iQ Real-time PCR Detection System, Bio-Rad Laboratories Inc., United States) using SYBR Green Real-time PCR Master Mix (Toyobo, Japan) in a total volume of 20 μL. Glyceraldehyde-3-phosphate dehydrogenase (GAPDH) was used as an internal standard to normalize the expression level of each mRNA. Primers were designed by Sangon Biotech (Shanghai, China). The target gene names and their primer sequences were shown as follows: forward primer 5′-CCCAAGTCCACACATCAAAG-3′, reverse primer 5′-GCAAGGCAGACTGTATGGAA-3′ for AT_1R; and forward primer 5′-AAGGTGGTGAAGCAGGCGGC-3′, reverse primer 5′-GAGCAATGCCAGCCCCAGCA-3′ for GAPDH. The PCR amplification consisted of 40 cycles of denaturation (94°C, 15 s), annealing (60°C, 30 s) and extension (72°C, 30 s). All the samples were assayed in one essay in our study. The relative quantification of gene expression was analyzed from the measured threshold cycles (CT) by using the $2-\Delta\Delta Ct$ method in the experiment.

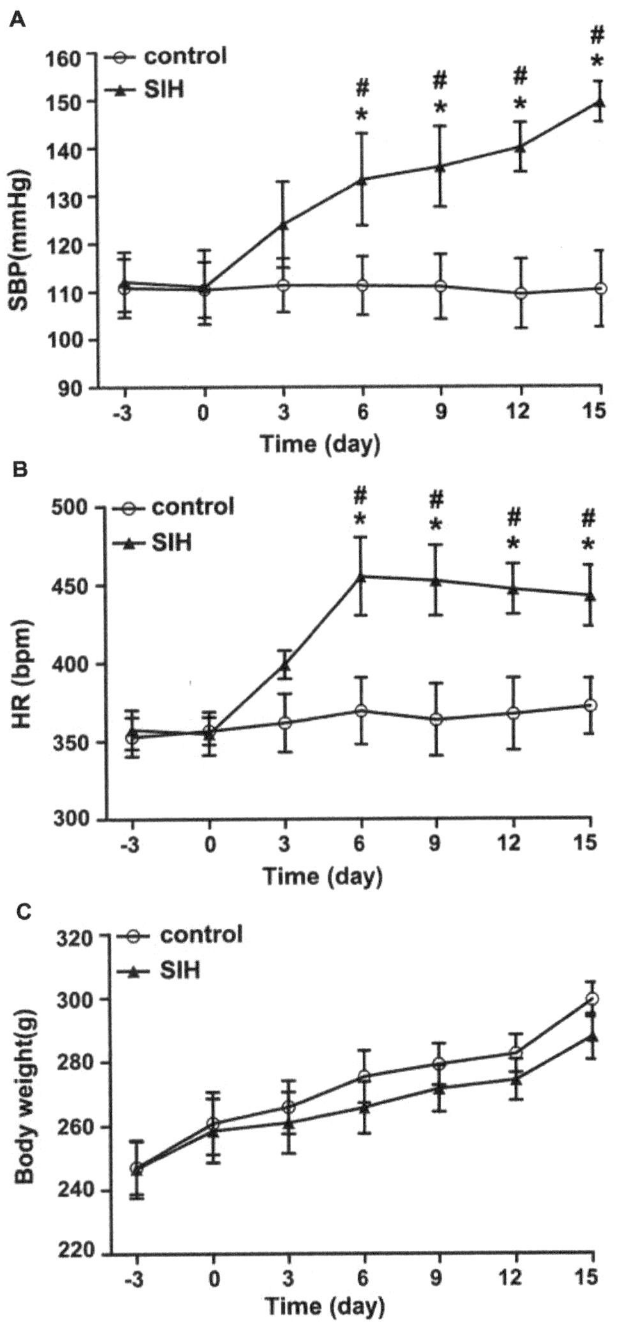

FIGURE 1 | The changes of systolic blood pressure (SBP) **(A)**, heart rate (HR) **(B)**, and body weight **(C)** in stress-induced hypertension (SIH) and control group. $n = 10$, $^*P < 0.05$ vs. control (Student's *t*-test); $^\#P < 0.05$ vs. baseline (paired *t*-test) (third day prior to stress).

Statistical Analysis

All of the data are presented as mean ± standard error (SE). Student's *t*-test, paired *t*-test, or analysis of variance (ANOVA) was performed as appropriate. Statistical analyses were performed using Statistical Package for the Social Sciences (SPSS) version 16.0. A $P < 0.05$ was considered statistically significant.

RESULTS

The Systolic Blood Pressure (SBP) and Heart Rate (HR) of the Stressed Rats Increase in a Time-Dependent Manner

Systolic blood pressure and HR of the stressed rats significantly increased from the 6th day compared with the control rats ($^{*}P < 0.05$). SBP and HR of stressed rats was also significantly different from the 6th day compared with baseline (3rd day prior to stress) ($^{\#}P < 0.05$), and stayed stable at a high level around the 15th day (**Figures 1A,B**). However, there was no discernible difference in body weight between the SIH and control group (**Figure 1C**).

AT_1R and VGLUT2 Co-localize in the RVLM and the Release of Glutamate Increases in the IML of SIHR

Figure 2A showed that AT_1R and VGLUT2 co-localized in the RVLM of SIHR, suggesting that AT_1R expressed in the glutamatergic neurons. To establish that the development of SIH is associated with the actions of glutamatergic neurons in the RVLM, we examined the concentration of amino acid neurotransmitters in the IML. We found the release of glutamate (Glu) neurotransmitter increased in SIHR (**Figure 2C**) than in the control rat (**Figure 2B**) ($n = 8$, $P < 0.05$, **Figure 2D**). These data reveal that the activated glutamatergic neurons of the RVLM release more glutamate neurotransmitter to the IML of SIHR.

Exogenous Ang II Activates SAPK/JNK, ERK1/2 and p38MAPK in the RVLM of SIHR

As **Figure 3** shows, SAPK/JNK, ERK1/2, and p38MAPK phosphorylation in the RVLM were much higher in SIHR than in control rats. RVLM microinjection of Ang II (50 pmol) increased SAPK/JNK, ERK1/2, and p38MAPK phosphorylation in SIHR at 15 min after application, and lasted at least 30 min; while total SAPK/JNK, ERK1/2, or p38MAPK levels were unchanged (**Figures 3A–C**).

Antagonist of AT_1R Decreases ROS Production and SAPK/JNK, ERK1/2, and p38MAPK Phosphorylation in the RVLM of SIHR

The production of ROS was significantly higher in the RVLM of SIHR (**Figure 4A**). Furthermore, the enhancement of ROS production and SAPK/JNK, ERK1/2, and p38MAPK phosphorylation were discernibly blunted (**Figures 4B,C**) by administration of candesartan (2 nmol, an AT_1R antagonist) to the RVLM, bilaterally. However, there was no discernible change elicited by microinjection of PD123319 (2 nmol, an AT_2R antagonist) to the RVLM, bilaterally (data not shown). These findings implicate that stress elevates phosphorylation of SAPK/JNK, ERK1/2, and p38MAPK and activates MAPK pathway via AT_1R.

NADPH Oxidase Inhibitor Inhibits the Activation of MAPK in the RVLM of SIHR

Bilateral administration of NADPH oxidase inhibitor APO (2 nmol) significantly inhibits SAPK/JNK, ERK1/2, or p38MAPK activation in the RVLM of SIHR (**Figures 5A–D**). These findings suggest that NADPH oxidase-derived ROS might be an upstream signaling molecule within the MAPK pathway.

Inhibitor of SAPK, but Not ERK1/2 or p38MAPK, Inhibits AT_1R Expression in the RVLM of SIHR

Both RT-PCR and Western blot studies showed that APO or SAPK inhibitor SP600125 led to a profound decrease in AT_1R mRNA and protein expression in the RVLM of SIHR, whereas ERK1/2 inhibitor U0126 or p38MAPK inhibitor SB203580 did not demonstrate a significant effect in AT_1R mRNA and protein expression in the RVLM of SIHR (**Figures 6A,B**).

Inhibitors of NADPH Oxidase and SAPK Decreased MABP of SIHR

Bilateral microinjection of the APO (2 nmol) or the SAPK inhibitor SP600125 (500 nmol) into the RVLM decreased MABP of SIHR. However, administration of the ERK1/2 inhibitor U0126 (500 nmol) or p38MAPK inhibitor SB203580 (500 nmol) into the RVLM did not obviously change the MABP of SIHR (**Figure 6C**). There was no obvious change in the HR of SIHR. In addition, microinjection of SP600125, U0126, or SB203580 into regions adjacent to the RVLM had no discernible change in the MABP or HR of SIHR. ICV infusion of the APO (0.45 mmol/L) or SP600125 (0.6 mmol/L) for 14 days decreased MABP in the SIHR, whereas U0126 (0.6 mmol/L) or SB203580 (0.6 mmol/L) did not obviously change the MABP of SIHR (**Figure 6D**).

DISCUSSION

Hypertension is a major risk factor for cardiovascular and cerebrovascular diseases, which affects over one billion individuals worldwide (Wu et al., 2015; Mills et al., 2016). SIH caused by chronic and excessive stress, is inflicted on an increasing number of people, including young adults. Therefore, it is necessary to understand the mechanism underlying SIH. The SIHR model is established by electric foot-shocks combined with interval noises (Xia et al., 2008; Xiao et al., 2013; Zhang et al., 2013). The present experiment revealed that this chronic stress in rats led to an increase in BP, implying the successful establishment of an SIHR model.

In the current study, we examined the roles of AT_1 R on cardiovascular modulation and the effects of NADPH oxidase-derived ROS-MAPK signaling in the glutamatergic neurons of the RVLM in SIHR. The primary findings of the present study are: (1) AT_1R expressed in the glutamatergic neurons of the RVLM of SIHR and the glutamate in the IML of the spinal cord is higher in SIHR than that in control rats. (2) Exogenous Ang II activates SAPK/JNK, ERK1/2, and p38MAPK in the RVLM of SIHR. AT_1R antagonist and NADPH oxidase inhibitor reduce the enhanced

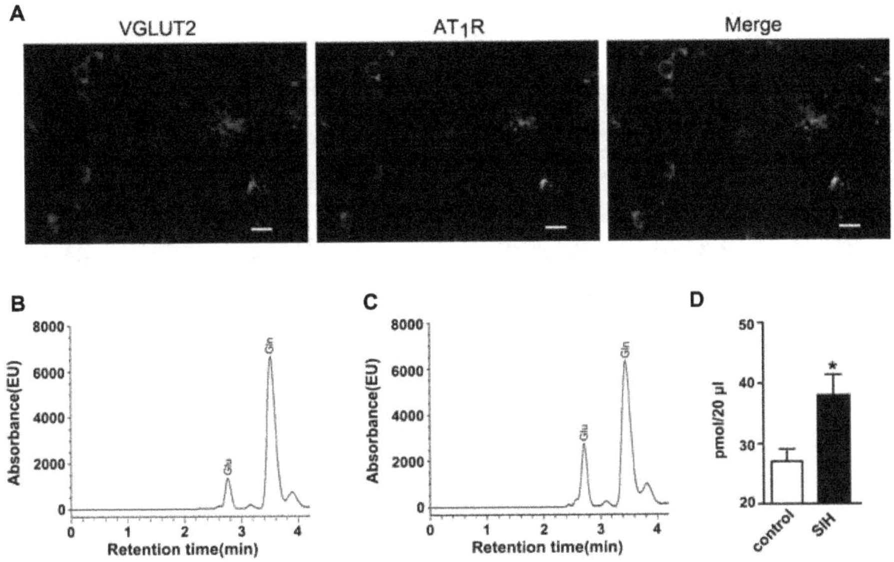

FIGURE 2 | Localization of AT_1R and VGLUT2 in the rostral ventrolateral medulla (RVLM) of SIH rat **(A)** and chromatogram of amino acids in the IML in control **(B)** and SIH rats **(C)** the red (cy3), green (FAM) areas represented the staining of glutamatergic neurons and AT_1R, respectively. Scale bars = 25 μm. The baseline release of glutamate increased in SIH rats compared with control rats **(D)**. $n = 8$, $^*P < 0.05$ vs. control (Student's *t*-test). Glu, glutamate; Gln, glutamine.

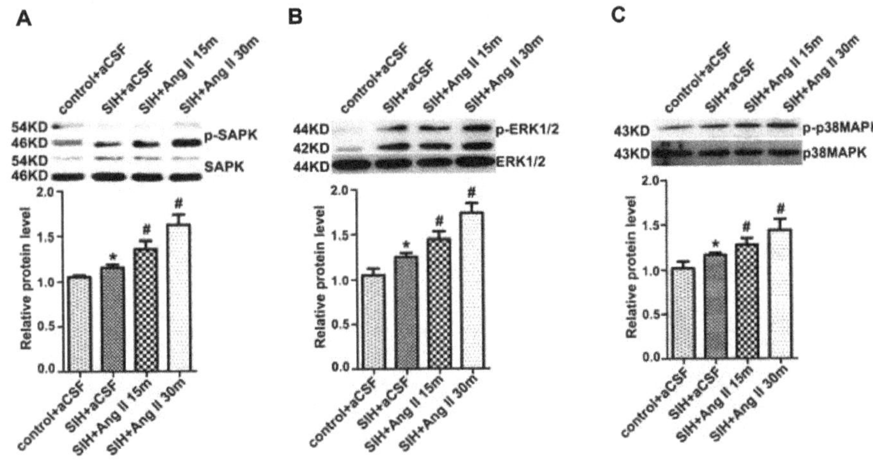

FIGURE 3 | The protein levels of phosphorylation or total SAPK/JNK **(A)**, ERK1/2 **(B)**, and p38MAPK **(C)** in the RVLM in the SIH group 15 and 30 min after RVLM microinjection of Ang II (50 pmol). Densitometry values were determined as indicated. $n = 4$, $^*P < 0.05$ vs. control; $^\#P < 0.05$ vs. SIH (one-way ANOVA with Tukey *post hoc* test).

production of ROS and the activation of SAPK/JNK, ERK1/2, and p38MAPK in the RVLM of SIHR. (3) Injection of the SAPK/JNK inhibitor, but not the p38MAPK or the ERK1/2 inhibitor, into the RVLM significantly decreases expression of AT_1R mRNA and MABP in SIHR. ICV infusion of the SAPK/JNK inhibitor for 14 days, but not the p38MAPK or the ERK1/2 inhibitor, significantly decreases the expression of AT_1R protein and MABP in SIHR.

First, we identified that AT_1R in glutamatergic neurons played a crucial role in the pathogenesis of SIH. Fluorescence *in situ* hybridization (FISH) analysis showed that the AT_1R and VGLUT2 co-localized in the RVLM of SIHR, which indicated that the activity that Ang II bands to AT_1R in the RVLM, is connected to the glutamatergic neurons. A majority of the glutamatergic neurons were co-localized with AT_1R in the RVLM of Wistar rats and SHR (Hu et al., 2002). In hypertensive Dahl salt-sensitive rats, the elevated BP response to AT_1R activation in the hypothalamic paraventricular nucleus (PVN) has been shown to be partly regulated by increased glutamate receptor activation (Gabor and Leenen, 2012). Ang II infusion increases co-localization of gp91^{phox}-containing NADPH oxidase and glutamate N-methyl-D-aspartate receptor (NMDAR) NR_1 subunit in the dendrites of PVN neurons, and augments baseline and NMDAR-induced production of ROS in PVN

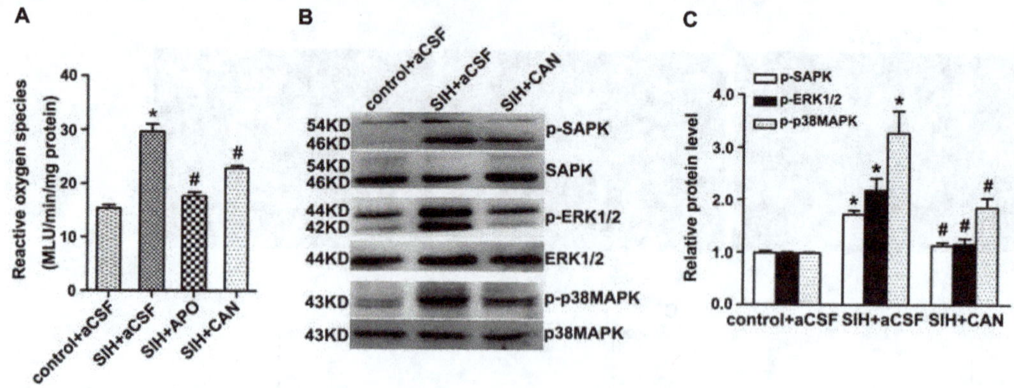

FIGURE 4 | Effects of candesartan (CAN) on the production of Reactive oxygen species (ROS) and phosphorylation of SAPK/JNK, ERK1/2, and p38MAPK in the RVLM in SIH and control groups. The production of ROS in the RVLM detected at 20 min after microinjection of apocynin APO (2 nmol) or CAN (2 nmol) into the RVLM **(A)**; $n = 6$. The protein levels of phosphorylated SAPK/JNK, ERK1/2, and p38MAPK were detected 30 min after microinjection of CAN (2 nmol) into the RVLM, bilaterally **(B,C)**; $n = 4$. $^{*}P < 0.05$ vs. control + aCSF; $^{\#}P < 0.05$ vs. SIH + aCSF (one-way ANOVA with Tukey *post hoc* test).

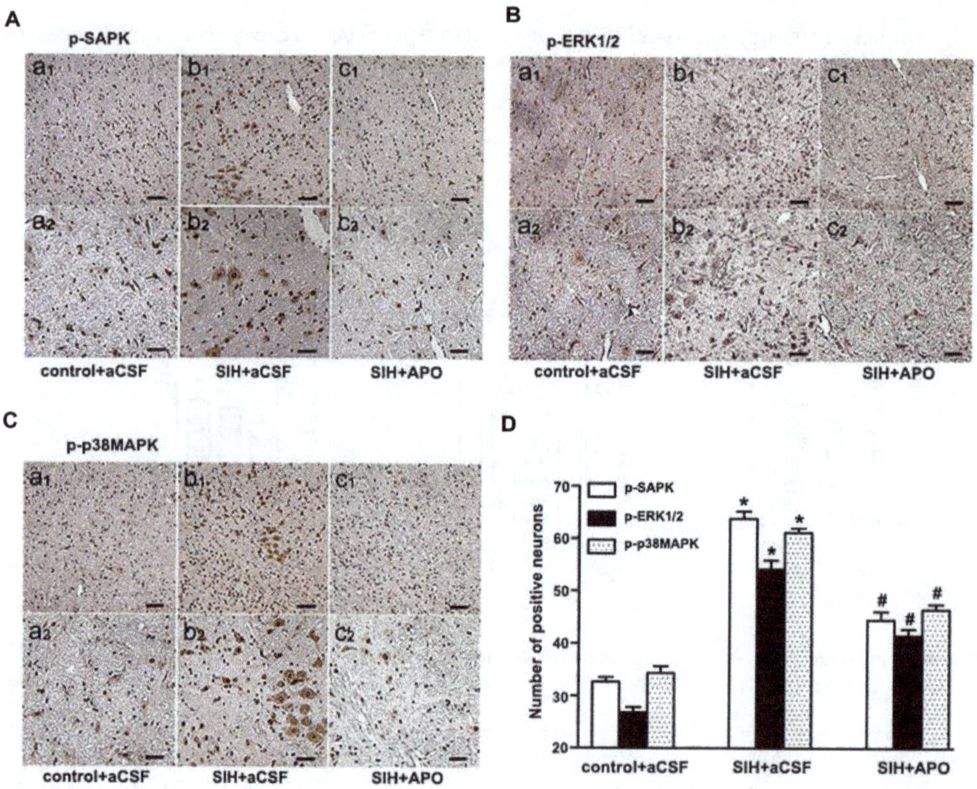

FIGURE 5 | Effects of APO on MAPK activation in the RVLM in the SIH and control group. Immunohistochemistry for p-SAPK/JNK **(A)**, p-ERK1/2 **(B)**, or p-p38MAPK **(C)** in control and SIH groups treated with or without APO **(D)**. Scale bars = 50 μm in a1, b1, c1; 25 μm in a2, b2, c2. $n = 4$, $^{*}P < 0.05$ vs. control + aCSF; $^{\#}P < 0.05$ vs. SIH + aCSF (one-way ANOVA with Tukey *post hoc* test).

cells and spinally projecting PVN neurons (Wang et al., 2013). Our findings provide evidence that AT_1R expressed in the glutamatergic neurons of the RVLM in SIHR, indicating that Ang II might evoke the activation of glutamatergic neurons via AT_1R in the RVLM of SIHR. Furthermore, HPLC analysis showed that the glutamate was increased in the IML of spinal cord. It has been shown that projections from the RVLM to the IML of spinal cord dominate preganglionic neurons resulting in the elevated BP and HR (Guyenet, 2006; Oshima et al., 2008). Our previous studies determined that Ang II-induced glutamate release in the spinal cord might arise from the AT_1R-containing glutamatergic spinally projecting neurons in the RVLM of SHR

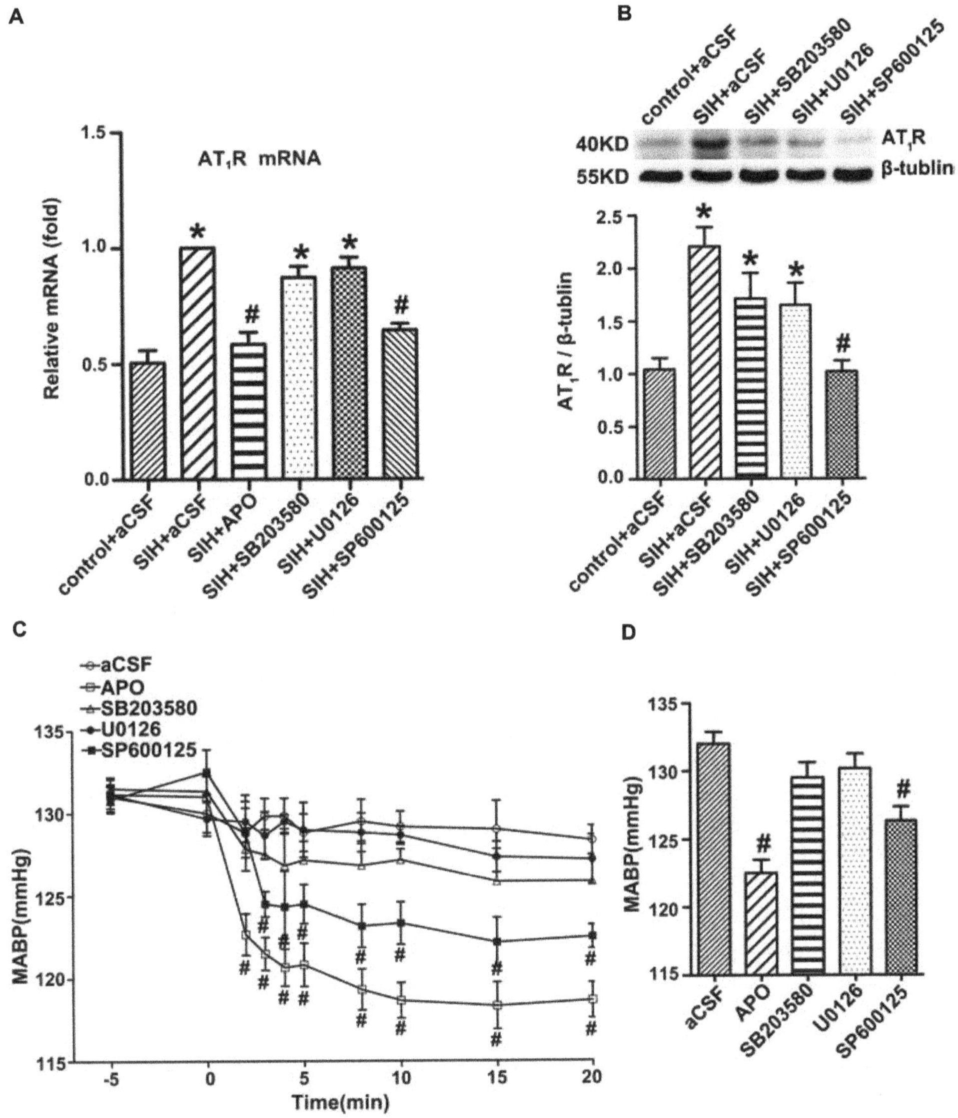

FIGURE 6 | Effects of the inhibitors of nicotinamide adenine dinucleotide phosphate (NADPH) oxidase, SAPK/JNK, ERK1/2, and p38MAPK on AT_1R expression in the RVLM and Mean arterial blood pressure (MABP) in rats with SIH. The mRNA levels of AT_1R in the RVLM (n = 4) **(A)**, and change in MABP (n = 6) **(C)** in response to microinjection of APO (2 nmol), SP600125 (500 nmol), U0126 (500 nmol), or SB203580 (500 nmol) into the RVLM of rats with SIH. Representative gels or densitometric analysis of AT_1R protein in the RVLM (n = 5) **(B)**, and change in MABP (n = 6) **(D)** of SIH group after intracerebroventricular infusion (ICV) of aCSF, APO (0.45 mol/L), SP600125 (0.6 mol/L), U0126 (0.6 mol/L), or SB203580 (0.6 mol/L) for 14 days in stress-induced hypertensive rats (SIHR). $^*P < 0.05$ vs. control + aCSF; $^\#P < 0.05$ vs. SIH + aCSF (one-way ANOVA with Tukey *post hoc* test, **A,B,D**; Student's t-test, **C**).

(Hu et al., 2002). Our present findings implicate that, in SIHR, the glutamatergic neurons of the RVLM are activated, which are associated with the binding of Ang II to AT_1R, and the further release of more glutamate neurotransmitter into the IML through projection fibers. The vesicular glutamate transporters (VGLUTs), capable of specifically packaging glutamate into presynaptic vesicles and promoting glutamate release (Liguz-Lecznar and Skangiel-Kramska, 2007), comprise three members, wherein VGLUT1 and VGLUT2 are considered as specific markers of canonical glutamatergic neurons. Additionally, VGLUT2-immunoreactivities were widely observed in the lower brainstem (Vigneault et al., 2015).

Chronic infusion of Ang II into the brain of normal rabbits resulted in sympathoexcitation and increased oxidative stress, as well as an upregulation of several of the protein subunits of NADPH oxidase, which have shown to be inhibited by losartan (Gao et al., 2005). In a study performed in rabbits with chronic heart failure, central administration of losartan, superoxide dismutase mimetic tempol, or NADPH oxidase inhibitor APO, reduced sympathetic nerve activity and oxidative stress (Gao et al., 2004). What is more, other models demonstrated similar findings, such as cardiac diastolic dysfunction (Li et al., 2013) and nitric oxide inhibition induced-hypertension (Rincón et al., 2015). In our experiments, ICV infusion for 14 days

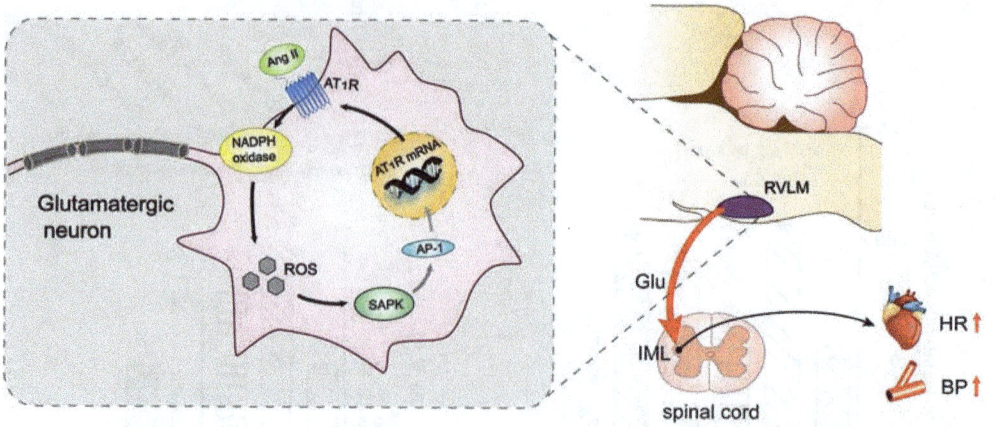

FIGURE 7 | Schematic diagram showing the mechanism by which AT_1R mediates pressor effect in the glutamatergic neurons of the RVLM of SIHR. Ang II triggers the activation of NADPH oxidase derived ROS-SAPK pathway via AT_1R in the glutamatergic neurons of the RVLM of SIHR, then may activate activator protein (AP)-1 to evoke gene transcription and increase AT_1R expression, which promotes the release of glutamate in the IML and eventually increases BP and HR.

or RVLM microinjection of NADPH oxidase inhibitor APO obviously decreased MABP in the SIHR. These results implicate that AT_1R and oxidative stress elicited by NADPH oxidase have an important effect on the regulation of sympathetic activities.

Secondly, we observed that the MAPK pathway was activated in SIHR and, specifically, that Ang II activated the MAPK pathway via AT_1R. The current data show that SAPK/JNK, ERK1/2, and p38MAPK phosphorylation in the RVLM were significantly higher in SIHR than in control rats. Additionally, exogenous Ang II application to the RVLM causes this increase in SAPK/JNK, ERK1/2, and p38MAPK phosphorylation in SIHR. The enhanced activation of MAPKs has been observed in pulmonary arterial hypertension and spontaneous hypertension (Cao et al., 2014; Awad et al., 2016). Importantly, we found that the activation of SAPK/JNK, ERK1/2, and p38MAPK in the RVLM was significantly inhibited by bilateral microinjection of AT_1R antagonist candesartan, which can cross the blood-brain barrier easily.

Our findings might not be consistent with previous studies noting that in normal rats, Ang II elicited ERK1/2 and p38MAPK phosphorylation, whereas SAPK/JNK was not activated in normal rats (Chan et al., 2005). The difference between the current study and these previous results is that SAPK/JNK, ERK1/2, and p38MAPK phosphorylation induced by Ang II administration may be related to the specialty of the current SIH model. Chronic and excessive stress can activate not only ERK1/2 and p38MAPK, but also the stress related proteins SAPK/JNK, to regulate sympathetic activity further.

Thirdly, we demonstrated that NADPH oxidase-derived ROS is the upstream messenger that mediated SAPK/JNK, ERK1/2, and p38MAPK activation induced by Ang II binding to AT_1R in the RVLM of SIHR. We identified that the production of ROS enhanced in SIHR compared with control rats. Microinjections of AT_1R antagonist candesartan and NADPH oxidase inhibitor APO into the RVLM partially inhibited ROS production and SAPK/JNK, ERK1/2, and p38MAPK phosphorylation in SIHR. APO also inhibited the elevation of MABP in SIHR. A previous study suggested that NADPH oxidase-derived ROS mediated the Ang II-evoked pressor effect via p38MAPK activation in the RVLM of normal rats (Chan et al., 2005). The present study suggests that in the RVLM of SIHR, NADPH oxidase-derived ROS has a crucial effect on SAPK/JNK, ERK1/2, and p38MAPK activation elicited by endogenous Ang II.

Finally, we noted that SAPK/JNK activation in the RVLM had important effects on AT_1R expression and the modulation of pressor response. The enhancement of AT_1R mRNA expression and MABP in SIHR were attenuated by the bilateral microinjection of SAPK/JNK inhibitor SP600125, but not ERK1/2 inhibitor U0126, or p38MAPK inhibitor SB203580. Besides, ICV infusion of the SAPK/JNK inhibitor, not ERK1/2, or p38MAPK inhibitor for 14 days decreased AT_1R protein expression and MABP in the SIHR, Our previous study demonstrated that endogenous Ang II production was increased in SIHR and AT_1R expression in the RVLM was much higher in SIHR than in control rats (Du et al., 2013). Hence, we suggested that SAPK/JNK played a major role in regulating the pressor effect.

The AT_1R expression was enhanced in the RVLM of normal rabbits infused with Ang II and rabbits with heart failure (Gao et al., 2005; Liu et al., 2006). It has been reported that Ang II induces MAPK signaling to upregulate AT_1R in PVN and contributes to AT_1R-mediated sympathetic excitation in heart failure (Wei et al., 2008). Ang II activates diverse nuclear transcription factors, such as activator protein-1 (AP-1) (Jia et al., 2008), some of which participate in AT_1R gene transcription. There was some evidence that Ang II promoted the upregulated transcription of AT_1R by oxidant stress and AP-1 activation in the intact brain of rabbits and cultured neuronal cells (Liu et al., 2008). The enhancement of AP-1 upregulated AT_1R expression in the RVLM of rabbits with heart failure, which was activated by the SAPK/JNK pathway (Liu et al., 2006). Furthermore, Ang II-evoked ERK1/2 phosphorylation also functioned in central sympathetic activities via transcription regulation. For example, the PKCb/NADPH oxidase/ERK1/2/CREB/c-fos signaling cascade modulates the long-term pressor effect induced by Ang II in the RVLM of normal rats (Chan et al., 2007). Our present findings indicate that SAPK/JNK, but not ERK1/2 or p38MAPK, has a crucial effect on the modulation of pressor response and AT_1R expression in the RVLM of SIHR. The findings reveal that Ang II upregulates its own receptors via positive feedback involving the AT_1R-ROS-SAPK/JNK pathway (**Figure 7**).

Overall, the present data show that AT_1R localizes in the glutamatergic neurons of the RVLM of SIHR. This localization results in the release of glutamate into the IML of the spinal cord, leading to the pressor response in SIHR. Further, the NADPH oxidase-ROS-SAPK/JNK pathway has an essential impact on the actions of glutamatergic neurons and promotes the expression of AT_1R in the RVLM of SIHR. Thus, this study reveals that Ang II modulates pressor effect through AT_1R-dependent activation of SAPK/JNK by NADPH oxidase-derived ROS in the glutamatergic neurons of the RVLM in SIHR. One limitation of the present study is that we didn't examine the expression of AP-1 and the role of AP-1 in SIHR, although it has been reported that AP-1 activation might participate in the upregulation of AT_1R in heart failure. This interesting possibility in SIHR will be investigated in our future study.

AUTHOR CONTRIBUTIONS

JinW designed the work. LJ, XZ, RG, and YX performed the experiments. XZ, JinW, and SM wrote the manuscript. HY drew the figures. JinW, JijW, LS, and DZ interpreted the data.

FUNDING

This study was supported by the National Natural Science Foundation of China (No. 31371155).

ACKNOWLEDGMENTS

We would like to thank Editage (www.editage.com) for English language editing.

REFERENCES

Awad, K. S., West, J. D., de Jesus, P. V., and MacLean, M. (2016). Novel signaling pathways in pulmonary arterial hypertension (2015 Grover Conference Series). *Pulm. Circ.* 6, 285–294. doi: 10.1086/688034

Bae, Y. S., Oh, H., Rhee, S. G., and Yoo, Y. D. (2011). Regulation of reactive oxygen species generation in cell signaling. *Mol. Cells* 32, 491–509. doi: 10.1007/s10059-011-0276-3

Bao, W., Behm, D. J., Nerurkar, S. S., Ao, Z., Bentley, R., Mirabile, R. C., et al. (2007). Effects of p38 MAPK inhibitor on angiotensin II-dependent hypertension, organ damage, and superoxide anion production. *J. Cardiovasc. Pharmacol.* 49, 362–368. doi: 10.1097/fjc.0b013e318046f34a

Campese, V. M., Shaohua, Y., and Huiquin, Z. (2005). Oxidative stress mediates angiotensin II-dependent stimulation of sympathetic nerve activity. *Hypertension* 46, 533–539. doi: 10.1161/01.hyp.0000179088.57586.26

Cao, Y., Zhang, Y., Wang, N., and He, L. (2014). Antioxidant effect of imperatorin from angelica dahurica in hypertension via inhibiting NADPH oxidase activation and MAPK pathway. *J. Am. Soc. Hypertens.* 8, 527–536. doi: 10.1016/j.jash.2014.04.006

Carvalho, T. H. F., Bergamaschi, C. T., Lopes, O. U., and Campos, R. R. (2003). Role of endogenous angiotensin II on glutamatergic actions in the rostral ventrolateral medulla in goldblatt hypertensive rats. *Hypertension* 42, 707–712. doi: 10.1161/01.hyp.0000086524.35251.2D

Chan, S. H., Hsu, K. S., Huang, C. C., Wang, L. L., Ou, C. C., and Chan, J. Y. (2005). NADPH oxidase-derived superoxide anion mediates angiotensin II-induced pressor effect via activation of p38 mitogen-activated protein kinase in the rostral ventrolateral medulla. *Circ. Res.* 97, 772–780. doi: 10.1161/01.res.0000185804.79157.C0

Chan, S. H., Wang, L. L., Tseng, H. L., and Chan, J. Y. (2007). Upregulation of AT1 receptor gene on activation of protein kinase C beta/nicotinamide adenine dinucleotide diphosphate oxidase/ERK1/2/c-fos signaling cascade mediates long-term pressor effect of angiotensin II in rostral ventrolateral medulla. *J. Hypertens.* 25, 1845–1861. doi: 10.1097/hjh.0b013e328217b286

Czikora, I., Feher, A., Lucas, R., Fulton, D. J., and Bagi, Z. (2015). Caveolin-1 prevents sustained angiotensin II-induced resistance artery constriction and obesity-induced high blood pressure. *Am. J. Physiol. Heart Circ. Physiol.* 308, H376–H385. doi: 10.1152/ajpheart.00649.2014

Dange, R. B., Agarwal, D., Masson, G. S., Vila, J., Wilson, B., Nair, A., et al. (2014). Central blockade of TLR4 improves cardiac function and attenuates myocardial inflammation in angiotensin II-induced hypertension. *Cardiovasc. Res.* 103, 17–27. doi: 10.1093/cvr/cvu067

Ding, K., Wang, Y., Jiang, W., Zhang, Y., Yin, H., and Fang, Z. (2015). Qian yang yu yin granule-containing serum inhibits angiotensin II-induced proliferation, reactive oxygen species production, and inflammation in human mesangial cells via an NADPH oxidase 4-dependent pathway. *BMC Complement. Altern. Med.* 15:81. doi: 10.1186/s12906-015-0619-2

Du, D., Chen, J., Liu, M., Zhu, M., Jing, H., Fang, J., et al. (2013). The effects of angiotensin II and angiotensin-(1-7) in the rostral ventrolateral medulla of rats on stress-induced hypertension. *PLoS One* 8:e70976. doi: 10.1371/journal.pone.0070976

Fang, X., Shu, G., Yu, J., Wang, L., Yang, J., Zeng, Q., et al. (2013). The anorexigenic effect of serotonin is mediated by the generation of NADPH oxidase-dependent ROS. *PLoS One* 8:e53142. doi: 10.1371/journal.pone.0053142

Gabor, A., and Leenen, F. H. H. (2012). Cardiovascular effects of angiotensin II and glutamate in the PVN of dahl salt-sensitive rats. *Brain Res.* 1447, 28–37. doi: 10.1016/j.brainres.2012.01.060

Gao, L., Wang, W., Li, Y. L., Schultz, H. D., Liu, D., Cornish, K. G., et al. (2004). Superoxide mediates sympathoexcitation in heart failure: roles of angiotensin II and NAD(P)H oxidase. *Circ. Res.* 95, 937–944. doi: 10.1161/01.res.0000146676.04359.64

Gao, L., Wang, W., Li, Y. L., Schultz, H. D., Liu, D., Cornish, K. G., et al. (2005). Sympathoexcitation by central ang II: roles for AT1 receptor upregulation and NAD(P)H oxidase in RVLM. *Am. J. Physiol. Heart Circ. Physiol.* 288, H2271–H2279. doi: 10.1152/ajpheart.00949.2004

Guyenet, P. G. (2006). The sympathetic control of blood pressure. *Nat. Rev. Neurosci.* 7, 335–346. doi: 10.1038/nrn1902

Hanna, I. R., Taniyama, Y., Szocs, K., Rocic, P., and Griendling, K. K. (2002). NAD(P)H oxidase-derived reactive oxygen species as mediators of angiotensin II signaling. *Antioxid. Redox. Signal.* 4, 899–914. doi: 10.1089/152308602762197443

Hausding, M., Jurk, K., Daub, S., Kröller-Schön, S., Stein, J., Schwenk, M., et al. (2013). CD40L contributes to angiotensin II-induced pro-thrombotic state, vascular inflammation, oxidative stress and endothelial dysfunction. *Basic Res. Cardiol.* 108:386. doi: 10.1007/s00395-013-0386-5

Hu, L., Zhu, D., Yu, Z., Wang, J. Q., Sun, Z., and Yao, T. (2002). Expression of angiotensin II type 1 (AT1) receptor in the rostral ventrolateral medulla in rats. *J. Appl. Physiol.* 92, 2153–2161. doi: 10.1152/japplphysiol.00261.2001

Jia, G., Cheng, G., Gangahar, D. M., and Agrawal, D. K. (2008). Involvement of connexin 43 in angiotensin II-induced migration and proliferation of saphenous vein smooth muscle cells via the MAPK-AP-1 signaling pathway. *J. Mol. Cell. Cardiol.* 44, 882–890. doi: 10.1016/j.yjmcc.2008.03.002

Lassegue, B., San, M. A., and Griendling, K. K. (2012). Biochemistry, physiology, and pathophysiology of NADPH oxidases in the cardiovascular system. *Circ. Res.* 110, 1364–1390. doi: 10.1161/circresaha.111.243972

Li, Y. Q., Li, X. B., Guo, S. J., Chu, S. L., Gao, P. J., Zhu, D. L., et al. (2013). Apocynin attenuates oxidative stress and cardiac fibrosis in angiotensin II-induced cardiac diastolic dysfunction in mice. *Acta Pharmacol. Sin.* 34, 352–359. doi: 10.1038/aps.2012.164

Liguz-Lecznar, M., and Skangiel-Kramska, J. (2007). Vesicular glutamate transporters (VGLUTs): the three musketeers of glutamatergic system. *Acta Neurobiol. Exp.* 67, 207–218.

Liu, D., Gao, L., Roy, S. K., Cornish, K. G., and Zucker, I. H. (2006). Neuronal angiotensin II type 1 receptor upregulation in heart failure: activation of activator protein 1 and jun N-terminal kinase. *Circ. Res.* 99, 1004–1011. doi: 10.1161/01.res.0000247066.19878.93

Liu, D., Gao, L., Roy, S. K., Cornish, K. G., and Zucker, I. H. (2008). Role of oxidant stress on AT1 receptor expression in neurons of rabbits with heart failure and in cultured neurons. *Circ. Res.* 103, 186–193. doi: 10.1161/circresaha.108.179408

Mills, K. T., Bundy, J. D., Kelly, T. N., Reed, J. E., Kearney, P. M., Reynolds, K., et al. (2016). Global disparities of hypertension prevalence and control: a systematic analysis of population-based studies from 90 countries. *Circulation* 134, 441–450. doi: 10.1161/circulationaha.115.018912

Minas, J. N., Thorwald, M. A., Conte, D., Vázquez-Medina, J., Nishiyama, A., and Ortiz, R. M. (2015). Angiotensin and mineralocorticoid receptor antagonism attenuates cardiac oxidative stress in angiotensin II-infused rats. *Clin. Exp. Pharmacol. Physiol.* 42, 1178–1188. doi: 10.1111/1440-1681.12473

Omura, T., Yoshiyama, M., Matsumoto, R., Kusuyama, T., Enomoto, S., Nishiya, D., et al. (2005). Role of c-jun NH2-terminal kinase in G-protein-coupled receptor agonist-induced cardiac plasminogen activator inhibitor-1 expression. *J. Mol. Cell. Cardiol.* 38, 583–592. doi: 10.1016/j.yjmcc.2005.01.008

Oshima, N., Kumagai, H., Onimaru, H., Kawai, A., Pilowsky, P. M., Iigaya, K., et al. (2008). Monosynaptic excitatory connection from the rostral ventrolateral medulla to sympathetic preganglionic neurons revealed by simultaneous recordings. *Hypertens. Res.* 31, 1445–1454. doi: 10.1291/hypres.31.1445

Pan, Y. X., Gao, L., Wang, W. Z., Zheng, H., Liu, D., Patel, K. P., et al. (2007). Exercise training prevents arterial baroreflex dysfunction in rats treated with central angiotensin II. *Hypertension* 49, 519–527. doi: 10.1161/01.hyp.0000256955.74461.93

Peng, J., Wang, Y. K., Wang, L. G., Yuan, W. J., Su, D. F., Ni, X., et al. (2009). Sympathoinhibitory mechanism of moxonidine: role of the inducible nitric oxide synthase in the rostral ventrolateral medulla. *Cardiovasc. Res.* 84, 283–291. doi: 10.1093/cvr/cvp202

Reja, V., Goodchild, A. K., Phillips, J. K., and Pilowsky, P. M. (2006). Upregulation of angiotensin AT1 receptor and intracellular kinase gene expression in hypertensive rats. *Clin. Exp. Pharmacol. Physiol.* 33, 690–695. doi: 10.1111/j.1440-1681.2006.04420.x

Rincón, J., Correia, D., Arcaya, J. L., Finol, E., Fernández, A., Pérez, M., et al. (2015). Role of angiotensin II type 1 receptor on renal NAD(P)H oxidase, oxidative stress and inflammation in nitric oxide inhibition induced-hypertension. *Life Sci.* 124, 81–90. doi: 10.1016/j.lfs.2015.01.005

Ross, C. A., Ruggiero, D. A., Park, D. H., Joh, T. H., Sved, A. F., Fernandez-Pardal, J., et al. (1984). Tonic vasomotor control by the rostral ventrolateral medulla: effect of electrical or chemical stimulation of the area containing C1 adrenaline neurons on arterial pressure, heart rate, and plasma catecholamines and vasopressin. *J. Neurosci.* 4, 474–494. doi: 10.1523/JNEUROSCI.04-02-00474.1984

Ushio-Fukai, M., and Alexander, R. W. (2004). Reactive oxygen species as mediators of angiogenesis signaling: role of NAD (P)H oxidase. *Mol. Cell. Biochem.* 264, 85–97. doi: 10.1023/B:MCBI.0000044378.09409.b5

Vigneault, E., Poirel, O., Riad, M., Prud'Homme, J., Dumas, S., Turecki, G., et al. (2015). Distribution of vesicular glutamate transporters in the human brain. *Front. Neuroanat.* 9:23. doi: 10.3389/fnana.2015.00023

Wakui, H., Dejima, T., Tamura, K., Uneda, K., Azuma, K., Maeda, A., et al. (2013). Activation of angiotensin II type 1 receptor-associated protein exerts an inhibitory effect on vascular hypertrophy and oxidative stress in angiotensin II-mediated hypertension. *Cardiovasc. Res.* 100, 511–519. doi: 10.1093/cvr/cvt225

Wang, G., Coleman, C. G., Chan, J., Faraco, G., Marques-Lopes, J., Milner, T. A., et al. (2013). Angiotensin II slow-pressor hypertension enhances NMDA currents and NOX2-dependent superoxide production in hypothalamic paraventricular neurons. *Am. J. Physiol. Regul. Integr. Comp. Physiol.* 304, R1096–R1106. doi: 10.1152/ajpregu.00367.2012

Wang, H. D., Johns, D. G., Xu, S., and Cohen, R. A. (2002). Role of superoxide anion in regulating pressor and vascular hypertrophic response to angiotensin II. *Am. J. Physiol. Heart Circ. Physiol.* 282, H1697–H1702. doi: 10.1152/ajpheart.00914.2001

Wang, M., Chen, D., Chen, L., Cao, G., Zhao, H., Liu, D., et al. (2018). Novel inhibitors of the cellular renin-angiotensin system components, poricoic acids, target Smad3 phosphorylation and Wnt/β-catenin pathway against renal fibrosis. *Br. J. Pharmacol.* 175, 2689–2708. doi: 10.1111/bph.14333

Wei, S. G., Yu, Y., Zhang, Z. H., Weiss, R. M., and Felder, R. B. (2008). Mitogen-activated protein kinases mediate upregulation of hypothalamic angiotensin II type 1 receptors in heart failure rats. *Hypertension* 52, 679–686. doi: 10.1161/hypertensionaha.108.113639

Wu, L., He, Y., Jiang, B., Sun, D., Wang, J., Liu, M., et al. (2015). Trends in prevalence, a wareness, treatment and control of hypertension during 2001-2010 in an urban elderly population of China. *PLoS One* 10:e0132814. doi: 10.1371/journal.pone.0132814

Xia, C., Shao, C., Xin, L., Wang, Y., Ding, C., Wang, J., et al. (2008). Effects of melatonin on blood pressure in stress-induced hypertension in rats. *Clin. Exp. Pharmacol. Physiol.* 35, 1258–1264. doi: 10.1111/j.1440-1681.2008.05000.x

Xiang, H. B., Liu, C., Liu, T. T., and Xiong, J. (2014). Central circuits regulating the sympathetic outflow to lumbar muscles in spinally transected mice by retrograde transsynaptic transport. *Int. J. Clin. Exp. Pathol.* 7, 2987–2997.

Xiao, F., Jiang, M., Du, D., Xia, C., Wang, J., Cao, Y., et al. (2013). Orexin A regulates cardiovascular responses in stress-induced hypertensive rats. *Neuropharmacology* 67, 16–24. doi: 10.1016/j.neuropharm.2012.10.021

Zha, Y. P., Wang, Y. K., Deng, Y., Zhang, R. W., Tan, X., Yuan, W. J., et al. (2013). Exercise training lowers the enhanced tonically active glutamatergic input to the rostral ventrolateral medulla in hypertensive rats. *CNS Neurosci. Ther.* 19, 244–251. doi: 10.1111/cns.12065

Zhang, C., Xia, C., Jiang, M., Zhu, M., Zhu, J., Du, D., et al. (2013). Repeated electroacupuncture attenuating of apelin expression and function in the rostral ventrolateral medulla in stress-induced hypertensive rats. *Brain Res. Bull.* 97, 53–62. doi: 10.1016/j.brainresbull.2013.05.013

Zhang, G. X., Lu, X. M., Kimura, S., and Nishiyama, A. (2007). Role of mitochondria in angiotensin II-induced reactive oxygen species and mitogen-activated protein kinase activation. *Cardiovasc. Res.* 76, 204–212. doi: 10.1016/j.cardiores.2007.07.014

13

Parameters of Surface Electromyogram Suggest that Dry Immersion Relieves Motor Symptoms in Patients with Parkinsonism

German G. Miroshnichenko[1], Alexander Yu Meigal[2], Irina V. Saenko[3], Liudmila I. Gerasimova-Meigal[4], Liudmila A. Chernikova[5], Natalia S. Subbotina[6], Saara M. Rissanen[1] and Pasi A. Karjalainen[1]*

[1] Biosignal Analysis and Medical Imaging Group, Department of Applied Physics, Faculty of Science and Forestry, University of Eastern Finland, Kuopio, Finland, [2] Laboratory for Novel Methods in Physiology, Institute of High-Tech Biomedical Solutions, Petrozavodsk State University, Petrozavodsk, Russia, [3] Laboratory of Gravitational Physiology of Sensorimotor System, Department of Sensorimotor Physiology and Countermeasure, Institute of BioMedical Problems, Russian Academy of Sciences, Moscow, Russia, [4] Department of Human and Animal Physiology, Physiopathology, Histology, Petrozavodsk State University, Petrozavodsk, Russia, [5] Department of Neurorehabilitation and Physiotherapy, Research Center of Neurology, Russian Academy of Medical Sciences, Moscow, Russia, [6] Department of Neurology, Psychiatry, and Microbiology, Petrozavodsk State University, Petrozavodsk, Russia

***Correspondence:**
German G. Miroshnichenko
germanmi@uef.fi

Dry immersion (DI) is acknowledged as a reliable space flight analog condition. At DI, subject is immersed in water being wrapped in a waterproof film to imitate microgravity (μG). Microgravity is known to decrease muscle tone due to deprivation of the sensory stimuli that activate the reflexes that keep up the muscle tone. In contrary, parkinsonian patients are characterized by elevated muscle tone, or rigidity, along with rest tremor and akinesia. We hypothesized that DI can diminish the elevated muscle tone and/or the tremor in parkinsonian patients. Fourteen patients with Parkinson's disease (PD, 10 males, 4 females, 47–73 years) and 5 patients with vascular parkinsonism (VP, 1 male, 4 females, 65–72 years) participated in the study. To evaluate the effect of DI on muscles' functioning, we compared parameters of surface electromyogram (sEMG) measured before and after a single 45-min long immersion session. The sEMG recordings were made from the biceps brachii muscle, bilaterally. Each recording was repeated with the following loading conditions: with arms hanging freely down, and with 0, 1, and 2 kg loading on each hand with elbows flexed to 90°. The sEMG parameters comprised of amplitude, median frequency, time of decay of mutual information, sample entropy, correlation dimension, recurrence rate, and determinism of sEMG. These parameters have earlier been proved to be sensitive to PD severity. We used the Wilcoxon test to decide which parameters were statistically significantly different before and after the dry immersion. Accepting the $p < 0.05$ significance level, amplitude, time of decay of mutual information, recurrence rate, and determinism tended to decrease, while median frequency and sample entropy of sEMG tended to increase after the DI. The most statistically significant change was for the determinism of sEMG from the left biceps with 1 kg loading, which decreased for 84% of the patients. The results suggest that DI can promptly relieve motor symptoms of parkinsonism. We conclude that DI has strong potential as a rehabilitation method for parkinsonian patients.

Keywords: parkinsonism, dry immersion, microgravity, rehabilitation, electromyogram, nonlinear dynamics, auto-mutual information, determinism

1. INTRODUCTION

Parkinson's disease (PD) is acknowledged as one of the major neurological problems due to its epidemiology (de Lau and Breteler, 2006), numerous motor and non-motor symptoms, and functional disability (Alves et al., 2005) in PD patients. From the patients' viewpoint, PD causes dramatic decrease in their safety, wellbeing, and quality of life (Boersma et al., 2016; Fan et al., 2016). From the society's viewpoint, PD patients have increased need for healthcare, which imposes notable economical burden on them, their families, and state (Noyes et al., 2006). PD is characterized by a classic triad of motor symptoms, which include rest tremor, elevated muscle tone, or rigidity, and akinesia. Motor symptoms worsen over time but respond to dopamine replenishment therapy (The Parkinson Study Group, 2004), deep brain stimulation (Vaillancourt et al., 2004), and transcranial magnetic stimulation (Zhu et al., 2015). Still, despite these medical therapies, PD patients develop progressive disability (Alves et al., 2005).

Varied physical interventions have been tried in an effort to find efficient, easy-to-perform, and no costly methods for rehabilitation of PD patients (Tomlinson et al., 2014). The techniques already tested include, e.g., resistance training (Scandalis et al., 2001), robotic-assisted therapy (Picelli et al., 2014), training by means of virtual reality (Yen et al., 2011), whole-body vibration (Ebersbach et al., 2008), and dancing (de Dreu et al., 2015). Also, such exotic therapies as Yoga (Ni et al., 2016), Tai Chi (Zhou et al., 2015), and music therapy (Bukowska et al., 2016) are reported to exert a positive effect on some symptoms of PD. Still, there is a strong need in a rehabilitation technique with a more clear link to pathophysiological mechanisms of parkinsonism. We assume that an unloading technique could be a relevant candidate. Indeed, various unloading techniques, such as weight support (Miyai et al., 2000) and water-related techniques, e.g., aquatic physical therapy (Katsura et al., 2010; Vivas et al., 2011; Volpe et al., 2014) have been reported to improve performance in PD patients.

The phenomenon of muscle tone appears as a commonly used, though often misunderstood concept (Needle et al., 2014). Muscle tone is defined as either the resistance of muscle being passively lengthened (Gordon, 1990), "state of readiness" (Davis et al., 2011), or unconscious "low-level steady-state muscle contraction at rest" (Needle et al., 2014). This prompts that muscle tone is comprised of several distinct components: (1) physical inertia of extremity, (2) the non-reflexive (mechanical-elastic) component, (3) peripheral reflexive muscle contraction, and (4) central neural mechanisms (Katz and Rymer, 1989; Ward, 2000; Needle et al., 2014). The non-reflexive component of muscle tone originates from intrinsic tension between molecules and cells and, correspondingly, it can be measured as a set of viscoelastic characteristics of the skeletal muscle (Demangel et al., 2017). The peripheral reflexive component of muscle tone originates from overactive tonic stretch reflex. On the level of CNS muscle tone is triggered and mediated through the reticular formation, brain stem, cerebellum, extrapyramidal pathways, with modifications from basal ganglia, gamma-motoneurones, and, finally, contraction of intrafusal fibers, which stretch spindle sensory organs, thus initiating activity of alpha-motoneurones via the stretch reflex (Needle et al., 2014). This reflexive activity is aimed at maximizing muscle responsiveness under stressful conditions (Davis et al., 2011). Inhibition from the cortical structures is needed to optimize muscle tone (Guyton and Hall, 2011). Due to complex origins, muscle tone has two different connotations in clinical and research practice. In clinics, muscle tone is used as an easy-to-do bedside measure performed with clinical scales, while for research purposes electromyography (EMG) is useful to assess muscle tone (Ward, 2000).

Two distinct types of exaggerated muscle tone—spasticity and rigidity—are known. Spasticity is hypertonicity caused by misbalance of supraspinal inhibitory and excitatory inputs directed to the spinal cord, leading to a state of disinhibition of the stretch reflex on one side of a joint (Dietz and Sinkjaer, 2007; Trompetto et al., 2014). Instead, rigidity is clinically defined as muscle hypertonicity that persists through the entire range of passive movement on both sides of a particular joint. Also, "unwilled" firing of slow-type motor units might be an important factor in the genesis of rigidity, which is seen as excessive EMG at rest (Cantello et al., 1995). Spasticity is very common in patients with the upper motoneurone lesion (stroke), cerebral palsy and multiply sclerosis (Rivelis and Morice, 2018), while rigidity is the characteristic of patients with Parkinson's disease (PD) and has distinctly different neurophysiological mechanisms (Baradaran et al., 2013).

It is well-known from space physiology that muscle tone in healthy subjects (cosmonauts/astronauts) dramatically decreases within even 1 day in real microgravity on orbit (Kozlovskaya et al., 1988). Tremor is also modified under conditions of space flight (Gallasch et al., 1994). Namely, frequency and amplitude of tremor decrease under weightlessness, presumably due to switch of main source of sensory information from load-dependent muscle reception to position-dependent joint reception (Gallasch et al., 1994). Therefore, we suppose that pathologically elevated muscle tone (rigidity) and tremor may be relieved in PD patients with the help of ground-based analog microgravity techniques. There are few microgravity analog environments: (i) dry immersion (DI), (ii) bed rest, (iii) parabolic airplane flight, (iv) free fall machine, (v) weight support. Among these, DI provides the best microgravity analog due to the following physical factors: (i) supportlessness, (ii) physical inactivity, (iii) whole-body hydrostatic compression (Navasiolava et al., 2011; Watenpaugh, 2016; Demangel et al., 2017).

Effects of DI on the viscoelastic component of muscle tone in healthy subjects are usually seen after 3 days staying at DI (Demangel et al., 2017). However, some studies have demonstrated a much faster effect of analog microgravity on muscles. For example, Schneider et al. (2015) have shown that muscle stiffness changes even after a few seconds of parabolic flight at zero G. Also, Cronin et al. (2016) have demonstrated that muscle spasticity has decreased after 5 min of water immersion due to diminished reflexivity. These data promise that even a short-term DI session, which would be more suitable for older people and PD patients, could exert rehabilitation effect on the motor system. Indeed, the program of several DI sessions with the same patient group as here has been recently reported to exert positive effect on some clinical metrics of PD patients, including scores of depressive mood, UPDRS-III (Unified Parkinson's disease rating scale, motor part), and the rigidity subtotal of the UPDRS-III (Meigal et al., 2018). Tremor subtotal of the UPDRS-III has also decreased, though insignificantly. Still, to date, no instrumented measurement has been conducted to evaluate the effect of a single one DI session on muscle function in PD patients.

Surface electromyography (sEMG) is an affordable, noninvasive, and high-throughput way to get information about muscle functioning. sEMG has been extensively used to examine either normal motor functioning or movement disorders in humans (Farina et al., 2014). Such classical parameters of sEMG as amplitude and spectral frequency allow some estimation of motor unit number and synchronization (Sturman et al., 2005). In recent years, recurrence quantification analysis, entropy and fractal analysis of sEMG provided additional insight in the underlying motor strategies. These parameters characterize a signal in terms of regularity, predictability and self-similarity (Riley and van Orden, 2005). Indeed, nonlinear dynamics based parameters of sEMG surpass the traditional spectral frequency metrics in detection of, for example, fatigue (Sung et al., 2008; Boccia et al., 2016). The nonlinear dynamics based parameters have already been applied for diagnostics of parkinsonism with promising results (Rissanen et al., 2008, 2011; Meigal et al., 2009; Ruonala et al., 2018). They also proved sensitive to neuroleptic-induced parkinsonism in patients with schizophrenia (Meigal et al., 2015). Taken together, nonlinear dynamics based parameters allow quantifying motor unit synchronization and estimating number of independent oscillators generating sEMG (Sturman et al., 2005). Thus, among cardinal motor symptoms of PD, tremor is most reliably characterized by sEMG parameters due to their sensitivity to "hidden rhythms" on electromyogram (Meigal et al., 2013; Oung et al., 2015). In contrary, muscle tone and, presumably, rigidity, are better described by the kinematic parameters collected by wearable inertial sensors (Sáchez-Ferro et al., 2016; di Biase et al., 2018) or by viscoelasticity parameters (Schneider et al., 2015). By using sEMG, rigidity can be seen at best as excessive muscle activity at rest condition (Cantello et al., 1995).

Several studies provide information on the characteristics of sEMG in healthy subjects during analog microgravity. For example, under the condition of 1–8 weeks bed rest, such sEMG parameters as amplitude, median frequency, muscle fiber conduction velocity, and entropy substantially decrease (Portero et al., 1996; Mulder et al., 2009; Cescon and Gazzoni, 2010; Buehring et al., 2011; Fu et al., 2016). Usually, bed rest experiments last for several weeks to simulate space flights of varied duration and lead to substantial impairment in muscle performance, structure, and fiber content (Watenpaugh, 2016). In that respect, bed rest, especially in its most perfect form (with 6° head tilt below horizontal) is likely not reliable for rehabilitation purposes. In contrast, the condition of dry immersion induces microgravity-specific modifications in skeletal muscles much faster than does the bed rest condition (Navasiolava et al., 2011; Watenpaugh, 2016; Demangel et al., 2017). Earlier it has been shown that even a 5 min period of water immersion in waterproof trousers can decrease peripheral reflex excitability after returning to dry land in both healthy controls and post-stroke patients (Cronin et al., 2016). That can be considered as a promise of non-pharmaceutical method of decreasing hyperreflexivity following stroke (Cronin et al., 2016). As such, the condition of short-term dry immersion can be regarded as a potentially reliable method to decrease excessive muscle tone also in PD patients, though neurophysiology of muscle rigidity and spasticity is clearly different.

Therefore, we hypothesize that application of a single one short-term session of DI can diminish tremor and muscle rigidity in PD patients seen as decreased amplitude and modified nonlinear dynamics based parameters of sEMG.

2. PATIENTS AND METHODS

2.1. Patients

The general inclusion criteria for the patients were that they had an earlier diagnosis of either Parkinson's disease (PD) or vascular parkinsonism (VP). The exclusion criteria are listed in **Table 1**. Twenty-six patients were clinically examined for participation in this study. Seven of the twenty-six patients were excluded because of elevated blood pressure or extrasystoles on their ECG before a pilot immersion. The remaining 19 of the 26 patients underwent the 15 min pilot dry immersion and further participated in the study. Six of the nineteen patients had controlled arterial hypertension (II–III stage). All the 19 patients gave their informed signed consent before the dry immersion.

Of the 19 patients, 14 had PD (10 males, 4 females, 47–73 years) and 5 had VP (1 male, 4 females, 65–72 years). Their anthropological data, medication, and disease characteristics: duration, form, stage of PD according to Hoehn and Yahr Rating Scale, and Unified Parkinson's disease Rating Scale (UPDRS) are presented in **Table 2**. All PD patients were recruited through the Department of Neurology, Psychiatry, and Microbiology, Petrozavodsk State University (Petrozavodsk,

TABLE 1 | Exclusion criteria for the patients.

Exclusion reason	Exclusion criteria
Masking or modification of parkinsonian symptoms	Other neurological disorder or injury that interferes motor function
	Osteoporosis
	Recent spinal fracture
	Metabolic disease (e.g., hyperthyreosis, diabetes)
Dry immersion absolute contraindications	Epilepsy
	Mental disorders
	Administration of muscle relaxants
	Cerebral palsy
Dry immersion relative contraindications (these pathologies are allowable during dry immersion when controlled properly, but we still excluded patients who had them)	Hypovolemia
	Myoma of uterus
	Atrial fibrillation
	Hemorrhage of various etiology
	Lung diseases in acute stage
	Oncologic problems
	Myocardial infarction
	Blood clotting disorders (e.g., phlebothrombosis or thrombophlebitis)

Russian Federation). This study was approved by Medical Ethic Committee of PetrSU and Ministry of health care and social development of Republic of Karelia.

2.2. Dry Immersion Procedure

For analog microgravity we utilized the medical system for imitation of weightlessness (MEDSIM, Institute of BioMedical Problems, Moscow, Russia). MEDSIM (**Figure 1**) appears as a bathtub filled with 2 m^3 of fresh water. The bathtub is covered by a thin waterproof film of a large size, which allows wrapping subject's body. On the bathtub floor, a motor driven raising platform is mounted. At the initial point the platform is positioned above the water level, enabling the subject to lie down on the film. When a dry immersion procedure starts, the platform lowers down into the water so that the subject stays immersed inside the bathtub wrapped in the film with face and upper part of thorax floating on the water surface. For further details of dry immersion (DI) physics and procedure see Navasiolava et al. (2011).

The patients were instructed to take their medicines at the same time (usually at 7 AM) to standardize conditions of DI and medication. The DI procedure started almost at the same time for each patient (at 9:30 a.m., ±10 min due to differences in time required for blood pressure stabilization). The temperature of water in the DI bathtub was set at 32°C, and it was also filtered and aerated. Before the procedure, the patients visited toilet to urinate, because DI has strong diuretic effect, and drunk a glass of fresh water (200 mL). Then the patients were allowed to adapt to experimental conditions for 10–15 min, lying on the platform wrapped in a cotton sheet to prevent body cooling. By the 10th min blood pressure (UA-767, A&D Company Ltd., Japan) was measured. If blood pressure was not higher than 140/80 mm Hg, the DI procedure was started. The patients were immersed in water in supine position for 45 min, with opportunity to stop the procedure by demand or clinical indications, which were ECG and blood pressure. ECG (Poly-Spectr VNS, Neirosoft Ltd., Ivanovo, Russia) was monitored in lead II to control heart rate and search for extrasystoles. Blood pressure was measured every 15 min (at 15th, 30th, and 45th min).

2.3. Measurements of Surface Electromyogram

The study corresponds to a common pre/post design: we compared surface electromyogram (sEMG) samples before and after a single dry immersion procedure. For our measurements, we used EMG device Neuro-MEP-4 and electrodes from Neurosoft Ltd. (Ivanovo, Russia). We measured sEMG bilaterally from *biceps brachii* muscle. The skin over the muscles was carefully cleaned with a cotton alcohol swab prior to electrodes placement. Abrasive products were not applied to prepare the skin because most of the subjects were older people. Due to the old age, many subjects also had obesity and big skin folds on their arms, which was the reason to choose bipolar plate-mounted electrodes, which have two relevant features. First, they provide closer positioning to the muscle due to their protruding leads. Second, they can be mounted by wrapping adhesive band around the arm, which prevents sliding of the electrode over the muscle. The electrodes were covered with conductive gel (Unimax, Geltek-Medica Company, Moscow, Russia) and applied to the muscle belly longitudinally between the innervation zone and cubital fossa. The electrodes were fixed with adhesive plaster to make sure that sEMG would be recorded from the same sites before and after the immersion. The electrodes were not removed between the pre- and post-immersion measurements. Reference electrode in the form of fabric wrist strap was moistened and attached to the right wrist. Prior to the testing, the subjects were carefully instructed to perform the test correctly, and they were allowed to practice shortly in order to get accustomed with the EMG device and the experimental setting. They were also allowed to warm up their muscles by performing several elbow flexions and extensions. Then we measured sEMG during a submaximal quasi-isometric holding test (Meigal et al., 2012). The recordings were made in standing position in four loading conditions: (1) with arms hanging freely along the trunk, (2) holding elbows flexed to 90° (forearm directed forward and parallel to floor) with palm open and directed upwards (0 kg), (3) with 1 kg, and (4) 2 kg load on each palm. Before each isometric holding, the patient was allowed to rest for a few seconds, after which the next load was introduced. In summary, for each patient we considered 2 body sides and 4 loading conditions and made the measurements before and after the immersion session, which made up at most 16 recordings per patient. Due to technical problems during the measurement, the recording from patient 3: 2 kg after the DI session and the recording from patient 9: 0 kg after the DI session were missing (the patients numbers are from **Table 2**).

Features and settings of the EMG device and properties of the electrodes were the following. The electrodes (Neurosoft

TABLE 2 | Information about the patients.

No.	Age (yr)	Gender	Height (cm), weight (kg)	Disease duration (yr)	UPDRS/ UPDRS-III	Stage by H & Y	Disease & symptoms	Antiparkinsonian medication
1	62	M	180, 69	7	70 / 37	2	PD, T	Piribedil 200 mg Levodopa 400 mg Carbidopa 62.5 mg Rasagiline 1.56 mg Amantadine 100 mg Entocapone 200 mg
2	64	F	160, 81	4	68 / 25	2	PD, T	Piribedil 20 mg Levodopa 250 mg Benserasid 62.5 mg
3	72	F	154, 66	8	98 / 48	2	VP, T	No medication (never administered)
4	68	M	169, 83	9	49 / 33	2.5	VP, T	Levodopa 975 mg Carbidopa 87.5 mg Amantadine 300 mg Piribedil 150 mg Benserasid 25 mg
5	71	M	170, 51	8	43 / 28	2	PD, T	Trihexyphenidyl 6 mg
6	68	F	164, 90	3	59 / 42	2.5	VP, T	Levodopa 225 mg Benserasid 25 mg Carbidopa 12.5 mg Piribedil 75 mg
7	73	M	172, 61	8	85 / 47	3	PD, T	Piribedil 100 mg Rasagiline 1.56 mg Levodopa 250 mg Carbidopa 25 mg
8	62	F	169, 81	4	41 / 26	2	PD, T	No medication (for 1 year*)
9	57	M	178, 63	6	65 / 48	2.5	PD, T	Piribedil 50 mg Amantadine 200 mg Levodopa 250 mg Carbidopa 25 mg
10	66	F	160, 67	2	21 / 13	2	VP, T	Levodopa 250 mg Carbidopa 25 mg Trihexyphenidyl 6 mg
11	66	F	156, 53	7	82 / 45	2	PD, T	Levodopa 250 mg Carbidopa 25 mg
12	53	M	171, 81	5	49 / 38	1.5	PD, AR	Piribedil 150 mg Amantadine 200 mg
13	70	M	176, 74	2	79 / 49	3	PD, T	Trihexyphenidyl 4 mg
14	68	M	167, 78	3	60 / 32	2	PD, AR	Levodopa 250 mg Carbidopa 25 mg Pramipexol 50 mg
15	66	F	172, 66	4	57 / 25	3	PD, AR	Levodopa 375 mg Carbidopa 37.5 mg Piribedil 50 mg
16	47	M	182, 81	3	45 / 16	3	PD, AR	No medication (for 1 month*)
17	58	M	170, 60	N/A	75 / 37	3	PD, T	Levodopa 300 mg Benserasid 75 mg Amantadine 200 mg

(Continued)

TABLE 2 | Continued

No.	Age (yr)	Gender	Height (cm), weight (kg)	Disease duration (yr)	UPDRS/ UPDRS-III	Stage by H & Y	Disease & symptoms	Antiparkinsonian medication
18	69	M	179, 69	4	60 / 32	3	PD, T	Piribedil 100 mg Levodopa 250 mg Carbidopa 25 mg
19	65	F	152, 78	7	51 / 15	1	VP, AR	Levodopa 500 mg Benserasid 100 mg Pramipexole 3 mg Amantadine 200 mg

*PD, Parkinson's disease; VP, vascular parkinsonism; UPDRS, Unified Parkinson's disease Rating Scale; UPDRS-III, UPDRS motor part III; H & Y, Hoehn and Yahr Rating Scale; T, tremor; AR, akinesia and rigidity; *these patients abandoned their therapy themselves.*

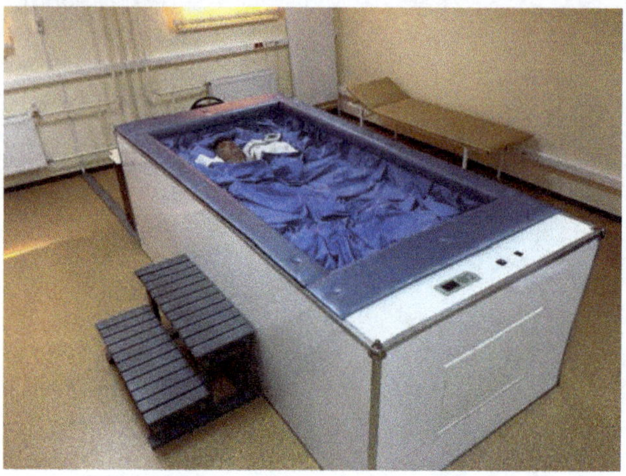

FIGURE 1 | The condition of dry immersion. © PetrSU/L. Gerasimova-Meigal.

Ltd., Ivanovo, Russia) were made of tin, disk-shaped (8 mm in diameter), with 20 mm spacing between the electrode centers. Input impedance was not less than 200 MΩ, and the measured impedance after electrode placement was not more 10 MΩ. The gain of differential amplifiers was set to 328, the ADC span was ±5 V, the ADC resolution was 16 bits, the peak-to-peak input-referred noise was not more than 5 μV, and the common mode rejection ratio (CMRR) was not less than 100 dB. Each sEMG recording was 3.5 s (70,000 samples) long. The sampling frequency was set to 20 kHz. The 50 Hz notch filter was enabled. The frequency bandwidth was 20–1,000 Hz, and the filters had 3 dB attenuation at the cutoff frequencies. The filters frequency responses corresponded to 1st order high-pass and 2nd order low-pass Butterworth filters.

2.4. Preprocessing of Surface Electromyogram

Data processing and analysis were made using Matlab software (MathWorks Inc., Natick, USA). Preprocessing of the data consisted of removal of power line interference, low-pass filtering, and detrending. Despite of the 50 Hz notch filter in the EMG device, we discovered sharp peaks at multiples of 50 Hz in the spectra of some sEMG recordings, so we applied Fourier interpolation (Mewett et al., 2004) to all the recordings in their frequency domain. The amplitudes in ±1 Hz range around the multiples of 50 Hz were replaced by interpolated values from the line drawn through two points adjacent to the range, while the phases were kept the same. The low-pass filtering was performed using a 14th order elliptic filter designed with Matlab `design` function (passband frequency 420 Hz, stopband frequency 500 Hz, passband ripple $2 \cdot 10^{-6}$ dB, stopband attenuation 80 dB, passband exact match). The filter was applied in both forward and reverse directions to avoid phase distortion. Then the recordings were detrended using the smoothness priors method (Tarvainen et al., 2002) to remove possible movement artifacts. The smoothness priors method is based on regularized least squares and operates as a time-varying FIR high-pass filter with the cutoff frequency gradually changing to zero near the beginning and the end of a signal. Higher values of the only parameter λ correspond to lower cutoff frequencies. We used $\lambda = 10^5$, which corresponds to attenuation of -40 dB at 10 Hz in the middle of a signal sampled at 20 kHz.

2.5. Parameters of Surface Electromyogram

2.5.1. Amplitude and Spectral Parameters

We calculated amplitude (root mean square) of the recordings and median frequency of power spectrum of the recordings. The power spectrum was calculated as Welch periodogram with segment length of 1 s and 50% segment overlap. The segments spectrum was obtained using fast Fourier transform (Matlab `fft` function). Hann window was applied to the segments prior to the spectrum calculation to eliminate spectrum distortion because of nonzero values at the segments edges.

2.5.2. Time Delay Embedding Transformation of Surface Electromyogram

In the nonlinear dynamics based analysis, it is assumed that the examined system is governed by a set of free variables, which follow a trajectory in their space. When the original free variables are unobtainable, the trajectory is replaced by a surrogate obtained from one-dimensional time series. This procedure is called phase space reconstruction and is justified by the embedding theorem (Mañé, 1981; Takens, 1981). As our sEMG recordings were one-dimensional, we applied the time delay embedding transformation to reconstruct the phase space trajectory. The one-dimensional sEMG time series $\{x_1, x_2, ..., x_n\}$ was transformed to sequences of vectors in m-dimensional space as in Equation (1).

$$X_i = (x_i, x_{i+L}, x_{i+2L}, ..., x_{i+(m-1)L})^T \quad (1)$$

The L parameter is called time lag. With properly chosen m and L parameters, the reconstruction produces a smooth m-dimensional trajectory that preserves some features of the presumed original trajectory in a space of free variables of the examined system.

L was chosen with the help of mutual information (MI) as advised by Celucci et al. (2003). The MI of a signal and the same signal shifted backwards in time on τ sampling periods was calculated with τ varying from 1 to 500 sampling periods, which produced a dependence MI(τ) for each sEMG recording. To calculate the MI of real-valued signals, we used the algorithm of Fraser and Swinney (1986). We slightly tuned the algorithm: recordings duration was not truncated to the nearest power of two, and the recursive splitting of the histogram bins was stopped when the number of points in a bin was less or equal to a preset value 547, which maximized smoothness of the MI(τ) dependencies. First minimum of MI(τ) (MI decay time) was converted to milliseconds and used as a separate signal parameter, and L was chosen as median MI decay time ($L = 54$ sampling periods). We used median instead of mean because the Kolmogorov-Smirnov test showed that the distribution of MI decay time was not normal.

We used false nearest neighbors (FNN) method to choose m (Kennel et al., 1992; Celucci et al., 2003). The dependence FNN(m) was calculated with m varying from 1 to 15, then the embedding dimension was chosen as the point where for all the recordings FNN dropped to 1% of the initial value or lower ($m = 6$).

2.5.3. Correlation Dimension and Sample Entropy

Correlation dimension was chosen as the slope of linear segment of the sEMG correlation integral in double logarithmic scale (Grassberger and Procaccia, 1983). The correlation integral was calculated with Theiler window $W_{CD} = 270$ ($W_{CD} = (m-1)L$, Gao and Zheng (1994)). We calculated sample entropy (Richman and Moorman, 2000) using Euclidean interpoint distances and the tolerance distance $r_{SampEn} = 1.15$. The measurements were normalized to unit standard deviation prior to the sample entropy calculation. The tolerance distance r_{SampEn} was fitted to maximize the difference between the maximum and minimum values of sample entropy. This fitting, on the one hand, does not imply any assumptions about the effect of dry immersion on sample entropy. On the other hand, it increases the differences of sample entropy between the recordings and, therefore, the potential of sample entropy to distinguish muscles' states.

2.5.4. Recurrence Quantification Analysis

Recurrence quantification analysis (RQA) parameters were calculated from recurrence plots (Marwan et al., 2007) of the recordings. Recurrence plot (Rec) is a tool for visualization of m-dimensional phase space trajectories on a plane. Rec is a square matrix of ones (black points) and zeros (white points) with a column i and a row j corresponding to the trajectory points X_i and X_j. Rec(i,j) is equal to one if the corresponding trajectory points X_i and X_j are not further apart from each other than the threshold distance ε and is equal to zero otherwise. Since consecutive ($i - j < W$) trajectory points tend to be close to each other, their proximity is not informative and is typically not shown on Rec, which produces a white strip along the main diagonal of Rec. Thus, Rec shows the periods of time when the trajectory passes close by its previous locations, which may be movement parallel to an earlier trajectory segment (diagonal lines) or enveloping movement perpendicularly to the segment (vertical lines). RQA quantifies the diagonal and vertical lines (we only quantified the diagonal lines). The recordings were normalized on mean Euclidean interpoint distance $\|X_i - X_j\|$, $i - j > 0$ prior to the RQA. Then we calculated recurrence rate (share of black points of Rec) and determinism (share of black points those form diagonal lines with the length not less than l_{min}). The auxiliary parameters ε, W, and minimum diagonal line length l_{min} were fitted to maximize the span of determinism similarly to sample entropy ($\varepsilon = 0.7$, $W = 270$, $l_{min} = 86$). However, in contrary to sample entropy, determinism may take saturated values 0 and 100%, which renders some sEMG recordings indistinguishable by their determinism because they share the same saturated value of it. Therefore, we fitted the auxiliary parameters so that to avoid the saturated values. We also limited the minimum index difference W so that $W \geq W_{CD}$.

2.6. Statistical Analysis

The statistical analysis was performed separately for each body side, each loading condition, and each parameter (2 sides $\times$ 4 conditions $\times$ 7 parameters = 56 statistical tests). The pre-immersion recordings from patients 3 and 4 those did not have the post-immersion counterpart were discarded from the statistical analysis. We used the Wilcoxon test to compare the parameters values before and after the dry immersion. This test quantifies within-subject differences for repeated measures. The reason to use a nonparametric test was that the distributions of the differences were not normal in most of the cases; the normality was tested using the Kolmogorov-Smirnov test. The p-values from the Wilcoxon test were compared to the significance level 0.05. We did not apply any correction for multiple comparisons because we had only one research question of whether dry immersion relieves motor symptoms, which are seen by sEMG in parkinsonian patients, so all the comparisons were complementary.

3. RESULTS

The general finding was that the post-immersion values of the surface electromyogram (sEMG) parameters tended to be different comparing to the pre-immersion values, excluding the correlation dimension. See the **Tables 3, 4** for median values and interquartile ranges of the parameters before and after the dry immersion, and for the percentages of patients for whom the parameters increased or decreased after the dry immersion. In the **Tables 3, 4**, the 2 pre-immersion recordings with missing post-immersion counterpart are not considered.

See **Figure 2** for changes of the determinism for each patient. One can trace the tendency of determinism to decrease, which is more visible for the left biceps. For half of the patients (No. 2, 4, 8, 10, 11, 12, 14, 16, and 18), the determinism of recordings from the left biceps decreased no matter of the loading. What comes to the right biceps, the determinism values were often close to those for the left biceps, and the determinism changes were approximately parallel to those for the left biceps, although some exceptions occured, especially for the "arms down" loading. One may also consider that the changes near the bottom limit of determinism (patients No. 5, 11, 17, 19: "arms down" loading) are not very informative since determinism inherently cannot decrease below zero. See **Figure 3** for general picture of changes of the amplitude, the median frequency, and the determinism. As for the determinism, the tendency of the amplitude to decrease and the tendency of the median frequency to increase were apparent for the left biceps only, so the pictures for the right biceps are not shown. See **Figure 4** for an example of sEMG before and after the immersion. One can visually observe the drop of signal regularity and hence determinism.

The statistical analysis revealed that the following changes of the sEMG parameters were statistically significant. The amplitude decreased for both arms with the "arms down" loading and for the left arm with the 1 and 2 kg loadings. The median frequency increased for the left arm with the 1 and 2 kg loadings. Mutual information decay time decreased for the left arm with the 0 and 2 kg loadings. Sample entropy increased for both arms with the "arms down" loading and for the left arm with the 1 kg loading. Recurrence rate decreased for both arms with the "arms down" loading and for the left arm with the 1 kg loading. Determinism decreased for both arms with the "arms down" loading and for the left arm with the 1 and 2 kg loadings. The most statistically significant ($p = 0.00084$) change was for the determinism from the left biceps with 1 kg loading, which decreased for 16 out of 19 patients.

As regards the multiplicity of the statistical tests applied, the number of their results with $p < 0.05$ was enough to make an overall conclusion that sEMG parameters changed after the dry immersion. Indeed, if all the null hypotheses had been true then we would have had $p < 0.05$ for 5% of the hypotheses, but we had $p < 0.05$ for 32% of the hypotheses.

4. DISCUSSION

The key hypothesis of this study postulated that a single one dry immersion (DI) exerts effect on the motor system in parkinsonian patients. Surface electromyogram (sEMG) signal during isometric contraction was assumed to be indicative of such effect. The major outcome of the present study was that the parameters of sEMG signal in parkinsonian patients indeed modified in the direction of improvement under a single DI session. Generally, we found that the amplitude and mutual information decay time of sEMG had decreased, while spectral frequencies had increased right after DI session. Among nonlinear dynamics based sEMG parameters, sample entropy had increased, while percent of determinism and recurrence rate had decreased after DI session. Correlation dimension proved insensitive to DI.

On one hand, the amplitude of sEMG is known to correlate with the number of active motor units and their firing rate (Farina et al., 2004). On the other hand, the rigidity in parkinsonian patients is often seen as "unwilled" muscle tension generated by uncontrolled firing of low-threshold (slow) motor units at rest (Cantello et al., 1995; Rossi et al., 1996). Therefore, we assume that lowered amplitude of sEMG in parkinsonian patients after DI session found in the present study may be attributed to decreased recruitment of these unconsciously active motor units, either at rest condition or under loading. Two neurophysiological mechanisms may have contributed to the decrease of sEMG amplitude after DI session.

First, sEMG amplitude may have decreased due to attenuation of the reflexive component of muscle tone. Such immersion-induced attenuation of the stretch reflex has been characteristic for another type of exaggerated muscle tone (spasticity) (Cronin et al., 2016). Similarly, in healthy subjects under a program of DI the reflex component of muscle tone has been diminished due to deprivation of excitatory tonic stimuli from the pacinian corpuscles of sole (Kozlovskaya et al., 1988; Navasiolava et al., 2011). In our recent study we have found that the rigidity subscore has indeed decreased under the program of short-term DI sessions (Meigal et al., 2018). However, the non-reflexive (mechano-elastic) component of muscle tone may also have contributed to the decrease of rigidity score. Further studying of the stretch reflex and viscoelasticity of muscles in PD patients under DI is needed to evaluate their contribution to hypotonic effect of DI.

Second, as muscle tone appears as muscle state of readiness to contraction (Davis et al., 2011) triggered by brainstem, basal ganglia, cerebellum, and cortical circuits in stressful conditions, we assume that central neural mechanisms might also have been involved in sEMG amplitude decreasing in PD patients during DI session. That is in good line with our earlier finding that after a program of DI the score of depression has significantly decreased (Meigal et al., 2018). As such, the DI condition has probably exerted its action on muscle hypertonicity (rigidity) via lowering the level of anxiety and thus relieving disinhibition of the stretch reflex. In an earlier study, Koryak (2002) have shown that electrically evoked maximal tetanic contraction force decreased by 8.2 after 7 days of DI, which suggests that most of the force loss was due to a reduction in motor drive. This supports the supraspinal application of DI action on sEMG parameters in PD patients. Similar decrease of central activation reflected in lower sEMG amplitude has been recently reported for the condition of hyperthermia (Coletta et al., 2018).

However, the amplitude of sEMG has decreased under DI at all loading conditions. That raises the question of whether sEMG amplitude in PD patients has decreased during DI due

TABLE 3 | Amplitude (RMS), median frequency, and mutual information (MI) decay time of surface electromyogram before and after the dry immersion (DI).

Muscle	Load	Electromyogram parameter	Median (IQR) before the DI	Median (IQR) after the DI	Drop (%)	Rise (%)	No change (%)	*p*-value
Right arm biceps	Arms down	Amplitude (μV)	1.7 (1.3, 2.1)	1.2 (0.66, 2.3)	79	21	0	0.024*
		Median frequency (Hz)	73 (36, 107)	90 (74, 111)	42	58	0	0.15
		MI decay time (ms)	4.2 (3.7, 7.2)	3.9 (2.4, 6)	58	37	5	0.21
	0 kg	Amplitude (μV)	15 (8, 25)	12 (8, 19)	67	33	0	0.18
		Median frequency (Hz)	96 (85, 101)	96 (89, 108)	44	56	0	0.25
		MI decay time (ms)	3 (2.6, 3.5)	2.7 (2.5, 3.1)	61	39	0	0.053
	1 kg	Amplitude (μV)	29 (15, 36)	21 (14, 40)	47	53	0	0.57
		Median frequency (Hz)	97 (87, 102)	101 (90, 105)	42	58	0	0.15
		MI decay time (ms)	2.7 (2.6, 3)	2.7 (2.5, 3)	52	37	11	0.32
	2 kg	Amplitude (μV)	34 (19, 56)	36 (21, 49)	50	50	0	0.88
		Median frequency (Hz)	95 (84, 100)	100 (85, 105)	28	72	0	0.053
		MI decay time (ms)	2.7 (2.5, 3.1)	2.6 (2.5, 3.1)	56	33	11	0.13
Left arm biceps	Arms down	Amplitude (μV)	1.6 (0.99, 2.9)	0.91 (0.53, 1.7)	79	21	0	0.016*
		Median frequency (Hz)	74 (27, 123)	114 (34, 175)	32	68	0	0.084
		MI decay time (ms)	4 (2, 11)	2 (1.4, 6.7)	63	26	11	0.062
	0 kg	Amplitude (μV)	14 (8, 21)	11 (4, 19)	78	22	0	0.071
		Median frequency (Hz)	104 (90, 112)	109 (96, 139)	39	61	0	0.064
		MI decay time (ms)	2.5 (2.4, 3)	2.3 (1.8, 3.1)	83	17	0	0.011*
	1 kg	Amplitude (μV)	24 (12, 33)	20 (7, 30)	68	32	0	0.024*
		Median frequency (Hz)	98 (88, 110)	108 (92, 130)	26	74	0	0.036*
		MI decay time (ms)	2.6 (2.3, 3)	2.4 (2, 2.9)	68	21	11	0.055
	2 kg	Amplitude (μV)	30 (16, 48)	24 (9, 36)	78	22	0	0.0029*
		Median frequency (Hz)	99 (82, 110)	111 (86, 125)	22	78	0	0.0057*
		MI decay time (ms)	2.7 (2.3, 3.3)	2.3 (2, 3)	72	28	0	0.02*

The picture of individual changes of a parameter is described with the percentages of patients for whom the parameter decreased (Drop), increased (Rise), or did not change. The p-values are the results of assessment of a parameter changes using the Wilcoxon test.
$^*p < 0.05$; IQR, interquartile range.

to inhibition of uncontrolled firing of "unwilled" motor units, or due to inhibition of voluntarily recruited motor units. The decrease of sEMG amplitude at loading was bigger in comparison with the decrease at the non-loading condition when arms were hanging down. Therefore, we assume that at loading conditions, besides these abnormally active "unwilled" motor units, some normally recruited motor units were also inhibited by DI. Passive heating has been already shown to inhibit spontaneous rest activity of motor units in PD patients (Meigal and Lupandin, 2005).

As for the nonlinear dynamics based sEMG parameters, several earlier studies have shown that in PD patients their values significantly differ from those in healthy controls. In particular, percent of recurrence rate and determinism of sEMG was higher in the PD group, while entropy and correlation dimension were lower in comparison to old and young healthy controls (Fattorini et al., 2005; Meigal et al., 2009). High percent of determinism reflects appearance of "recurrent fragments" on sEMG similar to one another, which is argued to originate from increased synchronization of motor units firing (Fattorini et al., 2005). In turn, such increased regularity of sEMG in PD indicates presence of mechanical tremor (Meigal et al., 2012). That is in line with growth of the spectral frequency of sEMG under certain loading conditions revealed in the present study, which may be associated with decreased synchronization of motor units (Fattorini et al., 2005). Therefore, shift of determinism and recurrence rate of sEMG after a single one DI session in the direction of lower values may be indicative of diminished synchronization of motor units firing and, hence, temporary inhibition of parkinsonian tremor. In our recent study we observed decrease of tremor score in some PD patients (Meigal et al., 2018). Still, direct accelerometric measurements are needed to validate that effect in a single DI session.

However, motor unit synchronization during muscle contraction is not a uniform phenomenon. Several forms of motor unit synchronization have been demonstrated (McAuley and Marsden, 2000). The first one is short-term synchronization (STS) that occurs within short time period (around 5 ms) as reflected with a narrow peak in the cross-correlogram (Kirkwood et al., 1982). The STS may either arise from the common axonal inputs to pairs of motoneurones (Sears and Stagg, 1976; Nordstrom et al., 1992) or be just an epiphenomenon of firing rate characteristics (Kline and de Luca, 2016). The other form of synchronization is long-term (or broad-peak) one (LTS) that

TABLE 4 | Nonlinear dynamics based parameters of surface electromyogram before and after the dry immersion (DI).

Muscle	Load	Electromyogram parameter	Median (IQR) before the DI	Median (IQR) after the DI	Drop (%)	Rise (%)	*p*-value
Right arm biceps	Arms down	Sample entropy	0.89 (0.73, 0.97)	0.96 (0.84, 1)	16	84	0.0089*
		Correlation dimension	6 (5.6, 6.2)	6 (5.5, 6.1)	53	47	0.81
		Recurrence rate (%)	11 (10, 16)	10 (9, 14)	89	11	0.0089*
		Determinism (%)	36 (21, 67)	20 (11, 54)	84	16	0.0079*
	0 kg	Sample entropy	0.9 (0.84, 0.92)	0.92 (0.85, 0.95)	33	67	0.18
		Correlation dimension	5.7 (5.2, 6.3)	5.6 (5.2, 5.8)	67	33	0.23
		Recurrence rate (%)	11 (10, 13)	10 (10, 13)	56	44	0.42
		Determinism (%)	49 (44, 60)	46 (37, 62)	56	44	0.1
	1 kg	Sample entropy	0.92 (0.87, 0.95)	0.92 (0.82, 0.94)	53	47	0.97
		Correlation dimension	6 (5.5, 6.4)	6.1 (5.6, 6.6)	42	58	0.57
		Recurrence rate (%)	10 (10, 13)	11 (10, 13)	47	53	0.69
		Determinism (%)	53 (41, 60)	51 (41, 61)	58	42	0.49
	2 kg	Sample entropy	0.93 (0.88, 0.95)	0.94 (0.89, 0.95)	50	50	0.88
		Correlation dimension	6.2 (5.7, 6.5)	5.7 (5, 6.2)	72	28	0.2
		Recurrence rate (%)	10 (9, 12)	10 (9, 12)	44	56	0.4
		Determinism (%)	44 (42, 53)	41 (38, 58)	67	33	0.33
Left arm biceps	Arms down	Sample entropy	0.89 (0.69, 0.97)	0.95 (0.88, 1)	26	74	0.0048*
		Correlation dimension	5.9 (5.6, 6.2)	6 (5.9, 6.3)	37	63	0.44
		Recurrence rate (%)	12 (10, 17)	10 (9, 13)	68	32	0.018*
		Determinism (%)	42 (19, 76)	27 (8, 43)	84	16	0.0062*
	0 kg	Sample entropy	0.92 (0.71, 0.96)	0.94 (0.81, 0.98)	28	72	0.085
		Correlation dimension	5.8 (5.5, 6.2)	5.9 (5.6, 6.2)	39	61	0.53
		Recurrence rate (%)	11 (10, 15)	11 (10, 15)	50	50	0.78
		Determinism (%)	46 (35, 58)	39 (26, 65)	78	22	0.11
	1 kg	Sample entropy	0.93 (0.85, 0.96)	0.96 (0.92, 0.99)	21	79	0.0033*
		Correlation dimension	6 (5.7, 6.2)	5.8 (5.6, 6.4)	53	47	0.69
		Recurrence rate (%)	11 (9, 12)	10 (9, 12)	68	32	0.049*
		Determinism (%)	40 (36, 53)	36 (23, 40)	84	16	0.00084*
	2 kg	Sample entropy	0.94 (0.91, 0.96)	0.96 (0.93, 0.98)	39	61	0.11
		Correlation dimension	5.9 (5.5, 6.5)	5.9 (5.6, 6.4)	44	56	0.78
		Recurrence rate (%)	10 (9, 12)	10 (9, 11)	44	56	0.81
		Determinism (%)	42 (34, 48)	35 (27, 43)	78	22	0.0065*

The picture of individual changes of a parameter is described with the percentages of patients for whom the parameter decreased (Drop) or increased (Rise). The p-values are the results of assessment of a parameter changes using the Wilcoxon test.
$^*p < 0.05$; IQR, interquartile range.

occurs within broader time band (> 20 ms) (Kirkwood et al., 1982; Freund, 1983). LTS comes into play when a large group of motoneurons starts to respond synchronically to a periodic synaptic input either of supraspinal or segmentary afferent origins (Kirkwood et al., 1982). Also, a tuned (or external) synchronization may arise when common inputs to a pair of motoneurones are themselves driven by a common input (McAuley and Marsden, 2000).

In PD, large part of motor units present specific firing pattern in a form of rhythmical groups of discharges (doublets and, occasionally, triplets). These groups are separated with longer interspike intervals and are associated with 4–6 Hz clustering on sEMG (Baker et al., 1992; Lupandin et al., 1993; Glendinning and Enoka, 1994). This pattern of firing is believed to largely contribute to generation of tremor in PD (Christakos et al., 2009). Doublets may also be associated with LTS that is seen as broad periodic correlations on cross-correlogram (Baker et al., 1992). As follows from these studies, both motor units synchrony and paired/tripled discharges may be responsible for greater values of determinism of sEMG in PD patients. STS has been shown to be greater in PD patients than in normal subjects but no evidence has been found that the higher incidence of STS in PD is a result of lower discharge rates of motor units or 4–6 Hz tremor that is the characteristic of PD patients (Baker et al., 1992).

Sample entropy has increased in some instances after the DI session. According to recent findings, sample entropy is higher when the motor units fire with higher variability of interspike intervals (Hwang et al., 2017).

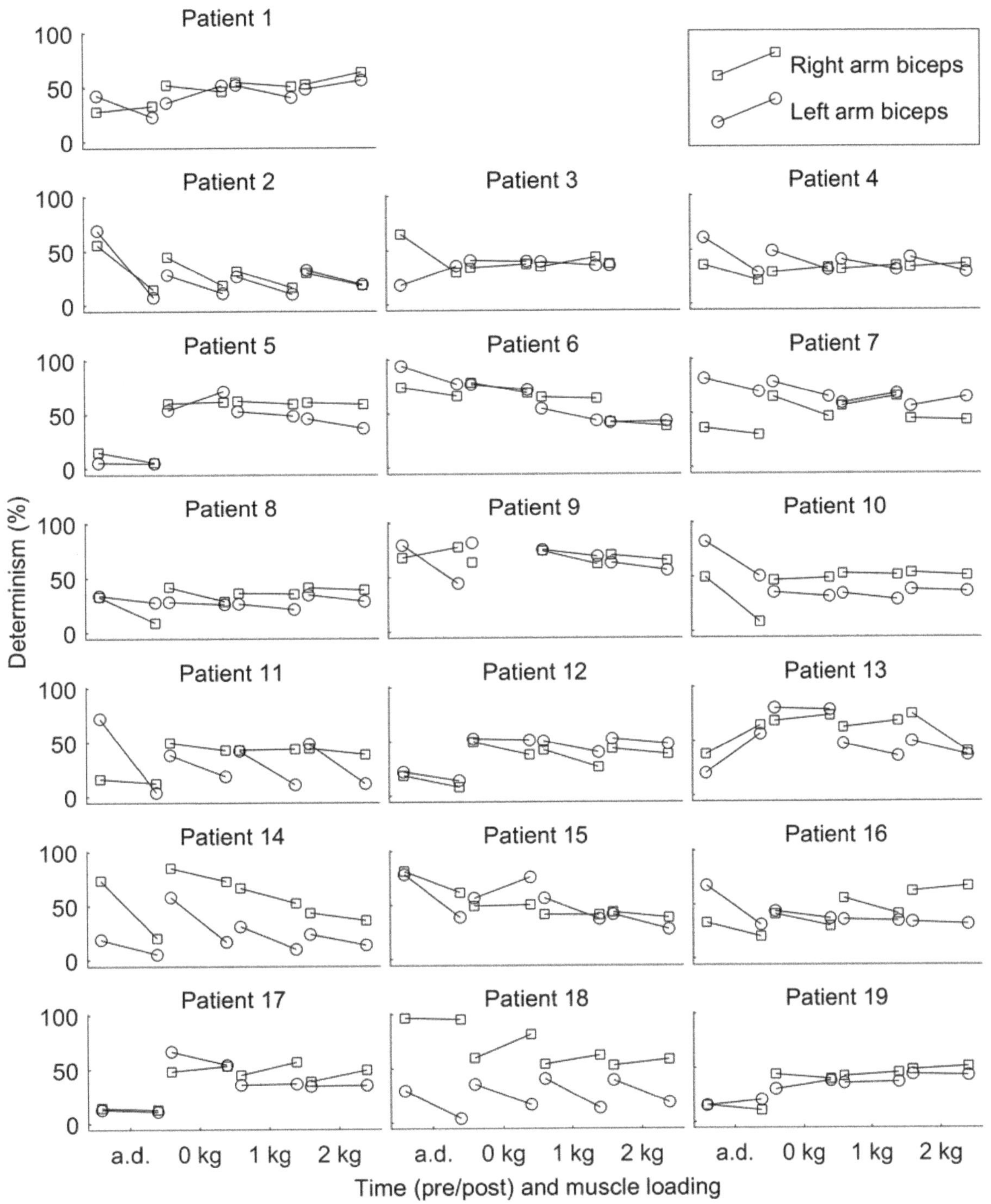

FIGURE 2 | Determinism of surface electromyogram for each patient before and after the dry immersion. The determinism tends to decrease after the dry immersion. Loading conditions are the following: arms down with no load (*a.d.*); 0, 1, and 2 kg loading on each hand with elbow being flexed to 90°.

The mutual information (MI) decay time, or first minimum of auto-mutual information function, quantifies how quickly information about a signal is lost as a function of time delay. MI decay time measures information transmission between a signal and its time shifted counterpart (Jeong et al., 2001) and, consequently, predictability of the signal (Ramanand et al., 2010). Also, MI decay time is regarded as a relevant estimator of irregularity of signal (Escudero et al., 2009). Though MI time decay has been already applied to measure information transmission within electroencephalographic signal (Jeong et al.,

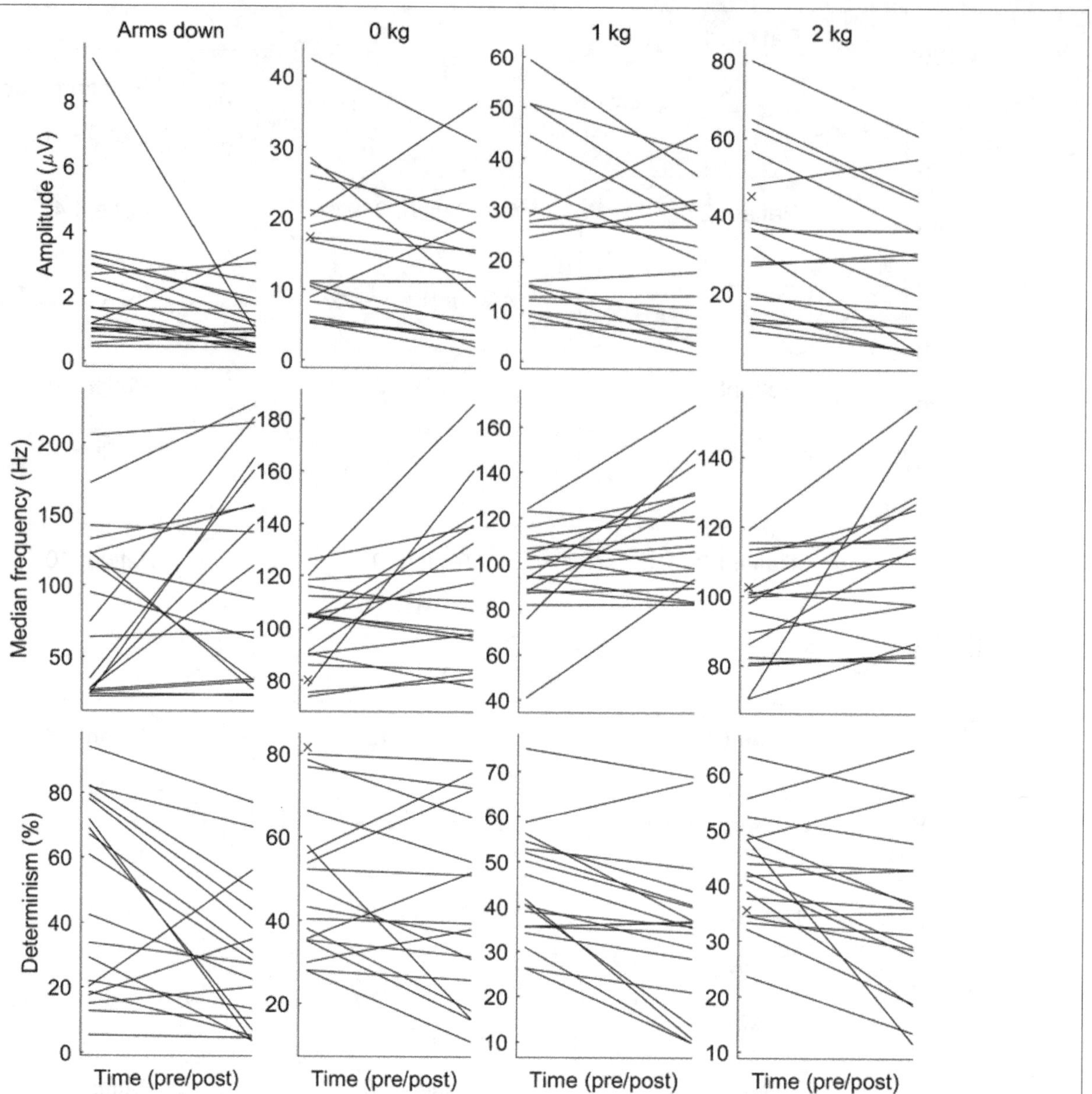

FIGURE 3 | The amplitude (RMS), the median frequency, and the determinism of surface electromyogram before and after the dry immersion. The amplitude and the determinism tend to decrease, while the median frequency tends to increase after the dry immersion. Each patient is denoted by a line. Each subplot corresponds to a combination of a parameter (the row) and a loading (the column). Loading conditions are the following: arms down without any load (*Arms down*); *0/1/2 kg* loading on each hand with elbow being flexed to 90°. The muscle is the biceps of the left arm. The pre-immersion values are marked with crosses when the post-immersion counterpart is missing.

2001; Ramanand et al., 2010) and heart rate (Hoyer et al., 2005), to the best of our knowledge it has not yet been used to characterize sEMG. Correspondingly, neurophysiology behind MI decay time for sEMG has not yet been well understood. In our study, the MI decay time lasted from 1 to 13 ms, and it had tendency to decrease after DI session. Visual inspection of sEMG records showed that those with lower MI decay time values had shorter turns of sEMG curve, while those with higher values of MI decay time had longer turns (see **Figure 4**). Therefore, we assume that MI decay time may correlate with average duration of signal turns or longer patterns those are typical for a particular sEMG recording. Also, duration of MI decay time overlaps with that of STS. That prompts hypothetic association between these two parameters, because STS has been shown to be characteristic of PD patients (Baker et al., 1992). As such, we speculate that DI might decrease STS during DI session.

From several studies it is known that percent of determinism of sEMG responds to certain anti-PD therapies. For example, under dopaminergic anti-PD treatment percent of determinism

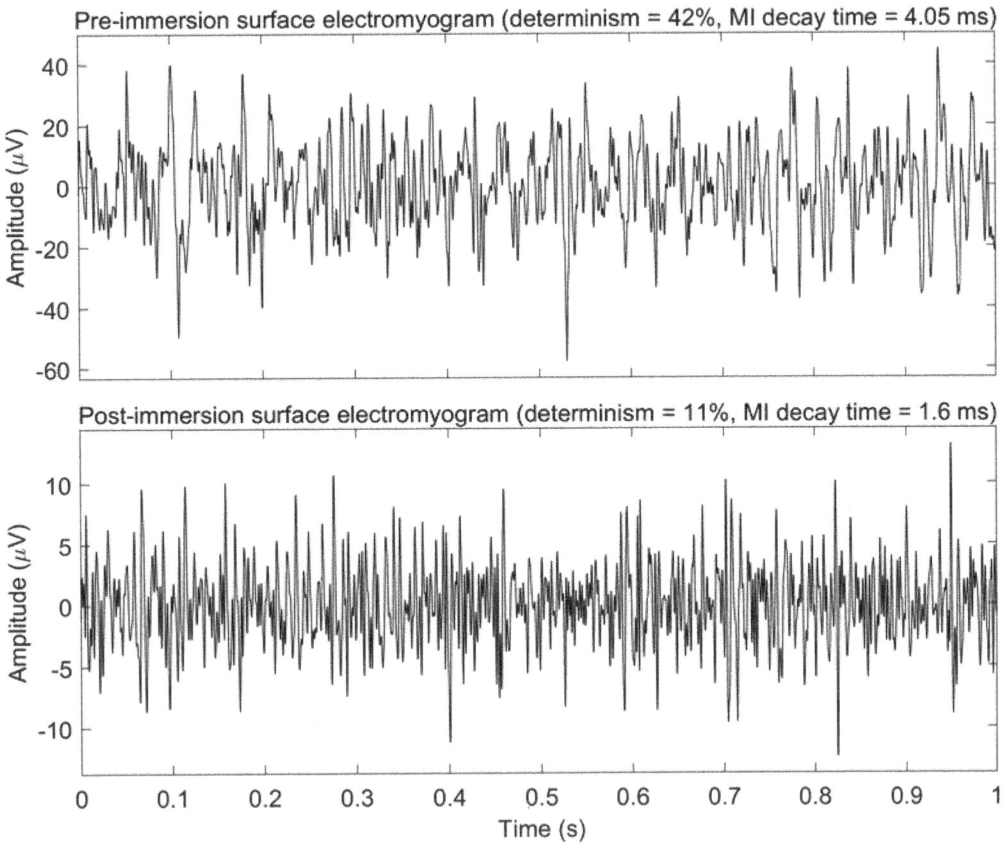

FIGURE 4 | Example of surface electromyogram before and after the dry immersion procedure (patient No. 11 in **Table 2**; 1 kg loading; left arm). Only first second of the electromyograms is shown. This example demonstrates drop of amplitude, mutual information (MI) decay time, and determinism of electromyogram signal after the dry immersion. MI decay time may be linked to typical duration of turns of electromyogram, and determinism may be linked to regularity of electromyogram.

of sEMG is decreased in comparison with the off-medication state (Rissanen et al., 2008; Ruonala et al., 2018). Similarly, after deep brain stimulation, sEMG signal characteristics turned more similar to the signal characteristics of the healthy controls (Rissanen et al., 2011). That is in good line with the result of the present study. We found only a few corresponding papers on the amount of motor unit synchrony after taking anti-PD medicine. In one, short-term synchrony was found to be irresponsible to taking levodopa (Baker et al., 1992). Therefore, we assume that analog microgravity induced by DI modulates the nonlinear dynamics based parameters of sEMG of parkinsonian patients by decreasing the long-term form of motor unit synchronization. We cannot exclude possible influence of DI also on the amount of motor unit doublets.

The most reliable neural site for effects of DI on motor unit synchrony and, hence, determinism of sEMG, presumably is located supraspinally, because (i) the above mentioned anti-PD therapies act directly on brain structures, and (ii) there is large corpus of data supporting the idea of supraspinal location of oscillatory circuits those generate the characteristic PD tremor (Timmermann et al., 2003). However, DI might also exerted certain peripheral action due to its well-documented unloading effect on muscles. We did not find corresponding data on nonlinear dynamics based parameters of sEMG during muscle contraction under the condition of real spaceflight. As for the physiological tremor, it is modified in the direction of lower frequency (as low as 4 Hz) and decreased amplitude by the 3rd day of space flight, presumably due to switch of main source of sensory information from load-dependent muscle reception to position-dependent joint reception (Gallasch et al., 1994). Thus, one may expect growth of regularity and decrease of amplitude of sEMG under the condition of real spaceflight. However, growth of determinism of sEMG was not the case in the present study. Several significant distinctions from real spaceflight condition could be figured out that probably contributed to such discrepancy. First, in our study, duration of analog microgravity was too short to induce the above said effect of microgravity on tremor. Second, arms under DI were not deprived of force-induced muscle afferent inputs. Additionally, in the present study, unlike to space based experiments, sEMG was collected under normal gravity, both before and after the session of DI. Thus, the condition of DI despite of its strong similarity with real microgravity cannot provide its absolute emulation.

The present study demonstrated large variance of sEMG parameters that might be associated with heterogeneity of clinical forms and severity of parkinsonism. Earlier, we demonstrated that percent of determinism of sEMG positively correlates with the UPDRS (part III) (Meigal et al., 2009) and tremor acceleration characteristic (Meigal et al., 2012). It means that with growing severity of PD tremor becomes more regular, while sEMG becomes more apparently clustered. We did not correlate percent of determinism of sEMG with the form of PD earlier, nor in this study due to insufficient number of parkinsonian patients with akinetic-rigid form. Further studies should have aimed on that.

4.1. Loading Conditions

In the present study the most readily seen modifications of sEMG parameters were the characteristic of the condition when arms were freely hanging down without any load. Earlier we found that the most significant differences between PD and control groups were observed when no additional loading was placed on hands during the isometric elbow flexion task (Meigal et al., 2009). We concluded that additional loading applied on hands most likely revealed "regular" postural muscle tonus. In a way, under loading, sEMG of parkinsonian patients may have become more "normal" in comparison to the unloading condition. However, the results for the condition with arms freely hanging down should be treated with caution, because the sEMG amplitude was comparable to typical level of the noise generated on a fully relaxed biceps (Piervirgili et al., 2014).

4.2. Limitations

The major methodological limitation in the present study was small number of subjects who met all inclusion criteria ($n = 19$). Such relatively small number of parkinsonian patients and big number of factors (disease duration, clinical form, stage of disease, age, sex, medication) presumably affecting the outcome restricted opportunities of statistical analysis. Earlier experiments with younger subjects showed that the most effect of microgravity on muscle tone is observed by 2 h of staying of healthy subjects under the DI environment (Navasiolava et al., 2011). In this study, average age of patients was around 65 years. That restricts their tolerance to the DI procedure, mostly for the reason of urge to urinate and, in some instances, due to unstable blood pressure. Also, staying in DI reportedly provokes some compensated neurological signs (Navasiolava et al., 2011). In older subjects, especially neurologically ill, such hidden symptoms may have taken place. However, a 45 min long DI session was still enough to exert effect on sEMG parameters in parkinsonian patients.

In that study we omitted measuring UPDRS scores right after the DI session due to highly probable inference of cardiovascular factors, such as DI-induced decrease of blood pressure and orthostatic reactions, on motor signs (gait, postural reactions, muscle tone) in PD patients. From our earlier study we know that muscle rigidity subtotal of UPDRS-III score and, to lesser degree, tremor subtotal, decrease across the program of DI (Meigal et al., 2018). In further studies, it would be wise to correlate sEMG parameters with clinical symptoms and scales that characterize parkinsonian patients for better understanding of the association between sEMG and motor symptoms. The idiopathic Parkinson's disease and vascular parkinsonism must be compared in their compliance to DI therapy. Additionally, it would be of interest to trace the net effect of several, rather than one, DI sessions on sEMG.

4.3. In Conclusion

The results presented here provide promising evidence that such analog microgravity environment as dry immersion exerts significant influence on the motor system in parkinsonian patients, as it is seen from surface electromyogram modification after a single short-term dry immersion session. The major outcome of the study was that the amplitude, mutual information decay time, recurrence rate, and determinism of surface electromyogram decreased whereas median frequency and sample entropy, in contrast, increased right after dry immersion. This evidences decreased rigidity and weakened tremor seen as synchronicity of motor unit activity.

AUTHOR CONTRIBUTIONS

GM has contributed by data analysis and interpretation, and by writing of the manuscript. AM has contributed by the research conception, design of the work, data acquisition and interpretation, and by writing of the manuscript. IS and LC have contributed by the research conception, design of the work, and by critical revision of the manuscript. LG-M has contributed by design of the work, data acquisition, and by writing of the manuscript. NS has contributed by design of the work, data acquisition, and by critical revision of the manuscript. SR and PK have contributed by data analysis and interpretation, and by critical revision of the manuscript. All the authors have read and approved the manuscript before the publication and agree to be accountable for all aspects of the research.

FUNDING

This study was financially supported by the University of Eastern Finland Doctoral Project funding to GM, by the Ministry of Higher Education and Science of Russian Federation (grants #761 and #17.7302.2017/VU to AM), and by Petrozavodsk State University Strategic Development Program (grant AAAA-A16-116093010011-5 to AM).

ACKNOWLEDGMENTS

We would like to thank CSC - IT CENTER FOR SCIENCE LTD. (Espoo, Finland) for giving us access to Taito supercluster, which helped to process our data rapidly.

REFERENCES

Alves, G., Wentzel-Larsen, T., Aarsland, D., and Larsen, J. P. (2005). Progression of motor impairment and disability in Parkinson disease: a population-based study. *Neurology* 65, 1436–1441. doi: 10.1212/01.wnl.0000183359.50822.f2

Baker, J. R., Davey, N. J., Ellaway, P. H., and Friediland, C. L. (1992). Short-term synchrony of motor unit discharge during weak isometric contraction in Parkinson's disease. *Brain* 115, 137–154. doi: 10.1093/brain/115.1.137

Baradaran, N., Tan, S. N., Liu, A., Ashoori, A., Palmer, S. J., Wang, Z. J., et al. (2013). Parkinson's disease rigidity: relation to brain connectivity and motor performance. *Front. Neurol.* 4:67. doi: 10.3389/fneur.2013.00067

Boccia, G., Dardanello, D., Beretta-Piccoli, M., Cescon, C., Coratella, G., Rinaldo, N., Barbero, M., et al. (2016). Muscle fiber conduction velocity and fractal dimension of EMG during fatiguing contraction of young and elderly active men. *Physiol. Meas.* 37, 162–174. doi: 10.1088/0967-3334/37/1/162

Boersma, I., Jones, J., Carter, J., Bekelman, D., Miyasaki, J., Kutner, J., et al. (2016). Parkinson disease patients' perspectives on palliative care needs: what are they telling us? *Neurol. Clin. Pract.* 6, 209–219. doi: 10.1212/CPJ.0000000000000233

Buehring, B., Belavý, D. L., Michaelis, I., Gast, U., Felsenberg, D., and Rittweger, J. (2011). Changes in lower extremity muscle function after 56 days of bed rest. *J. Appl. Physiol.* 111, 87–94. doi: 10.1152/japplphysiol.01294.2010

Bukowska, A. A., Krężałek, P., Mirek, E., Bujas, P., and Marchewka, A. (2016). Neurologic music therapy training for mobility and stability rehabilitation with Parkinson's disease – a pilot study. *Front. Hum. Neurosci.* 9:710. doi: 10.3389/fnhum.2015.00710

Cantello, R., Gianelli, M., Civardi, C., and Mutani, R. (1995). Parkinson's disease rigidity: EMG in a small hand muscle at "rest". *Electroencephalogr. Clin. Neurophysiol.* 97, 215–222. doi: 10.1016/0013-4694(95)93574-Q

Celucci, C. J., Albano, A. M., and Rapp, P. E. (2003). Comparative study of embedding methods. *Phys. Rev. E* 67:066210. doi: 10.1103/PhysRevE.67.066210

Cescon, C., and Gazzoni, M. (2010). Short term bed-rest reduces conduction velocity of individual motor units in leg muscles. *J. Electromyogr. Kines.* 20, 860–867. doi: 10.1016/j.jelekin.2010.03.008

Christakos, C. N., Erimaki, S., Anagnostou, E., and Anastasopoulos, D. (2009). Tremor-related motor unit firing in Parkinson's disease: implications for tremor genesis. *J. Physiol.* 587, 4811–4827. doi: 10.1113/jphysiol.2009.173989

Coletta, N. A., Mallette, M. M., Gabriel, D. A., Tyler, C. J., and Cheung, S. S. (2018). Core and skin temperature influences on the surface electromyographic responses to an isometric force and position task. *PLoS ONE* 13:e0195219. doi: 10.1371/journal.pone.0195219

Cronin, N. J., Valtonen, A. M., Waller, B., Pöyhönen, T., and Avela, J. (2016). Effects of short term water immersion on peripheral reflex excitability in hemiplegic and healthy individuals: a preliminary study. *J. Musculoskel. Neuron.* 16, 58–62. Available online at: http://www.ismni.org/jmni/pdf/63/V16I1_09CRONIN.pdf

Davis, J. R., Horslen, B. C., Nishikawa, K., Fukushima, K., Chua, R., Inglis, J. T., et al. (2011). Human proprioceptive adaptations during states of height-induced fear and anxiety. *J. Neurophysiol.* 106, 3082–3090. doi: 10.1152/jn.01030.2010

de Dreu, M. J., Kwakkel, G., and van Wegen, E. E. H. (2015). Partnered dancing to improve mobility for people with Parkinson's disease. *Front. Neurosci.* 9:444. doi: 10.3389/fnins.2015.00444

de Lau, L. M. L., and Breteler, M. M. B. (2006). Epidemiology of Parkinson's disease. *Lancet Neurol.* 5, 525–535. doi: 10.1016/S1474-4422(06)70471-9

Demangel, R., Treffel, L., Py, G., Brioche, T., Pagano, A. F., Bareille, M.-P., et al. (2017). Early structural and functional signature of 3-day human skeletal muscle disuse using the dry immersion model. *J. Physiol.* 595, 4301–4315. doi: 10.1113/JP273895

di Biase, L., Summa, S., Tosi, J., Taffoni, F., Marano, M., Rizzo, A. C., et al. (2018). Quantitative analysis of bradykinesia and rigidity in Parkinson's disease. *Front. Neurol.* 9:121. doi: 10.3389/fneur.2018.00121

Dietz, V., and Sinkjaer, T. (2007). Spastic movement disorder: impaired reflex function and altered muscle mechanic. *Lancet Neurol.* 6, 725–733. doi: 10.1016/S1474-4422(07)70193-X

Ebersbach, G., Edler, D., Kaufhold, O., and Wissel, J. (2008). Whole body vibration versus conventional physiotherapy to improve balance and gait in Parkinson's disease. *Arch. Phys. Med. Rehabil.* 89, 399–403. doi: 10.1016/j.apmr.2007.09.031

Escudero, J., Hornero, R., and Absolo, D. (2009). Interpretation of the auto-mutual information rate of decrease in the context of biomedical signal analysis. Application to electroencephalogram recordings. *Physiol. Meas.* 30, 187–199. doi: 10.1088/0967-3334/30/2/006

Fan, J.-Y., Chang, B.-L., and Wu, Y.-R. (2016). Relationships among depression, anxiety, sleep, and quality of life in patients with Parkinson's disease in Taiwan. *Parkinson's Dis.* 2016:4040185. doi: 10.1155/2016/4040185

Farina, D., Merletti, R., and Enoka, R. M. (2004). The extraction of neural strategies from the surface EMG. *J. Appl. Physiol.* 96, 1486–1495. doi: 10.1152/japplphysiol.01070.2003

Farina, D., Merletti, R., and Enoka, R. M. (2014). The extraction of neural strategies from the surface EMG: an update. *J. Appl. Physiol.* 117, 1215–1230. doi: 10.1152/japplphysiol.00162.2014

Fattorini, L., Felici, F., Filligoi, G. C., Traballesi, M., and Farina, D. (2005). Influence of high motor unit synchronization levels on non-linear and spectral variables of the surface EMG. *J. Neurosci. Methods* 143, 133–139. doi: 10.1016/j.jneumeth.2004.09.018

Fraser, A. M., and Swinney, H. L. (1986). Independent coordinates for strange attractors from mutual information. *Phys. Rev. A* 33, 1134–1140. doi: 10.1103/PhysRevA.33.1134

Freund, H. J. (1983). Motor unit and muscle activity in voluntary motor control. *Physiol. Rev.* 63, 387–436. doi: 10.1152/physrev.1983.63.2.387

Fu, A., Wang, C., Qi, H., Li, F., Wang, Z., He, F., et al. (2016). Electromyography-based analysis of human upper limbs during 45-day head-down bed-rest. *Acta Astronaut.* 120, 260–269. doi: 10.1016/j.actaastro.2015.12.007

Gallasch, E., Kozlovskaya, I., Löscher, W. N., Konev, A., and Kenner, T. (1994). Arm tremor and precision of hand force control in a short and long term flight on the Mir-Space-Station. *Acta Astronaut.* 33, 49–55. doi: 10.1016/0094-5765(94)90108-2

Gao, J. and Zheng, Z. (1994). Direct dynamical test for deterministic chaos and optimal embedding of a chaotic time series. *Phys. Rev. E* 49, 3807–3814. doi: 10.1103/PhysRevE.49.3807

Glendinning, D. S., and Enoka, R. M. (1994). Motor unit behavior in Parkinson's disease. *Phys. Ther.* 74, 61–70. doi: 10.1093/ptj/74.1.61

Gordon, J. (1990). "Disorders of motor control," in *Key Issues in Neurological Physiotherapy*, eds L. Ada and C. Canning (London: Heinemann), 35.

Grassberger, P., and Procaccia, I. (1983). Characterization of Strange Attractors. *Phys. Rev. Lett.* 50, 346–349. doi: 10.1103/PhysRevLett.50.346

Guyton, A. C., and Hall, J. E. (2011). *Textbook of Medical Physiology, 12th Edn.* Philadelphia, PA: Saunders Elsevier.

Hoyer, D., Pompe, B., Chon, K. H., Hardraht, H., Wicher, C., and Zwiener, U. (2005). Mutual information function assesses autonomic information flow of heart rate dynamics at different time scales. *IEEE Trans. Biomed. Eng.* 52, 584–592. doi: 10.1109/TBME.2005.844023

Hwang, I.-S., Lin, Y.-T., Huang, W.-M., Yang, Z.-R., Hu, C.-L., and Chen, Y.-C. (2017). Alterations in neural control of constant isometric contraction with the size of error feedback. *PLoS ONE* 12:e0170824. doi: 10.1371/journal.pone.0170824

Jeong, J., Gore, J. C., and Peterson, B. S. (2001). Mutual information analysis of the EEG in patients with Alzheimer's disease. *Clin. Neurophysiol.* 112, 827–835. doi: 10.1016/S1388-2457(01)00513-2

Katsura, Y., Yoshikawa, T., Ueda, S.-Y., Usui, T., Sotobayashi, D., Nakao, H., et al. (2010). Effects of aquatic exercise training using water-resistance equipment in elderly. *Eur. J. Appl. Physiol.* 108, 957–964. doi: 10.1007/s00421-009-1306-0

Katz, R. T., and Rymer, W. Z. (1989). Spastic hypertonia: mechanisms and measurement. *Arch. Phys. Med. Rehabil.* 70, 144–155.

Kennel, M. B., Brown, R., and Abarbanel, H. D. I. (1992). Determining embedding dimension for phase-space reconstruction using a geometrical construction. *Phys. Rev. A* 45, 3403–3411. doi: 10.1103/PhysRevA.45.3403

Kirkwood, P. A., Sears, T. A., Tuck, D. L., and Westgaard, R. H. (1982). Variations in the time course of the synchronization of intercostal motoneurones in the cat. *J. Physiol.* 327, 105–135. doi: 10.1113/jphysiol.1982.sp014223

Kline, J. C., and de Luca, C. J. (2016). Synchronization of motor unit firings: an epiphenomenon of firing rate characteristics not common inputs. *J. Neurophysiol.* 115, 178–192. doi: 10.1152/jn.00452.2015

Koryak, Y. A. (2002). Surface action potential and contractile properties of the human triceps surae muscle: effect of 'dry' water immersion. *Exp. Physiol.* 87, 101–111. doi: 10.1113/eph8702301

Kozlovskaya, I., Dmitrieva, I., Grigorieva, L., Kirenskaya, A., and Kreidich, Yu. (1988). "Gravitational mechanisms in the motor system. Studies in real and simulated weightlessness," in *Stance and Motion: Facts and Concepts*, eds V. S. Gurfinkel, M. E. Ioffe, J. Massion, and J. P. Roll (Boston, MA: Springer), 37–48.

Lupandin, Yu. V., Antonen, E. G., and Meigal, Yu. A. (1993). The patterns of bioelectrical activity of motor units in different forms of parkinsonism. *Zh. Nevrol. Psikhiatr. Im. S. S. Korsakova* 93, 30–34.

Mañé, R. (1981). "On the dimension of the compact invariant sets of certain nonlinear maps," in *Dynamical Systems and Turbulence, Lecture Notes in Mathematics*, vol. 898, eds D. A. Rand and L.-S. Young (Warwick: Springer-Verlag), 230–242.

Marwan, N., Romano, M. C., Thiel, M., and Kurths, J. (2007). Recurrence plots for the analysis of complex systems. *Phys. Rep.* 438, 237–329. doi: 10.1016/j.physrep.2006.11.001

McAuley, J. H., and Marsden, C. D. (2000). Physiological and pathological tremors and rhythmic central motor control. *Brain* 123, 1545–1567. doi: 10.1093/brain/123.8.1545

Meigal, A., Gerasimova-Meigal, L., Saenko, I., and Subbotina, N. (2018). Dry immersion as a novel physical therapeutic intervention for rehabilitation of Parkinson's disease patients: a feasibility study. *Phys. Med. Rehab. Kuror.* doi: 10.1055/a-0577-5139

Meigal, A., and Lupandin, Y. (2005). "Thermoregulation-dependent component" in pathophysiology of motor disorders in Parkinson's disease? *Pathophysiology* 11, 187–196. doi: 10.1016/j.pathophys.2005.02.001

Meigal, A., Miroshnichenko, G., Kuzmina, A., Rissanen, S., Georgiadis, S., and Karjalainen, P. (2015). Nonlinear parameters of surface EMG in schizophrenia patients depend on kind of antipsychotic therapy. *Front. Physiol.* 6:197. doi: 10.3389/fphys.2015.00197

Meigal, A. Yu., Rissanen, S., Tarvainen, M., Georgiadis, S. D., Karjalainen, P. A., Airaksinen, O., et al. (2012). Linear and nonlinear tremor acceleration characteristics in patients with Parkinson's disease. *Physiol. Meas.* 33, 395–412. doi: 10.1088/0967-3334/33/3/395

Meigal, A. Yu., Rissanen, S., Tarvainen, M., Kajalainen, P. A., Iudina-Vassel, I. A., Airaksinen, O., et al. (2009). Novel parameters of surface EMG in patients with Parkinson's disease and healthy young and old controls. *J. Electromyogr. Kines.* 19, e206–e213. doi: 10.1016/j.jelekin.2008.02.008

Meigal, A. Yu., Rissanen, S. M., Tarvainen, M. P., Airaksinen, O., Kankaanpää, M., and Karjalainen, P. A. (2013). Non-linear EMG parameters for differential and early diagnostics of Parkinson's disease. *Front. Neurol.* 4:135. doi: 10.3389/fneur.2013.00135

Mewett, D. T., Reynolds, K. J., and Nazeran, H. (2004). Reducing power line interference in digitised electromyogram recordings by spectrum interpolation. *Med. Biol. Eng. Comput.* 42, 524–531. doi: 10.1007/BF02350994

Miyai, I., Fujimoto, Y., Ueda, Y., Yamamoto, H., Nozaki, S., Saito, T., et al. (2000). Treadmill training with body weight support: its effect on Parkinson's disease. *Arch. Phys. Med. Rehabil.* 81, 849–852. doi: 10.1053/apmr.2000.4439

Mulder, E. R., Gerrits, K. H. L., Kleine, B. U., Rittweger, J., Felsenberg, D., de Haan, A., et al. (2009). High-density surface EMG study on the time course of central nervous and peripheral neuromuscular changes during 8 weeks of bed rest with or without resistive vibration exercise. *J. Electromyogr. Kines.* 19, 208–218. doi: 10.1016/j.jelekin.2007.04.002

Navasiolava, N. M., Custaud, M.-A., Tomilovskaya, E. S., Larina, I. M., Mano, T., Gauquelin-Koch, G., et al. (2011). Long-term dry immersion: review and prospects. *Eur. J. Appl. Physiol.* 111, 1235–1260. doi: 10.1007/s00421-010-1750-x

Needle, A. R., Baumeister, J., Kaminski, T. W., Higginson, J. S., Farquhar, W. B., and Swanik, C. B. (2014). Neuromechanical coupling in the regulation of muscle tone and joint stiffness. *Scand. J. Med. Sci. Sports* 24, 737–748. doi: 10.1111/sms.12181

Ni, M., Signorile, J. F., Mooney, K., Balachandran, A., Potiaumpai, M., Luca, C., et al. (2016). Comparative effect of power training and high-speed yoga on motor function in older patients with Parkinson disease. *Arch. Phys. Med. Rehabil.* 97, 345–354.e15. doi: 10.1016/j.apmr.2015.10.095

Nordstrom, M. A., Fuglevand, A. J., and Enoka, R. M. (1992). Estimating the strength of common input to human motoneurons from the cross-correlogram. *J. Physiol.* 453, 547–574. doi: 10.1113/jphysiol.1992.sp019244

Noyes, K., Liu, H., Li, Y., Holloway, R., and Dick, A. W. (2006). Economic burden associated with Parkinson's disease on elderly Medicare beneficiaries. *Mov. Disord.* 21, 362–372. doi: 10.1002/mds.20727

Oung, Q. W., Muthusamy, H., Lee, H. L., Basah, S. N., Yaacob, S., Sarillee, M., et al. (2015). Technologies for assessment of motor disorders in Parkinson's disease: a review. *Sensors* 15, 21710–21745. doi: 10.3390/s150921710

Picelli, A., Tamburin, S., Passuello, M., Waldner, A., and Smania, N. (2014). Robot-assisted arm training in patients with Parkinson's disease: a pilot study. *J. NeuroEng. Rehabil.* 11, 1–4. doi: 10.1186/1743-0003-11-28

Piervirgili, G., Petracca, F., and Merletti, R. (2014). A new method to assess skin treatments for lowering the impedance and noise of individual gelled Ag-AgCl electrodes. *Physiol. Meas.* 35, 2101–2118. doi: 10.1088/0967-3334/35/10/2101

Portero, P., Vanhoutte, C., and Goubel, F. (1996). Surface electromyogram power spectrum changes in human leg muscles following 4 weeks of simulated microgravity. *Eur. J. Appl. Physiol. O.* 73, 340–345. doi: 10.1007/BF02425496

Ramanand, P., Bruce, M. C., and Bruce, E. N. (2010). Mutual information analysis of EEG signals indicates age-related changes in cortical interdependence during sleep in middle-aged vs. elderly women. *J. Clin. Neurophysiol.* 27, 274–284. doi: 10.1097/WNP.0b013e3181eaa9f5

Richman, J. S., and Moorman, J. R. (2000). Physiological time-series analysis using approximate entropy and sample entropy. *Am. J. Physiol. Heart Circ. Physiol.* 278, H2039–H2049. doi: 10.1152/ajpheart.2000.278.6.H2039

Riley, M. A., and van Orden, G. C., editors (2005). *Tutorials in Contemporary Nonlinear Methods for the Behavioral Science*. Available online at: https://www.nsf.gov/pubs/2005/nsf05057/nmbs/nmbs.pdf (Accessed June 21, 2018).

Rissanen, S. M., Kankaanpää, M., Meigal, A., Tarvainen, M. P., Nuutinen, J., Tarkka, I. M., et al. (2008). Surface EMG and acceleration signals in Parkinson's disease: feature extraction and cluster analysis. *Med. Biol. Eng. Comput.* 46, 849–858. doi: 10.1007/s11517-008-0369-0

Rissanen, S. M., Kankaanpää, M., Tarvainen, M. P., Novak, V., Novak, P., Hu, K., et al. (2011). Analysis of EMG and acceleration signals for quantifying the effects of deep brain stimulation in Parkinson's disease. *IEEE Trans. Biomed. Eng.* 58, 2545–2553. doi: 10.1109/TBME.2011.2159380

Rivelis, Y., and Morice, K. (2018). "Spasticity," in *StatPearls [Internet]*. Treasure Island: StatPearls Publishing. Available online at: https://www.ncbi.nlm.nih.gov/books/NBK507869/ (Updated June 19, 2018).

Rossi, B., Siciliano, G., Carboncini, M. C., Manca, M. L., Massetani, R., Viacava, P., et al. (1996). Muscle modifications in Parkinson's disease: myoelectric manifestations. *Electroencephalogr. Clin. Neurophysiol.* 101, 211–218. doi: 10.1016/0924-980X(96)94672-X

Ruonala, V., Pekkonen, E., Airaksinen, O., Kankaanpää, M., Karjalainen, P. A., and Rissanen, S. M. (2018). Levodopa-induced changes in electromyographic patterns in patients with advanced Parkinson's disease. *Front. Neurol.* 9:35. doi: 10.3389/fneur.2018.00035

Sáchez-Ferro, Á., Elshehabi, M., Godinho, C., Salkovic, D., Hobert, M. A., Domingos, J., et al. (2016). New methods for the assessment of Parkinson's disease (2005 to 2015): a systematic review. *Movement Disord.* 31, 1283–1292. doi: 10.1002/mds.26723

Scandalis, T. A., Bosak, A., Berliner, J. C., Helman, L. L., and Wells, M. R. (2001). Resistance training and gait function in patients with Parkinson's disease. *Am. J. Phys. Med. Rehabil.* 80, 38–43. doi: 10.1097/00002060-200101000-00011

Schneider, S., Peipsi, A., Stokes, M., Knicker, A., and Abeln, V. (2015). Feasibility of monitoring muscle health in microgravity environments using Myoton technology. *Med. Biol. Eng. Comput.* 53, 57–66. doi: 10.1007/s11517-014-1211-5

Sears, T. A., and Stagg, D. (1976). Short-term synchronization of intercostal motoneurone activity. *J. Physiol.* 263, 357–381. doi: 10.1113/jphysiol.1976.sp011635

Sturman, M. M., Vaillancourt, D. E., and Corcos, D. M. (2005). Effects of aging on the regularity of physiological tremor. *J. Neurophysiol.* 93, 3064–3074. doi: 10.1152/jn.01218.2004

Sung, P. S., Zurcher, U., and Kaufman, M. (2008). Gender differences in spectral and entropic measures of erector spinae muscle fatigue. *J. Rehabil. Res. Dev.* 45, 1431–1440. doi: 10.1682/JRRD.2007.11.0196

Takens, F. (1981). "Detecting strange attractors in turbulence," in *Dynamical Systems and Turbulence, Lecture Notes in Mathematics*, vol. 898, eds D. A. Rand and L.-S. Young (Berlin; Heidelberg: Springer-Verlag), 366–381.

Tarvainen, M. P., Ranta-aho, P. O., and Karjalainen, P. A. (2002). An advanced detrending method with application to HRV analysis. *IEEE Trans. Biomed. Eng.* 49, 172–175. doi: 10.1109/10.979357

The Parkinson Study Group (2004). Levodopa and the progression of Parkinson's disease. *N. Engl. J. Med.* 351, 2498–2508. doi: 10.1056/NEJMoa033447

Timmermann, L., Gross, J., Dirks, M., Volkmann, J., Freund, H.-J., and Schnitzler, A. (2003). The cerebral oscillatory network of parkinsonian resting tremor. *Brain* 126, 199–212. doi: 10.1093/brain/awg022

Tomlinson, C. L., Herd, C. P., Clarke, C. E., Meek, C., Patel, S., Stowe, R., et al. (2014). Physiotherapy for Parkinson's disease: a comparison of techniques. *Cochrane Db. Syst. Rev.* 6:CD002815. doi: 10.1002/14651858.CD002815.pub2

Trompetto, C., Marinelli, L., Mori, L., Pelosin, E., Currà, A., Molfetta, L., et al. (2014). Pathophysiology of spasticity: implications for neurorehabilitation. *Biomed. Res. Int.* 2014:354906. doi: 10.1155/2014/354906

Vaillancourt, D. E., Prodoehl, J., Metman, L. V., Bakay, R. A., and Corcos, D. M. (2004). Effects of deep brain stimulation and medication on bradykinesia and muscle activation in Parkinson's disease. *Brain* 127, 491–504. doi: 10.1093/brain/awh057

Vivas, J., Arias, P., and Cudeiro, J. (2011). Aquatic therapy versus conventional land-based therapy for Parkinson's disease: an open-label pilot study. *Arch. Phys. Med. Rehabil.* 92, 1202–1210. doi: 10.1016/j.apmr.2011.03.017

Volpe, D., Giantin, M. G., Maestri, R., and Frazzitta, G. (2014). Comparing the effects of hydrotherapy and land-based therapy on balance in patients with Parkinson's disease: a randomized controlled pilot study. *Clin. Rehabil.* 28, 1210–1217. doi: 10.1177/0269215514536060

Ward, A. B. (2000). Assessment of muscle tone. *Age Ageing* 29, 385–386. doi: 10.1093/ageing/29.5.385

Watenpaugh, D. E. (2016). Analogs of microgravity: head-down tilt and water immersion. *J. Appl. Physiol.* 120, 904–914. doi: 10.1152/japplphysiol.00986.2015

Yen, C. Y., Lin, K. H., Hu, M. H., Wu, R. M., Lu, T. W., and Lin, C. H. (2011). Effects of virtual reality-augmented balance training on sensory organization and attentional demand for postural control in people with Parkinson disease: a randomized controlled trial. *Phys. Ther.* 91, 862–874. doi: 10.2522/ptj.20100050

Zhou, J., Yin, T., Gao, Q., and Yang, X. C. (2015). A meta-analysis on the efficacy of tai chi in patients with Parkinson's disease between 2008 and 2014. *Evid. Based Compl. Alt.* 2015:593263. doi: 10.1155/2015/593263

Zhu, H., Lu, Z., Jin, Y., Duan, X., Teng, J., and Duan, D. (2015). Low-frequency repetitive transcranial magnetic stimulation on Parkinson motor function: a meta-analysis of randomised controlled trials. *Acta Neuropsychiatr.* 27, 82–89. doi: 10.1017/neu.2014.43

14

Reticulospinal Systems for Tuning Motor Commands

Robert M. Brownstone* and Jeremy W. Chopek

Sobell Department of Motor Neuroscience and Movement Disorders, Institute of Neurology, University College London, London, United Kingdom

****Correspondence:***
Robert M. Brownstone
r.brownstone@ucl.ac.uk

The pontomedullary reticular formation (RF) is a key site responsible for integrating descending instructions to execute particular movements. The indiscrete nature of this region has led not only to some inconsistencies in nomenclature, but also to difficulties in understanding its role in the control of movement. In this review article, we first discuss nomenclature of the RF, and then examine the reticulospinal motor command system through evolution. These command neurons have direct monosynaptic connections with spinal interneurons and motoneurons. We next review their roles in postural adjustments, walking and sleep atonia, discussing their roles in movement activation or inhibition. We propose that knowledge of the internal organization of the RF is necessary to understand how the nervous system tunes motor commands, and that this knowledge will underlie strategies for motor functional recovery following neurological injuries or diseases.

Keywords: locomotion, mesencephalic locomotor region, reticular formation, microcircuits, sleep atonia

INTRODUCTION

As movement is necessary for the expression of all behavior, much of the vertebrate nervous system is involved in its production. A key site for integration of descending instructions to move is the reticular formation (RF), which is situated in the brain stem and comprised of multiple nuclei. The indiscrete nature of these regions combined with disparate neuronal types within each nucleus has led not only to some inconsistencies in nomenclature, but also to difficulties in understanding RF control of movement.

The RF is comprised of different neural types including monoaminergic, cholinergic, GABA/glycinergic and glutamatergic neurons, with glutamatergic reticulospinal neurons (RSNs) forming the key descending output. Axons of these neurons extend into the spinal cord such that RSN activity can lead to a variety of motor behaviors. Inputs to RSNs descend from diverse brain regions including the telencephalon, diencephalon and cerebellum, and ascend from the spinal cord. Local circuits within RF nuclei may also contribute to their output. RSNs therefore play a role in integrating and processing these diverse inputs in order to produce effective motor behaviors. Recent reviews have addressed the role of the RF in context specific locomotion (Kim et al., 2017) and the interaction of the control of posture and locomotion (Takakusaki et al., 2016). In this review, we will discuss glutamatergic RSN systems with a focus on their organization, connectivity with spinal neurons, control of hind limb movement, and the role of these systems in recovery of

Abbreviations: DTF, dorsal tegmental field; Gi, gigantocellular reticular nucleus; GiA, gigantocellular reticular nucleus, pars alpha; GRN, gigantocellular reticular nucleus; LPGi, lateral paragigantocellular nucleus; MdV, medulla reticular formation-ventral part; medRF, medulla reticular formation; MLR, mesencephalic locomotor region; PnC, pontine reticular formation, caudal part; PnO, pontine reticular formation, oral part; PPN, pedunculopontine nucleus; RF, reticular formation; RSN, reticulospinal neurons; SLDT, sublaterodorsal tegmental; VTF, ventral tegmental field.

function after neurological injury. Additionally, we address the lack of information regarding the internal organization of RF nuclei and why this knowledge is vital for understanding how RS output is refined.

RETICULAR FORMATION NOMENCLATURE

One difficulty in determining specific functions of the RF arises from the non-discrete boundaries between nuclei and the inconsistent nomenclature in the literature. In this review, we will use the terminology as set out by Paxinos and Franklin (2008). As different investigators have used different terms, in this section we have attempted to harmonize the nomenclature through assessment of the available anatomical sections provided in publications focussed on the role of RSNs in movement.

The RF extends through the mesencephalon, pons and medulla and is traditionally divided into three columns—median, medial and lateral. In this review, we will focus on RSNs involved in limb movement, which arise from the medial column in the pons and medulla. Descending neurons from the median column arise from the raphe nuclei and are responsible for serotoninergic neuromodulation (see review: Schmidt and Jordan, 2000). The neurons of the lateral column and those in the mesencephalic RF do not project to the spinal cord.

The medial pontine RF, from rostral to caudal, comprises the nucleus reticularis pontis oralis (PnO), from the decussation of the superior cerebellar peduncles to the trigeminal motor pool, and the nucleus reticularis pontis caudalis (PnC), overlapping with PnO and extending caudally to the facial nucleus. Situated dorsal to these nuclei are the pontine tegmental nuclei, divided into ventral (region referred to as the ventral tegmental field, or VTF), dorsal (region referred to as the dorsal tegmental field, or DTF), and lateral tegmental nuclei, as well as the sublaterodorsal tegmental (SLDT) nucleus. The dorsal tegmental nucleus extends caudally to lie dorsal to the gigantocellular reticular nucleus (GRN, *vide infra*), by which point the ventral and lateral tegmental nuclei merge to form the laterodorsal tegmental nucleus (LDT). In addition, rodents may have a ventral nucleus of the medial pontine RF (PnV, Liang et al., 2011) that contains a small population of RS neurons, although it has been suggested this is part of the rostral medullary GRN (see Sivertsen et al., 2016).

The rostral portion of the medial medullary RF (medRF) begins at the most caudal portion of the PnC, with the GRN lying ventral to PnC and extending from the facial nucleus to the obex. The GRN (sometimes referred to as Gi) is a large nucleus that contains the largest cells in the RF. Ventral to this is the pars alpha of the GRN (GiA), which merges with the Gi pars ventral (GiV) caudally. In the cat literature, the GRN is often referred to as the nucleus reticularis gigantocellularis (NRGc) or gigantocellular tegmental field (FTG), and the GiA/GiV as the nucleus reticularis magnocellularis (NRMc) or magnocellular tegmental field (FTM, see Noga et al., 1988; Takakusaki et al., 2016), with medullary sections 9 mm caudal to the junction of the superior and inferior colliculi (P9) in the cat corresponding approximately to Bregma −7 in the mouse (Paxinos and Franklin, 2008). The dorsal paragigantocellular nucleus (DPGi) is dorsal to the GRN, and the parvocellular reticular nucleus (PCRt) is dorsolateral to the GRN. The intermediate reticular zone (IRt) which contains the nucleus ambiguus, separates the GRN from the PCRt (Paxinos et al., 2012). The lateral paragigantocellular nucleus (LPGi), lies lateral to GiV and ventromedial to nucleus ambiguus. In the caudal medulla which lacks giant GRN neurons, the central nucleus can be subdivided into the medRF ventral part (MdV), and more cellular dorsal part (MdD), separated by the caudal IRt and located in the caudal medulla lateral to the medial longitudinal fasciculus.

It should be noted that the borders between these regions are somewhat indistinct, necessitating a degree of caution when interpreting experimental findings involving either electrical stimulation (Mori et al., 1978; Garcia-Rill and Skinner, 1987; Takakusaki et al., 2016) or local injections (Noga et al., 1988; Takakusaki et al., 2016; Capelli et al., 2017). The comparison of histological sections between studies is helpful, but co-labeling with antibodies against choline acetyltransferase would be helpful in aligning sections based on consistent cholinergic nuclei such as motor pools.

RETICULOSPINAL NEURONS ARE COMMAND NEURONS FOR MOVEMENT

RSNs Are Evolutionary Conserved Command Neurons

The reticulospinal (RS) system is a distributed network of neurons extending from the caudal midbrain through the pons and medulla (Peterson, 1984). RSNs receive inputs from rostral motor centers and have axons that descend through the ventrolateral funiculus of the spinal cord to form synapses with spinal interneurons and motoneurons that participate in movement. As RSNs are located between higher centers that select movement and spinal cord circuits where movement is organized, RSNs may be considered as command neurons.

Command neurons are widespread across invertebrate and vertebrate species. To be classified as a command neuron, a candidate neuron must satisfy the criteria of both sufficiency and necessity for initiating a given behavior (Kupfermann and Weiss, 1978). Command neurons in the brain stem have been identified in a number of vertebrate species in which they have been shown to be involved in motor behaviors such as escape and locomotion.

Dating back more than 500 million years, the early appearing agnathans, lampreys and hagfish, developed RS command neurons called Müller cells, that have axons that cross in the brainstem and descend the length of the spinal cord to evoke swimming (Shapovalov, 1972). Perhaps the prototypical RS command neuron, though, is the Mauthner cell, initially described in teleosts which arose ∼310 million years ago. Given that Mauthner cells were readily identifiable and that they share similar location, morphology, and synaptic connectivity across species, they have been well studied as command neurons (Sillar et al., 2016). Mauthner cells are likely present in lower vertebrates such as lamprey, but their function has mostly been studied in later-evolving fish as well as amphibians.

Two Mauthner cells, located directly opposite each other near the midline of the medulla can readily be identified in the RF based on their large cell size and location at the level of the 4th rhombomere (Sillar et al., 2016; Hildebrand et al., 2017). The axons of Mauthner cells cross in the brain stem and project through the spinal cord where they form glutamatergic, excitatory connections to large primary motoneurons and premotor excitatory interneurons (Fetcho and Faber, 1988; Faber et al., 1989; Fetcho, 1991). These interneurons have descending projections, are electrotonically coupled to large motoneurons, and form chemical synapses with small motoneurons (Fetcho, 1992). The Mauthner cell axon is also electrotonically coupled to glycinergic commissural interneurons that inhibit the large motoneurons and interneurons on the contralateral side (Yasargil and Sandri, 1990; Fetcho, 1991).

Mauthner cells receive multiple sensory inputs (Sillar et al., 2016). In response to acoustic stimuli (cf. startle response in humans below), Mauthner cells fire a single action potential (Zottoli, 1977). Based on the connectivity described above, this results in excitation of contralateral motoneurons and inhibition of ipsilateral motoneurons. This produces a fast and forceful C-start escape, arising from the initial C-bend, in which the fish moves away from the initial stimulus (Fetcho, 1992). Thus, Mauthner cell activation produces a conserved stereotypical C-start response that mediates escape (Eaton et al., 1988; Faber et al., 1989).

It is now recognized that the C-start escape response is not necessarily stereotypical, and that depending on the stimulus site and intensity, combinations of RSNs, including Mauthner cells, can produce variations of the escape response (Eaton et al., 2001). For example, it was recently demonstrated that Mauthner cells are involved in a second type of escape response, the S-start escape, when bilaterally activated (Liu and Hale, 2017). The selection of the S- vs. C-start was determined by the recruitment of segmental inhibitory neurons in spinal circuits, which would modify the response. The adaptability in behavioral responses mediated by the RS system indicates that responses to command neuron activity are variable and state-dependent.

With further study, it became apparent that the Mauthner cell has multiple smaller homologoues and that they are organized in a segmental plan, similar to the segmented organization seen in invertebrates (Kimmel, 1993). It was also demonstrated that there are additional command neurons in the teleost RS system, which comprises approximately 500 neurons (Prasada Rao et al., 1987). Thus, even in these relatively early appearing teleosts, complex descending systems were present.

As supraspinal systems developed to control limbed movement, the RS system remained a dominant system mediating movement. Across species including frog, turtle, rat, cat and rhesus monkey, RSNs project to and monosynaptically excite limb motoneurons (Shapovalov, 1972). It is noteworthy that, in addition to the RS system, other descending systems such as the vestibulospinal system appeared beginning in amphibians (Shapovalov, 1972). While these other systems evolved further in reptiles, the RS system also expanded and diversified to include, for example, inhibitory RSNs. With further evolution of corticospinal including corticomotoneuronal systems in primates, the RS system persisted, producing responses in spinal motoneurons similar to those seen in fish. Thus, the RS system remains conserved though evolution (Shapovalov, 1972), and plays an important role in vertebrate, including human, movement.

In fact, the RS system was not only conserved but it flourished in evolution. For instance, compared to the 500 RSNs in the fish, there are approximately 50,000 RSNs in the mouse. Of these, approximately 19,000 are located in the GRN alone (Liang et al., 2011). Based on a comparison of EPSPs and IPSPs across species, Shapovalov concluded "the basic similarity between reticulo-motoneuronal projections across all vertebrates investigated may evidently be attributable to the common origin of the reticulospinal system, which undergoes mainly quantitative changes in the course of evolution" (Shapovalov, 1972, p. 353). In other words, as behavior became more complex, so too did the RS system. But the fundamental architecture and role of the RS system persisted across species: RSNs are large cells with dense arborizations and large fast-conducting axons that descend in the spinal cord, forming synapses with interneurons and motoneurons in multiple segments in order to produce movement.

Reticulospinal Neurons Project to Spinal Interneurons and Motoneurons

The influence of the brainstem on posture was documented by Sherrington (1898) who noted that decerebration led to "decerebrate rigidity" or hyperactivity of extensor muscles, suggesting that there is an excitatory influence from sub-cerebral structures to the spinal cord. In the 1940s Rhines and Magoun demonstrated that following decerebration, stimulation of the ventral medulla could result in the complete loss of muscle tone, and cessation of stimulation led to the immediate return of hyperextensor activity, demonstrating that the RS system had both an excitatory and inhibitory influence on postural muscles (Magoun and Rhines, 1946; Rhines and Magoun, 1946). They also demonstrated that the RS system could either facilitate or inhibit spinal reflexes in the cat (Magoun, 1944; Magoun and Rhines, 1946; Rhines and Magoun, 1946), and found that the area responsible for inhibition resided in the ventral rostral medulla (Magoun and Rhines, 1946), whereas the excitatory regions extended through the pons and medulla (Rhines and Magoun, 1946). However, Sprague and Chamber (1954) found that in intact cats, for the most part, micro-stimulation of the RF led to reciprocal (flexion-extension as well as right-left) responses in the limbs rather than generalized facilitation or inhibition. Neurons in the caudal pons and GRN form either excitatory (Grillner and Lund, 1968) or inhibitory (Llinas and Terzuolo, 1964a,b) connections with flexor or extensor hindlimb motoneurons. In addition to the hindlimb responses, RS stimulation can produce direct excitation or inhibition of neck, back, and forelimb motoneurons (Wilson and Yoshida, 1969; Wilson et al., 1970; Peterson et al., 1978). In non-human primates, activation of movement by RS stimulation is achieved by both direct and indirect connectivity to motoneurons (Riddle et al., 2009). Thus, RSNs produce effects that are heterogeneous and widespread in the spinal cord.

It is important to note that, in contrast to other descending systems such as the lateral vestibulospinal and corticofugal systems, the RS system is not exclusively excitatory. A proportion of RSNs descending in the MLF are inhibitory (Du Beau et al., 2012), and approximately 20% of RS synaptic contacts on propriospinal and spinal commissural interneurons in the lumbar spinal cord are inhibitory (Mitchell et al., 2016). Recently it has been shown that glycinergic neurons located in the GRN descend to the lumbar spinal cord (Valencia Garcia et al., 2018; *vide infra*).

Within the RF, specific regions have been found to be responsible for specific responses (Drew and Rossignol, 1990). Ipsilateral projecting pontine RSNs outnumber contralateral projecting pontine RSNs three to one and are located throughout the pontine RF whereas the contralateral projecting neurons are concentrated in the rostral pontine RF (Sivertsen et al., 2016). In neonatal mice, medial neurons in the medRF predominantly activate lateral motor column (limb-innervating) MNs in the lumbar spinal cord, whereas lateral medRF neurons predominantly activate medial motor column (axial muscle-innervating) MNs (Szokol et al., 2008). In both cases, these actions may be mediated through polysynaptic pathways mediated by ipsilateral and contralateral descending spinal commissural interneurons (Szokol et al., 2011; Perreault and Glover, 2013).

Microstimulation within the RF can result in movement across multiple joints or limbs. For example, stimulation that produced forelimb movement was regularly accompanied by movement of the head or hindlimbs (Drew and Rossignol, 1990). Furthermore, homologous to Mauthner cell responses, motoneuron responses were not restricted to one side: microstimulation could evoke ipsilateral flexion and contralateral extension of the either the fore or hind limbs (Drew and Rossignol, 1990). These evoked movements are consistent with the axonal projections of RSNs, with 85% of axons extending to both the cervical and lumbar enlargements, and, at least in the cervical enlargement, axons projecting bilaterally (Peterson et al., 1975). Thus, RSNs have divergent spinal projections and are involved in multi-joint, multi-limb motor commands. In summary, the RS system in the mammal is functionally organized and acts to coordinate multiple movements including excitation and inhibition across joints and across limbs.

medRF Reticulospinal Neurons and Locomotion

The rhythm and pattern of locomotion are produced by spinal cord circuits in response to descending commands (Graham Brown, 1911; Jankowska et al., 1967). RF locomotor command neurons are activated by an upstream center called the mesencephalic locomotor region (MLR). MLR stimulation produces locomotion in decerebrate cats (Shik et al., 1966), rats (Skinner and Garcia-Rill, 1984), and mice (Roseberry et al., 2016; Stecina, 2017; Caggiano et al., 2018) through a pathway mediated by medRF RSNs (Noga et al., 2003). The medRF has been shown to be crucial for locomotion in a number of other species as well, including lamprey (McClellan and Grillner, 1984), ducks and geese (Steeves et al., 1987) and guinea pigs (Marlinskii and Voitenko, 1992). In the cat, medRF RSNs in the GRN are necessary for MLR-evoked locomotion, and are sufficient to induce locomotor activity through electrical (Jordan et al., 2008) or chemical stimulation (Noga et al., 1988). These "locomotor" medRF RSNs also receive input from the contralateral cerebellar locomotor region (Mori et al., 1998) and from the ipsilateral lateral hypothalamic area, termed the subthalamic locomotor region (Sinnamon and Stopford, 1987). Given the multitude of locomotor-related inputs, Orlovskii (1970) stated that "the invariable mediating link for initiating locomotion is the reticulospinal system."

Locomotor medRF RSNs are fast conducting (Orlovskii, 1970; Degtyarenko et al., 1998; Noga et al., 2003) and glutamatergic (Douglas et al., 1993; Jordan et al., 2008). They are phasically active during spontaneous locomotion in thalamic cats (Shimamura et al., 1982; Shimamura and Kogure, 1983), treadmill locomotion in unrestrained cats (Drew et al., 1986; Matsuyama and Drew, 2000), and spontaneous or MLR-evoked fictive locomotion in the absence of movement related feedback in decerebrate cats (Perreault et al., 1993). Locomotion-inducing RSN axons descend in the ventrolateral funiculus (Steeves and Jordan, 1980), may innervate the ipsi- or contra-lateral spinal cord (Matsuyama et al., 1988, 1999), and are known to innervate commissural interneurons in the lumbar spinal cord (Matsuyama et al., 2004; Jankowska, 2008). That is, RSNs in the medRF GRN provide extensive innervation to bilateral spinal motor regions, and seemingly fulfil the criteria of command neurons for locomotion.

While RSNs thus integrate inputs from multiple higher centers in order to send commands to the spinal cord, there may also be local processing of commands within the RF. Neurons within the RF have heterogeneous characteristics, leading to the suggestion that there may be local circuit processing of reticulospinal commands (Shimamura et al., 1980), but this has not been explored in detail. For example, a subset of neurons in this region in lamprey (Einum and Buchanan, 2004; Buchanan, 2011) and cat (Shimamura et al., 1980, 1982) receive inputs from the spinal cord. In the cat, it has been suggested that the phasic activity of RSNs during fictive locomotion may arise from inputs from the spinal cord (Perreault et al., 1993). This hypothesis is supported by the demonstrated phase-dependent modulation of RSN activity in response to cutaneous stimulation during locomotion (Drew et al., 1996). How these ascending inputs are processed and how they might affect the descending commands is not yet clear.

There is also evidence that some RSNs receive neuromodulatory input (Takakusaki et al., 1993a), indicating that their activity may be state dependent (Takakusaki et al., 2016). While there has been focus on modulation of RSNs by acetylcholine (Takakusaki et al., 1993b; Le Ray et al., 2010), serotonin also may play a role (Takakusaki et al., 1993a). Given the importance of serotoninergic activity in locomotion (Schmidt and Jordan, 2000), it is possible that this modulatory system is involved in both brain stem and spinal circuits for locomotion.

Pathways for different types of locomotor activity, such as escape vs. exploration, may differ (Sinnamon, 1993; Jordan, 1998). The MLR is comprised primarily of the cuneiform nucleus (Jordan, 1998), but recent evidence in the mouse suggests that while higher speed locomotion is mediated by the cuneiform nucleus, exploratory activity is initiated by a region just ventral to this, the pedunculopontine nucleus (PPN, Caggiano et al., 2018). The PPN has diverse projections to RF nuclei (Gi, GiV, GiA, LPGi, MdV), whereas the cuneiform projections are more restricted (LPGi, GiV, GiA but not the Gi or MdV, Caggiano et al., 2018). While cat studies have pointed towards the medial regions of the medRF as the command for locomotion (Noga et al., 2003), there has been a recent suggestion that in the mouse, LPGi activation is necessary for higher speed locomotion (Capelli et al., 2017). This suggests that there may be species differences in descending commands, a difference in the state of the circuits being studied across experiments, or that locomotor activity is initiated via indirect pathways in some experiments (see Noga et al., 2003). In summary, it is clear across multiple species that the medRF plays a key role in integrating and processing instructions for locomotion from more rostral centers.

In addition to their well-defined role in initiating locomotion, RSNs have recently been implicated in stopping locomotion. Optogenetic activation of a subset of glutamatergic neurons defined by expression of the transcription factor Chx10 located in the PnC and GRN regions can lead to cessation of locomotor activity in the mouse (Bouvier et al., 2015) and lamprey (Juvin et al., 2016). Three activity patterns in RSNs were seen in this region during swimming in lamprey: those that fired exclusively at the onset of swimming ("start" RSNs), those that fired throughout the swimming bout ("start and maintain" RSNs), and those that fired prior to the termination of locomotion ("stop" RSNs; Juvin et al., 2016). This indicates that there is a diversity of neuronal function within the RSN. In the mouse and possibly lamprey, the behavioral response from the stop RSNs is likely mediated by spinal inhibitory neurons targeted by these descending glutamatergic RSNs (Bouvier et al., 2015; Juvin et al., 2016).

The ability of RSNs in the medRF/GRN to act as command neurons for a variety of behaviors in addition to starting and stopping locomotion is highlighted by its involvement in a multitude of tasks ranging from, for example, maintaining posture during walking to atonia during sleep (*vide infra*).

Interaction of Reticulospinal Systems for Locomotion and Posture

In the late 1970s, it was shown that postural adjustments associated with locomotion originated in the caudal portion of the pontine RF (see Mori, 1987). Stimulation of the dorsal area of the caudal pontine tegmental field (DTF) resulted in the relaxation of extensor muscles, whereas stimulation of the ventral area of the caudal pontine tegmental field (VTF) resulted in activation or an increase in extensor muscle tone. More recently, it has been shown that injections of cholinergic and serotonergic agonists into the PnO resulted in atonia and hypertonia respectively. These effects were mediated through medRF RSNs, with atonia-related RSNs located in the dorsomedial part of the medRF and hypertonus-related RSNs located in the ventromedial part of the medRF (Takakusaki et al., 2016). Thus it is clear that RSNs, through excitation and inhibition of spinal circuits, regulate muscle tone (for review see Takakusaki et al., 2016).

Extensor muscle tone is necessary for locomotion as there must be adequate force production to support the body and propel limbs forward (Mori et al., 1978, 1982). The interplay of posture and locomotion was demonstrated during MLR evoked locomotion, when stimulation of the DTF halted locomotion and stimulation of the VTF resulted in enhanced locomotor activity or a change in gait pattern (Mori et al., 1978). In freely moving cats with electrodes implanted in the DTF or VTF and the MLR, DTF stimulation during walking (naturally or MLR induced) led to sequential postural reduction to a sitting then prone position, and VTF stimulation when lying led to a rise to stance followed by locomotion (Mori et al., 1986).

The co-expression of postural tone and locomotion is likely due to shared neural pathways. For example, in addition to projecting to locomotor neurons in the GRN, the MLR also projects to postural areas (DTF and VTF). About 70% of DTF neurons are activated by MLR stimulation, with most being tonically active but some demonstrating rhythmic activity (Kawahara et al., 1985). Thus the MLR through two DTF pathways may participate in both tonic regulation of posture for locomotion and phasic regulation contributing to step cycle timing.

Reticulospinal Neurons and Reaching

RSNs are involved in movements other than posture and locomotion. For example, some RSNs in the cat are active during the preparatory phase in anticipation of reaching, while others are active during the actual reaching task (Schepens, 2004). Anatomical evidence using viral tracing has demonstrated glutamatergic RSNs in the MdV that form synapses exclusively with forelimb and not hindlimb MNs, unlike other neurons, including those in the GRN, which form synapses with both forelimbs and hindlimb MNs (Esposito et al., 2014). Furthermore, these synapses are motor pool specific, appearing on biceps but not triceps motoneurons. Inhibition of these RSNs resulted in decreased ability of the mice to accurately reach and grasp during a food pellet challenge. Because these RSNs are not involved in hindlimb movement, we will not consider them further here.

Reticulospinal Neurons and Sleep Atonia

While descending commands can stop locomotion (*vide supra*), the prototypical "stop" command is that which produces sleep atonia, in which limb muscle tone is curtailed to prevent movement during REM sleep (Saper et al., 2010). This atonic command originates in the SLDT nucleus, which contains glutamatergic neurons that project both to GRN and to the spinal cord (Sastre et al., 1981; Chase et al., 1986; Saper et al., 2010). Both of these targets contribute to sleep atonia, but whether the direct descending command from the GRN is inhibitory and/or whether its inhibitory effects are mediated by spinal interneurons is not clear (Fuller et al., 2007; Arrigoni et al., 2016). Recent evidence, however, suggests that there is descending inhibitory input that produces sleep atonia (Valencia Garcia et al., 2018).

In cats, lesions to the subcoeruleus region (analogous to the SLDT) result in behavior in which the cats appear to act out their dreams during sleep (Mouret et al., 1967; Henley and Morrison, 1974). Similarly, lesions to the SLDT in rodents led to complex motor behaviors during REM sleep (Lu et al., 2006). These behaviors are akin to REM behavior disorder (RBD) in humans (Schenck and Mahowald, 1995). That RBD can be localized to the SLDT has been shown in a case report of a woman with a lesion in this region who suffered from RBD and somnambulism (Limousin et al., 2009). Interestingly, RSNs that are associated with specific movements during waking are also active during REM sleep (Siegel et al., 1981). This suggests that extraneous movements during RBD are produced by the same neurons as during wakefulness. RBD is perhaps an extreme example of pathological RSN circuit selection. Other examples could include other disorders affecting movement selection such as dystonic syndromes.

INTRINSIC ORGANIZATION OF THE RETICULAR FORMATION

Clearly, rostral centers must activate different populations of RSNs in order to produce selected movements. Given that there can be net inhibitory (sleep atonia) and net excitatory (locomotion) effects produced by RSNs, we propose that movement selection circuits activate smaller ensembles or microcircuits of RSNs in order to facilitate specific movements whilst inhibiting other movements. This concept is not unlike that of the direct and indirect pathways of the basal ganglia that cooperate in movement selection (Cui et al., 2013). This example also demonstrates that the control of moving and not moving are intimately intertwined, and that neurological disorders that alter either one or the other of these two classes of microcircuits can lead to significant impairment in quality of life. How these microcircuits interact with each other, however, is yet to be defined.

What determines the tuning of appropriate commands? As RSNs are involved in diverse movements and comprise a subset of RF neurons, it would be prudent to ask whether RSNs simply integrate and relay inputs from higher brain centers to the spinal cord, or whether local microcircuits participate in refining motor commands.

Whilst our knowledge of the functional and topographical organization of RSNs is increasing, little is known about the internal organization of the RF. Some neurons within these nuclei are inhibitory, presumably interneurons (Sivertsen et al., 2016), but there is little information about local connectivity. Several modeling studies have addressed this lack of understanding of the internal circuitry. One proposal is that the RF is a "small-world network" in which dense connectivity within small groups of nodes is responsible for appropriate action selection (Humphries et al., 2006). Individual nodes would comprise small diameter local interneurons, most likely inhibitory, that project medially and laterally and connect with larger projecting cells (likely RSNs) within their own node. Node to node connectivity would be via axon collaterals of the large projecting neurons which would form synapses at relatively short distances, allowing for nearby nodes to activate quickly and concurrently (Humphries et al., 2007).

Experimental data to support this model are in short supply to date. But it is clear that knowledge of the internal organization of the RF is critical to understand how the RF and RSNs are selected to produce a wide array of finely tuned motor commands.

RETICULOSPINAL NEURONS IN HUMANS AND THEIR ROLE IN RECOVERY OF MOTOR FUNCTION

The corticofugal system plays an important role in human movement (Lemon, 2008). Axon collaterals from descending corticospinal neurons have diffuse projections, including to the RF (Kita and Kita, 2012). It is of interest that, although there was a deficit in fractionated finger movements in monkeys following lesions of these tracts below the level of the collaterals to the RF, other movements including climbing and running persisted (Lawrence and Kuypers, 1968a,b). Furthermore, monosynaptic corticomotoneuronal synapses are not necessary for hand movements in non-human primates, which improved over time following pyramidal tract lesions (Sasaki et al., 2004). Similarly, rare reports of sectioning these tracts in humans have demonstrated initial hemiparesis followed by recovery, ultimately leaving patients with a relative lack of movement deficit (Bucy et al., 1964). These data suggest that other systems such as RSNs can play a prominent role in movement in primates, including humans.

RS systems have been studied in humans via the startle reflex. This reflex response is seen across species and been shown to originate in the caudal brainstem—most likely the PnC (Hammond, 1973; Leitner et al., 1980; Davis et al., 1982). The startle reflex is seen in response to a loud acoustic stimulus (cf. Mauthner cells, above), and is stereotypically comprised of activation of the sternocleidomastoid muscle, followed by cranial nerve innervated muscles and rectus abdominus, and finally forelimb and hindlimb muscles (Rothwell, 2006). Evidence for a brainstem origin for this response has come from electrophysiological studies. When the instruction to start voluntary movement was combined with a loud auditory cue, the time to movement onset was significantly reduced (Rothwell, 2006). For example, the onset to volitional arm movement was found to be 150 ms, whereas arm movement initiated by the startle response can occur in 80 ms. This reduced latency has also been associated with an increased rate of force development, as well as increased force output (Anzak et al., 2011). Moreover, in more complex movements involving sequential activation of agonist and antagonist muscles, auditory stimulation sped up the activation of movement without affecting the pattern of muscle activity (Valls-Solé et al., 1999). Together, these data all point towards a subcortical, and more specifically RS, origin for startle reflexes.

The startle response in humans integrates with voluntary movements and may thus facilitate a potential therapeutic approach for regaining volitional movement post neurological insults to the cortex such as stroke (Rothwell, 2006) or to enhance motor performance in diseases such as Parkinson's disease (Anzak et al., 2016). In stroke patients, when the startle response was combined with voluntary movement, the latency to EMG response was shorter and the response was much larger than when either was performed alone, leading to the suggestion that detail of voluntary movement can be stored in the brainstem and can be accessed to produce movement in the absence of descending inputs from the cerebral cortex (Rothwell, 2006).

Given that RSNs are important in movement, and that many neurological injuries occur above the level of the RF, it is reasonable to ask whether the RS system could be a therapeutic target for therapies aimed at recovery of motor function in neurological diseases and injuries such as stroke (Baker et al., 2015). Data from non-human primates supports this concept (Zaaimi et al., 2012). Presumably, intentional signals from higher centers would still need to reach the RF, but as noted above, there are many supramedullary inputs that converge on RSNs. For example, following unilateral stroke, there are non-crossed cortico-reticular inputs that could possibly harness the unaffected ipsilateral cortex to promote RF plasticity and motor functional recovery (Jankowska and Edgley, 2006). The RS system is well connected to play a key role in recovery from motor deficits, as it projects to all levels of the spinal cord including to key movement circuits.

Such RS-mediated functional recovery need not be limited to axial movement. Although initially proposed to be important for axial and proximal muscles, it is becoming clear from studies in non-human primates that RSNs are also involved in hand function (Riddle et al., 2009), and could thus be a substrate for functional recovery of hand movements following neurological injury (Baker, 2011). In support of this possibility, recent evidence from humans points to the RS system as being involved in gross hand function after spinal cord injury (Baker and Perez, 2017).

To promote RSN-mediated recovery of motor function, however, several challenges exist. It will be necessary to understand the functional organization of motor command circuits in the RF, including how nodes or microcircuits in the RF are engaged to produce movement, whether individual microcircuits participate in more than one motor behavior, how individual microcircuits are recruited by rostral circuits, whether these circuits are under neuromodulatory control, and whether "on" movement and "off" movement microcircuits are simultaneously recruited to refine motor commands. Understanding these concepts could form the foundation for future therapeutic strategies.

Ultimately, it is clear that our focus in understanding the RF should include not only an "integrate and relay" function, but also an understanding of the internal organization and processing that controls RSNs such that a great versatility of movements can be produced. This understanding will lead not only to improved knowledge of how we move, but potentially also to new experimental paradigms to understand motor system changes in injury and disease, and ultimately to the development of new therapeutic strategies aimed at improving motor functional recovery.

AUTHOR CONTRIBUTIONS

RB and JC conceived and wrote the manuscript.

FUNDING

RB was supported by Wellcome Trust (grant no. 110193) and Brain Research UK.

REFERENCES

Anzak, A., Tan, H., Pogosyan, A., and Brown, P. (2011). Doing better than your best: loud auditory stimulation yields improvements in maximal voluntary force. *Exp. Brain Res.* 208, 237–243. doi: 10.1007/s00221-010-2474-1

Anzak, A., Tan, H., Pogosyan, A., Khan, S., Javed, S., Gill, S. S., et al. (2016). Subcortical evoked activity and motor enhancement in Parkinson's disease. *Exp. Neurol.* 277, 19–26. doi: 10.1016/j.expneurol.2015.12.004

Arrigoni, E., Chen, M. C., and Fuller, P. M. (2016). The anatomical, cellular and synaptic basis of motor atonia during rapid eye movement sleep. *J. Physiol.* 594, 5391–5414. doi: 10.1113/JP271324

Baker, S. N. (2011). The primate reticulospinal tract, hand function and functional recovery. *J. Physiol.* 589, 5603–5612. doi: 10.1113/jphysiol.2011.215160

Baker, S. N., and Perez, M. A. (2017). Reticulospinal contributions to gross hand function after human spinal cord injury. *J. Neurosci.* 37, 9778–9784. doi: 10.1523/JNEUROSCI.3368-16.2017

Baker, S. N., Zaaimi, B., Fisher, K. M., Edgley, S. A., and Soteropoulos, D. S. (2015). Pathways mediating functional recovery. *Prog. Brain Res.* 218, 389–412. doi: 10.1016/bs.pbr.2014.12.010

Bouvier, J., Caggiano, V., Leiras, R., Caldeira, V., Bellardita, C., Balueva, K., et al. (2015). Descending command neurons in the brainstem that halt locomotion. *Cell* 163, 1191–1203. doi: 10.1016/j.cell.2015.10.074

Buchanan, J. T. (2011). Spinal locomotor inputs to individually identified reticulospinal neurons in the lamprey. *J. Neurophysiol.* 106, 2346–2357. doi: 10.1152/jn.01100.2010

Bucy, P. C., Keplinger, J. E., and Siqueira, E. B. (1964). Destruction of the 'pyramidal tract' in man. *J. Neurosurg.* 21, 285–298.

Caggiano, V., Leiras, R., Goñi-Erro, H., Masini, D., Bellardita, C., Bouvier, J., et al. (2018). Midbrain circuits that set locomotor speed and gait selection. *Nature* 553, 455–460. doi: 10.1038/nature25448

Capelli, P., Pivetta, C., Soledad Esposito, M., and Arber, S. (2017). Locomotor speed control circuits in the caudal brainstem. *Nature* 551, 373–377. doi: 10.1038/nature24064

Chase, M. H., Morales, F. R., Boxer, P. A., Fung, S. J., and Soja, P. J. (1986). Effect of stimulation of the nucleus reticularis gigantocellularis on the membrane potential of cat lumbar motoneurons during sleep and wakefulness. *Brain Res.* 386, 237–244. doi: 10.1016/0006-8993(86)90160-5

Cui, G., Jun, S. B., Jin, X., Pham, M. D., Vogel, S. S., Lovinger, D. M., et al. (2013). Concurrent activation of striatal direct and indirect pathways during action initiation. *Nature* 494, 238–242. doi: 10.1038/nature11846

Davis, M., Gendelman, D. S., Tischler, M. D., and Gendelman, P. M. (1982). A primary acoustic startle circuit: lesion and stimulation studies. *J. Neurosci.* 2, 791–805.

Degtyarenko, A. M., Simon, E. S., and Burke, R. E. (1998). Locomotor modulation of disynaptic EPSPs from the mesencephalic locomotor region in cat motoneurons. *J. Neurophysiol.* 80, 3284–3296. doi: 10.1152/jn.1998.80.6.3284

Douglas, J. R., Noga, B. R., Dai, X., and Jordan, L. M. (1993). The effects of intrathecal administration of excitatory amino-acid agonists and antagonists on the initiation of locomotion in the adult cat. *J. Neurosci.* 13, 990–1000.

Drew, T., Cabana, T., and Rossignol, S. (1996). Responses of medullary reticulospinal neurones to stimulation of cutaneous limb nerves during locomotion in intact cats. *Exp. Brain Res.* 111, 153–168. doi: 10.1007/bf00227294

Drew, T., Dubuc, R., and Rossignol, S. (1986). Discharge patterns of reticulospinal and other reticular neurons in chronic, unrestrained cats walking on a treadmill. *J. Neurophysiol.* 55, 375–401. doi: 10.1152/jn.1986.55.2.375

Drew, T., and Rossignol, S. (1990). Functional organization within the medullary reticular formation of intact unanesthetized cat. II. Electromyographic activity evoked by microstimulation. *J. Neurophysiol.* 64, 782–795. doi: 10.1152/jn.1990.64.3.782

Du Beau, A., Shakya Shrestha, S., Bannatyne, B. A., Jalicy, S. M., Linnen, S., and Maxwell, D. J. (2012). Neurotransmitter phenotypes of descending systems in the rat lumbar spinal cord. *Neuroscience* 227, 67–79. doi: 10.1016/j.neuroscience.2012.09.037

Eaton, R. C., DiDomenico, R., and Nissanov, J. (1988). Flexible body dynamics of the goldfish C-start: implications for reticulospinal command mechanisms. *J. Neurosci.* 8, 2758–2768.

Eaton, R. C., Lee, R. K. K., and Foreman, M. B. (2001). The Mauthner cell and other identified neurons of the brainstem escape network of fish. *Prog. Neurobiol.* 63, 467–485. doi: 10.1016/s0301-0082(00)00047-2

Einum, J. F., and Buchanan, J. T. (2004). Reticulospinal neurons receive direct spinobulbar inputs during locomotor activity in lamprey. *J. Neurophysiol.* 92, 1384–1390. doi: 10.1152/jn.00625.2003

Esposito, M. S., Capelli, P., and Arber, S. (2014). Brainstem nucleus MdV mediates skilled forelimb motor tasks. *Nature* 508, 351–356. doi: 10.1038/nature13023

Faber, D. S., Fetcho, J. R., and Korn, H. (1989). Neuronal networks underlying the escape response in goldfish. *Ann. N Y Acad. Sci.* 563, 11–33. doi: 10.1111/j.1749-6632.1989.tb42187.x

Fetcho, J. R. (1991). Spinal network of the Mauthner cell. *Brain Behav. Evol.* 37, 298–316. doi: 10.1159/000316094

Fetcho, J. R. (1992). The spinal motor system in early vertebrates and some of its evolutionary changes. *Brain Behav. Evol.* 40, 82–97. doi: 10.1159/000113905

Fetcho, J. R., and Faber, D. S. (1988). Identification of motoneurons and interneurons in the spinal network for escapes initiated by the mauthner cell in goldfish. *J. Neurosci.* 8, 4192–4213.

Fuller, P. M., Saper, C. B., and Lu, J. (2007). The pontine REM switch: past and present. *J. Physiol.* 584, 735–741. doi: 10.1113/jphysiol.2007.140160

Garcia-Rill, E., and Skinner, R. D. (1987). The mesencephalic locomotor region. I. Activation of a medullary projection site. *Brain Res.* 411, 1–12. doi: 10.1016/0006-8993(87)90675-5

Graham Brown, T. (1911). The intrinsic factors in the act of progression in the mammal. *Proc. R. Soc. B Biol. Sci.* 84, 308–319. doi: 10.1098/rspb.1911.0077

Grillner, S., and Lund, S. (1968). The origin of a descending pathway with monosynaptic action on flexor motoneurones. *Acta Physiol. Scand.* 74, 274–284. doi: 10.1111/j.1748-1716.1968.tb04236.x

Hammond, G. R. (1973). Lesions of pontine and medullary reticular formation and prestimulus inhibition of the acoustic startle reaction in rats. *Physiol. Behav.* 10, 239–243. doi: 10.1016/0031-9384(73)90304-1

Henley, K., and Morrison, A. R. (1974). A re-evaluation of the effects of lesions of the pontine tegmentum and locus coeruleus on phenomena of paradoxical sleep in the cat. *Acta Neurobiol. Exp.* 34, 215–232.

Hildebrand, D. G. C., Cicconet, M., Torres, R. M., Choi, W., Quan, T. M., Moon, J., et al. (2017). Whole-brain serial-section electron microscopy in larval zebrafish. *Nature* 545, 345–349. doi: 10.1038/nature22356

Humphries, M. D., Gurney, K., and Prescott, T. J. (2006). The brainstem reticular formation is a small-world, not scale-free, network. *Proc. R. Soc. B Biol. Sci.* 273, 503–511. doi: 10.1098/rspb.2005.3354

Humphries, M. D., Gurney, K., and Prescott, T. J. (2007). Is there a brainstem substrate for action selection? *Philos. Trans. R. Soc. London Ser. B Biol. Sci.* 362, 1627–1639. doi: 10.1098/rstb.2007.2057

Jankowska, E. (2008). Spinal interneuronal networks in the cat: elementary components. *Brain Res. Rev.* 57, 46–55. doi: 10.1016/j.brainresrev.2007.06.022

Jankowska, E., and Edgley, S. A. (2006). How can corticospinal tract neurons contribute to ipsilateral movements? A question with implications for recovery of motor functions. *Neuroscientist* 12, 67–79. doi: 10.1177/1073858405283392

Jankowska, E., Jukes, M., Lund, S., and Lundberg, A. (1967). The effect of DOPA on the spinal cord. 6. Half-centre organization of interneurones transmitting effects from the flexor reflex afferents. *Acta Physiol. Scand.* 70, 389–402. doi: 10.1111/j.1748-1716.1967.tb03637.x

Jordan, L. M. (1998). Initiation of locomotion in mammals. *Ann. N Y Acad. Sci.* 860, 83–93. doi: 10.1111/j.1749-6632.1998.tb09040.x

Jordan, L. M., Liu, J., Hedlund, P. B., Akay, T., and Pearson, K. G. (2008). Descending command systems for the initiation of locomotion in mammals. *Brain Res. Rev.* 57, 183–191. doi: 10.1016/j.brainresrev.2007.07.019

Juvin, L., Grätsch, S., Trillaud-Doppia, E., Gariépy, J. F., Büschges, A., and Dubuc, R. (2016). A specific population of reticulospinal neurons controls the termination of locomotion. *Cell Rep.* 15, 2377–2386. doi: 10.1016/j.celrep.2016.05.029

Kawahara, K., Mori, S., Tomiyama, T., and Kanaya, T. (1985). Discharges of neurons in the midpontine dorsal tegmentum of mesencephalic cat during locomotion. *Brain Res.* 341, 377–380. doi: 10.1016/0006-8993(85)91078-9

Kim, L. H., Sharma, S., Sharples, S. A., Mayr, K. A., Kwok, C. H. T., and Whelan, P. J. (2017). Integration of descending command systems for the generation of context-specific locomotor behaviors. *Front. Neurosci.* 11:581. doi: 10.3389/fnins.2017.00581

Kimmel, C. B. (1993). Patterning the brain of the zebrafish embryo. *Annu. Rev. Neurosci.* 16, 707–732. doi: 10.1146/annurev.neuro.16.1.707

Kita, T., and Kita, H. (2012). The subthalamic nucleus is one of multiple innervation sites for long-range corticofugal axons: a single-axon tracing study in the rat. *J. Neurosci.* 32, 5990–5999. doi: 10.1523/JNEUROSCI.5717-11.2012

Kupfermann, I., and Weiss, K. R. (1978). The command neuron concept. *Behav. Brain Sci.* 1, 3–10. doi: 10.1017/s0140525x00059057

Lawrence, D. G., and Kuypers, H. G. J. M. (1968a). The functional organization of the motor system in the monkey: I. The effects of bilateral pyramidal lesions. *Brain* 91, 1–14. doi: 10.1093/brain/91.1.1

Lawrence, D. G., and Kuypers, H. G. J. M. (1968b). The functional organization of the motor system in the monkey: II. The effects of lesions of the descending brain-stem pathways. *Brain* 91, 15–36. doi: 10.1093/brain/91.1.15

Leitner, D. S., Powers, A. S., and Hoffman, H. S. (1980). The neural substrate of the startle response. *Physiol. Behav.* 25, 291–297. doi: 10.1016/0031-9384(80)90219-x

Lemon, R. N. (2008). Descending pathways in motor control. *Annu. Rev. Neurosci.* 31, 195–218. doi: 10.1146/annurev.neuro.31.060407.125547

Le Ray, D., Juvin, L., Boutin, T., Auclair, F., and Dubuc, R. (2010). A neuronal substrate for a state-dependent modulation of sensory inputs in the brainstem. *Eur. J. Neurosci.* 32, 53–59. doi: 10.1111/j.1460-9568.2010.07276.x

Liang, H., Paxinos, G., and Watson, C. (2011). Projections from the brain to the spinal cord in the mouse. *Brain Struct. Funct.* 215, 159–186. doi: 10.1007/s00429-010-0281-x

Limousin, N., Dehais, C., Gout, O., Héran, F., Oudiette, D., and Arnulf, I. (2009). A brainstem inflammatory lesion causing REM sleep behavior disorder and sleepwalking (parasomnia overlap disorder). *Sleep Med.* 10, 1059–1062. doi: 10.1016/j.sleep.2008.12.006

Liu, Y. C., and Hale, M. E. (2017). Local spinal cord circuits and bilateral mauthner cell activity function together to drive alternative startle behaviors. *Curr. Biol.* 27, 697–704. doi: 10.1016/j.cub.2017.01.019

Llinas, R., and Terzuolo, C. (1964a). Mechanisms of supraspinal actions upon spinal cord activities. Reticular inhibitory mechanisms on alpha-extensor motoneurons. *J. Neurophysiol.* 27, 579–591. doi: 10.1152/jn.1964.27.4.579

Llinas, R., and Terzuolo, C. (1964b). Mechaniss of supraspinal actions upon spinal cord activities. Reticular inhibitory mechanisms upon flexor motoneurons. *J. Neurophysiol.* 28, 413–422. doi: 10.1152/jn.1965.28.2.413

Lu, J., Sherman, D., Devor, M., and Saper, C. B. (2006). A putative flip-flop switch for control of REM sleep. *Nature* 441, 589–594. doi: 10.1038/nature04767

Magoun, H. (1944). Bulbar inhibition and facilitation of motor activity. *Science* 100, 549–550. doi: 10.1126/science.100.2607.549

Magoun, H., and Rhines, R. (1946). An inhibitory mechanism in the bulbar reticular formation. *J. Neurophysiol.* 9, 165–171. doi: 10.1152/jn.1946.9.3.165

Marlinskii, V. V., and Voitenko, L. P. (1992). Participation of the medial reticular formation of the medulla oblongata in the supraspinal control of locomotor and postural activities in the guinea pig. *Neurosci. Behav. Physiol.* 22, 336–342. doi: 10.1007/bf01182876

Matsuyama, K., and Drew, T. (2000). Vestibulospinal and reticulospinal neuronal activity during locomotion in the intact cat. II. Walking on an inclined plane. *J. Neurophysiol.* 84, 2257–2276. doi: 10.1152/jn.2000.84.5.2257

Matsuyama, K., Mori, F., Kuze, B., and Mori, S. (1999). Morphology of single pontine reticulospinal axons in the lumbar enlargement of the cat: a study using the anterograde tracer PHA-L. *J. Comp. Neurol.* 410, 413–430. doi: 10.1002/(sici)1096-9861(19990802)410:3<413::aid-cne5>3.0.co;2-q

Matsuyama, K., Nakajima, K., Mori, F., Aoki, M., and Mori, S. (2004). Lumbar commissural interneurons with reticulospinal inputs in the cat: morphology and discharge patterns during fictive locomotion. *J. Comp. Neurol.* 474, 546–561. doi: 10.1002/cne.20131

Matsuyama, K., Ohta, Y., and Mori, S. (1988). Ascending and descending projections of the nucleus reticularis gigantocellularis in the cat demonstrated by the anterograde neural tracer, Phaseolus vulgaris leucoagglutinin (PHA-L). *Brain Res.* 460, 124–141. doi: 10.1016/0006-8993(88)91212-7

McClellan, A. D., and Grillner, S. (1984). Activation of 'fictive swimming' by electrical microstimulation of brainstem locomotor regions in an *in vitro* preparation of the lamprey central nervous system. *Brain Res.* 300, 357–361. doi: 10.1016/0006-8993(84)90846-1

Mitchell, E. J., McCallum, S., Dewar, D., and Maxwell, D. J. (2016). Corticospinal and reticulospinal contacts on cervical commissural and long descending propriospinal neurons in the adult rat spinal cord; evidence for powerful reticulospinal connections. *PLoS One* 11:e0155664. doi: 10.1371/journal.pone.0155664

Mori, S. (1987). Integration of posture and locomotion in acute decebrate cats and in a wake, freely moving cats. *Prog. Neurobiol.* 28, 161–195. doi: 10.1016/0301-0082(87)90010-4

Mori, S., Kawahara, K., Sakamoto, T., Aoki, M., and Tomiyama, T. (1982). Setting and resetting of level of postural muscle tone in decerebrate cat by stimulation of brain stem. *J. Neurophysiol.* 48, 737–748. doi: 10.1152/jn.1982.48.3.737

Mori, S., Matsui, T., Kuze, B., Asanome, M., Nakajima, K., and Matsuyama, K. (1998). Cerebellar-induced locomotion: reticulospinal control of spinal rhythm generating mechanism in cats. *Ann. N Y Acad. Sci.* 860, 94–105. doi: 10.1111/j.1749-6632.1998.tb09041.x

Mori, S., Nishimura, H., Kurakami, C., Yamamura, T., and Aoki, M. (1978). Controlled locomotion in the mesencephalic cat: distribution of facilitatory and inhibitory regions within pontine tegmentum. *J. Neurophysiol.* 41, 1580–1591. doi: 10.1152/jn.1978.41.6.1580

Mori, S., Ohta, Y., Matsuyama, K., and Takukuski, K. (1986). "The setting of postural muscle tone: its importance for behaviors in freely moving intact cats," in *Emotions: Neuronal and Chemical Control*, ed. Y. Oomura (Basel: Karger), 231–239.

Mouret, J., Delorme, F., and Jouvet, M. (1967). Lesions of the pontine tegmentum field. *Compt. Soc. Biol. Fil.* 161, 1603–1606.

Noga, B. R., Kettler, J., and Jordan, L. M. (1988). Locomotion produced in mesencephalic cats by injections of putative transmitter substances and antagonists into the medial reticular formation and the pontomedullary locomotor strip. *J. Neurosci.* 8, 2074–2086. doi: 10.1523/JNEUROSCI.08-06-02074.1988

Noga, B. R., Kriellaars, D. J., Brownstone, R. M., Jordan, L. M., Leiras, R., Velo, P., et al. (2003). Mechanism for activation of locomotor centers in the spinal cord by stimulation of the mesencephalic locomotor region mechanism for activation of locomotor centers in the spinal cord by stimulation of the mesencephalic locomotor region. *J. Neurophysiol.* 90, 1464–1478. doi: 10.1152/jn.00034.2003

Orlovskii, G. N. (1970). Work of the reticulo-spinal neurons during locomotion. *Biofizika* 15, 728–737.

Paxinos, G., and Franklin, B. (2008). *The Mouse Brain in Sterotaxic Coordinates.* 3rd Edn. Oxford: Academic Press.

Paxinos, G., Xu-Feng, H., Sengul, G., and Watson, C. (2012). "Organization of brainstem nuclei," in *The Huaman Nervous System*, eds J. K. Mai and G. Paxinos (Amsterdam: Elsevier Academic Press), 260–327.

Perreault, M. C., Drew, T., and Rossignol, S. (1993). Activity of medullary reticulospinal neurons during fictive locomotion. *J. Neurophysiol.* 69, 2232–2247. doi: 10.1152/jn.1993.69.6.2232

Perreault, M. C., and Glover, J. C. (2013). Glutamatergic reticulospinal neurons in the mouse: developmental origins, axon projections, and functional connectivity. *Ann. N Y Acad. Sci.* 1279, 80–89. doi: 10.1111/nyas.12054

Peterson, B. W. (1984). "The reticulospinal system and its role in the control of movement," in *Brainstem Control of Spinal Cord Function*, ed. C. D. Barnes (New York, NY: Academic Press), 27–86.

Peterson, B. W., Maunz, R. A., Pitts, N. G., and Mackel, R. G. (1975). Patterns of projection and branching of reticulospinal neurons. *Exp. Brain Res.* 23, 333–351. doi: 10.1007/bf00238019

Peterson, B. W., Pitts, N. G., Fukushima, K., and Mackel, R. (1978). Reticulospinal excitation and inhibition of neck motoneurons. *Exp. Brain Res.* 32, 471–489. doi: 10.1007/bf00239548

Prasada Rao, P. D., Jadhao, A. G., and Sharma, S. C. (1987). Descending projection neurons to the spinal cord of the goldfish, Carassius auratus. *J. Comp. Neurol.* 265, 96–108. doi: 10.1002/cne.902650107

Rhines, R., and Magoun, H. (1946). Brain stem facilitation of cortical motor response. *J. Neurophysiol.* 9, 219–229. doi: 10.1152/jn.1946.9.3.219

Riddle, C. N., Edgley, S. A., and Baker, S. N. (2009). Direct and indirect connections with upper limb motoneurons from the primate reticulospinal tract. *J. Neurosci.* 29, 4993–4999. doi: 10.1523/JNEUROSCI.3720-08.2009

Roseberry, T. K., Lee, A. M., Lalive, A. L., Wilbrecht, L., Bonci, A., and Kreitzer, A. C. (2016). Cell-type-specific control of brainstem locomotor circuits by basal ganglia. *Cell* 164, 526–537. doi: 10.1016/j.cell.2015.12.037

Rothwell, J. C. (2006). The startle reflex, voluntary movement, and the reticulospinal tract. *Suppl. Clin. Neurophysiol.* 58, 223–231. doi: 10.1016/s1567-424x(09)70071-6

Saper, C. B., Fuller, P. M., Pedersen, N. P., Lu, J., and Scammell, T. E. (2010). Sleep state switching. *Neuron* 68, 1023–1042. doi: 10.1016/j.neuron.2010.11.032

Sasaki, S., Isa, T., Pettersson, L. G., Alstermark, B., Naito, K., Yoshimura, K., et al. (2004). Dexterous finger movements in primate without monosynaptic corticomotoneuronal excitation. *J. Neurophysiol.* 92, 3142–3147. doi: 10.1152/jn.00342.2004

Sastre, J. P., Sakai, K., and Jouvet, M. (1981). Are the gigantocellular tegmental field neurons responsible for paradoxical sleep? *Brain Res.* 229, 147–161. doi: 10.1016/0006-8993(81)90752-6

Schenck, C. H., and Mahowald, M. W. (1995). A polysomnographically documented case of adult somnambulism with long-distance automobile driving and frequent nocturnal violence: parasomnia with continuing danger as a noninsane automatism? *Sleep* 18, 765–772. doi: 10.1093/sleep/18.9.765

Schepens, B. (2004). Independent and convergent signals from the pontomedullary reticular formation contribute to the control of posture and movement during reaching in the cat. *J. Neurophysiol.* 92, 2217–2238. doi: 10.1152/jn.01189.2003

Schmidt, B. J., and Jordan, L. M. (2000). The role of serotonin in reflex modulation and locomotor rhythm production in the mammalian spinal cord. *Brain Res. Bull.* 53, 689–710. doi: 10.1016/s0361-9230(00)00402-0

Shapovalov, A. (1972). Evolution of neuronal systems of suprasegmental motor control. *Neurophysiology* 4, 346–359. doi: 10.1007/bf01063005

Sherrington, C. S. (1898). Decerebrate rigidity and reflex coordination of movements. *J. Physiol.* 22, 319–332. doi: 10.1113/jphysiol.1898.sp000697

Shik, M. L., Severin, F. V., and Orlovskii, G. N. (1966). Control of walking and running by means of electrical stimulation of the midbrain. *Biofizika* 11, 659–666.

Shimamura, M., and Kogure, I. (1983). Discharge patterns of reticulospinal neurons corresponding with quadrupedal leg movements in thalamic cats. *Brain Res.* 260, 27–34. doi: 10.1016/0006-8993(83)90761-8

Shimamura, M., Kogure, I., and Wada, S. (1980). Three types of reticular neurons involved in the spinobulbo-spinal reflex of cats. *Brain Res.* 186, 99–113. doi: 10.1016/0006-8993(80)90258-9

Shimamura, M., Kogure, I., and Wada, S. I. (1982). Reticular neuron activities associated with locomotion in thalamic cats. *Brain Res.* 231, 51–62. doi: 10.1016/0006-8993(82)90006-3

Siegel, J. M., Nienhuis, R., Wheeler, R. L., McGinty, D. J., and Harper, R. M. (1981). Discharge pattern of reticular formation unit pairs in waking and REM sleep. *Exp. Neurol.* 74, 875–891. doi: 10.1016/0014-4886(81)90260-0

Sillar, K. T., Picton, L. D., and Heitler, W. J. (2016). *The Neuroethology of Predation and Escape.* 1st Edn. Oxford: Wiley-Blackwell.

Sinnamon, H. M. (1993). Preoptic and hypothalamic neurons and the initiation of locomotion in the anesthetized rat. *Prog. Neurobiol.* 41, 323–344. doi: 10.1016/0301-0082(93)90003-b

Sinnamon, H. M., and Stopford, C. K. (1987). Locomotion elicited by lateral hypothalamic stimulation in the anesthetized rat does not require the dorsal midbrain. *Brain Res.* 402, 78–86. doi: 10.1016/0006-8993(87)91049-3

Sivertsen, M. S., Perreault, M. C., and Glover, J. C. (2016). Pontine reticulospinal projections in the neonatal mouse: internal organization and axon trajectories. *J. Comp. Neurol.* 524, 1270–1291. doi: 10.1002/cne.23904

Skinner, R. D., and Garcia-Rill, E. (1984). The mesencephalic locomotor region (MLR) in the rat. *Brain Res.* 323, 385–389. doi: 10.1016/0006-8993(84)90319-6

Sprague, J. M., and Chamber, W. W. (1954). Control of posture by reticular formation and cerebellum in the intact, anesthetized and unanesthetized and in the decerebrated cat. *Am. J. Physiol.* 176, 52–64. doi: 10.1152/ajplegacy.1953.176.1.52

Stecina, K. (2017). Midbrain stimulation-evoked lumbar spinal activity in the adult decerebrate mouse. *J. Neurosci. Methods* 288, 99–105. doi: 10.1016/j.jneumeth.2017.06.015

Steeves, J. D., and Jordan, L. M. (1980). Localization of a descending pathway in the spinal cord which is necessary for controlled treadmill locomotion. *Neurosci. Lett.* 20, 282–288. doi: 10.1016/0304-3940(80)90161-5

Steeves, J. D., Sholomenko, G. N., and Webster, D. M. S. (1987). Stimulation of the pontomedullary reticular formation initiates locomotion in decerebrate birds. *Brain Res.* 401, 205–212. doi: 10.1016/0006-8993(87)91406-5

Szokol, K., Glover, J. C., and Perreault, M.-C. (2011). Organization of functional synaptic connections between medullary reticulospinal neurons and lumbar descending commissural interneurons in the neonatal mouse. *J. Neurosci.* 31, 4731–4742. doi: 10.1523/JNEUROSCI.5486-10.2011

Szokol, K., Glover, J. C., Perreault, M.-C., and Perreault, M.-C. (2008). Differential origin of reticulospinal drive to motoneurons innervating trunk and hindlimb muscles in the mouse revealed by optical recording. *J. Physiol.* 58621, 5259–5276. doi: 10.1113/jphysiol.2008.158105

Takakusaki, K., Chiba, R., Nozu, T., and Okumura, T. (2016). Brainstem control of locomotion and muscle tone with special reference to the role of the mesopontine tegmentum and medullary reticulospinal systems. *J. Neural Transm. (Vienna)* 123, 695–729. doi: 10.1007/s00702-015-1475-4

Takakusaki, K., Kohyama, J., Matsuyama, K., and Mori, S. (1993a). Synaptic mechanisms acting on lumbar motoneurons during postural augmentation induced by serotonin injection into the rostral pontine reticular formation in decerebrate cats. *Exp. Brain Res.* 93, 471–482. doi: 10.1007/bf00229362

Takakusaki, K., Matsuyama, K., Kobayashi, Y., Kohyama, J., and Mori, S. (1993b). Pontine microinjection of carbachol and critical zone for inducing postural atonia in reflexively standing decerebrate cats. *Neurosci. Lett.* 153, 185–188. doi: 10.1016/0304-3940(93)90318-f

Valencia Garcia, S., Brischoux, F., Clément, O., Libourel, P.-A., Arthaud, S., Lazarus, M., et al. (2018). Ventromedial medulla inhibitory neuron inactivation induces REM sleep without atonia and REM sleep behavior disorder. *Nat. Commun.* 9:504. doi: 10.1038/s41467-017-02761-0

Valls-Solé, J., Rothwell, J. C., Goulart, F., Cossu, G., and Muñoz, E. (1999). Patterned ballistic movements triggered by a startle in healthy humans. *J. Physiol.* 516, 931–938. doi: 10.1111/j.1469-7793.1999.0931u.x

Wilson, V. J., and Yoshida, M. (1969). Comparison of effects of stimulation of Deiters' nucleus and medial longitudinal fasciculus on neck, forelimb and hindlimb motoneurons. *J. Neurophysiol.* 32, 743–758. doi: 10.1152/jn.1969.32.5.743

Wilson, V. J., Yoshida, M., and Schor, R. H. (1970). Supraspinal monosynaptic excitation and inhibition of thoracic back motoneurons. *Exp. Brain Res.* 11, 282–295. doi: 10.1007/bf01474387

Yasargil, G. M., and Sandri, C. (1990). Topography and ultrastructure of commissural interneurons that may establish reciprocal inhibitory connections of the Mauthner axons in the spinal cord of the tench, Tinca tinca L. *J. Neurocytol.* 19, 111–126. doi: 10.1007/bf01188443

Zaaimi, B., Edgley, S. A., Soteropoulos, D. S., and Baker, S. N. (2012). Changes in descending motor pathway connectivity after corticospinal tract lesion in macaque monkey. *Brain* 135, 2277–2289. doi: 10.1093/brain/aws115

Zottoli, S. J. (1977). Correlation of the startle reflex and Mauthner cell auditory responses in unrestrained goldfish. *J. Exp. Biol.* 66, 243–254.

15

Optogenetic Activation of A11 Region Increases Motor Activity

*Kathrin Koblinger[1,2], Céline Jean-Xavier[1,2], Sandeep Sharma[1,2], Tamás Füzesi[1,3], Leanne Young[1,2], Shane E. A. Eaton[1,2], Charlie Hong Ting Kwok[1,2], Jaideep Singh Bains[1,3] and Patrick J. Whelan[1,2,3]**

[1] *Hotchkiss Brain Institute, University of Calgary, Calgary, AB, Canada,* [2] *Department of Comparative Biology and Experimental Medicine, University of Calgary, Calgary, AB, Canada,* [3] *Department of Physiology and Pharmacology, University of Calgary, Calgary, AB, Canada*

Correspondence:
Patrick J. Whelan
whelan@ucalgary.ca

Limbic brain regions drive goal-directed behaviors. These behaviors often require dynamic motor responses, but the functional connectome of limbic structures in the diencephalon that control locomotion is not well known. The A11 region, within the posterior diencephalon has been postulated to contribute to motor function and control of pain. Here we show that the A11 region initiates movement. Photostimulation of channelrhodopsin 2 (ChR2) transfected neurons in A11 slice preparations showed that neurons could follow stimulation at frequencies of 20 Hz. Our data show that photostimulation of ChR2 transfected neurons in the A11 region enhances motor activity often leading to locomotion. Using vGluT2-reporter and vGAT-reporter mice we show that the A11 tyrosine hydroxylase positive (TH) dopaminergic neurons are vGluT2 and vGAT negative. We find that in addition to dopaminergic neurons within the A11 region, there is another neuronal subtype which expresses the monoenzymatic aromatic L-amino acid decarboxylase (AADC), but not TH, a key enzyme involved in the synthesis of catecholamines including dopamine. This monoaminergic-based motor circuit may be involved in the control of motor behavior as part of a broader diencephalic motor region.

Keywords: spinal cord, dopamine, descending, motor activity, locomotion control

INTRODUCTION

Activation of the posterior hypothalamus, zona incerta or lateral hypothalamus can elicit a variety of motor behaviors, including locomotion (Shik and Orlovsky, 1976; Sinnamon et al., 1984; Sławińska and Kasicki, 1995; Young et al., 2009). A general finding was that the activity evoked from these areas was more complicated than the one elicited from motor regions of the brainstem (Mori et al., 1989), including the mesencephalic locomotor region and the medullary reticular formation (Kim et al., 2017). For example, stimulation of the lateral hypothalamus can result in varied responses ranging from feeding to predatory attack depending on context (Stuber and Wise, 2016; Kim et al., 2017). In this work, we focus on targeting diencephalic areas of the brain containing monoaminergic cells, with the goal of understanding their multifaceted motor function.

Dahlström and Fuxe (1964) identified a series of dopaminergic nuclei named A8-16. Some of these are well linked with motor functions such as the substantia nigra pars compacta (A9), while the role of others have been less well described. One of these nuclei is the A11 region which is located in the posterior diencephalon abutting the third ventricle (Björklund and Skagerberg, 1979; Barraud et al., 2010; Koblinger et al., 2014; Sharples et al., 2014). These neurons are non-canonical dopaminergic cells which lack the dopamine reuptake transporter in mouse (DAT) (Koblinger et al., 2014; Yip et al., 2017). The A11 cell group appears to be evolutionarily conserved from zebrafish (Ryu et al., 2007; Lambert et al., 2012) to mammals (Barraud et al., 2010). The broader connectome of the A11 has been under investigation; however, it has been shown to receive inputs from the parabrachial nucleus, infralimbic cortex, and the bed nucleus of the stria terminalis (Abrahamson and Moore, 2001; Qu et al., 2006). One of the primary efferent targets of the A11 is the spinal cord – sending collaterals at regular intervals into the gray matter, and has been proposed to be the primary source of spinal dopamine (Björklund and Skagerberg, 1979; Commissiong et al., 1979; Skagerberg and Lindvall, 1985). While the functions of the A11 are not fully understood, it appears to have both anti-nociceptive and pro-nociceptive properties (Fleetwood-Walker et al., 1988; Megat et al., 2018), pathologically it has been associated with Restless Legs Syndrome (RLS) (Clemens et al., 2006), and 6-OHDA lesions of the area are associated with an increase in motor function (Qu et al., 2007) possibly by actions on dopamine receptor type 3 (D_3) receptors (Clemens and Hochman, 2004; Qu et al., 2007).

One way in which A11 projections could control motor circuits is through direct modulation of spinal circuits, and indeed a sizable literature suggests that dopamine modulates the activity of motoneurons and interneurons within the lumbar spinal cord (Barrière et al., 2004; Madriaga et al., 2004; Han et al., 2007; Humphreys and Whelan, 2011; Gozal et al., 2014; Sharples et al., 2015; Sharples and Whelan, 2017). Specifically, dopamine can alter the frequency and pattern of locomotor activity, by increasing spiking frequency robustly, and decreasing both the first spike latency and after hyperpolarization amplitude (Han et al., 2007). The premotoneuronal excitatory drive onto motoneurons is also increased since dopamine can potentiate AMPA transmission in motoneurons by acting on D_1 receptors (Han and Whelan, 2009), and increase mEPSC frequency in motoneurons (Han et al., 2007). Finally, recent evidence suggests that dopamine acts on the sodium pump in motoneurons to directly increase an ultra-slow hyperpolarization (Picton et al., 2017). In sum, dopamine can modulate spinal motor function through an array of modulatory mechanisms. The larger family of monoamines (Kiehn et al., 1999; Madriaga et al., 2004; Liu and Jordan, 2005) and trace amines (Gozal et al., 2014; Hochman, 2015), can also sculpt the pattern of activity evoked from spinal cord circuits. Sources of these monoamines include supraspinal projections (Schmidt and Jordan, 2000; Sławińska et al., 2014).

Given the effects of monoamines on spinal motor circuits, this led to our hypothesis that activation of the A11 region in the freely behaving adult mouse would lead to changes in motor behavior. We found that photostimulation of the A11 region elicits motor behavior, and that dopamine neurons lacking DAT are present in the region (Ugrumov, 2009). Part of this work was reported in an abstract and in a mini-symposium (Koblinger et al., 2015; Whelan, 2017).

MATERIALS AND METHODS

Ethics Statement

All animal experiments were approved by the University of Calgary Health Sciences Animal Care Committee (Protocol: AC15-0016), following the Canadian Council for Animal Care guidelines. Animals were housed in a double-barrier facility for breeding.

Animals

TH-IRES-Cre knock-in mice were used (a gift from Dr. Antoine Adamantidis, Universität Bern, Switzerland – source; EM: 00254;B6.129X1-Thtm1(cre)Te/Kieg; European Mouse Mutant Archive) as well as DAT-IRES-Cre knock-in mice were obtained from Jackson labs [B6.SJL-Slc6a3tm1.1(cre)Bkmn/J]. Reporter mice were purchased from Jackson labs [tdTomato mice: B6.Cg-Gt(ROSA)26Sortm14(CAG-TdTomato)Hze/J (Ai14)]. vGluT2-Cre-tdTomato (gift from Dr. Marie-Claude Perreault, Slc17a7-IRES2-CRE, Jackson labs) and vGAT-ChR2-eYFP [B6.Cg-Tg(Slc32a1-COP4*H134R/EYFP)8Gfng/J, Jackson labs] mice were also used. We then crossed the different lines to obtain TH-IRES-Cre homozygous, TH-IRES-Cre tdTomato, and DAT-IRES-Cre tdTomato heterozygous mice. Pairs of homozygous TH-IRES-Cre (male), DAT-IRES-Cre (female) or Ai14 (male or female) genotypes were mated, and the resulting heterozygous TH-IRES-Cre; Ai14 and DAT-IRES-Cre; Ai14 male offspring were used in subsequent experiments. All mice were genotyped with DNA extracted from ear notches using the Kapa mouse genotyping kit (Kapa Biosystems, Wilmington, MA, United States) according to manufacturer's instructions. TH-IRES-Cre mice were genotyped using mixed primer PCR employing TH-IRES-Cre-F (CCTGGTCTGGACACAGTGC), TH-WT-F (CAAGCACTGAGTGCCATTAGC) and TH-Com-R (AGAGGCCAGGAACACTCCTG). Amplification of wild-type genomic DNA yielded a 298 bp PCR product whereas amplification from the mutant locus yielded a 453 bp PCR product. Genotyping of the TH-IRES-tdTomato and DAT-IRES-Cre mice was performed similarly, using the primers recommended by the supplier (Jackson Labs, Bar Harbor, ME, United States). Mice were housed on a 12:12 h light:dark schedule (lights on at 07:00 – off at 19:00) with *ad libitum* access to food and water. All behavioral experiments were performed in male mice between 8 and 16 weeks old.

Validation of TH-IRES-Cre Mice via Real Time qPCR

Total RNA was isolated from TH-IRES-Cre;CAG-LSL-tdTomato mouse microdissected brain regions (n = 7) A13, A11, and substantia nigra/ventral tegmental area (SN/VTA) using the RNeasy lipid tissue mini kit (Qiagen, Hilden, Germany) following manufacturer's recommendations. Reverse transcription was performed using the Superscript VILO IV kit (Thermo Fisher, Waltham, MA, United States). For the negative control groups, all components except the reverse transcriptase were included in the reaction mixtures. The primers for real time qPCR were mGAPD-F (GTGAAGGTCGGTGTGAACG) and mGAPD-R (TCGT TGATGGCAACAATCTC); TH-F (CCCAAGGGCTT CAGAAGAGC) and TH-R (ATCCTCGATGAGACTCTGCC); Cre-F (ACGCACTGATTTCGACCAGGTTCG) and Cre-R (CATTCTCCCACCGTCAGTACGTGAG). Real time qPCR was performed with PowerUp SYBR green master mix (Thermo Fisher, Waltham, MA, United States) and mouse GAPDH was utilized as the reference gene. The running protocol extended to 45 cycles in fast mode consisting of 95°C for 1 s, 60°C for 30 s using a Quantstudio 3 instrument (Thermo Fisher, Waltham, MA, United States). Standard curve experiments using control mouse brain RNA were determined using a 5 log range of cDNA concentrations yielding efficiencies ranging from 90 to 110% (Bustin et al., 2009). Control reactions and those containing cDNA from the various brain regions were performed with 10 ng of template per reaction. PCR specificity was checked by dissociation curve analysis. Template controls yielded no detectable fluorescence. The relative mRNA abundance of TH and Cre in each sample were normalized to the abundance of GAPDH mRNA.

Optogenetics

Under isoflurane anesthesia (1.5 %), mice were secured in a stereotaxic apparatus (Stoelting Co., Wood Dale, IL, United States), and glass capillaries were lowered into the brain of TH-IRES-Cre or TH-IRES-Cre; Ai14 mice (AP −2.3 mm; ML −0.1 mm from the bregma; DV −2.9 mm from the dura). Recombinant AAV carrying a fluorescently tagged channelrhodopsin 2, ChR2-eYFP (Addgene plasmid 20298, pAAV-EF1a-double floxed-hChR2(H134R)-eYFP-WPRE-HGHpA; titre: 3×10^{12} GC/ml; Virus Vector Core, UNC, Lot # AV4844B) or eYFP (Addgene plasmid 20296, pAAV-EF1a-double floxed-eYFP-WPRE-HGHpA; 4×10^{12} GC/ml; Virus Vector Core, UNC, Lot # AV4842C) were pressure injected using the Nanoject II apparatus (Drummond Scientific Company, Broomall, PA, United States). 210 nl of the virus were injected bilaterally, with a total volume of 420 nl per mouse.

Mice were returned to their home cage and left for at least 14 days to allow for transfection of the viral construct into A11 neurons. For optogenetic experiments, mono-fiber optic cannulas were stereotactically implanted into the A11 area (MF2.5-FLT, Doric, Quebec, QC, Canada) (AP −2.3 mm; ML, −0.1 mm from the bregma; DV −2.7 mm from the dura). Fiber optic cannulas were secured in place using dental cement (Metabond, Parkell, Brentwood, NY, United States and Dentsply, York, PA, United States). Mice were allowed to recover for at least 3 days before behavioral testing. We performed *post hoc* histology to confirm $A11^{ChR2}$ transfection and ferrule placement.

Whole Cell Patch Experiments

In a separate series of experiments, we measured inward currents and spike activity using *in vitro* slice preparations to examine the effectiveness of $A11^{ChR2}$ transfection. Young male TH-IRES-Cre; Ai14 mice (4–6 weeks postnatal) were deeply anesthetized with isoflurane and decapitated. Brains were then rapidly removed and immersed in 4°C slicing solution containing, in mM: 87 NaCl, 2.5 KCl, 0.5 $CaCl_2$, 7 $MgCl_2$, 25 $NaHCO_3$, 25 D-glucose, 1.25 NaH_2PO_4, 75 sucrose saturated with 95% O_2/5% CO_2. 250 μm coronal sections were obtained using a vibratome (Leica), and allowed to recover for 1 + h in 95% O_2/5% CO_2 saturated, 30°C artificial cerebrospinal fluid (aCSF) containing (in mM): 126 NaCl, 2.5 KCl, 26 $NaHCO_3$, 2.5 $CaCl_2$, 1.5 $MgCl_2$, 1.25 NaH_2PO_4, 10 glucose. All recordings took place in aCSF at 30–32°C perfused at a rate of 1 mL/min, with DNQX (10 μM, Tocris) or picrotoxin (100 μM, Sigma) applied via perfusion pump. Neurons were visualized with an upright microscope fitted with differential interference contrast and epifluorescence optics (UVICO, Rapp OptoElectronic) and camera (AxioCam MRm). Borosilicate pipettes (3–5 MΩ) were filled with internal solution containing (in mM) 108 K-gluconate, 2 $MgCl_2$, 8 Na-gluconate, 8 KCl, 1 K_2-EGTA, 4 K_2-ATP, 0.3 Na_3-GTP, 10 mM HEPES, 0.2 Alexa-488 hydrazide and 10 mg/mL biocytin. A fiber optic cable (105 μm core diameter) was placed 1–2 mm from the A11 using a manipulator to deliver light from a laser (473 nm, OptoGeni 473, IkeCool Corporation). Light intensity was measured by a Photodiode Power Sensor (Thorlabs). Maximally, 2.5 mW light was delivered to the tissue. Signals were amplified (Multiclamp 700B, Molecular Devices), low pass filtered at 1 kHz, digitized at 10 kHz (Digidata 1322, Molecular Devices, San Jose, CA, United States), and recorded (pClamp 9.2, Molecular Devices) for offline analysis of evoked or spontaneous synaptic currents (Clampfit, Molecular Devices; MiniAnalysis, Synaptosoft).

Behavior

For *in vivo* experiments the light source (473 nm, LRS-0473-GFM, Laserglow Technologies, Toronto, ON, Canada) was connected to an implanted ferrule with a fiber optic cable (200 μm core diameter, Doric Lenses, Quebec City, QC, Canada). The laser was controlled by TTL pulses delivered using a Master 8 pulse stimulator (A.M.P.I., Jerusalem, Israel). The blue light was delivered for 3 min (20 Hz, 10 ms pulse width, 15 mW).

Each mouse was tested for 9 min (3 min pre, 3 min light, 3 min post) for five consecutive days. Behavior was recorded using a vertically mounted video camera and *post hoc* analyzed with the TopScan video tracking software (Clever Sys Inc., Reston, VA, United States). For c-Fos immunolabelling, animals were sacrificed 2 h after light stimulation. Behavioral testing was performed in a 70 cm × 70 cm × 50 cm high open field chamber with opaque walls. Each mouse was habituated to the chamber for 3 days for 1 h per day before testing. On test days, mice were habituated for 30 min before testing and trials were performed at the same time of day. Mice were transferred to and from a behavioral testing room for day-to-day testing. Mice were housed singly in standard cages (SafeSeal Plus Mouse Green Line

GM500, Techniplast, Italy, 501 cm^2 floor) with no environmental enrichment.

The Clever Sys tracking software divided movement into three categories:

(1) Immobility/No movement: Immobility is defined by both speed and motion measures (animal body change in consecutive frames expressed as a percentage). Immobility bouts over 15 successive frames were estimated when speed was <60 mm/s and the change in motion was <1% change in animal body position.
(2) In Place Activity: Animal stays in one place with some observed activity such as grooming, sniffing, stretching, rearing, but the animal is not immobile.
(3) Locomotion. Distance traveled: The mouse physically moves or displaces itself from one location to another with a minimum prescribed speed of greater than 60 mm/s and a minimum distance of 100 mm. Locomotor bouts: the number of times animal moves from one place to another place. If the animal continuously moves, it is counted as one single bout. Locomotor duration: the amount of time the mouse spends in locomotion.

Immunohistochemistry

Mice were sacrificed with isoflurane (2%) and transcardially perfused with phosphate-buffered saline (PBS), followed by 10% formalin in PBS. Brains were placed in 10% formalin for 12 h followed by 30% sucrose phosphate buffer (PB) for cryoprotection. 30 μM coronal brain sections were obtained using a cryostat (Leica CM1850 UV, Leica Biosystems, Richmond Hill, ON, Canada). The sliced brain sections were collected in a staggered fashion and placed into four consecutive wells. Rinses were performed before and between incubations with 0.1 M PBS, followed by one 20 min wash in Tris-buffered saline containing Triton (TBSt; pH 7.4, with 0.1% TritonX-100). Sections were incubated in blocking solution (5% donkey and 5% goat serum in PBS) for 1 h, and blocking solution was used in subsequent antibody incubations. The primary antibodies used were rabbit anti-TH, sheep anti-TH (1:1000, Abcam Inc., Toronto, ON, Canada), chicken anti-GFP (1:1000, Aves Laboratories, Tigard, OR, United States), rabbit anti-c-Fos (1:1000, EMD Millipore, Billerica, MA, United States), rabbit anti-RFP (1:5000, Rockland Immunochemicals Inc, Limerick, PA, United States) and rabbit anti-AADC (1:250, Novus Biologicals, Littleton, CO, United States). The secondary antibodies used were Alexa-564-conjugated donkey anti-rabbit, Alexa-488-conjugated donkey anti-sheep, Alexa-488-conjugated goat anti-chicken, Alexa-647-conjugated donkey anti-sheep (1:1000, Molecular Probes, Burlington, ON, Canada), biotinylated donkey anti-rabbit and Cy3-conjugated streptavidin (1:500, Jackson Immuno Research, West Grove, PA, United States). Free-floating brain sections were then mounted onto Superfrost^{TM} slides, coated with Vectashield^{TM} (H-1000, Vector, Burlingame, CA, United States) and cover-slipped. Fluorescent images were collected using the following microscopes; Nikon Eclipse C1si spectral confocal microscope, Nikon A1R MP+ and Olympus BX51. The objectives used were 4X (NA 0.13), 20X PLAN APO DIC (NA 0.75), 20X PLAN FLUOR (NA 0.75), 60X PLAN APO IR (NA 1.27) for Nikon Eclipse C1si spectral confocal microscope. The lasers used were centered on 488 nm (515/30 nm emission filter) and 561 (590/50 nm emission filter). The objectives used were 10X DIC L N1 (NA 0.30), 20X PLAN FLUOR MImm DIC N2 (NA 0.75), 60X PLAN APO IR WI DIC N2 (1.27) for the Nikon A1R MP+ microscope. The lasers used were centered at 403 nm, (450 nm emission filter) 488 nm (525 nm emission filter), and 562 nm (595 nm emission filter), respectively using pinhole radius of 12.7–21.5 microns on Nikon A1R MP+ microscope. The 20X images were taken with z-step 0.5 or 1 μm, 60X with z-step 0.15 μm. Stacked images were acquired by averaging four frames with a resolution of 1024 × 1024 or 512 × 512. Some images were acquired using a Panoramic FLASH II digital slide scanner (3DHISTECH inc., provided by Quorum Technologies) equipped with a Lumencor SPECTRA light source and PCO.edge sCMOS camera. Off-line image processing included maximal intensity projections conducted using NIS-Elements Advanced Research Version 4.10 as well as adjustments of brightness and contrast in Adobe Photoshop. Cell counting was accomplished by a person blinded to the study using ImageJ (NIH Image, Bethesda, MD, United States). We counted five sections containing the area of interest per animal.

Data Analysis and Statistics

Statistical analyses were performed in GraphPad Prism 6. Unpaired Student's *t*-tests were conducted comparing between two independent groups (e.g., A11^{eYFP} vs. A11^{ChR2}). When assumptions of normality were violated, a Mann–Whitney test was performed instead of a *t*-test. A two-way repeated measures analysis of variance (ANOVA) was conducted to examine changes between two groups (i.e., A11^{eYFP} vs. A11^{ChR2}) across time. When a significant main effect or interaction was found, Tukey *post hoc* comparisons were conducted. When assumptions of normality were violated on the ANOVA, non-parametric Friedman tests were done with a Dunn's multiple comparison tests when significant main effects were found. Repeated measures one-way ANOVA (RM-ANOVA) tests were conducted to examine changes within a group (i.e., A11^{eYFP} vs. A11^{ChR2}) in different conditions (before, during, just after light-activation of the A11). When a significant main effect or interaction was found, Bonferroni multiple *post hoc* comparisons tests were conducted. Data are reported as the mean ± standard deviation (SD) and $P < 0.05$ values were considered significant. When data did not pass normality tests, the median is reported with 25–75% ranges. When histograms were used (**Figure 6**) both the median and mode were used to report data.

RESULTS

Classes of Cells Within the A11 Region

We used a viral approach to identify classes of cells within the A11. The viral transfection efficiency was confirmed by injecting an AAV-DIO-ChR2-eYFP construct into A11 region in TH-IRES-Cre-tdTomato reporter mice (**Figures 1A–C**, $n = 4$). We found that 96% (SD = 1.7%) of ChR2-eYFP neurons expressed

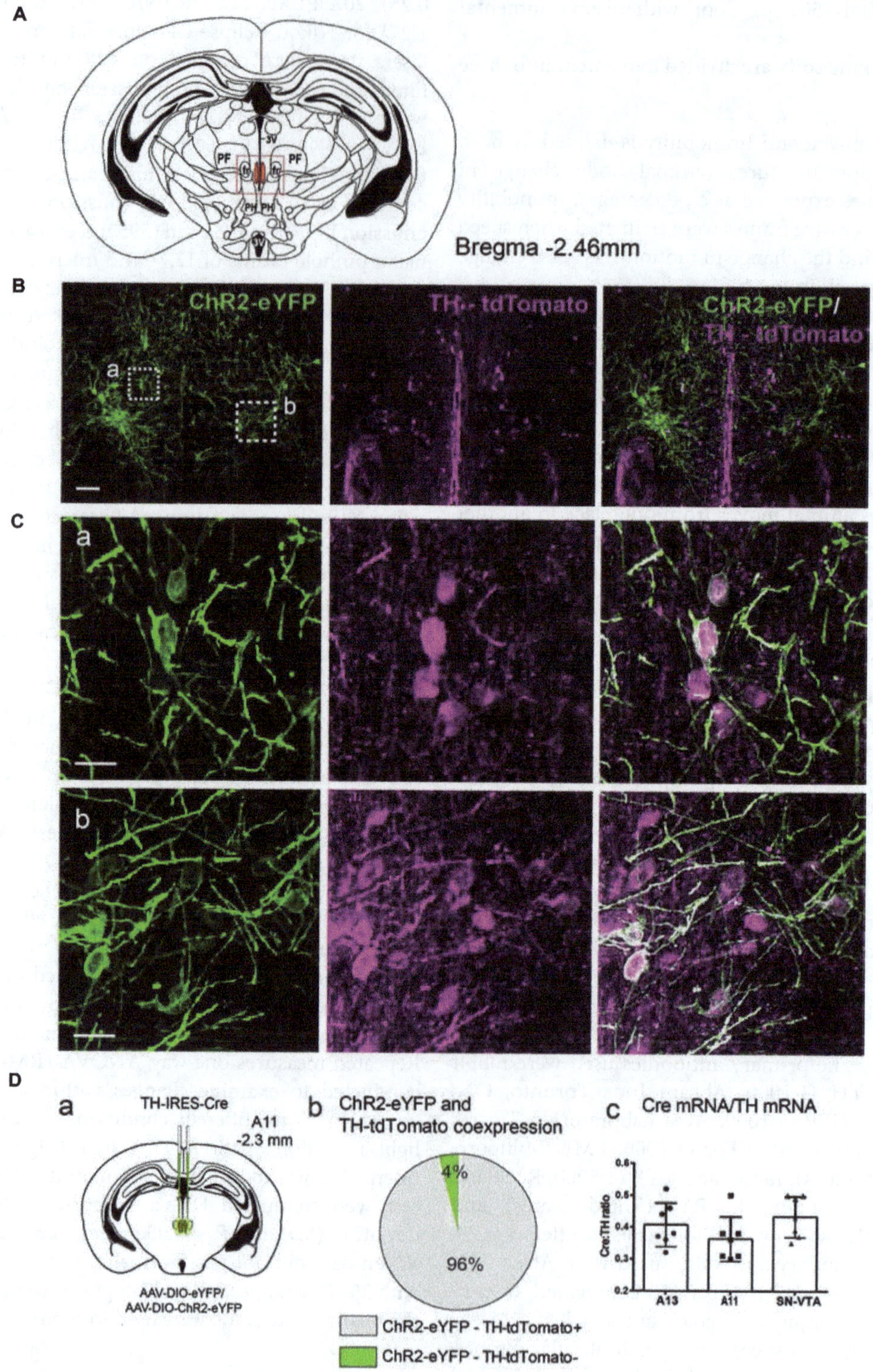

FIGURE 1 | Anatomical characterization of TH-IRES-Cre A11 neurons following transfection with AAV-DIO-ChR2-eYFP. **(A)** Diagram showing the middle region of the A11 area in the mouse (Bregma −2.46). The red frame represents the area where representative micrographs were taken. 3V, third ventricle; PF, parafascicular thalamic nucleus; fr, fasciculus retroflexus; PH, posterior hypothalamic nucleus. **(B)** TH-IRES-Cre tdTomato mice expressing channelrhodopsin-2 – enhanced yellow fluorescent protein (ChR2-eYFP) in A11. Confocal image showing A11 neurons expressing ChR2-eYFP bilaterally (stitched image consisting of 4 20X images). Scale bar 100 μm. **(C)** Higher magnification (60X zoom) of boxed areas **(a,b)** in **B**, Scale bar 20 μm. **(Da)** Schematic map showing the injection site of virus with the Cre-dependent ChR2 construct tagged with ChR2-eYFP or eYFP alone into the A11 of TH-IRES-Cre mice. **(Db)** Pie graph showing that 96% of ChR2-eYFP positive cells in A11 co-express tdTomato (*n* = 4). **(Dc)** Quantitative real-time PCR analysis of ratio of Cre mRNA to that of TH mRNA in A13, A11 and substantia nigra/ventral tegmental area (SN/VTA) brain regions.

TH-tdTomato (**Figure 1D**) in the A11 region. To confirm that Cre expression levels correlated with the expression levels of endogenous TH, real time qPCR analyses were performed on RNA isolated from TH-expressing brain regions A13 (A), A11 (B), and SN/VTA (C) (**Figure 1D**). Expression of TH and Cre, respectively, were normalized to the expression of the reference gene GAPDH. The normalized expression of Cre was consistently lower than that of TH, with levels ranging from 36 to 43%, depending on the brain region. All of the animals analyzed were heterozygous for the Cre transgene so the expected result was that Cre mRNA levels would be 50% of TH mRNA levels. Based on these results we expect that Cre mRNA levels will be close to TH mRNA levels in homozygous TH-IRES-Cre mice. Next, we confirmed in TH-IRES-Cre mice that the viral injections were restricted to the A11 region. **Figure 2** shows that the expression of ChR2-eYFP^{+} was spatially restricted to neurons from the A11 region (**Figure 2A**) following Cre-dependent viral expression. Other neighboring TH expressing regions, like the VTA, substantia nigra pars compacta and A13 did not show evidence of eYFP reporter expression (**Figures 2Ac,Ba–c,Ca–c**, respectively).

Next, we examined the co-localization of TH^{+}-IR cells with A11^{ChR2} cells to identify the neurotransmitter phenotype of the cells transfected within the A11 region of TH-IRES-Cre mice. Similar to recent reports (Lammel et al., 2015) we found that 54% of A11^{ChR2} expressing cells were co-localized with TH^{+}-IR (n = 4, ChR2 mean = 132, SD = 32.01, TH^{+}-IR mean = 105.5, SD = 11.03; co-localizing mean = 71.75, SD = 15.97, data not shown). In our previous work, we established that the large diameter cells which constitute the A11 region in mice are a non-canonical class of dopaminergic neurons that lack the Dopamine Transporter (DAT) (Koblinger et al., 2014) which was replicated in a report that used a DAT-GFP reporter line (Yip et al., 2017). We further confirmed these findings using our DAT-Cre-tdTomato reporter line (data not shown). We then tested for non-classical types of monoaminergic cells within the A11 region. These neurons only express the AADC enzyme and can produce various monoamines and trace amines (Ugrumov, 2009). We found evidence for AADC cells lacking TH in the A11 region (**Figure 3**) which suggest the presence of putative D-cells in the A11 region (Jaeger et al., 1983). In TH-tdTomato^{+} mice, we found that 35% of TH-tdTomato^{+}/TH^{-}-IR neurons were also AADC^{+} in the A11 region (n = 5, TH-tdTomato^{+}/TH^{-}-IR mean = 185.8, SD = 129.1, TH-tdTomato^{+}/TH^{-}-IR/AADC^{+} mean = 64.4, SD = 38.14; **Figure 3**). Taken together these results suggest that approximately 70% of transfected cells are capable of releasing dopamine and other monoamines such as serotonin (5-HT) or trace amines.

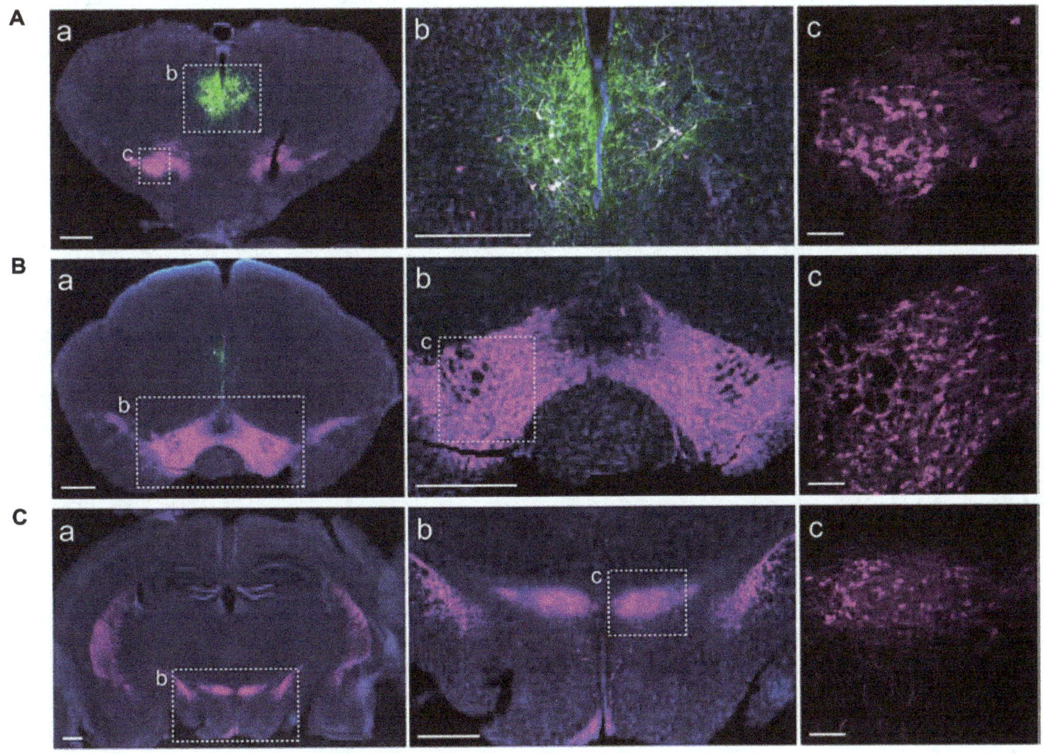

FIGURE 2 | ChR2-eYFP expression is restricted to A11 area. Immunohistochemistry targeted against eYFP (green) and TH (magenta) showing restricted ChR2-eYFP expression to A11. **(Aa,b)** ChR2-eYFP expression in A11 following Cre-dependent viral expression (DAPI, blue was used to label the cell nuclei). **(Ac)** Higher magnification (20X) of boxed TH^{+}-IR neurons in substantia nigra pars compacta. **(Ba,b,c)** No ChR2-eYFP expression in the ventral tegmental area (VTA). **(Ca,b,c)** No ChR2-eYFP expression in A13. Images **(Aa,b, Ba,b, Ca,b)** acquired with Olympus slide scanner 20X magnification, scale bar 500 μm; **(Ac, Bc, Cc)** Higher magnification confocal images of boxed area in **b (Ab, Bb, Cb)**, scale bar 100 μm.

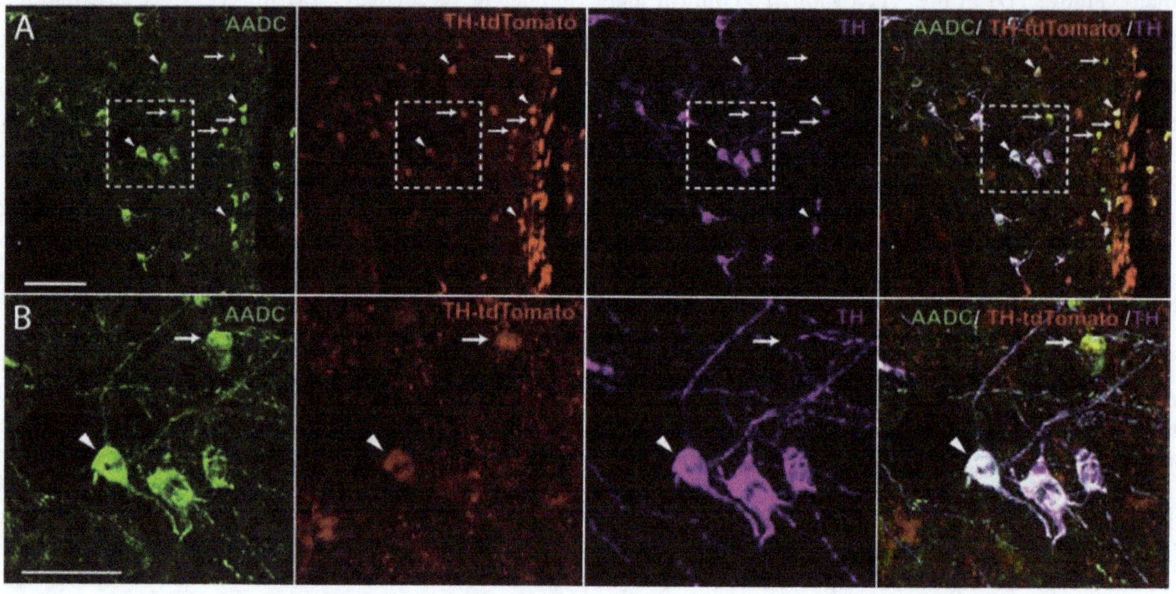

FIGURE 3 | Aromatic L-amino acid decarboxylase (AADC) expression in A11 TH-IR neurons. **(A)** Immunohistochemistry targeted against AADC (green) and TH^{+}-IR (magenta) as well as native TH-tdtomato (red) expression showing that a proportion of A11 $TH\text{-}tdTomato^{+}/TH^{-}$-IR neurons were also $AADC^{+}$ in TH-IRES-Cre tdTomato mice. 20X magnification, scale bar 100 μm. **(B)** Enlarged image showing $AADC^{+}/TH\text{-}tdTomato^{+}/TH^{-}$-IR (arrows) and $AADC^{+}/TH\text{-}tdTomato^{+}/TH^{+}$-IR neurons (arrowheads). 20X magnification, scale bar 50 μm.

Since there is evidence of localization of dopamine with co-transmitters such as peptides, glutamate or GABA, we asked whether co-localization of dopamine neurons in the A11 with GABA or glutamate could be detected. **Figure 4** illustrates there is evidence of a small number of $vGluT2^{+}$ cells within the A11 region. However, there was no $vGluT2^{+}$-TH^{+}-IR co-localization in the A11 region, compared to the arcuate nucleus of hypothalamus (**Figures 4A,B**). While vGluT2 was the most likely target subpopulation we also examined Allen Brain Atlas data and found strong expression of vGluT3, however, no evidence for vGluT1 staining in the A11 vicinity was found. Our data indicates a lack of vGAT colocalization in TH^{+} -IR neurons of A11 (**Figures 4C,D**). We did see evidence for some $vGAT^{+}$ somata within the A11 region.

Photostimulation of the A11 Region Increases Motor Activity

Given that the viral injections were restricted to the A11 region, we tested the feasibility of using TH-IRES-Cre mice as a tool to photostimulate A11 neurons.

First, we tested, using brain slices, if the $A11^{ChR2}$-cells could elicit sodium (Na^{+}) spikes or currents following photostimulation. Pulses of blue light (473 nm) were delivered via an optical fiber, which successfully elicited photocurrents in $A11^{ChR2}$ cells (**Figure 5**). We also determined that trains of Na^{+} spikes were reliably elicited at frequencies up to 20 Hz (**Figure 5Dc**), which was the frequency we adopted for *in vivo* studies.

We then asked whether light pulses directed to the A11 region *in vivo* could also successfully activate $A11^{ChR2}$-cells. We implanted a fiber optic cannula unilaterally 0.1 mm lateral to the midline just above A11 region to bilaterally stimulate A11. We photostimulated both $A11^{ChR2}$ or $A11^{eYFP}$ mice at 20 Hz for 3 min (same parameters as for behavior), sacrificed them 2 h later to allow for c-Fos expression and prepared brain slices to probe for $c\text{-}Fos^{+}$-expression, which is increased in neurons following depolarization (**Figures 5A,B**). We found that in 10 animals (ChR2 $n = 5$, eYFP $n = 5$) $A11^{ChR2}$-cells were more likely to be also $c\text{-}Fos^{+}$ compared to cells infected with control $eYFP^{+}$ construct (**Figure 5C**, ChR2 $n = 5$, eYFP $n = 5$, $U = 0$, $P = 0.004$, Mann-Whitney test). These data suggest that the $A11^{ChR2}$-cells can be photo-activated *in vitro* and *in vivo* and that the neurons from the A11 region that are infected with control $eYFP^{+}$ construct are not activated by the same light stimulation parameters.

Next, we addressed the functional role of A11 neuronal activation in freely moving mice. We assessed movement in the open field test in animals expressing $A11^{ChR2}$ or in $A11^{eYFP}$. The mice were habituated to the open field for 1 h daily for 3 days and then tested for a fixed period on each of five consecutive days. Prior to testing, mice were habituated to the open field for 30 min with optical fibers attached. We recorded baseline activity 3 min prior to light activation, directly followed by 3 min of 20 Hz, 10 ms pulse width of light (473 nm) and 3 min of post-light activation (**Figure 6A**).

In the $A11^{ChR2}$ cohort only, qualitatively we noticed that animals reacted immediately to the light by changing behavior in a variety of ways (e.g., postural changes, starting to groom, turning, sniffing, stretching, and rearing but the animal is neither locomoting nor immobile). Collectively, these behaviors were quantified as changes in "in-place activity." When we compared

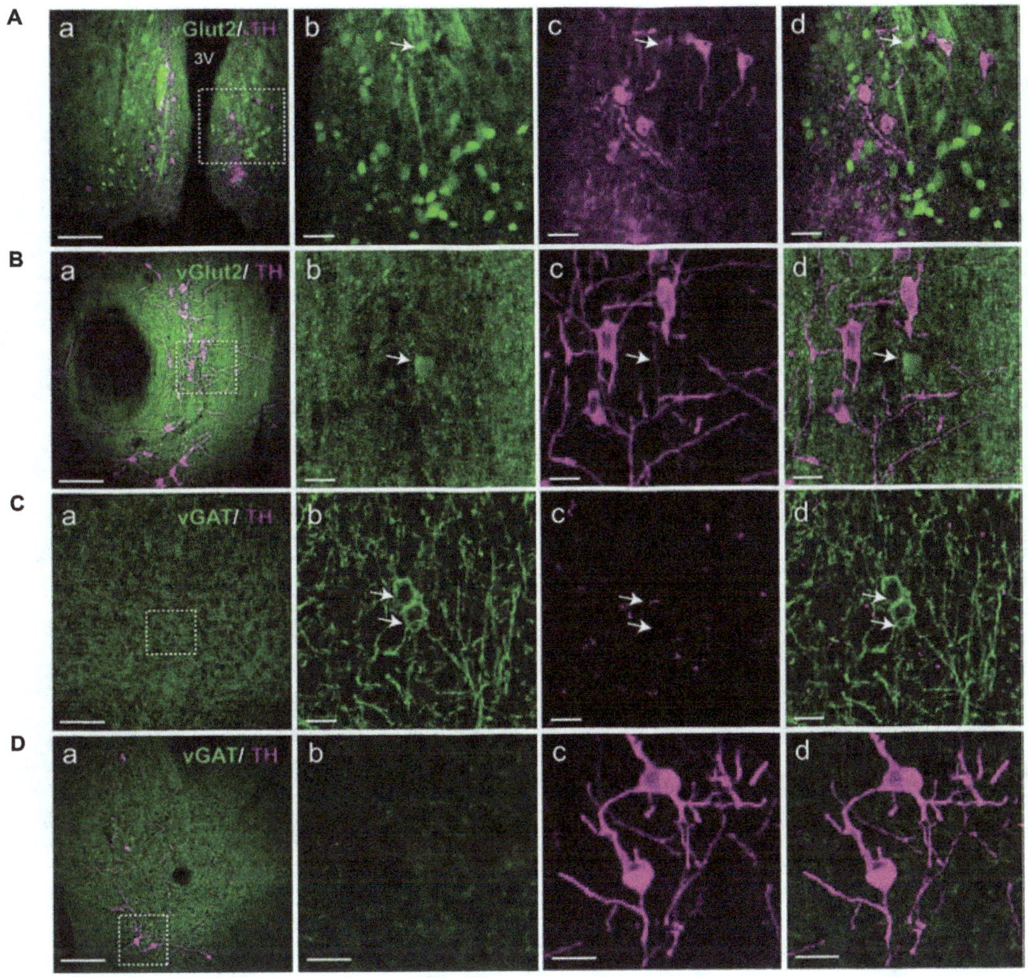

FIGURE 4 | A11 TH⁺-IR neurons lack vGluT2 and vGAT expression. **(A,B)** Immunohistochemistry targeted against TH (magenta) in a vGluT2-reporter (green) mouse. (Aa) vGluT2 expressing neurons are plentiful in the arcuate nucleus of hypothalamus, scale bar 200 μm. **(Ab–d)** Higher magnification of boxed area **(Aa)**, Scale bar 20 μm. vGluT2 is present in the arcuate nucleus of hypothalamus which served as a positive control. Arrow indicates a double positive TH⁺-IR A11 neuron expressing vGluT2. **(Ba)** TH⁺-IR neurons in A11 region, scale bar 200 μm. **(Bb–d)** Higher magnification of boxed area **(Ba)**, scale bar 10 μm. We observed a few vGluT2 expressing neurons in the A11 region but these neurons lacked TH⁺-IR (arrow). **(C,D)** Immunohistochemistry targeted against TH (magenta) in a vGAT-reporter (green) mouse. **(Ca)** Large number of vGAT expressing GABAergic interneurons are observed in cortex, scale bar 200 μm. **(Cb–d)** Higher magnification of boxed area **(Ca)**, scale bar 10 μm. Arrows indicate GABAergic interneurons expressing vGAT and TH⁺-IR fibers and puncta are also observed. **(Da)** TH⁺-IR neurons in A11 region, scale bar 200 μm. **(Db–d)** Higher magnification of boxed area **(Da)**, scale bar 10 μm. TH⁺-IR neurons in A11 region lack any vGAT expression.

the effect of light between the groups ($A11^{ChR2}$ and $A11^{eYFP}$, baseline corrected; difference = value - baseline) we found significant differences between the groups for in place activity ($A11^{ChR2}$ $n = 16$, 803 ± 741 mm; $A11^{eYFP}$ -391 ± 503 mm; $n = 7$, $U = 11$, $P = 0.0007$, Mann–Whitney test; data not shown).

These animals would then generally begin to locomote after engaging in these activities (see **Supplementary Video 1**). When we further examined these changes in the $A11^{ChR2}$ cohort, photostimulation increased the distance traveled by 86.0% (**Figure 6C**; $n = 16$, $Q = 18.9$, $P < 0.0001$, Friedman test) and the total number of locomotor bouts by 75.6% (**Figure 6D**; $n = 16$, $Q = 16.6$, $P = 0.0002$, Friedman test, see methods for definitions). In contrast, this was not observed in the $A11^{eYFP}$ control group (**Figure 6C**, $n = 7$, $Q = 2.0$, $P = 0.5$; **Figure 6D**, $n = 7$, $Q = 1.5$, $P = 0.5$, Friedman test). When we compared the effect of light between the groups ($A11^{ChR2}$ and $A11^{eYFP}$, baseline corrected, difference = value - baseline) we found significant differences for the following parameters: locomotion ($A11^{ChR2}$ $n = 16$, 1551 ± 1503 mm; $A11^{eYFP}$ -149 ± 665 mm; $n = 7$, $U = 10$, $P = 0.0005$, Mann–Whitney test), and bouts of locomotion ($A11^{ChR2}$, $n = 16$, 1.88 ± 4.09 bouts; $A11^{eYFP}$, -3.18 ± 3.36 bouts; $n = 7$, $U = 13$, $P = 0.001$, Mann–Whitney test). We did not observe an effect of day [2-way ANOVA with repeated measures, $F(4.6) = 0.04$, $P = 1$].

Next, we determined the latency for changes in movement behavior after photostimulation. For this, we averaged the data (distance in mm) into 10 s bins and set a threshold (mean of the pre-light distance traveled over 3 min, + two times SD) for

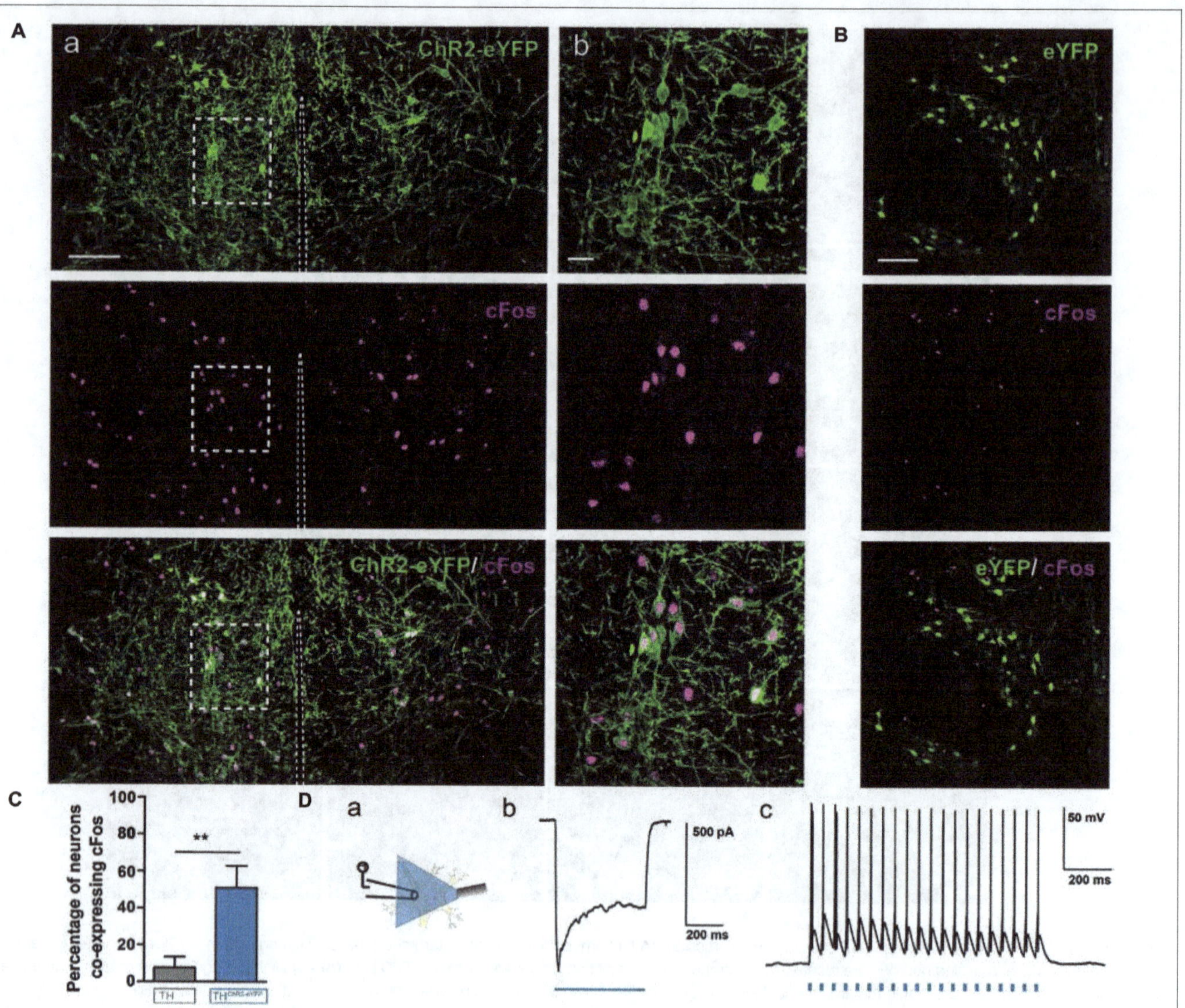

FIGURE 5 | Photostimulation of A11 cells induces c-Fos protein expression in A11 ChR2-eYFP neurons *in vivo* and action potentials *in vitro*. ChR2-eYFP expressing (n = 4) mice and eYFP control (n = 4) mice were stimulated with 473 nm light at 15 mW with 20 Hz, 10 ms pulses, 2 h prior to sacrifice. **(Aa)** A11 neurons from ChR2-eYFP light stimulated mouse (stitched image consisting of 4 20X images; scale bar 100 μm). **(Ab)** Higher magnification (60X zoom) of boxed area (scale bar 20 μm). **(B)** Photostimulation of A11 eYFP neurons (no ChR2) *in vivo* does not result in significant co-localization of c-Fos in A11-eYFP$^+$ cells (scale bar 100 μm). **(C)** Bar graph summarizing changes in the percentage of neurons co-expressing c-Fos in ChR2-eYFP (n = 4) versus eYFP (n = 4). **(D)** Real-time optical stimulation with 473 nm light reliably elicits spikes in A11 neurons *in vitro*. Example of a photocurrent recorded in voltage-clamp mode, elicited by 473 nm blue light **(Db)**. Trains of light pulses (10 ms pulse-width) at 20 Hz frequency evoked spike activity **(Dc)**. **(Da)** Schematic showing approach. $^{**}P < 0.01$.

each individual trial and determined the latency of crossing the threshold. We examined all trials (n = 80, all days, all animals) and found that 87.3% of the A11^{ChR2} trials crossed threshold during light activation with a median latency of 40 s (25–75% percentile 20–80, **Figure 6E**). In contrast, only 38.2% of the A11^{eYFP} mice trials (n = 35, all days, all animals) crossed threshold with a median latency of 60 s (25–75% percentile 48–130 **Figure 6E**).

When we examined all photostimulation trials on a trial-to-trial basis, there was no significant correlation between basal locomotor activity and the light mediated effect (distance traveled (mm); $r = -0.1$, $P = 0.1$) due to variability in the data (mean = 43.80 mm, SD = 272.2, median = 2.6 mm). Taken together our data suggest that photostimulation of A11 affects both the movement during locomotion as well as the in-place activity.

DISCUSSION

Previous work has shown that the diencephalic A11 cell group contains neurons that project to the spinal cord and its effects are associated with pain control (Fleetwood-Walker et al., 1988), migraine (Charbit et al., 2009), cataplexy (Okura et al., 2004), and possibly a role in RLS (Clemens et al., 2006). Our work provides

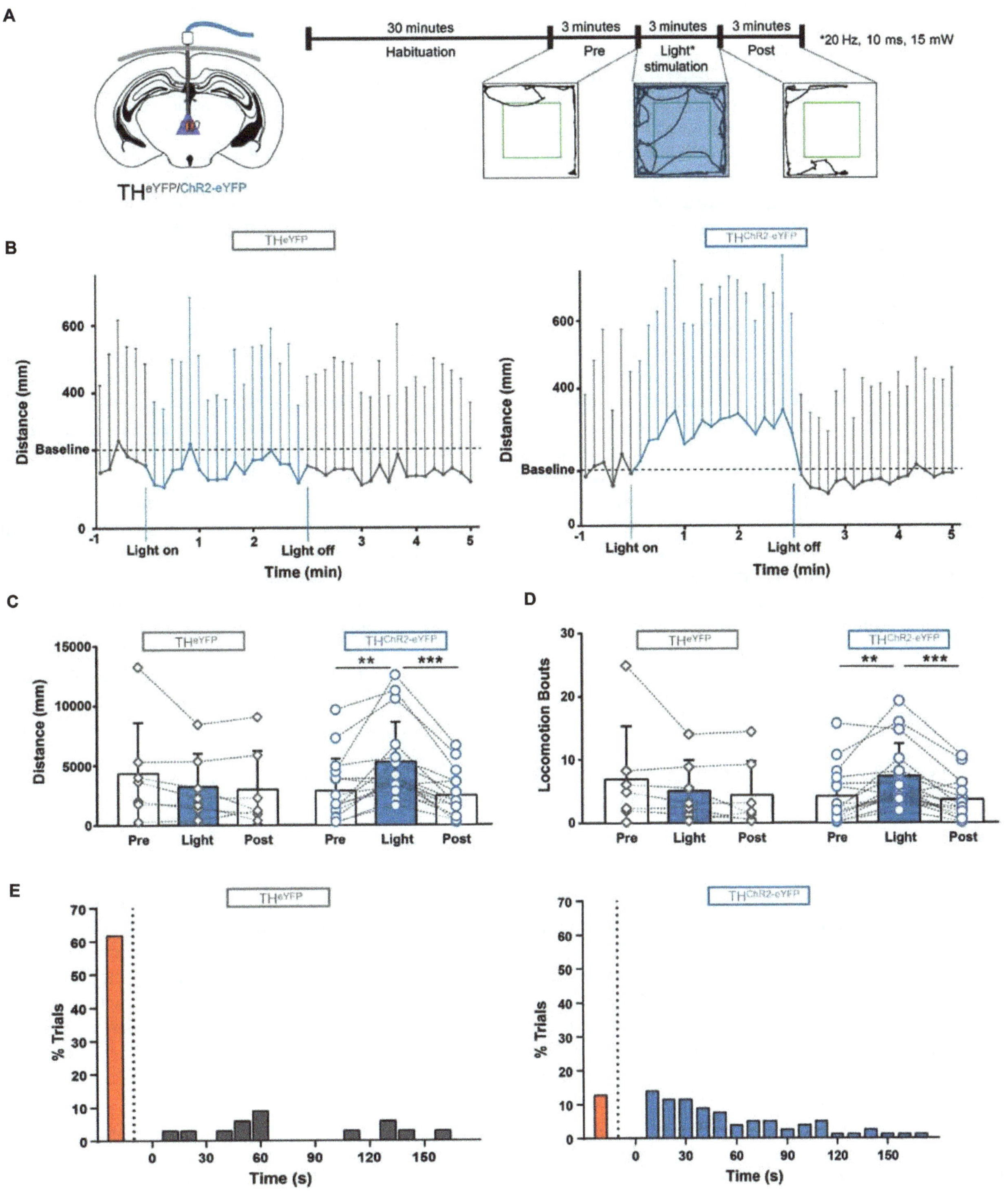

FIGURE 6 | Photostimulation of A11 in awake behaving mice initiates and modulates locomotion. **(A)** Schematic showing the implantation site of the light ferrule, along with a schematic of the experimental plan. **(B)** Locomotor distance was significantly increased during photostimulation in ChR2 animals compared to eYFP-control mice (averaged over 5 days). Baseline was corrected. **(C,D)** ChR2 mice displayed significantly more distance traveled **(C)** and locomotion bouts **(D)** during blue light stimulation compared with light-off conditions. There was no significant difference between the three conditions in eYFP control mice ($n = 7$) (average over 5 days). **(E)** 87.3% of ChR2 trials (blue bars) crossed the threshold during photostimulation while only 38.2% of the eYFP trials (gray bars) crossed the threshold (5 days, all trials), looking at individual trials the median time to cross the threshold was 40 s for ChR2 mice, and 60 s for eYFP mice. The red bars on the left of both graphs indicate the percentage of trials where the threshold was not crossed. These data suggest that photostimulation of A11 can initiate and modulate locomotion. $^{**}P < 0.01$; $^{***}P < 0.001$.

evidence that activation of A11 increases motor behavior, including locomotor and non-locomotor events. The A11 was shown to depress firing of dorsal horn neurons responding to noxious input (Fleetwood-Walker et al., 1988; Taniguchi et al., 2011), through a D_2 receptor-mediated mechanism (Tamae et al., 2005). Similar effects on trigeminal nociception have been also reported (Abdallah et al., 2015). But dopamine has also been shown to be pro-nociceptive through D_5 receptors expressed in the spinal cord (Megat et al., 2018). This complex sensorimotor role is shared with other monoamines such as 5-HT and noradrenaline (Schmidt and Jordan, 2000; Millan, 2002), and is partly dependent on the diversity of monoamine receptor subtypes. Indeed, this sensorimotor modulation may be related to expression of movement as hypothesized for RLS (Clemens et al., 2006). As outlined below, dopamine's actions on motor circuits are also diverse. This points to a role in both pain and motor function where the actions of dopamine can modulate multiple circuits within the spinal cord to fine-tune sensorimotor function. A further diversity of A11 actions could be linked to the sex of the animals. Our work used male mice and it is possible that results in females may differ, since work in rats has shown a sexual dimorphism in the A11 descending projections (Pappas et al., 2008, 2010) and recent work show spinal D_5 receptors in the dorsal horn contributing to hyperalgesia in male but not female mice (Megat et al., 2018). Since male rats have a greater density of A11 fibers in the ventral horn it is possible that A11 stimulation in males would show greater motor effects compared to females.

Mode of Action

Our previous work established that in mice, the A11 is primarily dopaminergic but lacks DAT (Koblinger et al., 2014) which has also been confirmed using DAT reporter mice (Yip et al., 2017). In the A11 system, this DAT^- mechanism may increase synaptic dopamine concentration, augmenting dopamine's actions within the spinal cord.

Data from the neonatal rat and mouse shows that bath application of dopamine restricted to the thoracolumbar spinal region modulates fictive locomotor patterns (Kiehn and Kjaerulff, 1996; Jiang et al., 1999; Whelan et al., 2000; Barrière et al., 2004; Christie and Whelan, 2005; Gordon and Whelan, 2006; Humphreys and Whelan, 2012; Sharples et al., 2015; Sharples and Whelan, 2017). This dopamine-evoked excitation of mammalian spinal locomotor circuits occurs through $D_{1/5}$ receptors (Maitra et al., 1993; Seth et al., 1993; Barrière et al., 2004; Madriaga et al., 2004; Gordon and Whelan, 2006; Han et al., 2007) although a role for $D_{2/3/4}$ receptors exists (Humphreys and Whelan, 2012). In particular, $D_{1/5}$ receptors appear to enhance the stability of ongoing locomotion but $D_{2/3/4}$ receptors appear to contribute to a slowing of the rhythm (Sharples et al., 2015), and may access part of the pattern generator through recurrent collaterals (Humphreys and Whelan, 2012). In adult spinalized mice, D_1 receptors appear to contribute more than D_5 receptors to locomotion, based on the use of D_5 receptors KO mice (Lapointe et al., 2009). Since this study used a mixed cohort of male and female mice, and recent evidence suggests that D_5 receptors are present in higher numbers in the spinal cord of male mice (Megat et al., 2018), a role for D_5 receptors in locomotion cannot be excluded. Dopamine fibers projecting from the diencephalon (A11 region) are present in the ventral horn of the mouse adult spinal cord, an area where dopamine receptors and motor circuits are located (Yoshida and Tanaka, 1988; Weil-Fugazza and Godefroy, 1993; Qu et al., 2006; Zhu et al., 2007). The release of dopamine and its metabolites occurs in the ventral horn of neonatal rats during fictive locomotion (Jordan and Schmidt, 2002) and in the spinal cord of adult rats following walking (Gerin and Privat, 1998). Moreover, administration of D_1 agonists in adult mice with a complete thoracic injury elicited bouts of stepping (Lapointe et al., 2009). Finally, the critical role played by dopamine transmission in locomotion is highlighted by the fact that L-DOPA-elicited air stepping in intact neonatal rats is blocked by intrathecally introduced dopamine receptor antagonists (Sickles et al., 1992; McCrea et al., 1997). Work by several groups (Fleetwood-Walker et al., 1988; Taniguchi et al., 2011) has shown that stimulation of A11 in adult animals has effects on nociception, acting both pre- and post-synaptically on neurons within the dorsal horn of the spinal cord (Taniguchi et al., 2011), and inhibited by dopaminergic antagonists. Taken together, these data suggest that A11 activation can influence spinal cord circuits via dopamine, and dopamine can have several actions on spinal motor circuits.

Like many nuclei the A11 is known to project to other areas of the brain, including the amygdala, prefrontal cortex (Takada et al., 1988; Takada, 1990, 1993), and dorsal raphe (Peyron et al., 1995). Indeed diencephalon-specific pathways to the brainstem, including the medullary reticular formation and the mesencephalic locomotor region have been shown in the past (Sinnamon and Stopford, 1987; Sinnamon et al., 1987). We expect therefore that the A11 connectome is more extensive than has been published. Therefore while spinal cord connections may be responsible for the observed effects, A11 collaterals projecting to other brain regions may also be involved. Within the A11 we found neurons that were positive for vGluT2 and negative for vGAT. But we did not find cells that co-localized dopamine and vGluT2. However, vGluT3 neurons are found in the A11 vicinity (Allen Brain Atlas) so it is possible that dopamine neurons could still contain glutamate. Our data show some $vGAT^+$ positive neurons in the A11 region, agreeing with data from the Allen Brain Atlas, and we saw no $vGAT^+$-TH^+-IR neurons.

Effects on Motor Activity

We found that photostimulation of the A11 region produced immediate responses that, although varied, always led to locomotion. The delay in the initiation of locomotion is consistent with early reports of stimulation of this region (Mori et al., 1989; Sławińska and Kasicki, 1995). There are several possibilities for this delay. The A11 network may form a reverberating positive-feedback local network resulting in an increase in spike output over time, and the fact that vGluT2 neurons are in the A11 region point to this being a possibility. We do not feel that the delay may be due to fast inhibitory neurons being recruited since our data do not show $vGAT^+$ somata within the A11. On the other hand, low concentrations of dopamine bind to high-affinity $D_{2/3/4}$ receptors, producing inhibition. At higher dopamine concentrations, expected with prolonged spiking within the A11, a switch to excitation could occur (Clemens et al., 2012). Alternatively, an interesting observation is that within the isolated spinal cord preparation of the rodent, bath application of dopamine produces a delayed activation of the network often being an order of magnitude slower compared to 5-HT application (Gozal et al., 2014). An action of dopamine on trace amine receptors (TAAR1) has been proposed to account for this delay in the rat (Bunzow et al., 2001; Gozal et al., 2014) and a similar mechanism operating *in vivo* could partly account for the delays noted here. A component of the A11 cells activated were presumably D-cells (Jaeger et al., 1983), which lack TH but contain AADC, based on the Allen Brain Atlas, and our own work. Little is known about the storage and release of dopamine (or other transmitters) from these cells. Work by Weihe et al. (2006) shows evidence of hypothalamic $AADC^{+}/TH^{-}$ cells that lack VMAT2. Therefore neurotransmitter release from D-cells likely occurs differently from the standard vesicular-based dopamine release. Recent evidence shows that the hypothalamic neurons containing glutamate, GABA, and dopamine cells can be subdivided into 62 distinct subpopulations where neuropeptides are co-localized in a distinct manner (Romanov et al., 2017). While our data show that the A11 contains a small number of vGluT2 neurons we did not see any co-expression with TH^{+} neurons, but vGluT3 expression was not tested here, and is observed in the A11 region, therefore glutamate co-localization in TH^{+} neurons may still be possible. Our RT-PCR data showed that the levels of Cre mRNA are between 36 and 41% of TH mRNA in heterozygous TH-tdTomato mice, which is close to our expectations of 50% levels. Slightly lower levels of Cre mRNA may be due to the possibility that the locus of TH transcription is more active than the locus of Cre transcription. On the other hand, this supports the idea of active transcription of TH mRNA in the absence of the translation of TH protein which was highlighted in a recent report (Meng et al., 2018). In this regard, we feel that future attempts using other techniques such as double fluorescent in situ hybridization or single cell RNA-seq may provide additional insights on molecular and cellular diversity in phenotypes of TH cells in the A11. The most conservative interpretation of our data is that at a minimum 54% of ChR2-TH^{+} neurons were dopaminergic, and a possibility remains that this percentage could be higher. Since we did not observe co-localization of vGAT or vGluT2 with TH^{+}-IR, we conclude that the stimulated population includes mainly dopaminergic neurons, D-cells, and an undefined neuronal population.

CONCLUSION

This is the first study to show that stimulation of the A11 has pro-locomotory effects. This adds to the hypothesized role of the A11 in RLS (Clemens et al., 2006; Qu et al., 2006, 2007), where patients suffer from an uncontrolled desire to move their limbs associated with modulation of D_3 receptors in the spinal cord (Maitra et al., 1993). Further clues to the role of the A11 in motor control will require selective activation and inactivation of spinally projecting axons to differentiate direct from indirect actions on spinal cord functions. Given the robust effects of dopamine on modulation of spinal circuits (Sharples et al., 2014) this would be an interesting target to investigate. A11 forms one of many nuclei in the diencephalon and midbrain that have motor effects and connect with nuclei in the brainstem and spinal cord (Kim et al., 2017; Brownstone and Chopek, 2018; Gatto and Goulding, 2018; Sharma et al., 2018). A more complete understanding of their role will require parallel recording and stimulation of these distinct regions during complex motor behavior.

AUTHOR CONTRIBUTIONS

KK performed the experiments, analyzed the data, and wrote and edited the paper. CJ-X participated in performing experiments, analyzed data, edited the paper, and participated in experimental design. SS participated in performing experiments, edited the paper, and participated in experimental design. TF edited the paper, analyzed the data, and participated in performing experiments. LY, SEAE, and CHTK performed experiments, analyzed data, and edited the paper. JB participated in experiment design and edited the paper. PW conceived the experiments, supervised the research, and edited and wrote the paper.

ACKNOWLEDGMENTS

We acknowledge grant support from the Canadian Institutes of Health Research and from the HALO initiative, HBI. KK and LY received studentship support from Alberta Innovates Health Solutions; KK also received support from the Fong studentship (Hotchkiss Brain Institute) and Eyes High (University of Calgary). We acknowledge technical assistance from Ms. Jillian Ejdrygiewicz, Ms. Claude Veillette, and Ms. Michelle Tran. We also acknowledge technical support from the RUN/HBI-AMP Core Microscopy, the HALO Behavioral Facility, and Dr. Frank Visser from the Molecular Core Facility at the University of Calgary. We acknowledge assistance from Dr. Luis de Lecea's lab (Stanford University) in ferrule implantation. The TH-IRES-Cre mice were a kind gift from Dr. Antoine Adamantidis (Universität Bern). The vGluT2 mice were a kind gift from Dr. Marie-Claude Perreault (Emory University).

REFERENCES

Abdallah, K., Monconduit, L., Artola, A., Luccarini, P., and Dallel, R. (2015). GABAAergic inhibition or dopamine denervation of the A11 hypothalamic nucleus induces trigeminal analgesia. *Pain* 156, 644–655. doi: 10.1097/j.pain.0000000000000091

Abrahamson, E. E., and Moore, R. Y. (2001). The posterior hypothalamic area: chemoarchitecture and afferent connections. *Brain Res.* 889, 1–22. doi: 10.1016/S0006-8993(00)03015-8

Barraud, Q., Obeid, I., Aubert, I., Barrière, G., Contamin, H., Mcguire, S., et al. (2010). Neuroanatomical study of the A11 diencephalospinal pathway in the non-human primate. *PLoS One* 5:e13306. doi: 10.1371/journal.pone.0013306

Barrière, G., Mellen, N., and Cazalets, J.-R. (2004). Neuromodulation of the locomotor network by dopamine in the isolated spinal cord of newborn rat. *Eur. J. Neurosci.* 19, 1325–1335. doi: 10.1111/j.1460-9568.2004.03210.x

Björklund, A., and Skagerberg, G. (1979). Evidence for a major spinal cord projection from the diencephalic A11 dopamine cell group in the rat using transmitter-specific fluorescent retrograde tracing. *Brain Res.* 177, 170–175. doi: 10.1016/0006-8993(79)90927-2

Brownstone, R. M., and Chopek, J. W. (2018). Reticulospinal systems for tuning motor commands. *Front. Neural Circuits* 12:30. doi: 10.3389/fncir.2018.00030

Bunzow, J. R., Sonders, M. S., Arttamangkul, S., Harrison, L. M., Zhang, G., Quigley, D. I., et al. (2001). Amphetamine, 3,4-methylenedioxymethamphetamine, lysergic acid diethylamide, and metabolites of the catecholamine neurotransmitters are agonists of a rat trace amine receptor. *Mol. Pharmacol.* 60, 1181–1188. doi: 10.1124/mol.60.6.1181

Bustin, S. A., Benes, V., Garson, J. A., Hellemans, J., Huggett, J., Kubista, M., et al. (2009). The MIQE guidelines: minimum information for publication of quantitative real-time PCR experiments. *Clin. Chem.* 55, 611–622. doi: 10.1373/clinchem.2008.112797

Charbit, A. R., Akerman, S., Holland, P. R., and Goadsby, P. J. (2009). Neurons of the dopaminergic/calcitonin gene-related peptide A11 cell group modulate neuronal firing in the trigeminocervical complex: an electrophysiological and immunohistochemical study. *J. Neurosci.* 29, 12532–12541. doi: 10.1523/JNEUROSCI.2887-09.2009

Christie, K. J., and Whelan, P. J. (2005). Monoaminergic establishment of rostrocaudal gradients of rhythmicity in the neonatal mouse spinal cord. *J. Neurophysiol.* 94, 1554–1564. doi: 10.1152/jn.00299.2005

Clemens, S., Belin-Rauscent, A., Simmers, J., and Combes, D. (2012). Opposing modulatory effects of D1- and D2-like receptor activation on a spinal central pattern generator. *J. Neurophysiol.* 107, 2250–2259. doi: 10.1152/jn.00366.2011

Clemens, S., and Hochman, S. (2004). Conversion of the modulatory actions of dopamine on spinal reflexes from depression to facilitation in D3 receptor knock-out mice. *J. Neurosci.* 24, 11337–11345. doi: 10.1523/JNEUROSCI.3698-04.2004

Clemens, S., Rye, D., and Hochman, S. (2006). Restless legs syndrome: revisiting the dopamine hypothesis from the spinal cord perspective. *Neurology* 67, 125–130. doi: 10.1212/01.wnl.0000223316.53428.c9

Commissiong, J. W., Gentleman, S., and Neff, N. H. (1979). Spinal cord dopaminergic neurons: evidence for an uncrossed nigrospinal pathway. *Neuropharmacology* 18, 565–568. doi: 10.1016/0028-3908(79)90102-3

Dahlström, A., and Fuxe, K. (1964). Evidence for the existence of monoamine-containing neurons in the central nervous system. I. Demonstration of monoamines in the cell bodies of brain stem neurons. *Acta Physiol. Scand. Suppl.* 232, 1–55.

Fleetwood-Walker, S. M., Hope, P. J., and Mitchell, R. (1988). Antinociceptive actions of descending dopaminergic tracts on cat and rat dorsal horn somatosensory neurones. *J. Physiol.* 399, 335–348. doi: 10.1113/jphysiol.1988.sp017084

Gatto, G., and Goulding, M. (2018). Locomotion control: brainstem circuits satisfy the need for speed. *Curr. Biol.* 28, R256–R259. doi: 10.1016/j.cub.2018.01.068

Gerin, C., and Privat, A. (1998). Direct evidence for the link between monoaminergic descending pathways and motor activity: II. A study with microdialysis probes implanted in the ventral horn of the spinal cord. *Brain Res.* 794, 169–173. doi: 10.1016/S0006-8993(98)00278-9

Gordon, I. T., and Whelan, P. J. (2006). Monoaminergic control of cauda-equina-evoked locomotion in the neonatal mouse spinal cord. *J. Neurophysiol.* 96, 3122–3129. doi: 10.1152/jn.00606.2006

Gozal, E. A., O'Neill, B. E., Sawchuk, M. A., Zhu, H., Halder, M., Chou, C.-C., et al. (2014). Anatomical and functional evidence for trace amines as unique modulators of locomotor function in the mammalian spinal cord. *Front. Neural Circuits* 8:134. doi: 10.3389/fncir.2014.00134

Han, P., Nakanishi, S. T., Tran, M. A., and Whelan, P. J. (2007). Dopaminergic modulation of spinal neuronal excitability. *J. Neurosci.* 27, 13192–13204. doi: 10.1523/JNEUROSCI.1279-07.2007

Han, P., and Whelan, P. J. (2009). Modulation of AMPA currents by D(1)-like but not D(2)-like receptors in spinal motoneurons. *Neuroscience* 158, 1699–1707. doi: 10.1016/j.neuroscience.2008.11.040

Hochman, S. (2015). Metabolic recruitment of spinal locomotion: intracellular neuromodulation by trace amines and their receptors. *Neural Regen. Res.* 10, 1940–1942. doi: 10.4103/1673-5374.169625

Humphreys, J., and Whelan, P. (2011). Dopamine exerts activation dependent modulation of spinal locomotor circuits in the mouse. *J. Neurophysiol.* 108, 3370–3381. doi: 10.1152/jn.00482.2012

Humphreys, J. M., and Whelan, P. J. (2012). Dopamine exerts activation-dependent modulation of spinal locomotor circuits in the neonatal mouse. *J. Neurophysiol.* 108, 3370–3381. doi: 10.1152/jn.00482.2012

Jaeger, C. B., Teitelman, G., Joh, T. H., Albert, V. R., Park, D. H., and Reis, D. J. (1983). Some neurons of the rat central nervous system contain aromatic-L-amino-acid decarboxylase but not monoamines. *Science* 219, 1233–1235. doi: 10.1126/science.6131537

Jiang, Z., Carlin, K. P., and Brownstone, R. M. (1999). An in vitro functionally mature mouse spinal cord preparation for the study of spinal motor networks. *Brain Res.* 816, 493–499. doi: 10.1016/S0006-8993(98)01199-8

Jordan, L. M., and Schmidt, B. J. (2002). Propriospinal neurons involved in the control of locomotion: potential targets for repair strategies? *Prog. Brain Res.* 137, 125–139. doi: 10.1016/S0079-6123(02)37012-2

Kiehn, O., and Kjaerulff, O. (1996). Spatiotemporal characteristics of 5-HT and dopamine-induced rhythmic hindlimb activity in the in vitro neonatal rat. *J. Neurophysiol.* 75, 1472–1482. doi: 10.1152/jn.1996.75.4.1472

Kiehn, O., Sillar, K. T., Kjaerulff, O., and McDearmid, J. R. (1999). Effects of noradrenaline on locomotor rhythm–generating networks in the isolated neonatal rat spinal cord. *J. Neurophysiol.* 82, 741–746. doi: 10.1152/jn.1999.82.2.741

Kim, L. H., Sharma, S., Sharples, S. A., Mayr, K. A., Kwok, C. H. T., and Whelan, P. J. (2017). Integration of descending command systems for the generation of context-specific locomotor behaviors. *Front. Neurosci.* 11:581. doi: 10.3389/fnins.2017.00581

Koblinger, K., Füzesi, T., Ejdrygiewicz, J., Krajacic, A., Bains, J. S., and Whelan, P. J. (2014). Characterization of a11 neurons projecting to the spinal cord of mice. *PLoS One* 9:e109636. doi: 10.1371/journal.pone.0109636

Koblinger, K., Jean-Xavier, C., Ejdrygiewicz, J., Fuzesi, T., Bains, J. S., and Whelan, P. J. (2015). "A11 optogenetic stimulation elicits locomotor activity in mice," in *Conference Society for Neuroscience*, Chicago, IL.

Lambert, A. M., Bonkowsky, J. L., and Masino, M. A. (2012). The conserved dopaminergic diencephalospinal tract mediates vertebrate locomotor development in zebrafish larvae. *J. Neurosci.* 32, 13488–13500. doi: 10.1523/JNEUROSCI.1638-12.2012

Lammel, S., Steinberg, E. E., Földy, C., Wall, N. R., Beier, K., Luo, L., et al. (2015). Diversity of transgenic mouse models for selective targeting of midbrain dopamine neurons. *Neuron* 85, 429–438. doi: 10.1016/j.neuron.2014.12.036

Lapointe, N. P., Rouleau, P., Ung, R.-V., and Guertin, P. A. (2009). Specific role of dopamine D1 receptors in spinal network activation and rhythmic movement induction in vertebrates. *J. Physiol.* 587, 1499–1511. doi: 10.1113/jphysiol.2008.166314

Liu, J., and Jordan, L. M. (2005). Stimulation of the parapyramidal region of the neonatal rat brain stem produces locomotor-like activity involving spinal 5-HT7 and 5-HT2A receptors. *J. Neurophysiol.* 94, 1392–1404. doi: 10.1152/jn.00136.2005

Madriaga, M. A., McPhee, L. C., Chersa, T., Christie, K. J., and Whelan, P. J. (2004). Modulation of locomotor activity by multiple 5-HT and dopaminergic receptor subtypes in the neonatal mouse spinal cord. *J. Neurophysiol.* 92, 1566–1576. doi: 10.1152/jn.01181.2003

Maitra, K. K., Seth, P., Thewissen, M., Ross, H. G., and Ganguly, D. K. (1993). Dopaminergic influence on the excitability of antidromically activated Renshaw cells in the lumbar spinal cord of the rat. *Acta Physiol. Scand.* 148, 101–107. doi: 10.1111/j.1748-1716.1993.tb09538.x

McCrea, A. E., Stehouwer, D. J., and van Hartesveldt, C. (1997). Dopamine D1 and D2 antagonists block L-DOPA-induced air-stepping in decerebrate neonatal rats. *Brain Res. Dev. Brain Res.* 100, 130–132. doi: 10.1016/S0165-3806(97)00027-8

Megat, S., Shiers, S., Moy, J. K., Barragan-Iglesias, P., Pradhan, G., Seal, R. P., et al. (2018). A critical role for dopamine d5 receptors in pain chronicity in male mice. *J. Neurosci.* 38, 379–397. doi: 10.1523/JNEUROSCI.2110-17.2017

Meng, D., Li, H.-Q., Deisseroth, K., Leutgeb, S., and Spitzer, N. C. (2018). Neuronal activity regulates neurotransmitter switching in the adult brain following light-induced stress. *Proc. Natl. Acad. Sci. U.S.A.* 115, 5064–5071. doi: 10.1073/pnas.1801598115

Millan, M. J. (2002). Descending control of pain. *Prog. Neurobiol.* 66, 355–474. doi: 10.1016/S0301-0082(02)00009-6

Mori, S., Sakamoto, T., Ohta, Y., Takakusaki, K., and Matsuyama, K. (1989). Site-specific postural and locomotor changes evoked in awake, freely moving intact cats by stimulating the brainstem. *Brain Res.* 505, 66–74. doi: 10.1016/0006-8993(89)90116-9

Okura, M., Fujiki, N., Kita, I., Honda, K., Yoshida, Y., Mignot, E., et al. (2004). The roles of midbrain and diencephalic dopamine cell groups in the regulation of cataplexy in narcoleptic Dobermans. *Neurobiol. Dis.* 16, 274–282. doi: 10.1016/j.nbd.2004.02.008

Pappas, S. S., Behrouz, B., Janis, K. L., Goudreau, J. L., and Lookingland, K. J. (2008). Lack of D2 receptor mediated regulation of dopamine synthesis in A11 diencephalospinal neurons in male and female mice. *Brain Res.* 1214, 1–10. doi: 10.1016/j.brainres.2008.03.010

Pappas, S. S., Tiernan, C. T., Behrouz, B., Jordan, C. L., Breedlove, S. M., Goudreau, J. L., et al. (2010). Neonatal androgen-dependent sex differences in lumbar spinal cord dopamine concentrations and the number of A11 diencephalospinal dopamine neurons. *J. Comp. Neurol.* 518, 2423–2436. doi: 10.1002/cne.22340

Peyron, C., Luppi, P. H., Kitahama, K., Fort, P., Hermann, D. M., and Jouvet, M. (1995). Origin of the dopaminergic innervation of the rat dorsal raphe nucleus. *Neuroreport* 6, 2527–2531. doi: 10.1097/00001756-199512150-00019

Picton, L. D., Nascimento, F., Broadhead, M. J., Sillar, K. T., and Miles, G. B. (2017). Sodium pumps mediate activity-dependent changes in mammalian motor networks. *J. Neurosci.* 37, 906–921. doi: 10.1523/JNEUROSCI.2005-16.2016

Qu, S., Le, W., Zhang, X., Xie, W., Zhang, A., and Ondo, W. G. (2007). Locomotion is increased in a11-lesioned mice with iron deprivation: a possible animal model for restless legs syndrome. *J. Neuropathol. Exp. Neurol.* 66, 383–388. doi: 10.1097/nen.0b013e3180517b5f

Qu, S., Ondo, W. G., Zhang, X., Xie, W. J., Pan, T. H., and Le, W. D. (2006). Projections of diencephalic dopamine neurons into the spinal cord in mice. *Exp. Brain Res.* 168, 152–156. doi: 10.1007/s00221-005-0075-1

Romanov, R. A., Zeisel, A., Bakker, J., Girach, F., Hellysaz, A., Tomer, R., et al. (2017). Molecular interrogation of hypothalamic organization reveals distinct dopamine neuronal subtypes. *Nat. Neurosci.* 20, 176–188. doi: 10.1038/nn.4462

Ryu, S., Mahler, J., Acampora, D., Holzschuh, J., Erhardt, S., Omodei, D., et al. (2007). Orthopedia homeodomain protein is essential for diencephalic dopaminergic neuron development. *Curr. Biol.* 17, 873–880. doi: 10.1016/j.cub.2007.04.003

Schmidt, B. J., and Jordan, L. M. (2000). The role of serotonin in reflex modulation and locomotor rhythm production in the mammalian spinal cord. *Brain Res. Bull.* 53, 689–710. doi: 10.1016/S0361-9230(00)00402-0

Seth, P., Gajendiran, M., Maitra, K. K., Ross, H. G., and Ganguly, D. K. (1993). Evidence for D1 dopamine receptor-mediated modulation of the synaptic transmission from motor axon collaterals to Renshaw cells in the rat spinal cord. *Neurosci. Lett.* 158, 217–220. doi: 10.1016/0304-3940(93)90268-P

Sharma, S., Kim, L. H., Mayr, K. A., Elliott, D. A., and Whelan, P. J. (2018). Parallel descending dopaminergic connectivity of A13 cells to the brainstem locomotor centers. *Sci. Rep.* 8:7972. doi: 10.1038/s41598-018-25908-5

Sharples, S. A., Humphreys, J. M., Jensen, A. M., Dhoopar, S., Delaloye, N., Clemens, S., et al. (2015). Dopaminergic modulation of locomotor network activity in the neonatal mouse spinal cord. *J. Neurophysiol.* 113, 2500–2510. doi: 10.1152/jn.00849.2014

Sharples, S. A., Koblinger, K., Humphreys, J. M., and Whelan, P. J. (2014). Dopamine: a parallel pathway for the modulation of spinal locomotor networks. *Front. Neural Circuits* 8:55. doi: 10.3389/fncir.2014.00055

Sharples, S. A., and Whelan, P. J. (2017). Modulation of rhythmic activity in mammalian spinal networks is dependent on excitability state. *eNeuro* 4:ENEURO.0368-16.2017. doi: 10.1523/ENEURO.0368-16.2017

Shik, M. L., and Orlovsky, G. N. (1976). Neurophysiology of locomotor automatism. *Physiol. Rev.* 56, 465–501. doi: 10.1152/physrev.1976.56.3.465

Sickles, A. E., Stehouwer, D. J., and van Hartesveldt, C. (1992). Dopamine D1 and D2 antagonists block L-dopa-elicited air-stepping in neonatal rats. *Brain Res. Dev. Brain Res.* 68, 17–22. doi: 10.1016/0165-3806(92)90243-P

Sinnamon, H. M., Ginzburg, R. N., and Kurose, G. A. (1987). Midbrain stimulation in the anesthetized rat: direct locomotor effects and modulation of locomotion produced by hypothalamic stimulation. *Neuroscience* 20, 695–707. doi: 10.1016/0306-4522(87)90120-5

Sinnamon, H. M., Lee, S. H., Adams, D. B., and Stopford, C. K. (1984). Locomotor stepping elicited by electrical stimulation of the lateral hypothalamus requires an ipsilateral descending pathway. *Physiol. Behav.* 33, 209–215. doi: 10.1016/0031-9384(84)90101-X

Sinnamon, H. M., and Stopford, C. K. (1987). Locomotion elicited by lateral hypothalamic stimulation in the anesthetized rat does not require the dorsal midbrain. *Brain Res.* 402, 78–86. doi: 10.1016/0006-8993(87)91049-3

Skagerberg, G., and Lindvall, O. (1985). Organization of diencephalic dopamine neurones projecting to the spinal cord in the rat. *Brain Res.* 342, 340–351. doi: 10.1016/0006-8993(85)91134-5

Sławińska, U., and Kasicki, S. (1995). Theta-like rhythm in depth EEG activity of hypothalamic areas during spontaneous or electrically induced locomotion in the rat. *Brain Res.* 678, 117–126. doi: 10.1016/0006-8993(95)00174-O

Sławińska, U., Miazga, K., and Jordan, L. M. (2014). The role of serotonin in the control of locomotor movements and strategies for restoring locomotion after spinal cord injury. *Acta Neurobiol. Exp.* 74, 172–187.

Stuber, G. D., and Wise, R. A. (2016). Lateral hypothalamic circuits for feeding and reward. *Nat. Neurosci.* 19, 198–205. doi: 10.1038/nn.4220

Takada, M. (1990). The A11 catecholamine cell group: another origin of the dopaminergic innervation of the amygdala. *Neurosci. Lett.* 118, 132–135. doi: 10.1016/0304-3940(90)90266-C

Takada, M. (1993). Widespread dopaminergic projections of the subparafascicular thalamic nucleus in the rat. *Brain Res. Bull.* 32, 301–309. doi: 10.1016/0361-9230(93)90191-D

Takada, M., Li, Z. K., and Hattori, T. (1988). Single thalamic dopaminergic neurons project to both the neocortex and spinal cord. *Brain Res.* 455, 346–352. doi: 10.1016/0006-8993(88)90093-5

Tamae, A., Nakatsuka, T., Koga, K., Kato, G., Furue, H., Katafuchi, T., et al. (2005). Direct inhibition of substantia gelatinosa neurones in the rat spinal cord by activation of dopamine D2-like receptors. *J. Physiol.* 568, 243–253. doi: 10.1113/jphysiol.2005.091843

Taniguchi, W., Nakatsuka, T., Miyazaki, N., Yamada, H., Takeda, D., Fujita, T., et al. (2011). In vivo patch-clamp analysis of dopaminergic antinociceptive actions on substantia gelatinosa neurons in the spinal cord. *Pain* 152, 95–105. doi: 10.1016/j.pain.2010.09.034

Ugrumov, M. V. (2009). Non-dopaminergic neurons partly expressing dopaminergic phenotype: distribution in the brain, development and functional significance. *J. Chem. Neuroanat.* 38, 241–256. doi: 10.1016/j.jchemneu.2009.08.004

Weihe, E., Depboylu, C., Schütz, B., Schäfer, M. K.-H., and Eiden, L. E. (2006). Three types of tyrosine hydroxylase-positive CNS neurons distinguished by dopa decarboxylase and VMAT2 co-expression. *Cell. Mol. Neurobiol.* 26, 659–678. doi: 10.1007/s10571-006-9053-9

Weil-Fugazza, J., and Godefroy, F. (1993). Dorsal and ventral dopaminergic innervation of the spinal cord: functional implications. *Brain Res. Bull.* 30, 319–324. doi: 10.1016/0361-9230(93)90259-E

Whelan, P., Bonnot, A., and O'Donovan, M. J. (2000). Properties of rhythmic activity generated by the isolated spinal cord of the neonatal mouse. *J. Neurophysiol.* 84, 2821–2833. doi: 10.1152/jn.2000.84.6.2821

Whelan, P. J. (2017). *Uncovering Parallel Pathways for Movement Control. Program No. 267.06. 2017 Neuroscience Meeting Planner*. Washington, DC: Society for Neuroscience.

Yip, S. H., York, J., Hyland, B., Bunn, S. J., and Grattan, D. R. (2017). Incomplete concordance of dopamine transporter Cre (DATIREScre)-mediated recombination and tyrosine hydroxylase immunoreactivity in the mouse forebrain. *J. Chem. Neuroanat.* 90, 40–48. doi: 10.1016/j.jchemneu.2017.12.002

Yoshida, M., and Tanaka, M. (1988). Existence of new dopaminergic terminal plexus in the rat spinal cord: assessment by immunohistochemistry using anti-dopamine serum. *Neurosci. Lett.* 94, 5–9. doi: 10.1016/0304-3940(88)90261-3

Young, C. K., Koke, S. J., Kiss, Z. H., and Bland, B. H. (2009). Deep brain stimulation of the posterior hypothalamic nucleus reverses akinesia in bilaterally 6-hydroxydopamine-lesioned rats. *Neuroscience* 162, 1–4. doi: 10.1016/j.neuroscience.2009.04.053

Zhu, H., Clemens, S., Sawchuk, M. A., and Hochman, S. (2007). Expression and distribution of all dopamine receptor subtypes (D(1)-D(5)) in the mouse lumbar spinal cord: a real-time polymerase chain reaction and non-autoradiographic in situ hybridization study. *Neuroscience* 149, 885–897. doi: 10.1016/j.neuroscience.2007.07.052

16

Monoaminergic Neuromodulation of Sensory Processing

Simon N. Jacob[1]* and Hendrikje Nienborg[2]*

[1] Department of Neurosurgery, Klinikum Rechts der Isar, Technical University of Munich, Munich, Germany,
[2] Werner Reichardt Centre for Integrative Neuroscience, University of Tübingen, Tübingen, Germany

****Correspondence:***
Simon N. Jacob
simon.jacob@tum.de
Hendrikje Nienborg
hendrikje.nienborg@cin.uni-tuebingen.de

All neuronal circuits are subject to neuromodulation. Modulatory effects on neuronal processing and resulting behavioral changes are most commonly reported for higher order cognitive brain functions. Comparatively little is known about how neuromodulators shape processing in sensory brain areas that provide the signals for downstream regions to operate on. In this article, we review the current knowledge about how the monoamine neuromodulators serotonin, dopamine and noradrenaline influence the representation of sensory stimuli in the mammalian sensory system. We review the functional organization of the monoaminergic brainstem neuromodulatory systems in relation to their role for sensory processing and summarize recent neurophysiological evidence showing that monoamines have diverse effects on early sensory processing, including changes in gain and in the precision of neuronal responses to sensory inputs. We also highlight the substantial evidence for complementarity between these neuromodulatory systems with different patterns of innervation across brain areas and cortical layers as well as distinct neuromodulatory actions. Studying the effects of neuromodulators at various target sites is a crucial step in the development of a mechanistic understanding of neuronal information processing in the healthy brain and in the generation and maintenance of mental diseases.

Keywords: serotonin, dopamine, noradrenaline, primary sensory cortex, primary visual cortex (V1), primary auditory cortex, early sensory processing

INTRODUCTION

Even at the earliest stages of sensory processing, the neuronal representation of external stimuli is modulated by internal brain states (Aston-Jones and Cohen, 2005; Harris and Thiele, 2011). While the evidence for such modulation is long-standing, the analysis of sensory representations has typically focused on the feed-forward stimulus-driven component while regarding the modulation by internal states as noise. However, recent results based on population recordings (Reimer et al., 2014; Rabinowitz et al., 2015; Schölvinck et al., 2015) that highlight the extent of brain-state dependent modulation of sensory processing, the discovery of substantial modulation of sensory activity with locomotion (Niell and Stryker, 2010; Polack et al., 2013), as well as novel tools to more selectively target modulatory circuit elements genetically have contributed to reviving the interest in the neuromodulation of sensory processing. Since the role of acetylcholine has received substantial attention and has been the subject of excellent recent reviews (Sarter et al., 2009; Harris and Thiele, 2011), we will focus here on the modulation by the monoamines dopamine (DA), noradrenaline (NA), and serotonin (5HT). For each of these modulatory systems, we will summarize anatomical data and electrophysiological findings to provide insights into their role in the modulation of sensory processing, placing an emphasis on studies in non-human primates and rodents, and highlighting the complementarity of these neuromodulatory systems (**Figure 1**). We will cover key classical studies and then shift our focus toward more recent work.

SEROTONERGIC MODULATION OF SENSORY PROCESSING

Serotonin Sources

Serotonin-synthesizing neurons are located in the brainstem in a small group of clusters [named B1–B9 after Dahlström and Fuxe (1964)]. These were first identified in the rat brain (Dahlström and Fuxe, 1964) but their anatomical localizations in mouse and primate species, e.g., Jacobowitz and MacLean (1978), have been found to be largely consistent with that in the rat. These clusters are typically divided into a caudal and a rostral group (Hornung, 2010). The caudal group, which consists of the raphe pallidus (B1), the raphe obscurus (B2), and raphe magnus (B3) (Lesch and Waider, 2012), projects mainly to the spinal cord and brain stem. The rostral group includes the dorsal raphe nucleus (B6, B7) and the median raphe nucleus (B5, B8, and B9) and projects to the cortex. Within this group, there is some topographic organization of the serotonergic innervation (Hornung, 2010) that reflects a rostral (frontal cortex) to caudal (occipital cortex) gradient (Wilson and Molliver, 1991b). Such topographical organization suggests that rather than reflecting a signal that is broadcasted uniformly throughout the brain, serotonergic projections to different areas are more specific and may serve different roles. Indeed, retrograde studies in rats support topographically specific projections, for example to the prefrontal cortex (PFC) (Chandler et al., 2013). Although serotonergic neurons represent only a very small number of the neurons in the brain [approx. 28,000 in the mouse (Ishimura et al., 1988) to several 100,000 in humans (Hornung, 2010)], they give rise to diverging projections to virtually all regions of the mammalian brain (Hornung, 2010). Here, we will focus on the serotonergic projections to primary sensory cortical areas and subcortical structures involved in sensory processing.

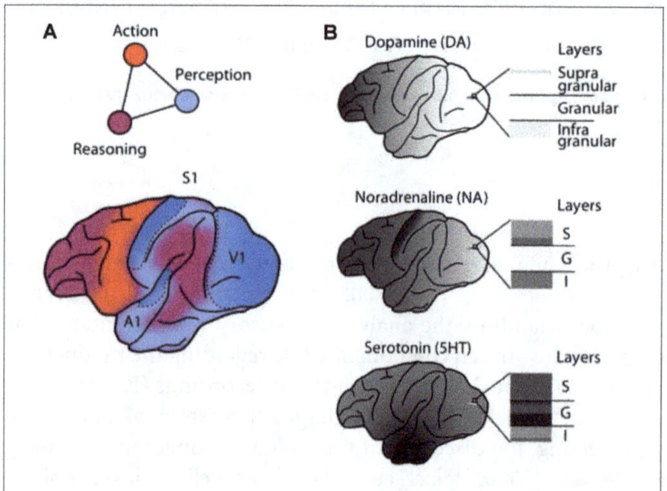

FIGURE 1 | Anatomical and functional complementarity of the monoaminergic neuromodulators. **(A)** Schematic illustrating the functional divisions of the perception-action-reasoning cycle projected onto the lateral surface of a macaque brain [after (Fuster, 2015)]. **(B)** The monoaminergic neuromodulators show pronounced differences in cortical regional [after Brown et al. (1979)] and laminar innervation patterns.

Serotonergic Projections to Early Sensory Areas

Anatomical studies in different rodent and monkey species have identified substantial serotonergic projections from the raphe nuclei to early sensory areas including the primary auditory, visual, and somatosensory areas, the olfactory bulb, and subcortical structures involved in sensory processing (**Table 1**). [Note that while in the auditory system, serotonergic innervation of the cochlear nucleus is established (Klepper and Herbert, 1991), serotonergic projections to the retina have been controversial (Schnyder and Künzle, 1984; Frazão et al., 2008)].

Comparisons of monoaminergic innervation found that the serotonergic innervation was substantially more pronounced than that for NA or DA in the macaque primary auditory cortex (Campbell et al., 1987) and in the macaque primary visual cortex (Morrison et al., 1982a; Kosofsky et al., 1984; Morrison and Foote, 1986; Lewis et al., 1987). This pattern mirrors early reports of regional differences in cortical monoaminergic distribution (Brown et al., 1979), with a pronounced decrease in DA from frontal to occipital cortex, a weaker gradient (interrupted by a peak in the somatosensory cortex) for NA, and a roughly uniform distribution for serotonin (**Figure 1B**).

Within primary sensory cortical areas, the distribution of serotonergic fibers in primates shows a characteristic laminar profile. In the primary visual cortex, anatomical data for different primate species agree that the distribution of serotonergic axons is highest in layer 4 (Kosofsky et al., 1984; Morrison and Foote, 1986). This suggests that the serotonergic modulation in the primary visual cortex is biased toward targeting the visual input stage. Serotonergic fibers are also consistently found in cortical layer 4 in the primary auditory cortex (Campbell et al., 1987) and somatosensory cortex (Wilson and Molliver, 1991a,b), although not preferentially.

This contrasts with the monoaminergic innervation of primary sensory areas by NA and DA (see below) that is typically sparse if not absent in layer 4 (**Figure 1B**). (Note that while a transient dominance of serotonergic input to layer 4 occurs during the early post-natal development in the rodent primary visual cortex and barrel cortex (Fujimiya et al., 1986; Dori et al., 1996), regional and laminar differences are less pronounced in rodents than in the primate species.)

Consistent serotonergic innervation is also found in subcortical structures involved in sensory processing such as the sensory thalamus (Vertes et al., 2010), the superior (Dori et al., 1998) and inferior (Klepper and Herbert, 1991) colliculi, and the cochlear nucleus (Klepper and Herbert, 1991). In the olfactory bulb, serotonergic fibers reach the glomerular layer, the primary input stage (Takeuchi et al., 1982). Together, the

TABLE 1 | Anatomical findings for the serotonin system in early sensory areas.

Sensory area	Species	Significance	Reference
V1	Squirrel monkey	V1 receives substantial projections from medial and dorsal raphe nucleus. Serotonergic fibers preferentially target layer 4 in V1.	Morrison et al., 1982a; Tigges et al., 1982
V1	Macaca fascicularis and nemestria	V1 receives substantial projections from the dorsal and medial raphe nuclei.	Doty, 1983
V1	Macaca fascicularis	Serotonergic fibers most pronounced in the layers 3–4Cα in V1 and overall denser than NA fibers	Kosofsky et al., 1984; de Lima et al., 1988
V1	Macaca fuscata	Serotonergic varicosities are densest in layer 4Cα, and in contact with stellate and pyramidal neurons.	Takeuchi and Sano, 1984
V1	Macaca fuscata and fascicularis	Detailed laminar profile of 5HT receptor expression. $5HT1_B$ and $5HT2_A$ are most pronounced. Expressed in layers 2–6, most pronounced in layer 4A and 4Cα/β.	Watakabe et al., 2009
V1	Rat	Transient increase during development in layer 4; later fairly uniform serotonergic innervation across layers.	Dori et al., 1996
V1	Rat	Serotonergic fibers in all layers but most pronounced in layer 4. Target pyramidal and interneurons. Among inhibitory interneurons, mostly somatostatin and NPY+ neurons but VIP+ interneurons are avoided.	Paspalas and Papadopoulos, 2001
LGN	Rat	Serotonergic projections identified using retrograde labeling; dense immunolabelling for the serotonin transporter (SERT), a sensitive marker for serotonergic fibers; most pronounced in the vLGN and IGL of the LGN complex	Villar et al., 1988; Papadopoulos and Parnavelas, 1990; Vertes et al., 2010
S1	Mouse	$5HT3_A$ receptor is expressed on most non-PV, non-SST inhibitory interneurons	Rudy et al., 2011
S1	Mouse	Innervation across all layers in the adult. Transient increase during postnatal development (~PD7). Similar to the rat.	Fujimiya et al., 1986
S1	Macaca fascicularis	(Areas 1, 2, 3) 5HT fibers across all layers but least pronounced in the lower part of layer 3 and layer 4.	DeFelipe and Jones, 1988
S1	Macaca mulatta and fascicularis	Fairly uniform distribution of serotonergic fibers across layers in S1.	Wilson and Molliver, 1991a,b
S1	Rat	5HT fibers are most pronounced superficially, but some controversy; 5HT concentration measured voltammetrically is highest in superficial layers and decreases toward deeper layers; Transient increase in layer 4 during development, later fairly uniform.	Fuxe, 1965; Beaudet and Descarries, 1976; Lamour et al., 1983; Dori et al., 1996
Inferior colliculus		Dense but complementary 5HT and NA projections in both IC and cochlear nucleus.	Klepper and Herbert, 1991
A1	Cat	5HT innervation mostly restricted to layers 1–3.	DeFelipe et al., 1991
A1	Macaca fascicularis	"Uniformly high density" across all layers.	Campbell et al., 1987
MGN	Rat	Homogenous serotonergic innervation.	Vertes et al., 2010
SC	Rat	Serotonergic fibers throughout, but more pronounced in the superficial than in the deep layers of the SC.	Villar et al., 1988; Dori et al., 1998
Olfactory bulb	Rat	Projections from dorsal and median raphe to all layers of olfactory bulb; most densely in glomerular layer, i.e., the input layer.	McLean and Shipley, 1987

extent of serotonergic innervation at the earliest stages of sensory processing makes this system well suited to directly modulate the incoming sensory information.

Serotonergic Synapses and Receptors

The serotonergic projections to the primary sensory areas consist of small varicose axons that are widely distributed (Hornung, 2010). Only a very small proportion of synaptic specializations, typically asymmetric, is found (Descarries et al., 2010), suggesting that serotonin predominantly acts by volume transmission from varicosities. Note, however, that the degree to which neuromodulatory systems rely on "wired" transmission, i.e., highly localized and typically synaptic, or "volume" transmission, i.e., more spatially diffuse, is subject to debate (e.g., Rice and Cragg, 2008; Sarter et al., 2009; Fuxe and Borroto-Escuela, 2016; Sulzer et al., 2016). In the mammalian brain, seven serotonin receptor families, most with several subtypes, have been identified to date and contribute to the functional diversity of serotonin (Mengod et al., 2010). A detailed overview is outside the scope of this review, but a few receptors should be highlighted. 5HT1A is expressed on cortical pyramidal neurons (DeFelipe et al., 2001). In the macaque primary visual cortex, the most densely expressed receptors are 5HT1B and 5HT2A (Watakabe et al., 2009), predominantly in layer 4. 5HT1B is also strongly expressed in the LGN, but only weakly in other cortical areas including the auditory and somatosensory cortex (Watakabe et al., 2009). In the mouse, GABAergic neurons that express the 5HT3A do not express the calcium binding protein parvalbumin or somatostatin and may form a third non-overlapping class of inhibitory interneurons (Rudy et al., 2011).

Serotonergic Modulation of Sensory Physiology

Given the complexity of the input to serotonergic neurons (Pollak Dorocic et al., 2014), the wide distribution of serotonergic projections in the brain and the diversity of serotonin receptors, it is unsurprising that serotonin has been implicated in a spectrum of brain functions. These include the sleep–wake cycle, hormonal regulation, regulation during development as well as affective, cognitive, and sensorimotor functions. Serotonergic neurons show tonic and phasic modes of discharge that are thought to signal different information. For example, in the mouse transient responses of putative serotonergic neurons in the dorsal raphe nucleus reflect a variety of behavioral, sensorimotor, and reward-linked information (Ranade and Mainen, 2009). Phasic and tonic response patterns of optogenetically identified serotonergic neurons in the mouse dorsal raphe have been proposed to reflect the contextual valence on different time-scales (Cohen et al., 2015). Serotonergic neurons have also been linked to signaling patience (Fonseca et al., 2015). But, even for the intensely studied links to reward signaling a simple computational account has proved challenging (Ranade et al., 2014; Dayan and Huys, 2015). Although it is unclear whether its modulatory role can be conceptualized by a simple overarching computational function, serotonin is thought to modulate sensory processing according to behavioral–motivational context.

In reviewing studies of serotonergic modulation of early sensory processing across modalities, consistencies are notable, which will be our focus here (**Table 2**). This focus contrasts with previous perspectives highlighting the diversity of findings (Hurley et al., 2004). (Note that we restricted this summary to studies of short-term sensory modulation and did not consider reports on adaptation or plasticity.) Some variability in the findings likely results from comparing results across anesthetized animals using different anesthetics or awake animals and different experimental approaches.

Despite this variability, most findings are consistent with an overall serotonin-mediated decrease of the sensory response. In the auditory system, a decrease of the extracellular response was observed for the majority of neurons both in the cochlear nucleus of the rat (Ebert and Ostwald, 1992) and the inferior colliculus (IC) of bats (Hurley and Pollak, 1999), although some variability of the effects between cells was observed. Behaviorally, a reduced startle response to auditory tones was observed for intraventricular injection of serotonin (Davis et al., 1980), which is consistent with reduced auditory response (but could also reflect downstream processing). Similarly, a reduced mechanosensory response was observed in behaving mice during optogenetic stimulation of serotonergic raphe neurons (Dugué et al., 2014), which could reflect downstream processing but would also be expected for a reduced sensory response in the somatosensory cortex as previously reported (Waterhouse et al., 1986).

For early visual processing, predominantly decreased responses were observed for the iontophoretic application of serotonin in the cat lateral geniculate nucleus (LGN) (Phillis et al., 1967) and rat V1 (Waterhouse et al., 1990). In the anesthetized macaque, when attempting to dissect the role of the two most strongly expressed receptors in V1, 5HT1B and 5HT2A, using receptor specific ligands, a diverse pattern and bi-directional modulation were observed for both (Watakabe et al., 2009). However, these effects were not compared to spontaneous variability of the responses resulting from the anesthesia or the iontophoretic application itself. For example, slow fluctuations in the neuronal responses have been shown to contribute to stimulus-independent co-variability ("noise correlations") between neurons (Ecker et al., 2014). When instead iontophoretically applying the endogenous ligand serotonin in awake macaques and comparing the effects against those of pH matched saline application, a recent study found an overall decrease of the sensory responses with serotonin (Seillier et al., 2017). While there was some variability across cells, consistent with the results of Watakabe et al. (2009), the inhibitory effect of serotonin was the dominant pattern across the sizeable neuronal population. This decrease was predominantly explained by a multiplicative change (gain change) of the neuronal tuning curves. Behaviorally, a recent study that systemically administered a serotonin-reuptake inhibitor to enhance the effect of serotonin while macaques performed a color discrimination task observed slowed reaction times as well as deteriorated perceptual performance (Costa et al., 2016), as expected for such reduced visual responses. Conversely, a gain reduction of the spontaneous response (Lottem et al., 2016), consistent with an increased signal-to-noise ratio (SNR), or a gain reduction of the tuning curves (Petzold et al., 2009) for serotonin was observed in the mouse olfactory bulb.

Taken together, a surprisingly consistent pattern of the serotonergic modulation of early sensory processing across modalities emerges. The decreased sensory response by serotonin – effectively lowering the salience of the sensory input – may reflect a sensory signature of how serotonin shapes behavior in downstream circuits, such as its proposed role as a behavioral inhibitor (Soubrie, 1986), to promote waiting (Miyazaki et al., 2014; Ranade et al., 2014; Fonseca et al., 2015) or persistence (Lottem et al., 2018).

NORADRENERGIC MODULATION OF SENSORY PROCESSING

Noradrenergic Sources

In rodents (Dahlström and Fuxe, 1964) and primates (Jacobowitz and MacLean, 1978), neurons that produce NA are located in the brainstem in clusters named A1–A7 after (Dahlström and Fuxe, 1964). Of these, the locus coeruleus (LC, A6) projects to most areas in the brain (Loughlin et al., 1986), except for to the basal ganglia [reviewed in Berridge and Waterhouse (2003)], and is the sole source of the noradrenergic innervation of the cerebral cortex (Jones et al., 1977; Moore and Bloom, 1979). Immunohistochemical evidence indicates that within the LC the vast majority of neurons are noradrenergic (Grzanna and Molliver, 1980). Similar to the serotonergic and dopaminergic systems, the absolute number of noradrenergic neurons in the LC is small [estimated between approx. 1500 per hemisphere in rodents and approx. 15,000 per hemisphere in humans, reviewed in Sara and Bouret (2012)], but the projections of these neurons are divergent and wide-spread throughout the brain. Despite these wide-spread projections recent findings indicate a modular organization of the LC in rats (Uematsu et al., 2017) and substantial anatomical specificity of the connections, for example

TABLE 2 | Findings related to sensory modulation by serotonin.

Sensory area	Species and anesthesia, if applicable	Significance	Reference
Cochlear nucleus	Urethane anesthetized rat	Mostly suppressive effect of iontophoretically applied 5HT on extracellular responses	Ebert and Ostwald, 1992
Inferior colliculus	Lightly anesthetized (ketamine/xylazine) Bat	Multiplicative decrease of response with iontophoretic 5HT application; weak increase in latency	Hurley and Pollak, 1999, 2005
Putative auditory contribution	Behaving rat	Startle response to auditory white noise is reduced by intraventricular 5HT application	Davis et al., 1980
V1	Anesthetized (isoflurane/droperidol/fentanyl) macaque	Variable bidirectional modulation of extracellular responses with application of $5HT1_B$ and $5HT2_A$ receptor selective agents	Watakabe et al., 2009
V1	Anesthetized (fentanyl/thiopental/succinylcholine chloride) macaque	Intracortical injection of $5HT1_A$ agonist decreases extracellularly recorded responses	Rauch et al., 2008
V1	Behaving macaque	Gain decrease of extracellular responses with iontophoretic 5HT application. Modest increase in response latency. No systematic effect on response variability, co-variability, or selectivity	Seillier et al., 2017
V1	Halothane anesthetized rat	Variable findings for iontophoretic 5HT application but mainly a decreased response across the population	Waterhouse et al., 1990
dLGN	Halothane/nitrous oxide anesthetized cat	Decrease of the extracellular responses for iontophoretic 5HT application	Phillis et al., 1967
S1	Halothane anesthetized rat	Suppression of response to tactile stimuli (forepaw touch), consistent with response gain decrease with iontophoretic 5HT application	Waterhouse et al., 1986
	Behaving mouse	Decreased mechanosensory response of mice during optogenetic activation of serotonergic raphe neurons	Dugué et al., 2014
	Behaving macaque	Blocking serotonin re-uptake slowed reaction times and worsened perceptual performance in a visual (color) discrimination task	Costa et al., 2016
Olfactory bulb	Ketamine/xylazine anesthetized mouse	Gain decrease for application of 5HT agonists, reversed for application of 5HT antagonist.	Petzold et al., 2009
Olfactory bulb	Urethane anesthetized mouse	Optogenetic activation of serotonergic neurons in the dorsal raphe lead to a gain decrease of spontaneous but not stimulus-driven extracellular response in the OB resulting in an increase in SNR	Lottem et al., 2016

to the prefrontal versus the motor cortex (Chandler et al., 2014), or different modules projecting to the amygdala compared to the medial PFC (mPFC) (Uematsu et al., 2017). It therefore seems likely that at least some degree of modularity is also characteristic of projections to sensory areas. In the following, we will again focus on the projections to the primary sensory areas and subcortical structures involved in early sensory processing.

Noradrenergic Projections to Early Sensory Areas

The LC sends divergent projections to the cortex and subcortical structures. Within the LC, these projections are roughly topographically organized [reviewed in Berridge and Waterhouse (2003)]. In the rat, cortex-projecting neurons are more prominent in the caudal portion of the LC and show some ventral (frontal cortex) to dorsal (occipital cortex) organization (Waterhouse et al., 1983). Despite the rough topography, a recent study combining retrograde labeling and optogenetic stimulation in the mouse found that the LC projections to primary sensory cortices are not modality-specific (Kim et al., 2016) (contrasting with these authors' findings for the cholinergic system). Nonetheless, projections from LC show clear regional differences (**Table 3**). Early studies in rats (Kehr et al., 1976) and macaques (Brown et al., 1979) observed an overall frontal (higher concentration) to occipital (lower concentration) gradient of NA throughout cortex, with the exception of somatosensory cortex where the concentration was highest (Brown et al., 1979). This gradient was weaker than that for DA and differed markedly from the absence of a gradient for serotonin (reviewed above and see **Figure 1**).

Within the primary sensory cortex, the noradrenergic innervation shows some laminar specialization, particularly in primates. In the primate somatosensory cortex, noradrenergic fibers are fairly uniform and dense throughout layers (Morrison et al., 1982b; Lewis et al., 1987). The innervation of the primary auditory cortex (Campbell et al., 1987) and primary visual cortex (Kosofsky et al., 1984; Morrison and Foote, 1986), in contrast, is sparser overall, and a "striking absence" (Foote and Morrison, 1987) of layer 4 innervation, particularly in V1, has been observed. Combined with the near absent innervation of the LGN (Morrison and Foote, 1986), which provides the dominant feed-forward visual input to V1, this suggests that – in contrast to the serotonergic system – noradrenergic modulation does not target the visual input stage. Interestingly, such complementarity between the serotonergic and noradrenergic innervation of the sensory input stage is also present in the rat olfactory bulb. While "virtually no label" was observed in the glomerular layer (the

TABLE 3 | Anatomical findings for the NA system in early sensory areas.

Structure	Species	Significance	Reference
V1	Squirrel monkey	Noradrenergic projections preferentially to layers 5 and 6 of V1	Morrison et al., 1982a; Lewis et al., 1987
V1	Macaca fascicularis	NA innervation much sparser than for 5HT, and least dense in layer 4C	Kosofsky et al., 1984
V1	Cynomolgus monkey	NA fibers less pronounced than 5HT. Weak in layers 1 and 2, and absent in layer 4Cβ	Kosofsky et al., 1984
V1	Rat	Decreasing fronto-occipital gradient of NA	Kehr et al., 1976
LGN	Squirrel monkeys and macaca fascicularis	Almost no noradrenergic innervation in the LGN	Morrison and Foote, 1986
LGN	Rat	NA fibers preferentially in the dLGN compared to vLGN and IGL (compared to 5HT fibers preferentially in the vLGN and IGL)	Papadopoulos and Parnavelas, 1990
S1	Squirrel monkey	Labeling in all layers	Morrison et al., 1982b; Lewis et al., 1987
S1	Rhesus monkeys	NA concentration highest in somatosensory cortex, lowest in V1	Brown et al., 1979
A1	Macaca fascicularis	Sparse innervation (substantially less dense than 5HT or Ach), lowest density in layer 4	Campbell et al., 1987
Olfactory bulb	Rat	Virtually no labeling fibers in the glomerular layer (first input stage) but fibers preferentially in the internal plexiform, granule cell, and external plexiform layers	McLean et al., 1989
IC, CN	Rat	LC heavily innervates both structures	Klepper and Herbert, 1991

site of the first synapse of the olfactory input) using anterograde tracer injections in the LC (McLean et al., 1989), this layer showed the densest serotonergic innervation (McLean and Shipley, 1987) (see above). Instead, pronounced noradrenergic innervation in the rat olfactory bulb was observed for the consecutive processing stages, the internal plexiform, granule, and external plexiform layers (McLean et al., 1989).

Noradrenergic Synapses and Receptors

Similar to the other monoaminergic systems, noradrenergic neurons in the LC show both tonic and phasic modes of activation [reviewed in Berridge and Waterhouse (2003)]. Their axons have characteristic NA-containing varicosities that can form synapses (e.g., Papadopoulos et al., 1989) and likely have non-synaptic release sites (Callado and Stamford, 2000). Three adrenergic receptor families are expressed in the brain (alpha 1, alpha 2, and beta 1–3), which have characteristic pre- and postsynaptic sites and laminar expression patterns across cortex (Berridge and Waterhouse, 2003). Noradrenaline has the highest affinity for the α2 receptors, intermediate for α1 receptors, and lowest affinity for the β adrenergic receptors [reviewed in Ramos and Arnsten (2007)]. In the primate PFC, these differences in affinity have been implicated in differentially modulating cognitive processes as a function of the level of noradrenergic tone (Ramos and Arnsten, 2007). They are likely also an important factor in the substantial diversity in modulation of sensory processing observed for NA (see below).

Noradrenergic Modulation of Sensory Physiology

The brain's noradrenergic system has long been linked to arousal (e.g., O'Hanlon, 1965; reviewed in, e.g., Berridge and Waterhouse, 2003; Sara and Bouret, 2012) and to adapting network activity for optimal, flexible behavior (Aston-Jones and Cohen, 2005; Bouret and Sara, 2005). Consistent with such a general function, NA has been shown to modulate sensory processing in complex ways (**Table 4**).

Earlier findings have been reviewed in detail (Berridge and Waterhouse, 2003). In brief, activating the LC or local application of NA has been found to result in a variety of effects, including inhibitory and/or facilitating modulation, selective gating, changes to a neuron's receptive field, and changes to its SNR. For example, iontophoretic application of NA was found to predominantly decrease responses in the dLGN, dorsal, and ventral thalamus of cats (Phillis et al., 1967; Phillis and Tebēcis, 1967), in A1 of squirrel monkeys (Foote et al., 1975) and of rats (Manunta and Edeline, 1997), and in rat S1 (Armstrong-James and Fox, 1983; Bassant et al., 1990). Conversely, a predominantly facilitating effect was observed for iontophoretic application of NA or LC stimulation in the rat dLGN (Rogawski and Aghajanian, 1980; Kayama et al., 1982) or V1 (Waterhouse et al., 1990), and for phasic LC stimulation in rat S1 (Waterhouse and Woodward, 1980; Waterhouse et al., 1980, 1998) or rat piriform cortex (Bouret and Sara, 2002). In cat V1 Sato and colleagues (Sato et al., 1989), observed a substantial layer-dependence of the response modulation with LC stimulation. It was predominantly inhibitory in layers 2–4, mostly α receptor mediated facilitation in layer 5 and approximately balanced in both directions in layer 6. These laminar differences likely reflect different receptor expression profiles across layers. The results suggest that some of the variability between studies may also reflect laminar differences between studies within the targeted structures in addition to, e.g., dose-dependent effects. Mirroring this variability, noradrenergic effects on the neuronal SNR differed between studies. While some reported an enhanced SNR (e.g., Foote et al., 1975; Waterhouse and Woodward, 1980; Kasamatsu and Heggelund, 1982) and others (Sato et al., 1989; Manunta and Edeline, 1997) reported no net effect on SNR across the population. In line with the notion of optimizing the

TABLE 4 | Findings related to sensory modulation by NA.

Sensory area	Species and anesthesia (if applicable)	Significance	Reference
dLGN	Chloral hydrate/urethane anesthetized rat	NA or LC activation facilitates responses in dLGN; the facilitation of LGN response to LC stimulation is blocked by α1 but not β receptor antagonists	Rogawski and Aghajanian, 1980; Kayama et al., 1982
dLGN, dorsal, and ventral thalamus	Halothane anesthetized cat	Predominantly depression of responses by iontophoretic application of NA	Phillis et al., 1967; Phillis and Tebĕcis, 1967
V1	Nitrous oxide anesthetized cat	Bi-directional modulation. Enhanced SNR for modulated neurons	Kasamatsu and Heggelund, 1982
V1	Halothane anesthetized/nitrous oxide cat	LC stimulation results in both facilitation and inhibition of extracellular responses in V1, which vary by layer. Results from α1, α2, and β antagonists suggest that α receptors facilitate the responses while β receptor activation results in bi-directional modulation. No change in SNR	Sato et al., 1989
V1	Thiopental anesthetized cat	Iontophoretic NA application results in variable modulation of the responses and affects receptive field properties	McLean and Waterhouse, 1994
V1	Awake mouse	NA was found necessary for tonic depolarization with locomotion of layer 2/3 excitatory neurons	Polack et al., 2013
V1	Urethane anesthetized rat	LC activity precedes increases in cortical excitability	Safaai et al., 2015
V1	Halothane anesthetized rat	Iontophoretic application of NA enhances visual responses	Waterhouse et al., 1990
A1	Awake squirrel monkey	Iontophoretic NA application decreases evoked and spontaneous extracellular activity consistent with an increased SNR	Foote et al., 1975
A1	Urethane-anesthetized rat	Iontophoretic NA application induces bi-directional modulation, with the dominant effect a response decrease, α1-receptor mediated. No net change in SNR across the population	Manunta and Edeline, 1997
CN	Awake bat	Enhances "temporal contrast," i.e., the temporal precision of the response	Kössl and Vater, 1989
S1 and ventral posteriomedial thalamus	Awake rat	Tonic vs. phasic activation differentially modulates responses in the somatosensory processing hierarchy	Devilbiss and Waterhouse, 2011
S1	Isoflurane anesthetized rat	Intracellular recordings *in vivo*: NA blockage reduces up-states in neurons	Constantinople and Bruno, 2011
S1	Urethane anesthetized and awake rat	Iontophoretic NA application suppresses spontaneous and glutamate evoked activity	Armstrong-James and Fox, 1983; Bassant et al., 1990
S1	Halothane anesthetized rat	Variable effects on rates and SNR for iontophoretic NA application; phasic LC stimulation predominantly enhances responses. NA depletion abolishes this modulation	Waterhouse and Woodward, 1980; Waterhouse et al., 1980, 1998
Piriform cortex	Urethane anesthetized rat	Mainly enhancement of odor responses in piriform cortex with LC stimulation	Bouret and Sara, 2002
Olfactory bulb	Urethane anesthetized rat	Infusion of NA and stimulation of the LC decreases responses at low and high levels but not intermediate levels of stimulation/NA	Manella et al., 2017

neuronal gain for behavior (Aston-Jones and Cohen, 2005), this variability may reflect the noradrenergic role in different states of a dynamical system.

Indeed, simultaneous recordings in the LC and barrel cortex of anesthetized rats combined with dynamical systems modeling showed that activity in the LC was highly predictive of dynamic changes in cortical excitability (Safaai et al., 2015). Moreover, phasic responses in the LC or urethane anesthetized rats were elicited by aversive somatosensory stimuli and modulated the stimulus-induced gamma oscillations in the mPFC, suggesting a corresponding modulation of somatosensory processing (Neves et al., 2018). In awake mice, visual responses have been found to be substantially enhanced during phases when the animals were running compared to no locomotion (Niell and Stryker, 2010). Intriguingly, intracellular recordings showed that this effect was accompanied by a depolarization of the membrane potential in layer 2/3 neurons, which in turn was blocked by noradrenergic antagonists (Polack et al., 2013). Indeed, both noradrenergic and cholinergic mechanisms were linked to this locomotion-dependent modulation, with partially complementary functions (Polack et al., 2013; Reimer et al., 2016). These findings align with the notion of a noradrenergic role in adapting sensory circuits for optimal behavior (Aston-Jones and Cohen, 2005). Additionally, they highlight the importance of interactions between neuromodulatory systems that go beyond the scope of this review.

DOPAMINERGIC MODULATION OF SENSORY PROCESSING

Dopamine Sources

Dopamine synthesizing neurons represent a comparatively small population of neurons in the mammalian brain (Bentivoglio and Morelli, 2005). The majority of DA neurons are found in three cell groups in the ventral midbrain (mesencephalon) (Dahlström and Fuxe, 1964). Based on cytoarchitectonic features, most dopaminergic cells reside in the substantia nigra (SN) pars compacta (SNc, A9), the ventral tegmental area (VTA, A10) medial to the SN and in the retrorubral area (RRA; A8), which lies caudal and dorsal to the SN. Other, smaller dopaminergic cell groups are present in the periaqueductal gray matter (PAG; A11) and in the hypothalamus (A12–A15), the lateral parabrachial nucleus, the olfactory bulb (A16), and in the retina (A17) (Sánchez-González et al., 2005).

The most frequently used marker for identifying dopaminergic neurons is tyrosine hydroxylase (TH), the rate-limiting enzyme of DA synthesis. For TH-immunopositive neurons, the A8 group comprises approx. 5% of cells, while A9 and A10 account for the remaining 95% with a slight dominance of A9 over A10 (Bentivoglio and Morelli, 2005). The DA system undergoes considerable expansion from rodents to primates (Berger et al., 1991). By immunostaining for TH, the number of mesencephalic DA neurons has been estimated at approx. 20,000–30,000 in total in mice (Nelson et al., 1996), 45,000 in rats (German and Manaye, 1993), 110,000–220,000 in the SN in rhesus monkeys (Emborg et al., 1998), and between 230,000 and 430,000 in the human SN (Chu et al., 2002). Thus, a large dopaminergic A9 group is a distinctive feature of the primate brain.

Tyrosine hydroxylase labeling to identify dopaminergic neurons has been called into question because of a lack of specificity (Lammel et al., 2015). Staining for the dopamine transporter (DAT), which removes DA from the extracellular space and is largely responsible for the termination of dopaminergic neurotransmission, is more specific and is not detected, e.g., in noradrenergic cells (Ciliax et al., 1995). However, DAT is not expressed in all DA neurons. For example, it cannot be used to label the diencephalic (hypothalamic) cell groups (Sánchez-González et al., 2005). The subgroup of VTA DA neurons that project to the PFC also contains very little DAT (Lammel et al., 2008). Distinct expression profiles of TH and DAT can therefore be exploited to trace independent populations among dopaminergic neurons.

There is mounting evidence that DA is also released from terminals of LC neurons as a co-transmitter of NA (Devoto et al., 2001, 2003, 2005). These important findings underscore the potential caveats of using cellular protein markers instead of the transmitter receptor or the transmitter itself to investigate monoaminergic neurotransmission. Considerable complexity within the monoaminergic system is therefore likely to shape sensory and higher-order cognitive processing (Takeuchi et al., 2016).

Dopamine Projections

A variety of different techniques has been used to investigate dopaminergic innervation of target structures, including direct (e.g., photometric or autoradiographic) neurotransmitter measurements (Brown et al., 1979; Descarries et al., 1987), immunostaining for TH in comparison to staining for DA-β hydroxylase (Lewis et al., 1987) and DAT (Sánchez-González et al., 2005), DA receptor autoradiography (Lidow et al., 1991), and DA receptor mRNA assays (Weiner et al., 1991; Hurd et al., 2001; Santana et al., 2009). It is important to keep in mind that these methods differ not just with regard to their sensitivity and specificity, but that they also target distinct stages of DA production and neurotransmission. This is a likely source of variability and even discrepancy in the literature. Ultimately, functional evidence is required that local DA modulates neuronal processing in target areas. Physiological studies are therefore the gold-standard for demonstrating effective dopaminergic innervation (see below).

The DA system projects extensively to many subcortical and cortical structures of the brain, albeit with a clear concentration. Lewis et al. (1987) noted, summarizing their work on the cortical distribution of dopaminergic afferents in the non-human primate, that "dopaminergic fibers preferentially innervate motor over sensory regions, sensory association over primary sensory regions, and auditory association over visual association regions."

The dopaminergic projections from the midbrain are typically subdivided into the mesostriatal pathway and the mesocorticolimbic pathway. The striatum is the major target of mesencephalic DA neurons (Bentivoglio and Morelli, 2005). Ipsilateral projections to the dorsal striatum mainly arise from the SNc (nigrostriatal pathway). Limbic efferents including projections to the ventral striatum (nucleus accumbens) emanate largely from the VTA.

The mesocortical pathways target in particular the motor cortex, the prefrontal, the anterior cingulate, and the rhinal cortices in rodents (Descarries et al., 1987) and in the non-human primate (Berger et al., 1988; Lidow et al., 1991). Similar to the number of dopaminergic midbrain neurons, however, the density of cortical DA terminals varies considerably from species to species, reaching a maximum in primates (Berger et al., 1991). Unlike NA and, especially, serotonin, cortical levels of DA in the macaque brain exhibit a prominent gradient with a strong decrease along the fronto-occipital axis and only minimal amounts detectable in visual cortex (Brown et al., 1979; see **Figure 1B**).

Mesocortical projections originate from all major cell groups in the ventral mesencephalon, with a looser organization compared to the mesostriatal system. A clear topographical relationship, however, has been described for the most densely innervated frontal lobe. Dopaminergic projections to the dorsolateral PFC in the macaque brain arise from the dorsal and lateral regions of three midbrain cell groups A8, A9, and A10, whereas the ventromedial regions of the PFC receive projections from the medial parabrachial pigmented nucleus and the midline nuclei of the VTA (Williams and Goldman-Rakic, 1998). A similar medial–lateral arrangement has been found in rats (Loughlin and Fallon, 1984). Here, most of the dopaminergic innervation of the medial frontal cortex comes from VTA neurons that project to the deep layers 5 and 6 of the mPFC and in particular to the orbitofrontal cortex (Chandler et al., 2013), with substantially fewer cells from the SNc innervating predominately the superficial mPFC layers (Berger et al., 1991). SNc DA neurons preferentially target the lateral frontal cortex, e.g., the premotor areas (Loughlin and Fallon, 1984; Muller et al., 2014).

Overall, VTA dopaminergic neurons show little collateralization to extensive terminal fields, somewhat in contrast to SNc cells (Loughlin and Fallon, 1984; Chandler et al., 2013). This suggests that, in light of the topographical arrangement described above, discrete, anatomically circumscribed dopaminergic subsystems exist that could modulate selected target regions.

Dopamine Synapses and Receptors

Dopamine-containing varicosities can form multiple synaptic contacts along the course of an axonal fiber. In frontal cortex, these terminals establish conventional, symmetric synapses with postsynaptic dendritic shafts and spines, preferentially on pyramidal neurons (Berger et al., 1991). At the ultrastructural level, dopaminergic afferents form synaptic triads with postsynaptic spines that receive a second, presumably glutamatergic input (Goldman-Rakic et al., 1989). This configuration would allow DA to modulate ongoing neuronal transmission both pre- and postsynaptically.

Dopamine receptors are expressed by pyramidal neurons and GABAergic interneurons alike, indicating that DA modulates excitatory and inhibitory synaptic transmission (Santana et al., 2009). Dopamine receptors are categorized into two major families: the D1 family comprising the D_1 and D_5 receptors, and the D2 family comprising the D_2, D_3, and D_4 receptors. Both D1 and D2 families of receptors are G protein-coupled receptors, which initiate intracellular signaling cascades rather than directly inducing postsynaptic currents (Missale et al., 1998; Bentivoglio and Morelli, 2005). D1 and D2 receptors are largely expressed in different cell populations (Vincent et al., 1993). In most rat brain structures except for the VTA and some midbrain cell groups, D1 receptors outnumber D2 receptors (Boyson et al., 1986; Weiner et al., 1991). In the human brain, D1 receptor mRNA clearly dominates over D2 receptor mRNA in the cortical mantle, whereas D2 receptor mRNA is more abundant in the hippocampal formation, brainstem, and in subcortical structures such as the thalamus (Hurd et al., 2001). Of note, a high proportion of DA (D1) receptors are found at extrasynaptic sites, suggesting that DA might also exert its effects via diffusion in the neuropil (volume transmission) (Smiley et al., 1994).

Cortical DA receptors show a laminar-specific distribution profile. D1 receptors are expressed in all cortical layers in the primate frontal brain (Lidow et al., 1991; Huntley et al., 1992), often with a bilaminar infra-supragranular pattern with a relative paucity in layer 4 (Lewis et al., 1987) and a predilection for deeper layers. D2 receptors, in contrast, are typically confined to cortical layer 5 (Weiner et al., 1991; Lidow et al., 1998).

Dopaminergic Innervation of Sensory Brain Structures

Compared to the densely innervated frontal cortex, the sensory cortices receive very sparse dopaminergic afferents (**Table 5**). In both rat and primate studies, the primary visual cortex shows the lowest DA fiber density of all investigated cortical structures (Descarries et al., 1987; Lidow et al., 1991). TH immunoreactivity in primate primary visual cortex V1 is restricted to layer 1, and few fibers reach layer 6 as well in V2 (Lewis et al., 1987; Berger et al., 1988). The same layers are targeted by dopaminergic fibers in the rat primary visual cortex (Phillipson et al., 1987).

A slight increase in fiber density is seen in primary auditory cortex. In the gerbil, D1 receptors are found in infragranular layers mainly associated with pyramidal neurons (Schicknick et al., 2008). TH positive fibers loosely innervate auditory cortex layers 1 and 6 in primates (Lewis et al., 1987). In primary somatosensory cortex, labeled fibers are also found in layer 5. A further increase in dopaminergic innervation is then observed in the association cortices of the temporal, parietal, and frontal lobe, where the aforementioned bilaminar profile emerges (Lewis et al., 1987).

Dopaminergic fibers have also been reported to innervate subcortical structures that are involved in processing sensory stimuli. Dopamine axons reach the LGN of the thalamus (LGN, visual nucleus) (Papadopoulos and Parnavelas, 1990). Here, D1 and D2 receptors are found in excitatory relay neurons and in inhibitory local interneurons (Albrecht et al., 1996; Zhao et al., 2002; Munsch et al., 2005). D2 receptors are also present in the thalamic medial geniculate nucleus (MGN, auditory nucleus) (Hurd et al., 2001; Chun et al., 2014) and in the ventrobasal complex (VB, somatosensory nucleus) (Govindaiah et al., 2010b).

While these first-order thalamic nuclei mainly relay sensory input to the cortex, the second-order thalamic nuclei are part of cortico–thalamo–cortical loops and could support higher brain functions operating on sensory information (Sherman, 2016). The second-order thalamus is more strongly innervated by DA neurons than its first-order counterpart, reaching the levels of highest cortical density in some nuclei (Sánchez-González et al., 2005). Thalamic DA fibers are much denser in primates than in rodents (García-Cabezas et al., 2009). Dopaminergic afferents in the thalamus stem from multiple sources including the hypothalamus, ventral mesencephalon, the PAG, and the lateral parabrachial nucleus, possibly hinting at the existence of a distinct "thalamic dopaminergic system" (Groenewegen, 1988; Sánchez-González et al., 2005). Interestingly, the densest dopaminergic projections to the thalamus are found in those second-order nuclei that are linked to frontal and limbic cortex, e.g., the mediodorsal (MD) nucleus and the midline nuclei (García-Cabezas et al., 2007). In fact, these DA projections share many anatomical features with the strong meso-prefrontal DA system (Melchitzky et al., 2006). These findings suggest that DA could modulate higher-order frontal lobe functions both at the cortical level and by controlling its associated thalamic nuclei (Varela, 2014). Finally, it has been noted that VTA axon terminals and terminals from thalamic MD neurons converge in mPFC layer 5, forming a synaptic triad as described above (Kuroda et al., 1996). Thus, dopaminergic modulation of thalamic function might also have extra-thalamic components.

The main auditory midbrain nucleus, the IC, is targeted by TH-immunoreactive nerve terminals arising from the subparafascicular thalamic nucleus (Tong et al., 2005; Nevue et al., 2015), and the IC has been shown to express D2 receptors (Weiner et al., 1991). Dopaminergic afferents to the superior colliculus, a crucial midbrain structure for oculomotor and visual processing, are sparser in comparison (Weiner et al., 1991).

TABLE 5 | Anatomical findings for the DA system in early sensory areas.

Structure	Species	Significance	Reference
V1	Rhesus monkey and rat	Lowest density of dopaminergic innervation across cortical mantle	Brown et al., 1979; Descarries et al., 1987; Lidow et al., 1991
V1	Cynomolgus monkey	TH immunoreactive fibers restricted to layer 1	Berger et al., 1988
V1	Rat	Dopaminergic innervation in infragranular layers and weaker in layer 1	Phillipson et al., 1987
A1	Gerbil	D1 receptors in infragranular layers	Schicknick et al., 2008
A1	Cynomolgus and squirrel monkey	TH immunoreactive fibers in layers 1 and 6	Lewis et al., 1987
S1	Cynomolgus and squirrel monkey	TH immunoreactive fibers in supra- and infragranular layers	Lewis et al., 1987
LGN	Rat	Dopaminergic innervation of all LGN subdivisions	Papadopoulos and Parnavelas, 1990
LGN and MGN	Human	Moderate levels of D2 receptor mRNA	Hurd et al., 2001
Inferior colliculus	Rat and mouse	Innervation by TH immunoreactive fibers	Tong et al., 2005; Nevue et al., 2015
Inferior colliculus	Rat	D2 receptors present at moderate levels	Weiner et al., 1991
Superior colliculus	Rat	D2 receptors present at low levels	Weiner et al., 1991

TABLE 6 | Findings related to sensory modulation by DA.

Structure	Species and anesthesia (if applicable)	Significance	Reference
V1	Remifentanil anesthetized rhesus monkey	Systemic administration of L-DOPA increases supragranular oscillatory activity encoding visual information, but failure to induce changes in neuronal activity by local DA application	Zaldivar et al., 2018, 2014
dLGN	Urethane anesthetized rat and ketamine or halothane anesthetized cat	D1 receptors inhibit and D2 receptors excite extracellularly recorded relay neurons	Phillis et al., 1967; Albrecht et al., 1996; Zhao et al., 2002
dLGN	Rat and mouse (brain slices)	D1 receptors depolarize and D2 receptors inhibit intracellularly recorded neurons	Govindaiah and Cox, 2005; Munsch et al., 2005
A1	Awake gerbil	D1 receptors modulate auditory discrimination learning	Schicknick et al., 2012; Happel et al., 2014
MGN	Mouse (brain slices)	D2 receptors modulate synaptic transmission at thalamocortical afferents in A1	Chun et al., 2014
Inferior colliculus	Awake mouse	Dopamine inhibits neuronal activity	Gittelman et al., 2013
S1	Awake rat	Dopamine inhibits neuronal activity	Bassant et al., 1990
Ventrobasal thalamus	Rat (brain slices)	Dopamine increases excitability of intracellularly recorded neurons	Govindaiah et al., 2010a

Dopaminergic Modulation of Sensory Physiology

Dopamine neuron activity is classically described as being time locked to the presentation of rewarding stimuli. Phasic firing of action potentials by DA neurons especially in the medial mesencephalon communicates a reward prediction error that scales with the difference between predicted and actual reward (Schultz, 2007). These neurophysiological findings form the basis for the large number of studies that have investigated DA's role in motivation, appetence, and reward-related learning ("motivational salience"). More recent experiments have revealed the existence of functionally distinct subgroups of DA neurons in particular in the lateral midbrain that are activated both by rewarding and aversive events (Matsumoto and Hikosaka, 2009; Matsumoto et al., 2013). This suggests that these neurons are responsive to a more general group of sensory stimuli that are behaviorally relevant and should trigger an appropriate coordinated response ("cognitive salience"). The physiological effects of DA on sensory information processing, however, are not yet well understood. Given the sparse innervation of sensory structures, comparatively few studies have addressed the role of DA in directly modulating sensory inputs (**Table 6**).

In rat and cat dorsal LGN, *in vivo* iontophoretic activation of D1 receptors produced inhibition, whereas engagement of D2 receptors resulted in excitation of extracellularly recorded relay neurons (Phillis et al., 1967; Albrecht et al., 1996; Zhao et al., 2002). Intracellular recordings in rat and mouse LGN slices, however, found that D1 receptors lead to an excitatory membrane depolarization in relay neurons (Govindaiah and Cox, 2005), whereas D2 receptors on local GABAergic interneurons produced inhibition in postsynaptic neurons (Munsch et al., 2005), in complete contrast to the *in vivo* results. It is currently unclear whether these diverging findings reflect dose-dependent effects, where application of small and large drug concentrations often yields opposite effects (Zhao et al., 2002), or rather result from network mechanisms that differ in the *in vivo* and *in vitro* preparation.

In primate primary visual cortex (V1), oscillatory activity (local field potentials) containing information about animated visual stimuli (movie clips) was enhanced in particular in supragranular layers following systemic administration of the DA precursor L-DOPA (Zaldivar et al., 2018). However, focal application of DA failed to induce changes in neuronal activity (Zaldivar et al., 2014), possibly reflecting the very sparse dopaminergic innervation of the occipital pole. In accordance with the notion that dopaminergic effects on visual processing are not mediated by early primary visual regions but possibly by higher-order brain areas, visually induced neuronal responses were directly modulated by DA in the monkey lateral PFC (Jacob et al., 2013). Here, iontophoretically applied DA affected two distinct neuronal populations involved in encoding behaviorally relevant visual stimuli. In putative interneurons, DA inhibited activity in form of a subtractive shift in response levels with unchanged SNR. In putative pyramidal neurons, DA increased excitability in form of a multiplication in gain and enhanced SNR through a reduction of response variability across trials (Jacob et al., 2013). By increasing the coding strength of sensory signals, DA could play a crucial role in how sensory information is represented, memorized, and interpreted in PFC (Ott et al., 2014; Jacob et al., 2016).

Acting on cognitive brain centers, DA might influence visual cortical processing (Arsenault et al., 2013) by long-range interactions originating, e.g., in frontal cortex. Support for this hypothesis comes from exploring DA's modulatory influence on PFC-guided allocation of visual attention in the macaque monkey (Noudoost and Moore, 2011). D1R were blocked by local antagonist injections into sites of the frontal eye fields (FEFs) that represented the same region of visual space (the "response field") as simultaneously recorded neurons in visual cortex area V4. Prefrontal D1R antagonism caused the animals to saccade more frequently toward FEF response field targets, meaning this part of the visual field had grasped their attention. The response properties of V4 neurons were changed in a way that is consistent with a multiplicative increase in gain: first, there was an enhancement in the magnitude of responses to visual stimulation; second, the visual responses became more selective to stimulus orientation; third, the visual responses became less variable across trials (Noudoost and Moore, 2011). Thus, prefrontal top-down control over visual cortical neurons during visual attention is under the influence of D1 receptors.

In the auditory system, both inhibitory and – less frequently – excitatory responses in IC neurons were observed after local iontophoretic application of DA in awake mice (Gittelman et al., 2013). The importance of subcortical DA for auditory information processing was underscored by showing that overexpressed MGN D2 receptors in a schizophrenia mouse model reduce the efficiency of synaptic transmission of excitatory thalamocortical afferents in auditory cortex (Chun et al., 2014). These changes were accompanied by behavioral deficits in auditory perception (acoustic startle response). Because thalamocortical afferents in visual or somatosensory cortex were not affected, studying this mouse model might help to provide a neuronal mechanism that links dopaminergic dysfunction to the generation of auditory hallucinations in schizophrenia (Chun et al., 2014). Auditory processing is modulated by cortical DA receptors as well. Systemic administration of D1 receptor antagonists or local injections directly into auditory cortex of gerbils impaired discrimination learning of acoustic stimuli, while D1 receptor agonists improved the animals' performance (Schicknick et al., 2012; Happel et al., 2014).

Finally, the representation of somatosensory information is also strengthened by DA: *in vivo* depletion of DA in mouse striatum worsened the laterality coding of whisker deflections in medium spiny neurons, i.e., the projection neurons of this structure, indicating that tactile acuity requires dopaminergic input (Ketzef et al., 2017). Intracellular recordings in rat VB thalamic slices showed that DA increases neuronal excitability in two different ways: activation of D1 receptors leads to membrane depolarization, whereas D2 receptors facilitate action potential discharge (Govindaiah et al., 2010b). In contrast, in rat S1, iontophoretic DA application produced inhibitory effects on neuronal firing (Bassant et al., 1990).

Putting It All Together: Monoaminergic Neuromodulation of Sensory Processing

The discussed studies provide compelling evidence that the representation and processing of sensory information is heavily regulated by the brain's monoamine transmitters. Despite their widespread cortical and subcortical targeting, the monoaminergic systems are by no means blurry, brain-wide modulators of neuronal activity. They send regionally and laminar-specific projections, which may allow them to control both feed-forward and feed-back influences (Cumming and Nienborg, 2016) on sensory signaling by distinct mechanisms. These regional and laminar differences are particularly pronounced in the macaque brain (**Figure 1**).

The indolamine serotonin has prominent projections to the primary sensory areas and innervates all cortical layers including the thalamo-cortical input layer 4. Serotonin is well suited to regulate the sensory input stages by acting in these primary sensory areas and in the first-order thalamic relay nuclei. Despite some degree of variability between studies on the serotonergic modulation of sensory processing, the emerging pattern is that it dampens neuronal responses and reduces gain. The reduction in gain may reduce the salience of a sensory stimulus (Seillier et al., 2017). Alternatively, if it only affects the spontaneous but not the stimulus-driven response (Lottem et al., 2016), it may increase a neuron's SNR and hence effectively increase stimulus salience. Probing the serotonergic modulation of sensory processing during perceptually driven behavior may resolve this seeming discrepancy. In general, however, the experimental data show that serotonin directly modulates sensory processing as early as the feed-forward sensory input stage.

In contrast to serotonin the catecholamine DA has a pronounced fronto-occipital gradient (**Figure 1**), is less abundant in sensory cortices, particularly sparse in the primary visual cortex, and only weakly active in granular layers. This suggests that dopaminergic effects on sensory processing are not mediated primarily by local modulation of early sensory input stages (e.g., Zaldivar et al., 2014) but instead by modulating long-range recurrent cortico-cortical and cortico-bulbar interactions originating in the strongly innervated supragranular and infragranular layers, respectively, e.g., of the frontal lobe cognitive control centers (Lewis et al., 1987; Noudoost and Moore, 2011; Jacob et al., 2013). Its modulatory effects stem from a variable and complex combination of inhibition and excitation in the targeted circuits. The net result is likely an increase in SNR, which is based both on additive operations, e.g., predominant suppression of responses to non-preferred stimuli ("sculpting inhibition") (Vijayraghavan et al., 2007), and on multiplicative operations, e.g., increase in gain and response reliability (reduction of trial-to-trial variability) (Noudoost and Moore, 2011; Jacob et al., 2013). Thus, the role of DA could primarily be to adapt the read-out of sensory circuits to best serve task demands and behavioral goals.

The catecholamine NA, conversely, may play a role in between these two extremes. It has a less pronounced fronto-occipital gradient than DA and, like serotonin, substantial projections to the primary sensory cortices, including the primary visual cortex. But in contrast to serotonin, the innervation of the granular layers is relatively sparse (**Figure 1**). The modulatory effects of NA on sensory processing are diverse. This variability may reflect adaptable modulation depending on the behavioral state of the animal, in line with the notion of optimizing the neuronal gain for behavior (Aston-Jones and Cohen, 2005).

Taken together, the current literature argues for a prominent complementarity in sensory neuromodulation by monoamines. This complementarity is prominent anatomically (**Figure 1B**), resulting in both direct bottom-up and indirect top-down control over sensory signaling by the indolamine serotonin and the catecholamines NA and DA, respectively (Papadopoulos and Parnavelas, 1991). One of the main challenges will now be to dissect the individual contributions of the anatomically and functionally separable monoamine subsystems in shaping how sensory information is represented, processed, and evaluated by the brain's sensory, cognitive, and motivational networks (**Figure 1A**). We believe that key to such insights will be the combination of increased specificity and precision when targeting these neuromodulatory systems with well characterized behavior (Krakauer et al., 2017).

AUTHOR CONTRIBUTIONS

All authors listed have made a substantial, direct and intellectual contribution to the work, and approved it for publication.

FUNDING

SJ acknowledges support by the German Research Foundation (DFG JA1999/3-1), the German Federal Ministry of Education and Research (01ZX1404C) and the Berlin Institute of Health (TRG 1.2.4). HN acknowledges support by a Starting Independent Researcher Grant from the European Research Council (NEUROOPTOGEN), and by funds from the German Research Foundation awarded to the Centre for Integrative Neuroscience (DFG EXC 307).

REFERENCES

Albrecht, D., Quäschling, U., Zippel, U., and Davidowa, H. (1996). Effects of dopamine on neurons of the lateral geniculate nucleus: an iontophoretic study. *Synapse* 23, 70–78. doi: 10.1002/(SICI)1098-2396(199606)23:2<70::AID-SYN2>3.0.CO;2-D

Armstrong-James, M., and Fox, K. (1983). Effects of ionophoresed noradrenaline on the spontaneous activity of neurones in rat primary somatosensory cortex. *J. Physiol.* 335, 427–447. doi: 10.1113/jphysiol.1983.sp014542

Arsenault, J. T., Nelissen, K., Jarraya, B., and Vanduffel, W. (2013). Dopaminergic reward signals selectively decrease fMRI activity in primate visual cortex. *Neuron* 77, 1174–1186. doi: 10.1016/j.neuron.2013.01.008

Aston-Jones, G., and Cohen, J. D. (2005). Adaptive gain and the role of the locus coeruleus-norepinephrine system in optimal performance. *J. Comp. Neurol.* 493, 99–110. doi: 10.1002/cne.20723

Bassant, M. H., Ennouri, K., and Lamour, Y. (1990). Effects of iontophoretically applied monoamines on somatosensory cortical neurons of unanesthetized rats. *Neuroscience* 39, 431–439. doi: 10.1016/0306-4522(90)90279-D

Beaudet, A., and Descarries, L. (1976). Quantitative data on serotonin nerve terminals in adult rat neocortex. *Brain Res.* 111, 301–309. doi: 10.1016/0006-8993(76)90775-7

Bentivoglio, M., and Morelli, M. (2005). "Chapter I The organization and circuits of mesencephalic dopaminergic neurons and the distribution of dopamine receptors in the brain," in *Dopamine: Handbook of Chemical Neuroanal*, Vol. 21, eds S. B. Dunnett, M. Bentivoglio, A. Bjorklund, and T. Hokfelt (Amsterdam: Elsevier), 1–107. doi: 10.1016/S0924-8196(05)80005-3

Berger, B., Gaspar, P., and Verney, C. (1991). Dopaminergic innervation of the cerebral cortex: unexpected differences between rodents and primates. *Trends Neurosci.* 14, 21–27. doi: 10.1016/0166-2236(91)90179-X

Berger, B., Trottier, S., Verney, C., Gaspar, P., and Alvarez, C. (1988). Regional and laminar distribution of the dopamine and serotonin innervation in the macaque cerebral cortex: a radioautographic study. *J. Comp. Neurol.* 273, 99–119. doi: 10.1002/cne.902730109

Berridge, C. W., and Waterhouse, B. D. (2003). The locus coeruleus-noradrenergic system: modulation of behavioral state and state-dependent cognitive processes. *Brain Res. Brain Res. Rev.* 42, 33–84. doi: 10.1016/S0165-0173(03)00143-7

Bouret, S., and Sara, S. J. (2002). Locus coeruleus activation modulates firing rate and temporal organization of odour-induced single-cell responses in rat piriform cortex. *Eur. J. Neurosci.* 16, 2371–2382. doi: 10.1046/j.1460-9568.2002.02413.x

Bouret, S., and Sara, S. J. (2005). Network reset: a simplified overarching theory of locus coeruleus noradrenaline function. *Trends Neurosci.* 28, 574–582. doi: 10.1016/j.tins.2005.09.002

Boyson, S. J., McGonigle, P., and Molinoff, P. B. (1986). Quantitative autoradiographic localization of the D1 and D2 subtypes of dopamine receptors in rat brain. *J. Neurosci.* 6, 3177–3188. doi: 10.1523/JNEUROSCI.06-11-03177.1986

Brown, R. M., Crane, A. M., and Goldman, P. S. (1979). Regional distribution of monoamines in the cerebral cortex and subcortical structures of the rhesus monkey: concentrations and in vivo synthesis rates. *Brain Res.* 168, 133–150. doi: 10.1016/0006-8993(79)90132-X

Callado, L. F., and Stamford, J. A. (2000). Spatiotemporal interaction of alpha(2) autoreceptors and noradrenaline transporters in the rat locus coeruleus: implications for volume transmission. *J. Neurochem.* 74, 2350–2358. doi: 10.1046/j.1471-4159.2000.0742350.x

Campbell, M. J., Lewis, D. A., Foote, S. L., and Morrison, J. H. (1987). Distribution of choline acetyltransferase-, serotonin-, dopamine-beta-hydroxylase-, tyrosine hydroxylase-immunoreactive fibers in monkey primary auditory cortex. *J. Comp. Neurol.* 261, 209–220. doi: 10.1002/cne.902610204

Chandler, D. J., Gao, W. J., and Waterhouse, B. D. (2014). Heterogeneous organization of the locus coeruleus projections to prefrontal and motor cortices. *Proc. Natl. Acad. Sci. U.S.A.* 111, 6816–6821. doi: 10.1073/pnas.1320827111

Chandler, D. J., Lamperski, C. S., and Waterhouse, B. D. (2013). Identification and distribution of projections from monoaminergic and cholinergic nuclei to functionally differentiated subregions of prefrontal cortex. *Brain Res.* 1522, 38–58. doi: 10.1016/j.brainres.2013.04.057

Chu, Y., Kompoliti, K., Cochran, E. J., Mufson, E. J., and Kordower, J. H. (2002). Age-related decreases in Nurrl immunoreactivity in the human substantia nigra. *J. Comp. Neurol.* 450, 203–214. doi: 10.1002/cne.10261

Chun, S., Westmoreland, J. J., Bayazitov, I. T., Eddins, D., Pani, A. K., Smeyne, R. J., et al. (2014). Specific disruption of thalamic inputs to the auditory cortex in schizophrenia models. *Science* 344, 1178–1182. doi: 10.1126/science.125 3895

Ciliax, B. J., Heilman, C., Demchyshyn, L. L., Pristupa, Z. B., Ince, E., Hersch, S. M., et al. (1995). The dopamine transporter: immunochemical characterization and localization in brain. *J. Neurosci.* 15(3 Pt 1), 1714–1723. doi: 10.1523/JNEUROSCI.15-03-01714.1995

Cohen, J. Y., Amoroso, M. W., and Uchida, N. (2015). Serotonergic neurons signal reward and punishment on multiple timescales. *eLife* 4:e06346. doi: 10.7554/eLife.06346

Constantinople, C. M., and Bruno, R. M. (2011). Effects and mechanisms of wakefulness on local cortical networks. *Neuron* 69, 1061–1068. doi: 10.1016/j.neuron.2011.02.040

Costa, V. D., Kakalios, L. C., and Averbeck, B. B. (2016). Blocking serotonin but not dopamine reuptake alters neural processing during perceptual decision making. *Behav. Neurosci.* 130, 461–468. doi: 10.1037/bne0000162

Cumming, B. G., and Nienborg, H. (2016). Feedforward and feedback sources of choice probability in neural population responses. *Curr. Opin. Neurobiol.* 37, 126–132. doi: 10.1016/j.conb.2016.01.009

Dahlström, A., and Fuxe, K. (1964). Localization of monoamines in the lower brain stem. *Experientia* 20, 398–399. doi: 10.1007/BF02147990

Davis, M., Strachan, D. I., and Kass, E. (1980). Excitatory and inhibitory effects of serotonin on sensorimotor reactivity measured with acoustic startle. *Science* 209, 521–523. doi: 10.1126/science.7394520

Dayan, P., and Huys, Q. (2015). Serotonin's many meanings elude simple theories. *eLife* 4:e07390. doi: 10.7554/eLife.07390

de Lima, A. D., Bloom, F. E., and Morrison, J. H. (1988). Synaptic organization of serotonin-immunoreactive fibers in primary visual cortex of the macaque monkey. *J. Comp. Neurol.* 274, 280–294. doi: 10.1002/cne.902740211

DeFelipe, J., Arellano, J. I., Gómez, A., Azmitia, E. C., and Muñoz, A. (2001). Pyramidal cell axons show a local specialization for GABA and 5-HT inputs in monkey and human cerebral cortex. *J. Comp. Neurol.* 433, 148–155. doi: 10.1002/cne.1132

DeFelipe, J., Hendry, S. H., Hashikawa, T., and Jones, E. G. (1991). Synaptic relationships of serotonin-immunoreactive terminal baskets on GABA neurons in the cat auditory cortex. *Cereb. Cortex* 1, 117–133. doi: 10.1093/cercor/1.2.117

DeFelipe, J., and Jones, E. G. (1988). A light and electron microscopic study of serotonin-immunoreactive fibers and terminals in the monkey sensory-motor cortex. *Exp. Brain Res.* 71, 171–182. doi: 10.1007/BF0024 7532

Descarries, L., Lemay, B., Doucet, G., and Berger, B. (1987). Regional and laminar density of the dopamine innervation in adult rat cerebral cortex. *Neuroscience* 21, 807–824. doi: 10.1016/0306-4522(87)90038-8

Descarries, L., Riad, M., and Parent, M. (2010). "Ultrastructure of the serotonin innervation in the mammalian central nervous system," in *Handbook of the Behavioral Neurobiology of Serotonin*, eds C. P. Mueller and B. L. Jacobs (London: Academic Press), 82–119.

Devilbiss, D. M., and Waterhouse, B. D. (2011). Phasic and tonic patterns of locus coeruleus output differentially modulate sensory network function in the awake rat. *J. Neurophysiol.* 105, 69–87. doi: 10.1152/jn.00445.2010

Devoto, P., Flore, G., Longu, G., Pira, L., and Gessa, G. L. (2003). Origin of extracellular dopamine from dopamine and noradrenaline neurons in the medial prefrontal and occipital cortex. *Synapse* 50, 200–205. doi: 10.1002/syn.10264

Devoto, P., Flore, G., Pani, L., and Gessa, G. L. (2001). Evidence for co-release of noradrenaline and dopamine from noradrenergic neurons in the cerebral cortex. *Mol. Psychiatry* 6, 657–664. doi: 10.1038/sj.mp.4000904

Devoto, P., Flore, G., Saba, P., Fà, M., and Gessa, G. L. (2005). Stimulation of the locus coeruleus elicits noradrenaline and dopamine release in the medial prefrontal and parietal cortex. *J. Neurochem.* 92, 368–374. doi: 10.1111/j.1471-4159.2004.02866.x

Dori, I., Dinopoulos, A., Blue, M. E., and Parnavelas, J. G. (1996). Regional differences in the ontogeny of the serotonergic projection to the cerebral cortex. *Exp. Neurol.* 138, 1–14. doi: 10.1006/exnr.1996.0041

Dori, I. E., Dinopoulos, A., and Parnavelas, J. G. (1998). The development of the synaptic organization of the serotonergic system differs in brain areas with different functions. *Exp. Neurol.* 154, 113–125. doi: 10.1006/exnr.1998.6937

Doty, R. W. (1983). Nongeniculate afferents to striate cortex in macaques. *J. Comp. Neurol.* 218, 159–173. doi: 10.1002/cne.902180204

Dugué, G. P., Lörincz, M. L., Lottem, E., Audero, E., Matias, S., Correia, P. A., et al. (2014). Optogenetic recruitment of dorsal raphe serotonergic neurons acutely decreases mechanosensory responsivity in behaving mice. *PLoS One* 9:e105941. doi: 10.1371/journal.pone.0105941

Ebert, U., and Ostwald, J. (1992). Serotonin modulates auditory information processing in the cochlear nucleus of the rat. *Neurosci. Lett.* 145, 51–54. doi: 10.1016/0304-3940(92)90201-H

Ecker, A. S., Berens, P., Cotton, R. J., Subramaniyan, M., Denfield, G. H., Cadwell, C. R., et al. (2014). State dependence of noise correlations in macaque primary visual cortex. *Neuron* 82, 235–248. doi: 10.1016/j.neuron.2014.02.006

Emborg, M. E., Ma, S. Y., Mufson, E. J., Levey, A. I., Taylor, M. D., Brown, W. D., et al. (1998). Age-related declines in nigral neuronal function correlate with motor impairments in rhesus monkeys. *J. Comp. Neurol.* 401, 253–265. doi: 10.1002/(SICI)1096-9861(19981116)401:2<253::AID-CNE7>3.0.CO;2-X

Fonseca, M. S., Murakami, M., and Mainen, Z. F. (2015). Activation of dorsal raphe serotonergic neurons promotes waiting but is not reinforcing. *Curr. Biol.* 25, 306–315. doi: 10.1016/j.cub.2014.12.002

Foote, S. L., Freedman, R., and Oliver, A. P. (1975). Effects of putative neurotransmitters on neuronal activity in monkey auditory cortex. *Brain Res.* 86, 229–242. doi: 10.1016/0006-8993(75)90699-X

Foote, S. L., and Morrison, J. H. (1987). Extrathalamic modulation of cortical function. *Annu. Rev. Neurosci.* 10, 67–95. doi: 10.1146/annurev.ne.10.030187.000435

Frazão, R., Pinato, L., da Silva, A. V., Britto, L. R., Oliveira, J. A., and Nogueira, M. I. (2008). Evidence of reciprocal connections between the dorsal raphe nucleus and the retina in the monkey *Cebus apella*. *Neurosci. Lett.* 430, 119–123. doi: 10.1016/j.neulet.2007.10.032

Fujimiya, M., Kimura, H., and Maeda, T. (1986). Postnatal development of serotonin nerve fibers in the somatosensory cortex of mice studied by immunohistochemistry. *J. Comp. Neurol.* 246, 191–201. doi: 10.1002/cne.902460205

Fuster, J. (2015). *The Prefrontal Cortex*, 5th Edn. Cambridge, MA: Academic Press.

Fuxe, K. (1965). Evidence for the existence of monoamine neurons in the central nervous system. IV. Distribution of monoamine nerve terminals in the central nervous system. *Acta Physiol. Scand. Suppl.* 247:37. doi: 10.1007/BF00337069

Fuxe, K., and Borroto-Escuela, D. O. (2016). Volume transmission and receptor-receptor interactions in heteroreceptor complexes: understanding the role of new concepts for brain communication. *Neural Regen. Res.* 11, 1220–1223. doi: 10.4103/1673-5374.189168

García-Cabezas, M. A., Martínez-Sánchez, P., Sánchez-González, M. A., Garzón, M., and Cavada, C. (2009). Dopamine innervation in the thalamus: monkey versus rat. *Cereb. Cortex* 19, 424–434. doi: 10.1093/cercor/bhn093

García-Cabezas, M. A., Rico, B., Sánchez-González, M. A., and Cavada, C. (2007). Distribution of the dopamine innervation in the macaque and human thalamus. *Neuroimage* 34, 965–984. doi: 10.1016/j.neuroimage.2006.07.032

German, D. C., and Manaye, K. F. (1993). Midbrain dopaminergic neurons (nuclei A8, A9, and A10): three-dimensional reconstruction in the rat. *J. Comp. Neurol.* 331, 297–309. doi: 10.1002/cne.903310302

Gittelman, J. X., Perkel, D. J., and Portfors, C. V. (2013). Dopamine modulates auditory responses in the inferior colliculus in a heterogeneous manner. *J. Assoc. Res. Otolaryngol.* 14, 719–729. doi: 10.1007/s10162-013-0405-0

Goldman-Rakic, P. S., Leranth, C., Williams, S. M., Mons, N., and Geffard, M. (1989). Dopamine synaptic complex with pyramidal neurons in primate cerebral cortex. *Proc. Natl. Acad. Sci. U.S.A.* 86, 9015–9019. doi: 10.1073/pnas.86.22.9015

Govindaiah, G., and Cox, C. L. (2005). Excitatory actions of dopamine via D1-like receptors in the rat lateral geniculate nucleus. *J. Neurophysiol.* 94, 3708–3718. doi: 10.1152/jn.00583.2005

Govindaiah, G., Wang, Y., and Cox, C. L. (2010a). Dopamine enhances the excitability of somatosensory thalamocortical neurons. *Neuroscience* 170, 981–991. doi: 10.1016/j.neuroscience.2010.08.043

Govindaiah, G., Wang, T., Gillette, M. U., Crandall, S. R., and Cox, C. L. (2010b). Regulation of inhibitory synapses by presynaptic D_4 dopamine receptors in thalamus. *J. Neurophysiol.* 104, 2757–2765. doi: 10.1152/jn.00361.2010

Groenewegen, H. J. (1988). Organization of the afferent connections of the mediodorsal thalamic nucleus in the rat, related to the mediodorsal-prefrontal topography. *Neuroscience* 24, 379–431. doi: 10.1016/0306-4522(88)90339-9

Grzanna, R., and Molliver, M. E. (1980). The locus coeruleus in the rat: an immunohistochemical delineation. *Neuroscience* 5, 21–40. doi: 10.1016/0306-4522(80)90068-8

Happel, M. F. K., Deliano, M., Handschuh, J., and Ohl, F. W. (2014). Dopamine-modulated recurrent corticoefferent feedback in primary sensory cortex promotes detection of behaviorally relevant stimuli. *J. Neurosci.* 34, 1234–1247. doi: 10.1523/JNEUROSCI.1990-13.2014

Harris, K. D., and Thiele, A. (2011). Cortical state and attention. *Nat. Rev. Neurosci.* 12, 509–523. doi: 10.1038/nrn3084

Hornung, J. P. (2010). "The neuroanatomy of the serotonergic system," in *Handbook of the Behavioral Neurobiology of Serotonin*, eds C. P. Mueller and B. L. Jacobs (London: Academic Press), 68–81.

Huntley, G. W., Morrison, J. H., Prikhozhan, A., and Sealfon, S. C. (1992). Localization of multiple dopamine receptor subtype mRNAs in human and monkey motor cortex and striatum. *Brain Res. Mol. Brain Res.* 15, 181–188. doi: 10.1016/0169-328X(92)90107-M

Hurd, Y. L., Suzuki, M., and Sedvall, G. C. (2001). D1 and D2 dopamine receptor mRNA expression in whole hemisphere sections of the human brain. *J. Chem. Neuroanat.* 22, 127–137. doi: 10.1016/S0891-0618(01)00122-3

Hurley, L. M., Devilbiss, D. M., and Waterhouse, B. D. (2004). A matter of focus: monoaminergic modulation of stimulus coding in mammalian sensory networks. *Curr. Opin. Neurobiol.* 14, 488–495. doi: 10.1016/j.conb.2004.06.007

Hurley, L. M., and Pollak, G. D. (1999). Serotonin differentially modulates responses to tones and frequency-modulated sweeps in the inferior colliculus. *J. Neurosci.* 19, 8071–8082. doi: 10.1523/JNEUROSCI.19-18-08071.1999

Hurley, L. M., and Pollak, G. D. (2005). Serotonin shifts first-spike latencies of inferior colliculus neurons. *J. Neurosci.* 25, 7876–7886. doi: 10.1523/JNEUROSCI.1178-05.2005

Ishimura, K., Takeuchi, Y., Fujiwara, K., Tominaga, M., Yoshioka, H., and Sawada, T. (1988). Quantitative analysis of the distribution of serotonin-immunoreactive cell bodies in the mouse brain. *Neurosci. Lett.* 91, 265–270. doi: 10.1016/0304-3940(88)90691-X

Jacob, S. N., Ott, T., and Nieder, A. (2013). Dopamine regulates two classes of primate prefrontal neurons that represent sensory signals. *J. Neurosci.* 33, 13724–13734. doi: 10.1523/JNEUROSCI.0210-13.2013

Jacob, S. N., Stalter, M., and Nieder, A. (2016). Cell-type-specific modulation of targets and distractors by dopamine D1 receptors in primate prefrontal cortex. *Nat. Commun.* 7:13218. doi: 10.1038/ncomms13218

Jacobowitz, D. M., and MacLean, P. D. (1978). A brainstem atlas of catecholaminergic neurons and serotonergic perikarya in a pygmy primate (*Cebuella pygmaea*). *J. Comp. Neurol.* 177, 397–416. doi: 10.1002/cne.901770304

Jones, B. E., Halaris, A. E., McIlhany, M., and Moore, R. Y. (1977). Ascending projections of the locus coeruleus in the rat. I. Axonal transport in central noradrenaline neurons. *Brain Res.* 127, 1–21. doi: 10.1016/0006-8993(77)90377-8

Kasamatsu, T., and Heggelund, P. (1982). Single cell responses in cat visual cortex to visual stimulation during iontophoresis of noradrenaline. *Exp. Brain Res.* 45, 317–327. doi: 10.1007/BF01208591

Kayama, Y., Negi, T., Sugitani, M., and Iwama, K. (1982). Effects of locus coeruleus stimulation on neuronal activities of dorsal lateral geniculate nucleus and perigeniculate reticular nucleus of the rat. *Neuroscience* 7, 655–666. doi: 10.1016/0306-4522(82)90071-9

Kehr, W., Lindqvist, M., and Carlsson, A. (1976). Distribution of dopamine in the rat cerebral cortex. *J. Neural Transm.* 38, 173–180. doi: 10.1007/BF01249437

Ketzef, M., Spigolon, G., Johansson, Y., Bonito-Oliva, A., Fisone, G., and Silberberg, G. (2017). Dopamine depletion impairs bilateral sensory processing in the striatum in a pathway-dependent manner. *Neuron* 94, 855–865. doi: 10.1016/j.neuron.2017.05.004

Kim, J. H., Jung, A. H., Jeong, D., Choi, I., Kim, K., Shin, S., et al. (2016). Selectivity of neuromodulatory projections from the basal forebrain and locus ceruleus to primary sensory cortices. *J. Neurosci.* 36, 5314–5327. doi: 10.1523/JNEUROSCI.4333-15.2016

Klepper, A., and Herbert, H. (1991). Distribution and origin of noradrenergic and serotonergic fibers in the cochlear nucleus and inferior colliculus of the rat. *Brain Res.* 557, 190–201. doi: 10.1016/0006-8993(91)90134-H

Kosofsky, B. E., Molliver, M. E., Morrison, J. H., and Foote, S. L. (1984). The serotonin and norepinephrine innervation of primary visual cortex in the cynomolgus monkey (*Macaca fascicularis*). *J. Comp. Neurol.* 230, 168–178. doi: 10.1002/cne.902300203

Kössl, M., and Vater, M. (1989). Noradrenaline enhances temporal auditory contrast and neuronal timing precision in the cochlear nucleus of the mustached bat. *J. Neurosci.* 9, 4169–4178. doi: 10.1523/JNEUROSCI.09-12-04169.1989

Krakauer, J. W., Ghazanfar, A. A., Gomez-Marin, A., MacIver, M. A., and Poeppel, D. (2017). Neuroscience needs behavior: correcting a reductionist bias. *Neuron* 93, 480–490. doi: 10.1016/j.neuron.2016.12.041

Kuroda, M., Murakami, K., Igarashi, H., and Okada, A. (1996). The convergence of axon terminals from the mediodorsal thalamic nucleus and ventral tegmental area on pyramidal cells in layer V of the rat prelimbic cortex. *Eur. J. Neurosci.* 8, 1340–1349. doi: 10.1111/j.1460-9568.1996.tb01596.x

Lammel, S., Hetzel, A., Häckel, O., Jones, I., Liss, B., and Roeper, J. (2008). Unique properties of mesoprefrontal neurons within a dual mesocorticolimbic dopamine system. *Neuron* 57, 760–773. doi: 10.1016/j.neuron.2008.01.022

Lammel, S., Steinberg, E. E., Földy, C., Wall, N. R., Beier, K., Luo, L., et al. (2015). Diversity of transgenic mouse models for selective targeting of midbrain dopamine neurons. *Neuron* 85, 429–438. doi: 10.1016/j.neuron.2014.12.036

Lamour, Y., Rivot, J. P., Pointis, D., and Ory-Lavollee, L. (1983). Laminar distribution of serotonergic innervation in rat somatosensory cortex, as determined by in vivo electrochemical detection. *Brain Res.* 259, 163–166. doi: 10.1016/0006-8993(83)91082-X

Lesch, K. P., and Waider, J. (2012). Serotonin in the modulation of neural plasticity and networks: implications for neurodevelopmental disorders. *Neuron* 76, 175–191. doi: 10.1016/j.neuron.2012.09.013

Lewis, D. A., Campbell, M. J., Foote, S. L., Goldstein, M., and Morrison, J. H. (1987). The distribution of tyrosine hydroxylase-immunoreactive fibers in primate neocortex is widespread but regionally specific. *J. Neurosci.* 7, 279–290. doi: 10.1523/JNEUROSCI.07-01-00279.1987

Lidow, M. S., Goldman-Rakic, P. S., Gallager, D. W., and Rakic, P. (1991). Distribution of dopaminergic receptors in the primate cerebral cortex: quantitative autoradiographic analysis using [3H]raclopride, [3H]spiperone and [3H]SCH23390. *Neuroscience* 40, 657–671. doi: 10.1016/0306-4522(91)90003-7

Lidow, M. S., Wang, F., Cao, Y., and Goldman-Rakic, P. S. (1998). Layer V neurons bear the majority of mRNAs encoding the five distinct dopamine receptor subtypes in the primate prefrontal cortex. *Synapse* 28, 10–20. doi: 10.1002/(SICI)1098-2396(199801)28:1<10::AID-SYN2>3.0.CO;2-F

Lottem, E., Banerjee, D., Vertechi, P., Sarra, D., Lohuis, M. O., and Mainen, Z. F. (2018). Activation of serotonin neurons promotes active persistence in a probabilistic foraging task. *Nat. Commun.* 9:1000. doi: 10.1038/s41467-018-03438-y

Lottem, E., Lörincz, M. L., and Mainen, Z. F. (2016). Optogenetic activation of dorsal raphe serotonin neurons rapidly inhibits spontaneous but not odor-evoked activity in olfactory cortex. *J. Neurosci.* 36, 7–18. doi: 10.1523/JNEUROSCI.3008-15.2016

Loughlin, S. E., and Fallon, J. H. (1984). Substantia nigra and ventral tegmental area projections to cortex: topography and collateralization. *Neuroscience* 11, 425–435. doi: 10.1016/0306-4522(84)90034-4

Loughlin, S. E., Foote, S. L., and Bloom, F. E. (1986). Efferent projections of nucleus locus coeruleus: topographic organization of cells of origin demonstrated by three-dimensional reconstruction. *Neuroscience* 18, 291–306. doi: 10.1016/0306-4522(86)90155-7

Manella, L. C., Petersen, N., and Linster, C. (2017). Stimulation of the locus ceruleus modulates signal-to-noise ratio in the olfactory bulb. *J. Neurosci.* 37, 11605–11615. doi: 10.1523/JNEUROSCI.2026-17.2017

Manunta, Y., and Edeline, J. M. (1997). Effects of noradrenaline on frequency tuning of rat auditory cortex neurons. *Eur. J. Neurosci.* 9, 833–847. doi: 10.1111/j.1460-9568.1997.tb01433.x

Matsumoto, M., and Hikosaka, O. (2009). Two types of dopamine neuron distinctly convey positive and negative motivational signals. *Nature* 459, 837–841. doi: 10.1038/nature08028

Matsumoto, M., Matsumoto, M., Takada, M., and Takada, M. (2013). Distinct representations of cognitive and motivational signals in midbrain dopamine neurons. *Neuron* 79, 1011–1024. doi: 10.1016/j.neuron.2013.07.002

McLean, J., and Waterhouse, B. D. (1994). Noradrenergic modulation of cat area 17 neuronal responses to moving visual stimuli. *Brain Res.* 667, 83–97. doi: 10.1016/0006-8993(94)91716-7

McLean, J. H., and Shipley, M. T. (1987). Serotonergic afferents to the rat olfactory bulb: I. Origins and laminar specificity of serotonergic inputs in the adult rat. *J. Neurosci.* 7, 3016–3028. doi: 10.1523/JNEUROSCI.07-10-03016.1987

McLean, J. H., Shipley, M. T., Nickell, W. T., Aston-Jones, G., and Reyher, C. K. (1989). Chemoanatomical organization of the noradrenergic input from locus coeruleus to the olfactory bulb of the adult rat. *J. Comp. Neurol.* 285, 339–349. doi: 10.1002/cne.902850305

Melchitzky, D. S., Erickson, S. L., and Lewis, D. A. (2006). Dopamine innervation of the monkey mediodorsal thalamus: location of projection neurons and ultrastructural characteristics of axon terminals. *Neuroscience* 143, 1021–1030. doi: 10.1016/j.neuroscience.2006.08.056

Mengod, G., Cortes, R., Vilaro, M. T., and Hoyer, D. (2010). "Distribution of 5-HT receptors in the central nervous system," in *Handbook of the Behavioral Neurobiology of Serotonin*, eds C. P. Mueller and B. L. Jacobs (London: Academic Press), 140–155.

Missale, C., Nash, S. R., Robinson, S. W., Jaber, M., and Caron, M. G. (1998). Dopamine receptors: from structure to function. *Physiol. Rev.* 78, 189–225. doi: 10.1152/physrev.1998.78.1.189

Miyazaki, K. W., Miyazaki, K., Tanaka, K. F., Yamanaka, A., Takahashi, A., Tabuchi, S., et al. (2014). Optogenetic activation of dorsal raphe serotonin neurons enhances patience for future rewards. *Curr. Biol.* 24, 2033–2040. doi: 10.1016/j.cub.2014.07.041

Moore, R. Y., and Bloom, F. E. (1979). Central catecholamine neuron systems: anatomy and physiology of the norepinephrine and epinephrine systems. *Annu. Rev. Neurosci.* 2, 113–168. doi: 10.1146/annurev.ne.02.030179.000553

Morrison, J. H., and Foote, S. L. (1986). Noradrenergic and serotoninergic innervation of cortical, thalamic, and tectal visual structures in Old and New World monkeys. *J. Comp. Neurol.* 243, 117–138. doi: 10.1002/cne.902430110

Morrison, J. H., Foote, S. L., Molliver, M. E., Bloom, F. E., and Lidov, H. G. (1982a). Noradrenergic and serotonergic fibers innervate complementary layers in monkey primary visual cortex: an immunohistochemical study. *Proc. Natl. Acad. Sci. U.S.A.* 79, 2401–2405.

Morrison, J. H., Foote, S. L., O'Connor, D., and Bloom, F. E. (1982b). Laminar, tangential and regional organization of the noradrenergic innervation of monkey cortex: dopamine-beta-hydroxylase immunohistochemistry. *Brain Res. Bull.* 9, 309–319.

Muller, A., Joseph, V., Slesinger, P. A., and Kleinfeld, D. (2014). Cell-based reporters reveal in vivo dynamics of dopamine and norepinephrine release in murine cortex. *Nat. Methods* 11, 1245–1252. doi: 10.1038/nmeth.3151

Munsch, T., Yanagawa, Y., Obata, K., and Pape, H.-C. (2005). Dopaminergic control of local interneuron activity in the thalamus. *Eur. J. Neurosci.* 21, 290–294. doi: 10.1111/j.1460-9568.2004.03842.x

Nelson, E. L., Liang, C. L., Sinton, C. M., and German, D. C. (1996). Midbrain dopaminergic neurons in the mouse: computer-assisted mapping. *J. Comp. Neurol.* 369, 361–371. doi: 10.1002/(SICI)1096-9861(19960603)369:3<361::AID-CNE3>3.0.CO;2-3

Neves, R. M., van Keulen, S., Yang, M., Logothetis, N. K., and Eschenko, O. (2018). Locus coeruleus phasic discharge is essential for stimulus-induced gamma oscillations in the prefrontal cortex. *J. Neurophysiol.* 119, 904–920. doi: 10.1152/jn.00552.2017

Nevue, A. A., Elde, C. J., Perkel, D. J., and Portfors, C. V. (2015). Dopaminergic input to the inferior colliculus in mice. *Front. Neuroanat.* 9:168. doi: 10.3389/fnana.2015.00168

Niell, C. M., and Stryker, M. P. (2010). Modulation of visual responses by behavioral state in mouse visual cortex. *Neuron* 65, 472–479. doi: 10.1016/j.neuron.2010.01.033

Noudoost, B., and Moore, T. (2011). Control of visual cortical signals by prefrontal dopamine. *Nature* 474, 372–375. doi: 10.1038/nature09995

O'Hanlon, J. F. (1965). Adrenaline and noradrenaline: relation to performance in a visual vigilance task. *Science* 150, 507–509. doi: 10.1126/science.150.3695.507

Ott, T., Jacob, S. N., and Nieder, A. (2014). Dopamine receptors differentially enhance rule coding in primate prefrontal cortex neurons. *Neuron* 84, 1317–1328. doi: 10.1016/j.neuron.2014.11.012

Papadopoulos, G. C., and Parnavelas, J. G. (1990). Distribution and synaptic organization of dopaminergic axons in the lateral geniculate nucleus of the rat. *J. Comp. Neurol.* 294, 356–361. doi: 10.1002/cne.902940305

Papadopoulos, G. C., and Parnavelas, J. G. (1991). Monoamine systems in the cerebral cortex: evidence for anatomical specificity. *Prog. Neurobiol.* 36, 195–200. doi: 10.1016/0301-0082(91)90030-5

Papadopoulos, G. C., Parnavelas, J. G., and Buijs, R. M. (1989). Light and electron microscopic immunocytochemical analysis of the noradrenaline innervation of the rat visual cortex. *J. Neurocytol.* 18, 1–10. doi: 10.1007/BF01188418

Paspalas, C. D., and Papadopoulos, G. C. (2001). Serotoninergic afferents preferentially innervate distinct subclasses of peptidergic interneurons in the rat visual cortex. *Brain Res.* 891, 158–167. doi: 10.1016/S0006-8993(00)03193-0

Petzold, G. C., Hagiwara, A., and Murthy, V. N. (2009). Serotonergic modulation of odor input to the mammalian olfactory bulb. *Nat. Neurosci.* 12, 784–791. doi: 10.1038/nn.2335

Phillipson, O. T., Kilpatrick, I. C., and Jones, M. W. (1987). Dopaminergic innervation of the primary visual cortex in the rat, and some correlations with human cortex. *Brain Res. Bull.* 18, 621–633. doi: 10.1016/0361-9230(87)90132-8

Phillis, J. W., and Teběcis, A. K. (1967). The responses of thalamic neurons to iontophoretically applied monoamines. *J. Physiol.* 192, 715–745. doi: 10.1113/jphysiol.1967.sp008327

Phillis, J. W., Teběcis, A. K., and York, D. H. (1967). The inhibitory action of monoamines on lateral geniculate neurones. *J. Physiol.* 190, 563–581. doi: 10.1113/jphysiol.1967.sp008228

Polack, P. O., Friedman, J., and Golshani, P. (2013). Cellular mechanisms of brain state-dependent gain modulation in visual cortex. *Nat. Neurosci.* 16, 1331–1339. doi: 10.1038/nn.3464

Pollak Dorocic, I., Fürth, D., Xuan, Y., Johansson, Y., Pozzi, L., Silberberg, G., et al. (2014). A whole-brain atlas of inputs to serotonergic neurons of the dorsal and median raphe nuclei. *Neuron* 83, 663–678. doi: 10.1016/j.neuron.2014.07.002

Rabinowitz, N. C., Goris, R. L., Cohen, M., and Simoncelli, E. (2015). Attention stabilizes the shared gain of V4 populations. *eLife* 4:e08998. doi: 10.7554/eLife.08998

Ramos, B. P., and Arnsten, A. F. (2007). Adrenergic pharmacology and cognition: focus on the prefrontal cortex. *Pharmacol. Ther.* 113, 523–536. doi: 10.1016/j.pharmthera.2006.11.006

Ranade, S., Pi, H. J., and Kepecs, A. (2014). Neuroscience: waiting for serotonin. *Curr. Biol.* 24, R803–R805. doi: 10.1016/j.cub.2014.07.024

Ranade, S. P., and Mainen, Z. F. (2009). Transient firing of dorsal raphe neurons encodes diverse and specific sensory, motor, and reward events. *J. Neurophysiol.* 102, 3026–3037. doi: 10.1152/jn.00507.2009

Rauch, A., Rainer, G., and Logothetis, N. K. (2008). The effect of a serotonin-induced dissociation between spiking and perisynaptic activity on BOLD functional MRI. *Proc. Natl. Acad. Sci. U.S.A.* 105, 6759–6764. doi: 10.1073/pnas.0800312105

Reimer, J., Froudarakis, E., Cadwell, C. R., Yatsenko, D., Denfield, G. H., and Tolias, A. S. (2014). Pupil fluctuations track fast switching of cortical states during quiet wakefulness. *Neuron* 84, 355–362. doi: 10.1016/j.neuron.2014.09.033

Reimer, J., McGinley, M. J., Liu, Y., Rodenkirch, C., Wang, Q., McCormick, D. A., et al. (2016). Pupil fluctuations track rapid changes in adrenergic and cholinergic activity in cortex. *Nat. Commun.* 7:13289. doi: 10.1038/ncomms13289

Rice, M. E., and Cragg, S. J. (2008). Dopamine spillover after quantal release: rethinking dopamine transmission in the nigrostriatal pathway. *Brain Res. Rev.* 58, 303–313. doi: 10.1016/j.brainresrev.2008.02.004

Rogawski, M. A., and Aghajanian, G. K. (1980). Modulation of lateral geniculate neurone excitability by noradrenaline microiontophoresis or locus coeruleus stimulation. *Nature* 287, 731–734. doi: 10.1038/287731a0

Rudy, B., Fishell, G., Lee, S., and Hjerling-Leffler, J. (2011). Three groups of interneurons account for nearly 100% of neocortical GABAergic neurons. *Dev. Neurobiol.* 71, 45–61. doi: 10.1002/dneu.20853

Safaai, H., Neves, R., Eschenko, O., Logothetis, N. K., and Panzeri, S. (2015). Modeling the effect of locus coeruleus firing on cortical state dynamics and single-trial sensory processing. *Proc. Natl. Acad. Sci. U.S.A.* 112, 12834–12839. doi: 10.1073/pnas.1516539112

Sánchez-González, M. A., García-Cabezas, M. A., Rico, B., and Cavada, C. (2005). The primate thalamus is a key target for brain dopamine. *J. Neurosci.* 25, 6076–6083. doi: 10.1523/JNEUROSCI.0968-05.2005

Santana, N., Mengod, G., and Artigas, F. (2009). Quantitative analysis of the expression of dopamine D1 and D2 receptors in pyramidal and GABAergic neurons of the rat prefrontal cortex. *Cereb. Cortex* 19, 849–860. doi: 10.1093/cercor/bhn134

Sara, S. J., and Bouret, S. (2012). Orienting and reorienting: the locus coeruleus mediates cognition through arousal. *Neuron* 76, 130–141. doi: 10.1016/j.neuron.2012.09.011

Sarter, M., Parikh, V., and Howe, W. M. (2009). Phasic acetylcholine release and the volume transmission hypothesis: time to move on. *Nat. Rev. Neurosci.* 10, 383–390. doi: 10.1038/nrn2635

Sato, H., Fox, K., and Daw, N. W. (1989). Effect of electrical stimulation of locus coeruleus on the activity of neurons in the cat visual cortex. *J. Neurophysiol.* 62, 946–958. doi: 10.1152/jn.1989.62.4.946

Schicknick, H., Reichenbach, N., Smalla, K.-H., Scheich, H., Gundelfinger, E. D., and Tischmeyer, W. (2012). Dopamine modulates memory consolidation of discrimination learning in the auditory cortex. *Eur. J. Neurosci.* 35, 763–774. doi: 10.1111/j.1460-9568.2012.07994.x

Schicknick, H., Schott, B. H., Budinger, E., Smalla, K.-H., Riedel, A., Seidenbecher, C. I., et al. (2008). Dopaminergic modulation of auditory cortex-dependent memory consolidation through mTOR. *Cereb. Cortex* 18, 2646–2658. doi: 10.1093/cercor/bhn026

Schnyder, H., and Künzle, H. (1984). Is there a retinopetal system in the rat. *Exp. Brain Res.* 56, 502–508. doi: 10.1007/BF00237991

Schölvinck, M. L., Saleem, A. B., Benucci, A., Harris, K. D., and Carandini, M. (2015). Cortical state determines global variability and correlations in visual cortex. *J. Neurosci.* 35, 170–178. doi: 10.1523/JNEUROSCI.4994-13.2015

Schultz, W. (2007). Multiple dopamine functions at different time courses. *Annu. Rev. Neurosci.* 30, 259–288. doi: 10.1146/annurev.neuro.28.061604.135722

Seillier, L., Lorenz, C., Kawaguchi, K., Ott, T., Nieder, A., Pourriahi, P., et al. (2017). Serotonin decreases the gain of visual responses in awake macaque V1. *J. Neurosci.* 37, 11390–11405. doi: 10.1523/JNEUROSCI.1339-17.2017

Sherman, S. M. (2016). Thalamus plays a central role in ongoing cortical functioning. *Nat. Neurosci.* 19, 533–541. doi: 10.1038/nn.4269

Smiley, J. F., Levey, A. I., Ciliax, B. J., and Goldman-Rakic, P. S. (1994). D1 dopamine receptor immunoreactivity in human and monkey cerebral cortex: predominant and extrasynaptic localization in dendritic spines. *Proc. Natl. Acad. Sci. U.S.A.* 91, 5720–5724. doi: 10.1073/pnas.91.12.5720

Soubrie, P. (1986). Reconciling the role of central serotonin neurons in human and animal behavior. *Behav. Brain Sci.* 9, 319–335. doi: 10.1017/S0140525X00022871

Sulzer, D., Cragg, S. J., and Rice, M. E. (2016). Striatal dopamine neurotransmission: regulation of release and uptake. *Basal Ganglia* 6, 123–148. doi: 10.1016/j.baga.2016.02.001

Takeuchi, T., Duszkiewicz, A. J., Sonneborn, A., Spooner, P. A., Yamasaki, M., Watanabe, M., et al. (2016). Locus coeruleus and dopaminergic consolidation of everyday memory. *Nature* 537, 357–362. doi: 10.1038/nature19325

Takeuchi, Y., Kimura, H., and Sano, Y. (1982). Immunohistochemical demonstration of serotonin nerve fibers in the olfactory bulb of the rat, cat and monkey. *Histochemistry* 75, 461–471.

Takeuchi, Y., and Sano, Y. (1984). Serotonin nerve fibers in the primary visual cortex of the monkey. Quantitative and immunoelectronmicroscopical analysis. *Anat. Embryol.* 169, 1–8. doi: 10.1007/BF00300581

Tigges, J., Tigges, M., Cross, N. A., McBride, R. L., Letbetter, W. D., and Anschel, S. (1982). Subcortical structures projecting to visual cortical areas in squirrel monkey. *J. Comp. Neurol.* 209, 29–40. doi: 10.1002/cne.902090104

Tong, L., Altschuler, R. A., and Holt, A. G. (2005). Tyrosine hydroxylase in rat auditory midbrain: distribution and changes following deafness. *Hear. Res.* 206, 28–41. doi: 10.1016/j.heares.2005.03.006

Uematsu, A., Tan, B. Z., Ycu, E. A., Cuevas, J. S., Koivumaa, J., Junyent, F., et al. (2017). Modular organization of the brainstem noradrenaline system coordinates opposing learning states. *Nat. Neurosci.* 20, 1602–1611. doi: 10.1038/nn.4642

Varela, C. (2014). Thalamic neuromodulation and its implications for executive networks. *Front. Neural Circuits* 8:69. doi: 10.3389/fncir.2014.00069

Vertes, R. P., Linley, S. B., and Hoover, W. B. (2010). Pattern of distribution of serotonergic fibers to the thalamus of the rat. *Brain Struct. Funct.* 215, 1–28. doi: 10.1007/s00429-010-0249-x

Vijayraghavan, S., Wang, M., Birnbaum, S. G., von Williams, G., and Arnsten, A. F. T. (2007). Inverted-U dopamine D1 receptor actions on prefrontal neurons engaged in working memory. *Nat. Neurosci.* 10, 376–384. doi: 10.1038/nn1846

Villar, M. J., Vitale, M. L., Hökfelt, T., and Verhofstad, A. A. (1988). Dorsal raphe serotoninergic branching neurons projecting both to the lateral geniculate body and superior colliculus: a combined retrograde tracing-immunohistochemical study in the rat. *J. Comp. Neurol.* 277, 126–140. doi: 10.1002/cne.902770109

Vincent, S. L., Khan, Y., and Benes, F. M. (1993). Cellular distribution of dopamine D1 and D2 receptors in rat medial prefrontal cortex. *J. Neurosci.* 13, 2551–2564. doi: 10.1523/JNEUROSCI.13-06-02551.1993

Watakabe, A., Komatsu, Y., Sadakane, O., Shimegi, S., Takahata, T., Higo, N., et al. (2009). Enriched expression of serotonin 1B and 2A receptor genes in macaque visual cortex and their bidirectional modulatory effects on neuronal responses. *Cereb. Cortex* 19, 1915–1928. doi: 10.1093/cercor/bhn219

Waterhouse, B. D., Azizi, S. A., Burne, R. A., and Woodward, D. J. (1990). Modulation of rat cortical area 17 neuronal responses to moving visual stimuli during norepinephrine and serotonin microiontophoresis. *Brain Res.* 514, 276–292. doi: 10.1016/0006-8993(90)91422-D

Waterhouse, B. D., Lin, C. S., Burne, R. A., and Woodward, D. J. (1983). The distribution of neocortical projection neurons in the locus coeruleus. *J. Comp. Neurol.* 217, 418–431. doi: 10.1002/cne.902170406

Waterhouse, B. D., Moises, H. C., and Woodward, D. J. (1980). Noradrenergic modulation of somatosensory cortical neuronal responses to iontophoretically applied putative neurotransmitters. *Exp. Neurol.* 69, 30–49. doi: 10.1016/0014-4886(80)90141-7

Waterhouse, B. D., Moises, H. C., and Woodward, D. J. (1986). Interaction of serotonin with somatosensory cortical neuronal responses to afferent synaptic inputs and putative neurotransmitters. *Brain Res. Bull.* 17, 507–518. doi: 10.1016/0361-9230(86)90218-2

Waterhouse, B. D., Moises, H. C., and Woodward, D. J. (1998). Phasic activation of the locus coeruleus enhances responses of primary sensory cortical neurons to peripheral receptive field stimulation. *Brain Res.* 790, 33–44. doi: 10.1016/S0006-8993(98)00117-6

Waterhouse, B. D., and Woodward, D. J. (1980). Interaction of norepinephrine with cerebrocortical activity evoked by stimulation of somatosensory afferent pathways in the rat. *Exp. Neurol.* 67, 11–34. doi: 10.1016/0014-4886(80)90159-4

Weiner, D. M., Levey, A. I., Sunahara, R. K., Niznik, H. B., O'Dowd, B. F., Seeman, P., et al. (1991). D1 and D2 dopamine receptor mRNA in rat brain. *Proc. Natl. Acad. Sci. U.S.A.* 88, 1859–1863. doi: 10.1073/pnas.88.5.1859

Williams, S. M., and Goldman-Rakic, P. S. (1998). Widespread origin of the primate mesofrontal dopamine system. *Cereb. Cortex* 8, 321–345. doi: 10.1093/cercor/8.4.321

Wilson, M. A., and Molliver, M. E. (1991a). The organization of serotonergic projections to cerebral cortex in primates: regional distribution of axon terminals. *Neuroscience* 44, 537–553.

Wilson, M. A., and Molliver, M. E. (1991b). The organization of serotonergic projections to cerebral cortex in primates: retrograde transport studies. *Neuroscience* 44, 555–570.

Zaldivar, D., Goense, J., Lowe, S. C., Logothetis, N. K., and Panzeri, S. (2018). Dopamine is signaled by mid-frequency oscillations and boosts output layers visual information in visual cortex. *Curr. Biol.* 28, 224.e5–235.e5. doi: 10.1016/j.cub.2017.12.006

Zaldivar, D., Rauch, A., Whittingstall, K., Logothetis, N. K., and Goense, J. (2014). Dopamine-induced dissociation of BOLD and neural activity in macaque visual cortex. *Curr. Biol.* 24, 2805–2811. doi: 10.1016/j.cub.2014.10.006

Zhao, Y., Kerscher, N., Eysel, U., and Funke, K. (2002). D1 and D2 receptor-mediated dopaminergic modulation of visual responses in cat dorsal lateral geniculate nucleus. *J. Physiol.* 539(Pt 1), 223–238.

17

Effective Stimulation Type and Waveform for Force Control of the Motor Unit System: Implications for Intraspinal Microstimulation

Hojeong Kim[1]* and Youngchang Ju[2]

[1] *Division of Biotechnology, DGIST, Daegu, South Korea,*

[2] *Department of Brain and Cognitive Sciences, DGIST, Daegu, South Korea*

***Correspondence:**
Hojeong Kim
hojeong.kim03@gmail.com

The input–output properties of spinal motoneurons and muscle fibers comprising motor units are highly non-linear. The goal of this study was to investigate the stimulation type (continuous versus discrete) and waveform (linear versus non-linear) controlling force production at the motor unit level under intraspinal microstimulation. We constructed a physiological model of the motor unit with computer software enabling virtual experiments on single motor units under a wide range of input conditions, including intracellular and synaptic stimulation of the motoneuron and variation in the muscle length under neuromodulatory inputs originating from the brainstem. Continuous current intensity and impulse current frequency waveforms were inversely estimated such that the motor unit could linearly develop and relax the muscle force within a broad range of contraction speeds and levels during isometric contraction at various muscle lengths. Under both continuous and discrete stimulation, the stimulation waveform non-linearity increased with increasing speed and level of force production and with decreasing muscle length. Only discrete stimulation could control force relaxation at all muscle lengths. In contrast, continuous stimulation could not control force relaxation at high contraction levels in shorter-than-optimal muscles due to persistent inward current saturation on the motoneuron dendrites. These results indicate that non-linear adjustment of the stimulation waveform is more effective in regard to varying the force profile and muscle length and that the discrete stimulation protocol is a more robust approach for designing stimulation patterns aimed at neural interfaces for precise movement control under pathological conditions.

Keywords: stimulation waveform, force control, motor unit, neuromodulation, intraspinal microstimulation, stimulation type

---

Abbreviations: VI, voltage–current; IV, current–voltage; VODE, variable-coefficient ordinary differential equation; LSODE, livermore solver for ordinary differential equations; PIC, persistent inward current; PyMUS, python-based motor unit simulator.

INTRODUCTION

Recent advances in neural interface technology have allowed the direct modulation of nervous system functions by injecting currents into specific compartments of individual neurons (Holsheimer, 1998; Radivojevic et al., 2016). In regard to neuromuscular systems, individual motor units, consisting of a single motoneuron and its innervating muscle fibers (i.e., the muscle unit), could represent a target modulated at the spinal cord to accurately evoke proper movements (Wagner et al., 2018). However, the prediction of stimulation patterns and their effects on force control have remained difficult, mainly due to the non-linearities inherited in the fundamental elements comprising neuromuscular systems (Heckman and Enoka, 2012).

The input–output relationship of spinal motoneurons is highly non-linear in various species, including rats, mice, cats, and turtles (Heckman et al., 2003). The firing mode of the motoneuron may transition from quiescent to regular firing or from low- to high-frequency firing in response to brief excitatory current injection at the soma, thereby revealing the occurrence of bistability (Hounsgaard et al., 1988). While slowly increasing and decreasing current injection at the soma, low-threshold motoneurons (presumably slow-type motoneurons) tend to exhibit notable counterclockwise hysteresis and a self-sustaining firing behavior below the firing initiation threshold in the descending stimulation phase, whereas high-threshold motoneurons (presumably fast-type motoneurons) tend to exhibit slight clockwise hysteresis under the absence of self-sustaining firing behavior (Lee and Heckman, 1998b). The underlying mechanism of this non-linear input–output relationship has been suggested as the spatiotemporal interaction between action potential-producing membrane mechanisms at the soma and plateau potential-generating calcium channels in dendritic areas (i.e., 300–800 μm from the soma) (Kim et al., 2014). These dendritic calcium channels (presumably L-type $Ca_V1.3$ channels) are actively involved through monoaminergic neuromodulation due to the brainstem regarding normal motor behavior and through endogenous monoamines in regard to spinal cord injury (Heckmann et al., 2005).

The input–output relationship of muscle fibers has also been demonstrated to be highly non-linear in frogs, rats, and cats (Mrowczynski et al., 2006). Compared to its low frequency, a greater muscle force is produced in response to high-frequency current stimulation, resulting in a sigmoid curve of the relationship between the stimulation frequency and force output. In addition, the muscle force is maximized at the optimal muscle length over smaller and larger muscle lengths, thereby revealing a bell-shaped relationship between the muscle length and force output during isometric contraction (Winters et al., 2011). This non-linear relationship is attributable to the complex interactions between calcium dynamics, cross-bridge formation, and length variation in the sarcoplasm of muscle fibers (Kim et al., 2015). In summary, the dynamics of muscle activation are non-linearly related to both the stimulation frequency and muscle length and greatly decrease under shorter-than-optimal lengths at the physiological stimulation frequency (i.e., <20 Hz) (Perreault et al., 2003).

Intraspinal microstimulation exhibits the capability of activating a specific set of neurons within the spinal cord to modulate muscle activity in different body parts, including the hindlimb (Mushahwar and Horch, 1998), forelimb (Sunshine et al., 2013), and respiratory system (Sunshine et al., 2018). Recently, the relationship between current stimulation and motoneuron firing has been investigated *via* the direct application of direct or pulsed current injection to the spinal cord. The intradural region of the spinal cord in mice has been targeted for direct current stimulation purposes to elucidate the influence of the stimulation polarity on the firing outputs of hindlimb motoneurons (Ahmed, 2016). Computational and imaging studies have further demonstrated that the asymmetric waveform of a biphasic stimulus current pulse may enhance the target selectivity, and the stimulus frequency may alter the neuronal output (McIntyre and Grill, 2000; Wang et al., 2012). However, little is known regarding the stimulation pattern to produce desired force profiles *via* skeletal muscles at the motor unit level, which is the smallest element underlying all movements.

Here, we theoretically investigated the effective waveforms during intraspinal microstimulation to control the muscle force under two types of stimulation protocols, namely, continuous and discrete (or impulse) current stimulation protocols, during isometric muscle contraction within a full physiological range of the muscle length and force level. The present study focused on the direct activation of a spinal motoneuron with a microelectrode in close proximity to its initial segment and cell body. Extracellular microstimulation of other components, such as axons or dendrites, was not involved in the current analysis. We hypothesize (1) that non-linear stimulation waveforms are needed to elicit linear force generation at the motor unit level and (2) that the discrete current stimulation protocol more effectively prevents the non-linearities induced by the active channels in motoneuron dendrites, including muscle afferent inputs due to muscle length variation. Simulation analysis demonstrated the systematic stimulation waveform non-linearity depending on the stimulation type, muscle length, and force profile. These simulation results provide a basis for the design of stimulation patterns for neural interfaces to enhance motor precision control under pathological conditions.

MATERIALS AND METHODS

Motor Unit Model

Stimulation waveforms were investigated in regard to extracellular microstimulation with a sharp-tipped electrode near the initial segment and cell body of a spinal motoneuron (**Figure 1**). A motor unit model comprising a two-compartment motoneuron model and a three-module muscle unit model was physiologically constructed and simulated in Python-based Motor Unit Simulator (PyMUS) software, which was developed for virtual experiments on single motor units under a wide range of physiological conditions (Kim and Kim, 2018).

Briefly, in terms of the reduced motoneuron model, one compartment (referred to as the somatic compartment)

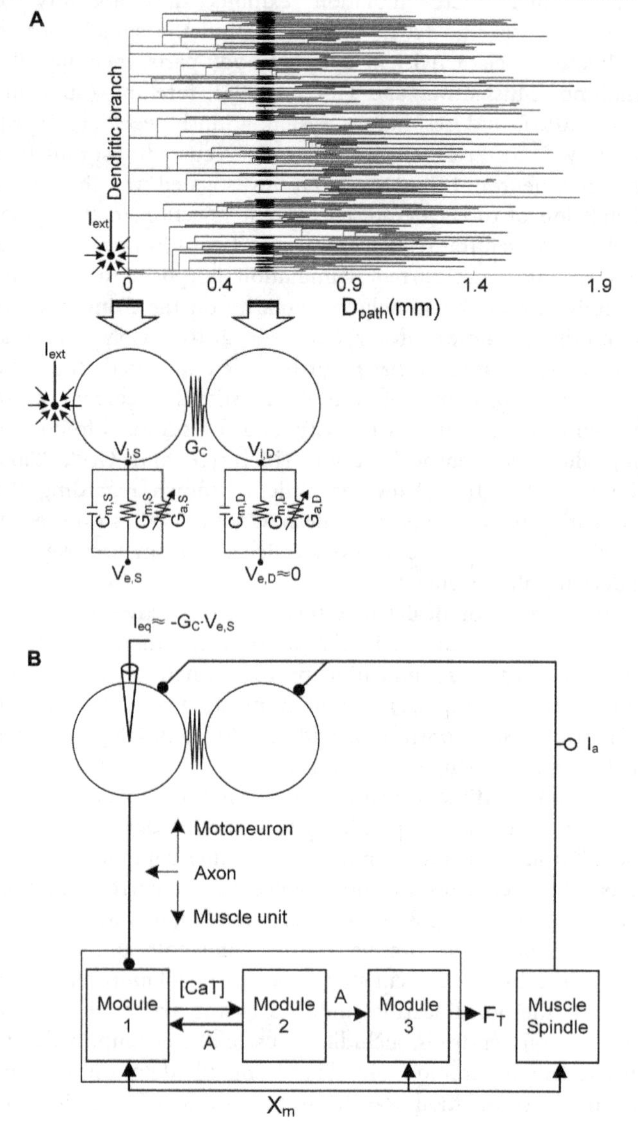

FIGURE 1 | Simulation setup. **(A)** Reduction in the anatomical motoneuron (*top*, dendrogram) into a two-compartment framework (*bottom*) as a function of the path length (D_{path}) from the center of the cell body (D_{path} = 0). The left arrow indicates the mapping of the soma/axonal hillock/initial segment of the anatomical model into the somatic compartment of the reduced model. The right arrow indicates the mapping of all points over the narrow band (a mean value of 0.6 mm) of the anatomical dendrites into the dendritic compartment of the reduced model. C_m, G_m, G_a G_C, V_i, and V_e indicate the membrane capacitance, leak conductance, voltage-gated conductance, coupling conductance, and intracellular and extracellular potentials, respectively. The subscripts S and D indicate the somatic and dendritic compartments, respectively. I_{ext}, the current passing through the microelectrode, is located close to the initial segment and cell body. In the current analysis, $V_{e,S}$ is determined by I_{ext}, while the influence of I_{ext} on $V_{e,D}$ is assumed to be negligible. **(B)** Model motor unit comprising the two-compartment motoneuron model and three-module muscle unit along with the muscle spindle afferent (I_a). I_{eq} is the equivalent current intracellularly injected at the somatic compartment of the motoneuron to evoke the same transmembrane potential induced by I_{ext}. [CaT], A, F_T, and X_m indicate the concentration of calcium bound to troponin, the muscle activation level, the force output, and the muscle length, respectively.

represents the soma and axonal hillock/initial segment, and the other compartment (denoted as the dendritic compartment) represents the dendritic regions, including persistent inward current-generating voltage-gated channels (Booth et al., 1997). These two compartments are connected *via* the coupling conductance, representing the electrical distance between the soma and dendritic regions. Five passive parameters, including the specific membrane conductance and capacitance (i.e., $G_{m,S}$ and $C_{m,S}$ of the somatic compartment, $G_{m,D}$ and $C_{m,D}$ of the dendritic compartment, and G_C in regard to the coupling conductance between these two compartments), were analytically determined to capture five electrotonical properties, including the somatic input resistance (i.e., $R_{N,S}$), system time constant (i.e., τ_m), and three voltage attenuation factors between the soma and all dendritic sites separated by a similar path length (i.e., D_{path}) (i.e., VA_{SD}^{DC} and VA_{SD}^{AC} describing soma-to-dendrite propagation of direct and alternative currents and VA_{DS}^{DC} describing dendrite-to-soma propagation of a direct current). Action and plateau potentials were generated in the somatic and dendritic compartments *via* the incorporation of Hodgkin–Huxley-style active channels [i.e., G_{Naf}, G_{Nap}, G_{Kdr}, $G_{K(Ca)}$, and G_{Can}, with dynamic changes in the calcium reversal potential of the soma, and G_{Cal}, with a constant calcium reversal potential of the dendrites]. The passive parameter values were first determined to capture the passive properties [$R_{N,S}$ = 1.29 MΩ, τ_m = 7.2 ms, $VA_{SD}^{DC}(D_{path}$ = 0.6 mm) = 0.76, $VA_{SD}^{AC}(D_{path}$ = 0.6 mm) = 0.27, and $VA_{DS}^{DC}(D_{path}$ = 0.6 mm) = 0.75] measured at the soma and dendrites as previously reported in Zengel et al. (1985); Spruston et al. (1994), and Kim et al. (2014). Then, the active parameters were determined to replicate the active properties (spike height = 92.3 mV, rheobase current = 10.5 nA, afterhyperpolarization duration = 98.5 ms, and depth = 3.1 mV under passive dendrites, and effective persistent inward current = −22 nA under active dendrites) obtained from the cell body as previously mentioned in Zengel et al. (1985); Hochman and McCrea (1994), and Hornby et al. (2002). The voltage–current (i.e., VI) and current–voltage (i.e., IV) properties of the model motoneuron were validated *via* a comparison to those of an anatomically reconstructed motoneuron model that reproduces non-linear behaviors observed from *in vivo* cat α-motoneurons with low thresholds during voltage- and current-clamping at the cell body (Kim et al., 2014) (please refer to **Figure 2A** for non-linear behavior of the model motoneuron).

Regarding the modular muscle unit model, the muscle force was produced through three physiological procedures in response to action potentials originating from the motoneuron. Module 1 transforms neural signals into dynamics of the calcium concentration (i.e., Ca_{SP}) in the sarcoplasm, including calcium release and uptake of the sarcoplasmic reticulum, calcium-buffering proteins, and calcium-bound troponin complex. Module 2 then transforms the concentration dynamics of calcium-bound troponin (i.e., $Ca_{SP}T$) into the degree of cross-bridge formation, representing muscle activation dynamics (i.e., A). Finally, module 3 transforms the above muscle activation dynamics into force based on Hill-type muscle–tendon mechanics, reflecting length–and velocity–tension relationships.

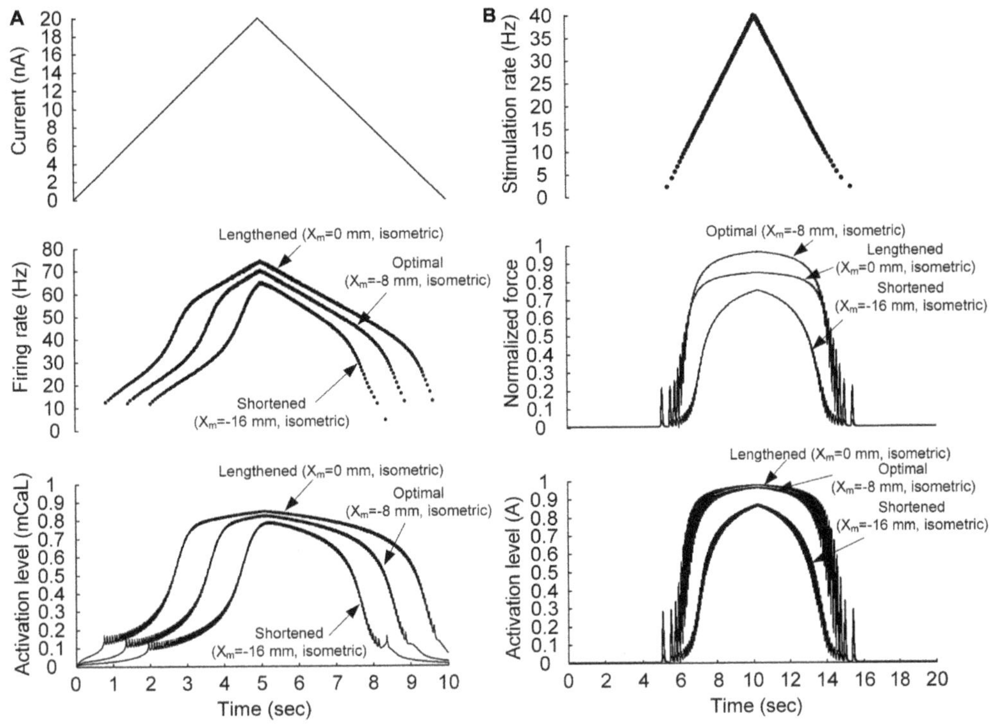

FIGURE 2 | Non-linear behavior of the motoneuron **(A)** and motor unit **(B)**. **(A)** Current stimulation applied to the somatic compartment of the motoneuron model (*top*), instantaneous firing rate (*middle*), and dynamics of the PIC activation level in the motoneuron dendrite (*bottom*). The arrows indicate the responses at the three muscle lengths (minimal length with $X_m = -16$ mm, optimal length with $X_m = -8$ mm, and maximal length with $X_m = 0$ mm). **(B)** Frequency of impulse current stimulation applied to the muscle unit model (*top*), force normalized with the peak force at the optimal length (*middle*), and dynamics of the muscle activation level (*bottom*). The arrows indicate the responses at the three muscle lengths (minimal length with $X_m = -16$ mm, optimal length with $X_m = -8$ mm, and maximal length with $X_m = 0$ mm).

Model parameter values were determined for each module to reproduce the force generation process. These values reflect sarcoplasmic calcium dynamics (Westerblad and Allen, 1994) in module 1, calcium–force relationship (Shames et al., 1996) in module 2, length–and velocity–tension properties (Scott et al., 1996) in module 3, and muscle activation dependence on muscle length variation (Sandercock and Heckman, 1997) in modules 1 and 3. The input–output properties of the model muscle unit have been validated through a comparison to those of adult cat soleus muscles within a full physiological range of stimulation rates (i.e., 1–100 Hz) and muscle lengths (i.e., approximately -16 to 0 mm) during isometric, isokinetic, and dynamic contractions (Kim et al., 2015) (please refer to **Figure 2B** for non-linear behavior of the model muscle unit).

The axonal nerve coupling the motoneuron with the muscle unit was modeled *via* a single parameter representing the delay time (~10 ms) required for the transmission of action potentials from the motoneuron to the muscle unit, assuming perfect action potential transmission from the motoneuron to the muscle unit (Kim, 2017). The overall input–output properties of the model motor unit were validated by comparison to those of a physiologically reconstructed model for an adult cat slow-type motor unit in the previous study [please refer to Figures 8, 9 in Kim and Kim (2018) for non-linear behavior of the model motor unit]. The system equations and parameter values used for this study are presented as supplementary material (**Supplementary File 1**).

Stimulation Protocols

The non-linearity of the input-output relationship was investigated separately for the motoneuron and muscle unit. In regard to the motoneuron, a linearly ascending and descending current with a peak value of 20 nA over 10 s was injected at the soma of the motoneuron (as shown in **Figure 2A**). In regard to the muscle unit, a train of current impulses was applied such that the stimulation frequency increased and decreased according to a triangular shape with a peak value of 40 Hz over 10 s (see **Figure 2B**). The peak stimulation frequency was selected to ensure that the model muscle unit produced the maximal force during isometric contraction at the optimal muscle length.

In the present study, stimulation waveforms were investigated under extracellular motoneuron microstimulation with a sharp-tipped electrode near the initial segment and cell body (**Figure 1**). Under these conditions, the extracellular potential (i.e., $V_{e,S}$) at the soma is determined by the current (i.e., I_{ext}) passing through the microelectrode, whereas the extracellular potential (i.e., $V_{e,D}$) across the dendritic area (i.e., $D_{path} > 0.6$ mm) distal to the soma tends to not depend on I_{ext} (McIntyre and Grill, 2002). The variation in transmembrane potential (i.e., V_S) at the soma due to I_{ext} was simulated *via* intracellular injection of

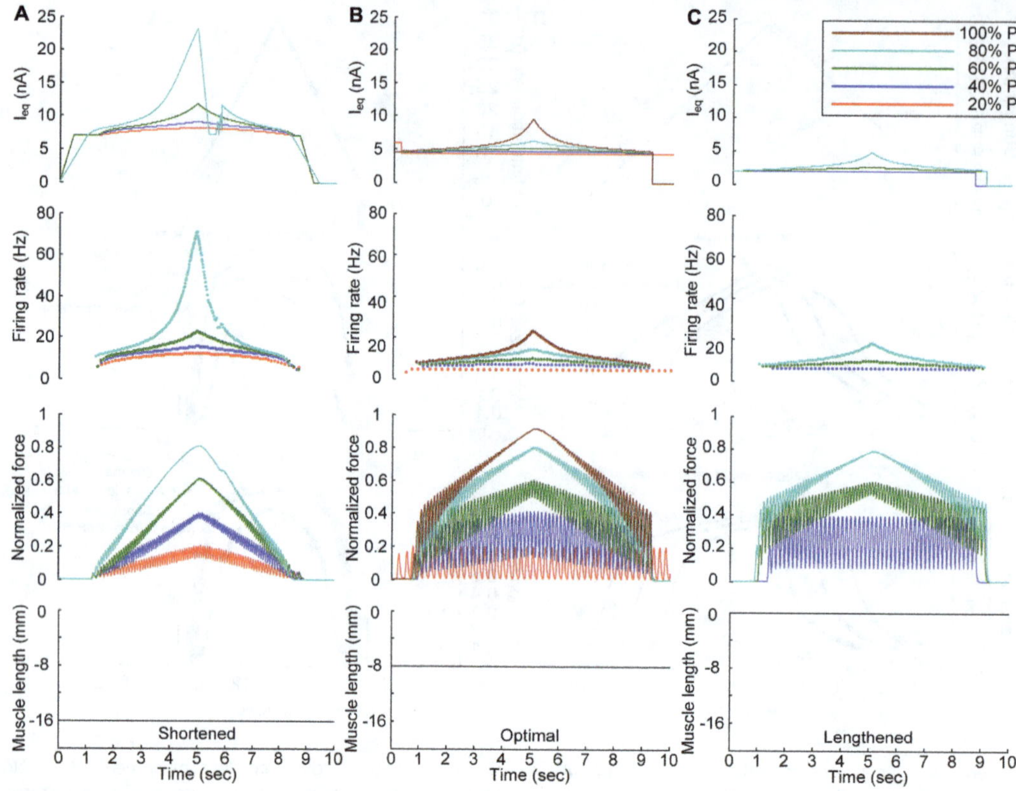

FIGURE 3 | Continuous stimulation waveforms for linear force production. Intensities of continuous current stimulation (I_{eq}) applied to the somatic compartment (*top*), instantaneous firing rate (*upper middle*) in the motoneuron, and normalized muscle force (*lower middle*) produced by the muscle unit at the three muscle lengths (*bottom*): physiologically minimum **(A)**, optimal **(B)**, and maximum muscle lengths **(C)**. The level of force production produced by the motor unit is denoted as a percentage of the maximal isometric force (P_0) at the optimal muscle length and indicated with different colors.

the equivalent current (i.e., I_{eq}) at the soma, as proposed in a previous study (Warman et al., 1992). With the application of Kirchhoff's current law to the somatic compartment of the two-compartment model in addition to approximation of $V_{e,D}$ as zero under passive membrane conditions, I_{eq} can be derived as the following analytical form:

$$I_{eq} = C_{m,S} \cdot dV_S/dt + G_{m,S} \cdot V_S + G_C \cdot V_S = -G_C \cdot V_{e,S}$$

Where V_S is the potential difference between the intracellular ($V_{i,S}$) and extracellular sides ($V_{e,S}$) of the somatic compartment in the two-compartment neuron model.

Linear force production of the motor unit was induced considering two types (continuous and discrete) of current stimulation (i.e., I_{eq}) in the somatic compartment of the motoneuron model over 10 s. The shape and amplitude of continuous current stimulation were first determined with a linear function in a piecewise manner so that the force linearly increased and decreased at the various speeds over 10 s. Then, piecewise linear functions were fitted with a continuous function ensuring linear force production by the motor unit (please refer to **Table 1**). In the case of discrete current stimulation, the timing and amplitude of the current pulses were adjusted such that the discrete current simulation process reproduced the temporal evolution of force production induced under continuous current stimulation condition. In this study, the amplitude of the current pulses indicated the minimal current intensity yielding a desired force profile. The width of the current pulse was set to 0.5 ms, ensuring a one-to-one stimulus-firing reaction at the stimulus amplitude threshold. To compare the different states between the various muscle lengths, all muscle forces induced under current stimulation in the somatic compartment of the motoneuron model were normalized based on the maximum force (i.e., P_0) actively produced by the model motor unit during isometric contraction at the optimal muscle length. In the present study, the simulation data are not shown when the model motor unit could not produce the desired peak force (i.e., 20–100% of P_0).

Muscle Length Variation

The stimulation patterns required for triangular force production by the motor unit during isometric contraction were predicted under three different modes of the muscle length: physiologically minimal ($X_m = -16$ mm), optimal ($X_m = -8$ mm), and maximal ($X_m = 0$ mm) muscle lengths. The physiological range of the variation in muscle length was determined based on the locomotor data of adult cats reported in a previous study (Goslow et al., 1973). The variation in muscle length influences both the motoneuron and muscle unit by transmitting muscle spindle signals to the motoneuron and adjusting a certain kinetic

TABLE 1 | Piecewise equations for the time courses of continuous current stimulation (i.e., I_{eq}) presented in **Figures 3**, **5**, **7**.

Muscle length	Target force level	Figure 3	Figure 5	Figure 7
$X_m = -16$ mm	80% P_0	• $0 < t \leq 1{,}000$: $I_{eq} = 7.015{\cdot}10^{-3}\ t$ • $1{,}000 < t \leq 4{,}950$ $I_{eq} = 28.99{\cdot}\sin[7.766{\cdot}10^{-4}{\cdot}(t-1{,}000) - 0.318] + 123.5{\cdot}\sin[1.445{\cdot}10^{-3}{\cdot}(t-1{,}000) + 1.768] + 105.7{\cdot}\sin[1.502{\cdot}10^{-3}{\cdot}(t-1{,}000) + 4.822] + 0.042$ • $4{,}950 < t \leq 5{,}350$: $I_{eq} = -0.04{\cdot}(t-4{,}950) + 23.153$ • $5{,}350 < t \leq 5{,}600$: $I_{eq} = 7.157$ • $5{,}600 < t \leq 5{,}650$: $I_{eq} = 0.04{\cdot}(t-5{,}600) + 7.197$ • $5{,}650 < t \leq 5{,}700$: $I_{eq} = -0.04{\cdot}(t-5{,}650) + 9.193$ • $5{,}700 < t \leq 5{,}750$: $I_{eq} = 0.06{\cdot}(t-5{,}700) + 7.157$ • $5{,}750 < t \leq 5{,}800$: $I_{eq} = -0.04{\cdot}(t-5{,}750) + 10.153$ • $5{,}800 < t \leq 8{,}400$: $I_{eq} = 28.99{\cdot}\sin[7.766{\cdot}10^{-3}{\cdot}(8{,}400-t) - 0.318] + 123.5{\cdot}\sin[1.445{\cdot}10^{-3}{\cdot}(8{,}400-t) + 1.768] + 105.7{\cdot}\sin[1.502{\cdot}10^{-3}{\cdot}(8{,}400-t) + 4.822] + 0.042$ • $8{,}400 < t \leq 9{,}400$: $I_{eq} = 7.015{\cdot}10^{-3}{\cdot}(9{,}400-t)$ • $9{,}400 < t \leq 10{,}000$: $I_{eq} = 0$	• $0 < t \leq 5{,}000$: $I_{eq} = 10.81{\cdot}\exp[4.379{\cdot}10^{-5}{\cdot}(2{\cdot}t - 1{,}250.1)] + 3.544{\cdot}10^{-3}{\cdot}\exp[1.008{\cdot}10^{-3}{\cdot}(2{\cdot}t - 1{,}250.1)]$ • $5{,}000 < t \leq 10{,}000$: $I_{eq} = 10.81{\cdot}\exp\{4.379{\cdot}10^{-5}{\cdot}[2{\cdot}(10{,}000 - t) - 1{,}250.1]\} + 3.544{\cdot}10^{-3}{\cdot}\exp\{1.008{\cdot}10^{-3}{\cdot}[2{\cdot}(10{,}000 - t) - 1{,}250.1]\}$	
	60% P_0	• $0 < t \leq 500$: $I_{eq} = 1.403{\cdot}10^{-2}{\cdot}t$ • $500 < t \leq 1{,}380$: $I_{eq} = 7.015$ • $1{,}380 < t \leq 4{,}950$: $I_{eq} = 28.99{\cdot}\sin[5.726{\cdot}10^{-4}{\cdot}(t-1{,}380) - 0.318] + 123.5{\cdot}\sin[1.064{\cdot}10^{-3}{\cdot}(t-1{,}380) + 1.768] + 105.7{\cdot}\sin[1.108{\cdot}10^{-3}{\cdot}(t-1{,}380) + 4.822] + 0.042$ • $4{,}950 < t \leq 8{,}520$: $I_{eq} = 28.99{\cdot}\sin[5.726{\cdot}10^{-4}{\cdot}(8{,}520-t) - 0.318] + 123.5{\cdot}\sin[1.064{\cdot}10^{-3}{\cdot}(8{,}520-t) + 1.768] + 105.7{\cdot}\sin[1.108{\cdot}10^{-3}{\cdot}(8{,}520-t) + 4.822] + 0.042$ • $8{,}520 < t \leq 8{,}700$: $I_{eq} = 7.015$ • $8{,}700 < t \leq 9{,}200$: $I_{eq} = 1.403{\cdot}10^{-2}{\cdot}(9{,}200-t)$ • $9{,}200 < t \leq 10{,}000$: $I_{eq} = 0$	• $0 < t \leq 5{,}000$: $I_{eq} = 10.81{\cdot}\exp[4.379{\cdot}10^{-5}{\cdot}(1.5{\cdot}t - 1{,}250.1)] + 3.544{\cdot}10^{-3}{\cdot}\exp[1.008{\cdot}10^{-3}{\cdot}(1.5{\cdot}t - 1{,}250.1)]$ • $5{,}000 < t \leq 10{,}000$: $I_{eq} = 10.81{\cdot}\exp\{4.379{\cdot}10^{-5}{\cdot}[1.5{\cdot}(10{,}000 - t) - 1{,}250.1]\} + 3.544{\cdot}10^{-3}{\cdot}\exp\{1.008{\cdot}10^{-3}{\cdot}[1.5{\cdot}(10{,}000 - t) - 1{,}250.1]\}$	
	40% P_0	• $0 < t \leq 500$: $I_{eq} = 1.403{\cdot}10^{-2}{\cdot}t$ • $500 < t \leq 1{,}380$: $I_{eq} = 7.015$ • $1{,}380 < t \leq 4{,}950$: $I_{eq} = 28.99{\cdot}\sin[3.507{\cdot}10^{-4}{\cdot}(t-1{,}380) - 0.318] + 123.5{\cdot}\sin[0.652{\cdot}10^{-3}{\cdot}(t-1{,}380) + 1.768] + 105.7{\cdot}\sin[0.678{\cdot}10^{-3}{\cdot}(t-1{,}380) + 4.822] + 0.042$ • $4{,}950 < t \leq 8{,}520$: $I_{eq} = 28.99{\cdot}\sin[3.507{\cdot}10^{-4}{\cdot}(8{,}520-t) - 0.318] + 123.5{\cdot}\sin[0.652{\cdot}10^{-3}{\cdot}(8{,}520-t) + 1.768] + 105.7{\cdot}\sin[0.678{\cdot}10^{-3}{\cdot}(8{,}520-t) + 4.822] + 0.042$ • $8{,}520 < t \leq 8{,}700$: $I_{eq} = 7.015$ • $8{,}700 < t \leq 9{,}200$: $I_{eq} = 1.403{\cdot}10^{-2}{\cdot}(9{,}200-t)$ • $9{,}200 < t \leq 10{,}000$: $I_{eq} = 0$	• $0 < t \leq 5{,}000$: $I_{eq} = 10.81{\cdot}\exp[4.379{\cdot}10^{-5}{\cdot}(0.94{\cdot}t - 1{,}250.1)] + 3.544{\cdot}10^{-3}{\cdot}\exp[1.008{\cdot}10^{-3}{\cdot}(0.94{\cdot}t - 1{,}250.1)]$ • $5{,}000 < t \leq 10{,}000$: $I_{eq} = 10.81{\cdot}\exp[4.379{\cdot}10^{-5}{\cdot}(0.94{\cdot}(10{,}000 - t) - 1{,}250.1)] + 3.544{\cdot}10^{-3}{\cdot}\exp[1.008{\cdot}10^{-3}{\cdot}(0.94{\cdot}(10{,}000 - t) - 1{,}250.1)]$	

(Continued)

TABLE 1 | Continued

Muscle length	Target force level	Figure 3	Figure 5	Figure 7
	20% P_0	• $0 < t \le 500$: $l_{eq} = 1.403 \cdot 10^{-2} \cdot t$ • $500 < t \le 1{,}380$: $l_{eq} = 7.015$ • $1{,}380 < t \le 4{,}950$: $l_{eq} = 28.99 \cdot \sin[1.432 \cdot 10^{-4} \cdot (t - 1{,}380) - 0.318] + 123.5 \cdot \sin[0.266 \cdot 10^{-3} \cdot (t - 1{,}380) + 1.768] + 105.7 \cdot \sin[0.277 \cdot 10^{-3} \cdot (t - 1{,}380) + 4.822] + 0.042$ • $4{,}950 < t \le 8{,}520$: $l_{eq} = 28.99 \cdot \sin[1.432 \cdot 10^{-4} \cdot (8{,}520 - t) - 0.318] + 123.5 \cdot \sin[0.266 \cdot 10^{-3} \cdot (8{,}520 - t) + 1.768] + 105.7 \cdot \sin[0.277 \cdot 10^{-3} \cdot (8{,}520 - t) + 4.822] + 0.042$ • $8{,}520 < t \le 8{,}700$: $l_{eq} = 7.015$ • $8{,}700 < t \le 9{,}200$: $l_{eq} = 1.403 \cdot 10^{-2} \cdot (9{,}200 - t)$ • $9{,}200 < t \le 10{,}000$: $l_{eq} = 0$	• $0 < t \le 5{,}000$: $l_{eq} = 10.55 + 1.864 \cdot 10^{-4} \cdot t$ • $5{,}000 < t \le 10{,}000$: $l_{eq} = 10.55 + 1.864 \cdot 10^{-4} \cdot (10{,}000 - t)$	
X_m = -8 mm	100% P_0	• $0 < t \le 5{,}000$: $l_{eq} = 3.827 \cdot \exp[4.696 \cdot 10^{-5} \cdot (1.3 \cdot t + 3{,}500)] + 6.883 \cdot 10^{-7} \cdot \exp[1.545 \cdot 10^{-3} \cdot (1.3 \cdot t + 3{,}500)]$ • $5{,}000 < t \le 9{,}250$: $l_{eq} = 3.827 \cdot \exp[4.696 \cdot 10^{-5} \cdot (1.3 \cdot (10{,}000 - t) + 3{,}500)] + 6.883 \cdot 10^{-7} \cdot \exp[1.545 \cdot 10^{-3} \cdot (1.3 \cdot (10{,}000 - t) + 3{,}500)]$ • $9{,}250 < t \le 10{,}000$: $l_{eq} = 0$	• $0 < t \le 2{,}000$: $l_{eq} = 8.684 \cdot \exp(-4.554 \cdot 10^{-6} \cdot t) + 0.03 \cdot \exp(1.03 \cdot 10^{-3} \cdot t)$ • $2{,}000 < t \le 5{,}000$: $l_{eq} = 8.543 \cdot \exp(2.704 \cdot 10^{-5} \cdot t) + 2.749 \cdot 10^{-5} \cdot \exp(2.772 \cdot 10^{-3} \cdot t) - 0.18$ • $5{,}000 < t \le 8{,}000$: $l_{eq} = 8.543 \cdot \exp[2.704 \cdot 10^{-5} \cdot (10{,}000 - t)] + 2.749 \cdot 10^{-5} \cdot \exp[2.772 \cdot 10^{-3} \cdot (10{,}000 - t)] - 0.18$ • $8{,}000 < t \le 10{,}000$: $l_{eq} = 8.684 \cdot \exp[-4.554 \cdot 10^{-6} \cdot (10{,}000 - t)] + 0.03 \cdot \exp[1.03 \cdot 10^{-3} \cdot (10{,}000 - t)]$	• $0 < t \le 4{,}750$: $l_{eq} = 6.85 \cdot \exp(3.54 \cdot 10^{-5} \cdot t) + 1.097 \cdot 10^{-5} \cdot \exp(2.778 \cdot 10^{-3} \cdot t)$ • $4{,}750 < t \le 5{,}050$: $l_{eq} = 14.006$ • $5{,}050 < t \le 8{,}900$: $l_{eq} = 6.85 \cdot \exp[3.54 \cdot 10^{-5} \cdot (9{,}800 - t)] + 1.097 \cdot 10^{-5} \cdot \exp[2.778 \cdot 10^{-3} \cdot (9{,}800 - t)]$ • $8{,}900 < t \le 10{,}000$: $l_{eq} = 0$
	80% P_0	• $0 < t \le 5{,}000$: $l_{eq} = 3.827 \cdot \exp[4.696 \cdot 10^{-5} \cdot (1.053 \cdot t + 3{,}500)] + 6.883 \cdot 10^{-7} \cdot \exp[1.545 \cdot 10^{-3} \cdot (1.053 \cdot t + 3{,}500)]$ • $5{,}000 < t \le 9{,}250$: $l_{eq} = 3.827 \cdot \exp\{4.696 \cdot 10^{-5} \cdot [1.053 \cdot (10{,}000 - t) + 3{,}500]\} + 6.883 \cdot 10^{-7} \cdot \exp\{1.545 \cdot 10^{-3} \cdot [1.053 \cdot (10{,}000 - t) + 3{,}500]\}$ • $9{,}250 < t \le 10{,}000$: $l_{eq} = 0$	• $0 < t \le 2{,}000$: $l_{eq} = 8.684 \cdot \exp(-3.416 \cdot 10^{-6} \cdot t) + 0.03 \cdot \exp(0.773 \cdot 10^{-3} \cdot t)$ • $2{,}000 < t \le 5{,}000$: $l_{eq} = 8.543 \cdot \exp(2.028 \cdot 10^{-5} \cdot t) + 2.749 \cdot 10^{-5} \cdot \exp(2.079 \cdot 10^{-3} \cdot t) - 0.132$ • $5{,}000 < t \le 8{,}000$: $l_{eq} = 8.543 \cdot \exp[2.028 \cdot 10^{-5} \cdot (10{,}000 - t)] + 2.749 \cdot 10^{-5} \cdot \exp[2.079 \cdot 10^{-3} \cdot (10{,}000 - t)] - 0.132$ • $8{,}000 < t \le 10{,}000$: $l_{eq} = 8.684 \cdot \exp[-3.416 \cdot 10^{-6} \cdot (10{,}000 - t)] + 0.03 \cdot \exp[0.773 \cdot 10^{-3} \cdot (10{,}000 - t)]$	• $0 < t \le 5{,}000$: $l_{eq} = 6.85 \cdot \exp(1.416 \cdot 10^{-5} \cdot t) + 1.097 \cdot 10^{-5} \cdot \exp(1.111 \cdot 10^{-3} \cdot t)$ • $5{,}000 < t \le 8{,}800$: $l_{eq} = 6.85 \cdot \exp[1.416 \cdot 10^{-5} \cdot (10{,}000 - t)] + 1.097 \cdot 10^{-5} \cdot \exp[1.111 \cdot 10^{-3} \cdot (10{,}000 - t)]$ • $8{,}800 < t \le 10{,}000$: $l_{eq} = 0$
	60% P_0	• $0 < t \le 5{,}000$: $l_{eq} = 3.827 \cdot \exp[4.696 \cdot 10^{-5} \cdot (0.59 \cdot t + 3{,}500)] + 6.883 \cdot 10^{-7} \cdot \exp[1.545 \cdot 10^{-3} \cdot (0.59 \cdot t + 3{,}500)]$ • $5{,}000 < t \le 9{,}250$: $l_{eq} = 3.827 \cdot \exp\{4.696 \cdot 10^{-5} \cdot [0.59 \cdot (10{,}000 - t) + 3{,}500]\} + 6.883 \cdot 10^{-7} \cdot \exp\{1.545 \cdot 10^{-3} \cdot [0.59 \cdot (10{,}000 - t) + 3{,}500]\}$ • $9{,}250 < t \le 10{,}000$: $l_{eq} = 0$	• $0 < t \le 5{,}000$: $l_{eq} = 8.53 \cdot \exp(-5.754 \cdot 10^{-6} \cdot t) + 0.186 \cdot \exp(2.562 \cdot 10^{-4} \cdot t)$ • $5{,}000 < t \le 10{,}000$: $l_{eq} = 8.53 \cdot \exp[-5.754 \cdot 10^{-6} \cdot (10{,}000 - t)] + 0.186 \cdot \exp[2.562 \cdot 10^{-4} \cdot (10{,}000 - t)]$	• $0 < t \le 5{,}000$: $l_{eq} = 6.85 \cdot \exp(1.77 \cdot 10^{-5} \cdot 0.6 \cdot t) + 1.097 \cdot 10^{-5} \cdot \exp(0.833 \cdot 10^{-3} \cdot t)$ • $5{,}000 < t \le 8{,}700$: $l_{eq} = 6.85 \cdot \exp[1.062 \cdot 10^{-5} \cdot (10{,}000 - t)] + 1.097 \cdot 10^{-5} \cdot \exp[0.833 \cdot 10^{-3} \cdot (10{,}000 - t)]$ • $8{,}700 < t \le 10{,}000$: $l_{eq} = 0$

(Continued)

TABLE 1 | Continued

Muscle length	Target force level	Figure 3	Figure 5	Figure 7
	40% P_O	• $0 < t \le 5{,}000$: $l_{eq} = 3.827\cdot\exp[4.7\cdot10^{-5}\cdot(0.212\cdot t + 3{,}500)] + 6.883\cdot10^{-7}\cdot\exp[1.545\cdot10^{-3}\cdot(0.212\cdot t + 3{,}500)]$ • $5{,}000 < t \le 9{,}250$: $l_{eq} = 3.827\cdot\exp\{4.696\cdot10^{-5}\cdot[0.212\cdot(10{,}000 - t) + 3{,}500]\} + 6.883\cdot10^{-7}\cdot\exp\{1.545\cdot10^{-3}\cdot[0.212\cdot(10{,}000 - t) + 3{,}500]\}$ • $9{,}250 < t \le 10{,}000$: $l_{eq} = 0$	• $0 < t \le 10{,}000$: $l_{eq} = 8.732$	• $0 < t \le 5{,}000$: $l_{eq} = 6.85\cdot\exp(0.708\cdot10^{-5}\cdot t) + 1.097\cdot10^{-5}\cdot\exp(0.556\cdot10^{-3}\cdot t)$ • $5{,}000 < t \le 8{,}500$: $l_{eq} = 6.85\cdot\exp[0.708\cdot10^{-5}\cdot(10{,}000 - t)] + 1.097\cdot10^{-5}\cdot\exp[0.556\cdot10^{-3}\cdot(10{,}000 - t)]$ • $8{,}500 < t \le 10{,}000$: $l_{eq} = 0$
	20% P_O	• $0 < t \le 262$: $l_{eq} = 6$ • $262 < t \le 10{,}000$: $l_{eq} = 4.354$		• $0 < t \le 8{,}500$: $l_{eq} = 6.92$ • $8{,}500 < t \le 10{,}000$: $l_{eq} = 0$
$X_m = 0$ mm	80% P_O	• $0 < t \le 5{,}000$: $l_{eq} = 1.166\cdot\exp[1.058\cdot10^{-4}\cdot(t + 5{,}000)] + 1.033\cdot10^{-8}\cdot\exp[1.881\cdot10^{-3}\cdot(t + 5{,}000)]$ • $5{,}000 < t \le 9{,}100$: $l_{eq} = 1.166\cdot\exp[1.058\cdot10^{-4}\cdot(15{,}000 - t)] + 1.033\cdot10^{-8}\cdot\exp[1.881\cdot10^{-3}\cdot(15{,}000 - t)]$ • $9{,}100 < t \le 10{,}000$: $l_{eq} = 0$	• $0 < t \le 2{,}000$: $l_{eq} = 6.249\cdot\exp(-2.269\cdot10^{-5}\cdot t) + 0.519\cdot\exp(2.798\cdot10^{-4}\cdot t)$ • $2{,}000 < t \le 5{,}000$: $l_{eq} = 6.719\cdot\exp(1.239\cdot10^{-5}\cdot t) + 5.718\cdot10^{-4}\cdot\exp(1.709\cdot10^{-3}\cdot t) - 0.026$ • $5{,}000 < t \le 8{,}000$: $l_{eq} = 6.719\cdot\exp[1.239\cdot10^{-5}\cdot(10{,}000 - t)] + 5.718\cdot10^{-4}\cdot\exp[1.709\cdot10^{-3}\cdot(10{,}000 - t)] - 0.026$ • $8{,}000 < t \le 10{,}000$: $l_{eq} = 6.249\cdot\exp[-2.269\cdot10^{-5}\cdot(10{,}000 - t)] + 0.519\cdot\exp[2.798\cdot10^{-4}\cdot(10{,}000 - t)]$	• $0 < t \le 5{,}000$: $l_{eq} = 6.926\cdot\exp(3.115\cdot10^{-5}\cdot t) + 1.461\cdot10^{-4}\cdot\exp(1.903\cdot10^{-3}\cdot t)$ • $5{,}000 < t \le 9{,}000$: $l_{eq} = 6.926\cdot\exp[3.115\cdot10^{-5}\cdot(10{,}000 - t)] + 1.461\cdot10^{-4}\cdot\exp[1.903\cdot10^{-3}\cdot(10{,}000 - t)]$ • $9{,}000 < t \le 10{,}000$: $l_{eq} = 0$
	60% P_O	• $0 < t \le 5{,}000$: $l_{eq} = 1.166\cdot\exp[1.058\cdot10^{-4}\cdot(0.506\cdot t + 5{,}000)] + 1.033\cdot10^{-8}\cdot\exp[1.881\cdot10^{-3}\cdot(0.506\cdot t + 5{,}000)]$ • $5{,}000 < t \le 9{,}100$: $l_{eq} = 1.166\cdot\exp[1.058\cdot10^{-4}\cdot(10{,}060 - 0.506\cdot t)] + 1.033\cdot10^{-8}\cdot\exp[1.881\cdot10^{-3}\cdot(10{,}060 - 0.506\cdot t)]$ • $9{,}100 < t \le 10{,}000$: $l_{eq} = 0$	• $0 < t \le 5{,}000$: $l_{eq} = 6.554\cdot\exp(-5.482\cdot10^{-6}\cdot t) + 0.213\cdot\exp(2.105\cdot10^{-4}\cdot t)$ • $5{,}000 < t \le 10{,}000$: $l_{eq} = 6.554\cdot\exp[-5.482\cdot10^{-6}\cdot(10{,}000 - t)] + 0.213\cdot\exp[2.105\cdot10^{-4}\cdot(10{,}000 - t)]$	• $0 < t \le 5{,}000$: $l_{eq} = 6.926\cdot\exp(1.767\cdot10^{-5}\cdot t) + 1.461\cdot10^{-4}\cdot\exp(1.081\cdot10^{-3}\cdot t)$ • $5{,}000 < t \le 9{,}000$: $l_{eq} = 6.926\cdot\exp[1.767\cdot10^{-5}\cdot(10{,}000 - t)] + 1.461\cdot10^{-4}\cdot\exp[1.081\cdot10^{-3}\cdot(10{,}000 - t)]$ • $9{,}000 < t \le 10{,}000$: $l_{eq} = 0$
	40% P_O	• $0 < t \le 8{,}700$: $l_{eq} = 1.95$ • $8{,}700 < t \le 10{,}000$: $l_{eq} = 0$	• $0 < t \le 10{,}000$: $l_{eq} = 6.768$	• $0 < t \le 5{,}000$: $l_{eq} = 6.926\cdot\exp(0.623\cdot10^{-5}\cdot t) + 1.461\cdot10^{-4}\cdot\exp(0.381\cdot10^{-3}\cdot t)$ • $5{,}000 < t \le 9{,}000$: $l_{eq} = 6.926\cdot\exp[0.623\cdot10^{-5}\cdot(10{,}000 - t)] + 1.461\cdot10^{-4}\cdot\exp[0.381\cdot10^{-3}\cdot(10{,}000 - t)]$ • $9{,}000 < t \le 10{,}000$: $l_{eq} = 0$

The unit of time is a millisecond. ● Indicates individual time intervals and piecewise equations.

parameter [i.e., K5 in Kim et al. (2015)] of the formation of calcium-binding troponin in the sarcoplasm of the muscle unit model as a function of the muscle length.

Muscle Afferent Signals

The feedback signals originating from the muscle spindle were simulated by summing the excitatory synaptic inputs (i.e., G_{esyn})

over both the soma and dendrite (Segev et al., 1990). Under passive membrane conditions, the peak conductance for muscle afferent inputs was determined to match the current (i.e., $I_{N,PASS}$) experimentally measured during voltage clamping over the soma under a 10-mV hyperpolarized potential below the resting potential while slowly varying the muscle length from the physiologically minimum length to the maximum length (Lee et al., 2003). The peak conductance for muscle afferent inputs was set to 0 mS/cm^2 to yield an $I_{N,PASS}$ value of 0 nA at −16 mm, 0.0064 mS/cm^2 to yield an $I_{N,PASS}$ value of 2.5 nA at −8 mm, and 0.0128 mS/cm^2 to yield an $I_{N,PASS}$ value of 5 nA at 0 mm under isometric conditions.

Simulations

All simulations were performed in the PyMUS software environment (version 2.0.1) *via* the Python integration method (a Variable-coefficient Ordinary Differential Equation (VODE) was applied to the motoneuron, and the Livermore Solver for Ordinary Differential Equations (LSODE) was applied to the muscle unit) at a fixed time step (0.1 ms) on a desktop computer operated by 64-bit Microsoft Windows 10. Default values of the model parameters and simulation conditions were implemented unless noted otherwise in the text. The computer codes of the models and simulations in this study are presented in the supplementary information (**Supplementary File 2**) and are publicly available from the public repository of GitHub[1]. The data employed for the estimation of the stimulation waveforms required for force production by the motor unit at the various speeds and levels in the present study are presented in the supplementary material (**Supplementary File 3**).

RESULTS

Non-linear Input–Output Relationship of the Motoneuron and Muscle Unit

We first evaluated whether the model motor unit captures the non-linearity of the input–output function of the motoneuron and muscle unit. **Figure 2** shows the non-linear response of the motoneuron and muscle unit under linearly increasing and decreasing excitation effects. The model motoneuron suitably replicated experimental observations of non-linear firing of spinal motoneurons during triangular current injection at the cell body [please refer to Figure 3 in Hounsgaard et al. (1984)]. In particular, the firing rate was enhanced at a current intensity higher than the recruitment threshold in the ascending stimulation phase, and firing was sustained below the recruitment threshold in the descending stimulation phase (as shown in the top and middle panels of **Figure 2A**). This result was mainly attributed to the activation of persistent inward current (PIC)-generating calcium channels at the dendrite underlying the non-linear input–output relationship of the motoneuron (as shown in the bottom panel of **Figure 2A**). In terms of the model muscle unit, a non-linear relationship of the stimulation frequency and force genesis has been experimentally verified during electrical stimulation of soleus muscles in adult cat preparations [please refer to Figure 8 in Rack and Westbury (1969)]. The muscle unit model reproduced the sigmoidal shape of force production well when slowly increasing and decreasing the stimulation rate (as shown in the top and middle panels, respectively, of **Figure 2B**). This was mainly attributed to the non-linear dynamics of muscle activation (as shown in the bottom panel of **Figure 2B**). Furthermore, the non-linear input–output relationship of the motoneuron and muscle unit was modulated by the variation in muscle length, indicating the influence of the muscle afferent inputs and the length dependence of muscle activation. These results indicate that the stimulation waveforms required for the motoneuron to control the muscle force may strongly depend on the muscle length.

Continuous Stimulation Waveforms for Force Control at the Various Muscle Lengths

Figure 3 shows the waveforms under continuous current stimulation in regard to linear force generation at the various speeds and levels during isometric contraction at the minimal, optimal, and maximal muscle lengths. Overall, the current intensity exponentially increased and decreased in regard to linear force development and relaxation, respectively, at all muscle lengths. The current stimulation amplitude increased with increasing force speed and magnitude and with decreasing muscle length. The length dependence of the stimulation amplitude was attributed to the reduction in muscle afferent inputs and muscle activation level with decreasing muscle length from the physiologically maximal length. In accordance, the peak firing rate of the motoneuron was the highest at the highest speed and largest magnitude of force production in the shortened muscle state.

In terms of the shortened muscle, the motor unit produced various force levels ranging from 20 to 80% of the maximal force (i.e., P_0) generated at the optimal muscle length (**Figure 3A**). The 100% P_0 level was not achievable due to the bell-shaped length-tension muscle properties, indicating a force decline with decreasing or increasing muscle length from the optimal length. The stimulation waveforms were almost symmetric up to 60% of P_0. At 80% of P_0, however, the stimulation intensity rapidly decreased near the recruitment threshold to achieve linear force relaxation in the descending stimulation phase. This was required to prevent the full activation of the PIC channels located across the motoneuron dendrite in the descending stimulation phase. At the optimal muscle length, the current threshold for firing initiation was lower than that in the shortened muscle case due to the excitatory muscle afferent inputs to the motoneuron (**Figure 3B**). Brief injection of an excitatory step current at the beginning of current stimulation was required to slowly produce force up to 20% of P_0. This result indicates that the PIC may partially be activated and slowly oscillate, leading to slow firing at the motoneuron. Notably, the model motor unit could not fully reach the maximal force level due to the limitation of the stimulation intensity to prevent full PIC activation in the motoneuron. Once the PIC was fully activated in the ascending

[1]https://github.com/NMSL-DGIST/PyMUS

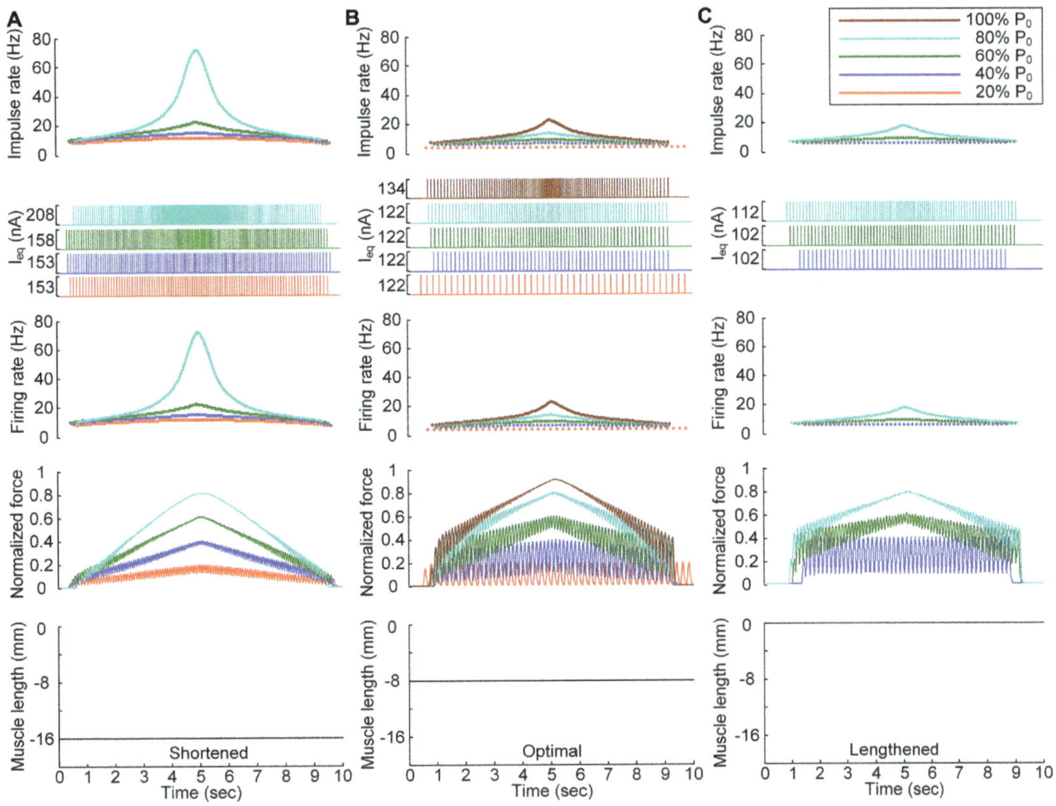

FIGURE 4 | Discrete stimulation waveforms for linear force production. Frequency and amplitude (two *top panels*) of impulse current stimulation (I_{eq}) applied to the somatic compartment, instantaneous firing rate (*upper middle*) in the motoneuron, and normalized muscle force (*lower middle*) produced by the muscle unit at the three muscle lengths (*bottom*): physiologically minimum **(A)**, optimal **(B)**, and maximum muscle lengths **(C)**. The level of force production produced by the motor unit is denoted as a percentage of the maximal isometric force (P_0) at the optimal muscle length and indicated with different colors.

stimulation phase, the deactivation of PIC channels became uncontrollable, resulting in difficulty in achieving linear force relaxation in the descending stimulation phase. This result could be attributed to the severe attenuation of the electrical signals generated near the cell body when transmitted to distal dendritic areas in the motoneuron. In terms of the lengthened muscle, the current threshold for firing initiation further decreased due to the increase in excitatory muscle afferent inputs to the motoneuron (**Figure 3C**). Force production was realized from the peak level of 40% of P_0 to 80% of P_0 owing to the twitch force greater than 20% of P_0 and the bell-shaped length-tension muscle properties.

All these results suggest that the exponential waveform under a continuous current intensity effectively controlled linear force production and that the continuous type of current stimulation could limit the range of force generation in shorter-than-optimal muscles.

Discrete Stimulation Waveforms for Force Control at the Various Muscle Lengths

After stimulation waveform estimation under continuous stimulation conditions, the stimulation waveforms required for force production were assessed under discrete stimulation conditions (**Figure 4**). In general, the rate of current impulse stimulation should exponentially increase and then decrease to produce forces according to a triangular shape at all muscle lengths. Similar to the continuous stimulation case, the amplitude and peak rate of the current impulses increased with increasing speed and magnitude of force production and with decreasing muscle length. The length dependence of the stimulation amplitude and rate was attributed to the increase in muscle afferent inputs and muscle activation level with increasing muscle length from the shortened state. In accordance, the peak firing rate of the motoneuron was the highest at the minimal muscle length and the highest speed and level of force production. However, in contrast to the continuous stimulation case, the stimulation waveforms were almost symmetric at all force production levels during isometric contraction at the minimal muscle length (see **Figure 4A**). Furthermore, the model motor unit fully produced the maximum force at the optimal muscle length without full activation of the PIC channels across the motoneuron (**Supplementary File 4**).

All these results indicate that the exponential waveform due to the current impulse frequency is effective in regard to linear production of the muscle force and that the discrete type of current stimulation is suitable for the full range of force generation and muscle length levels.

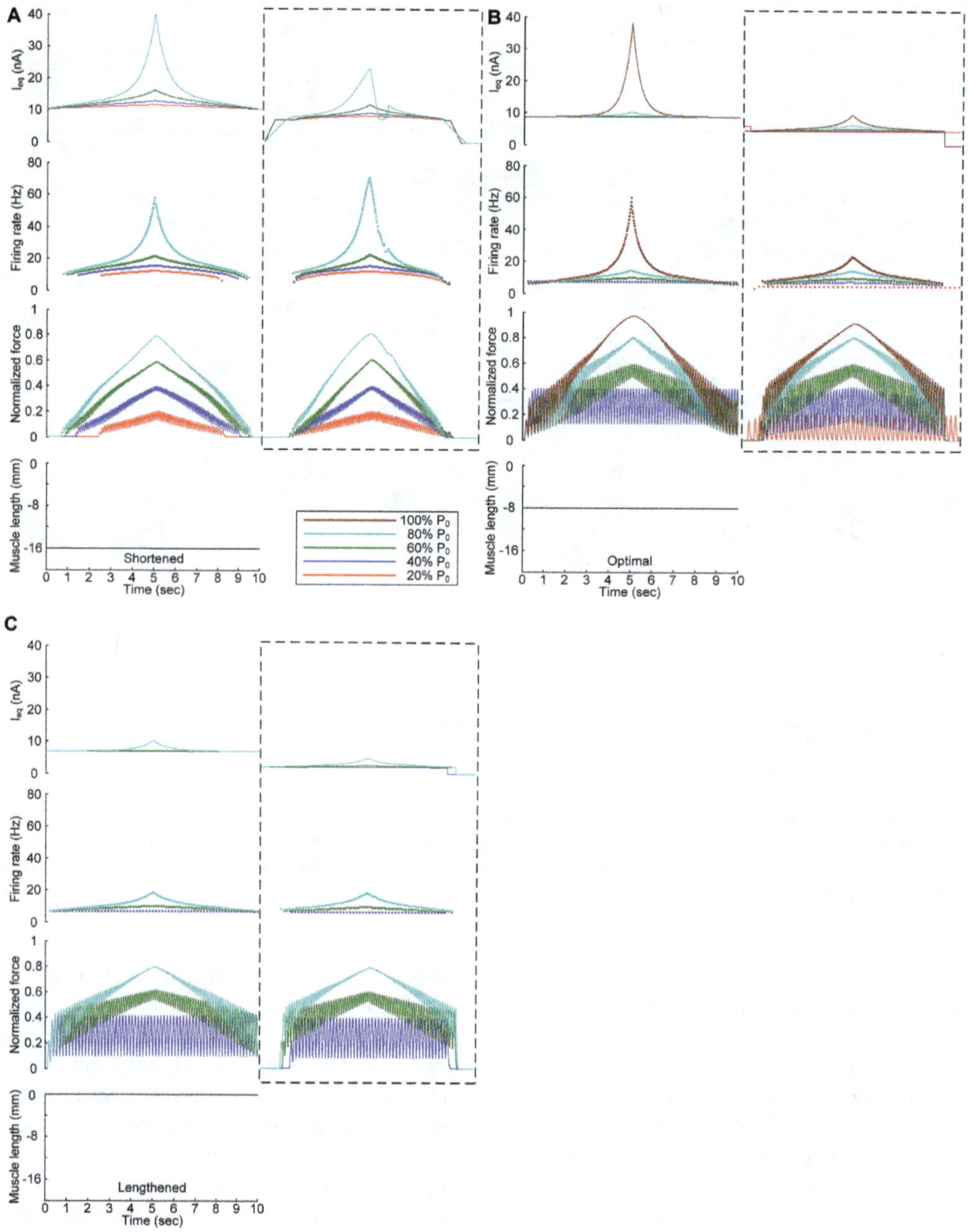

FIGURE 5 | Influence of the PIC on the stimulation waveforms under the continuous conditions. Intensities of continuous current stimulation (I_{eq}) applied to the somatic compartment (*top*), instantaneous firing rate (*upper middle*) in the motoneuron, and normalized muscle force (*lower middle*) generated by the muscle unit at the three muscle lengths (*bottom*): physiologically minimum **(A)**, optimal **(B)**, and maximum muscle lengths **(C)**. The level of force production produced by the motor unit is denoted as a percentage of the maximal isometric force (P_0) at the optimal muscle length and indicated with different colors. The dashed-line rectangles indicate the simulation results with the motoneuron PIC channels, as shown in **Figure 3**, for the purpose of comparison.

Influence of the PICs Over the Motoneuron Dendrites on the Stimulation Waveforms

We further investigated the influence of the PIC channels responsible for the plateau potentials over the motoneuron dendrites on the stimulation waveforms required for force control. To this end, we compared the stimulation waveforms obtained with and without PIC channels over the dendritic compartment of the motoneuron model, as shown in **Figures 3, 4**, respectively. **Figure 5** shows the stimulation waveforms under continuous stimulation conditions without PIC channels over the motoneuron. Overall, the current stimulation amplitude increased to compensate for the lack of an intrinsic PIC current in the motoneuron when the motoneuron PICs were excluded at all muscle lengths. In contrast to the case involving PIC channels

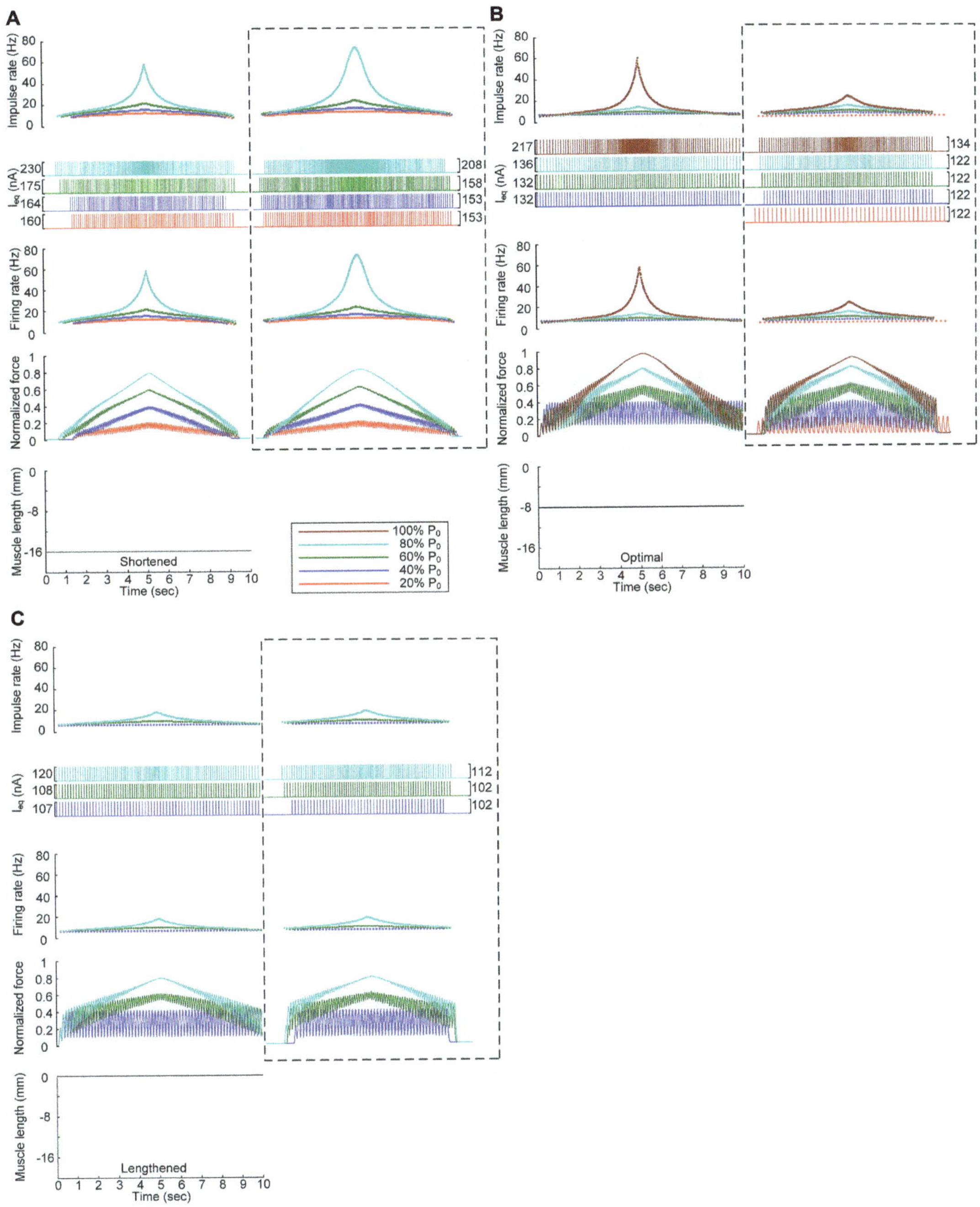

FIGURE 6 | Influence of the PIC on the stimulation waveforms under discrete conditions. Frequency and amplitude (two *top panels*) of impulse current stimulation (I_{eq}) applied to the somatic compartment, instantaneous firing rate (*upper middle*) in the motoneuron, and normalized muscle force (*lower middle*) produced by the muscle unit at the three muscle lengths (*bottom*): physiologically minimum **(A)**, optimal **(B)**, and maximum muscle lengths **(C)**. The level of force production by the motor unit is denoted as a percentage of the maximal isometric force (P_0) at the optimal muscle length and indicated with different colors. The dashed-line rectangles indicate the simulation results with the motoneuron PIC channels, as shown in **Figure 4**, for the purpose of comparison.

over the motoneuron dendrite (please refer to the dashed-line boxes in **Figure 5**), the stimulation waveforms were symmetric between the ascending and descending force production phases at all muscle lengths (**Figure 5A**). Notably, the model motor unit without PIC channels over the motoneuron fully reached the maximal force level at the optimal muscle length during linear force development (**Figure 5B**). However, the force level of 20% of P_0 was unattainable because of the increase in the recruitment threshold and firing rate in the absence of motoneuron PIC channels (**Figure 5B**).

The comparison analysis results revealed the causal relationship of PIC saturation over the motoneuron dendrites

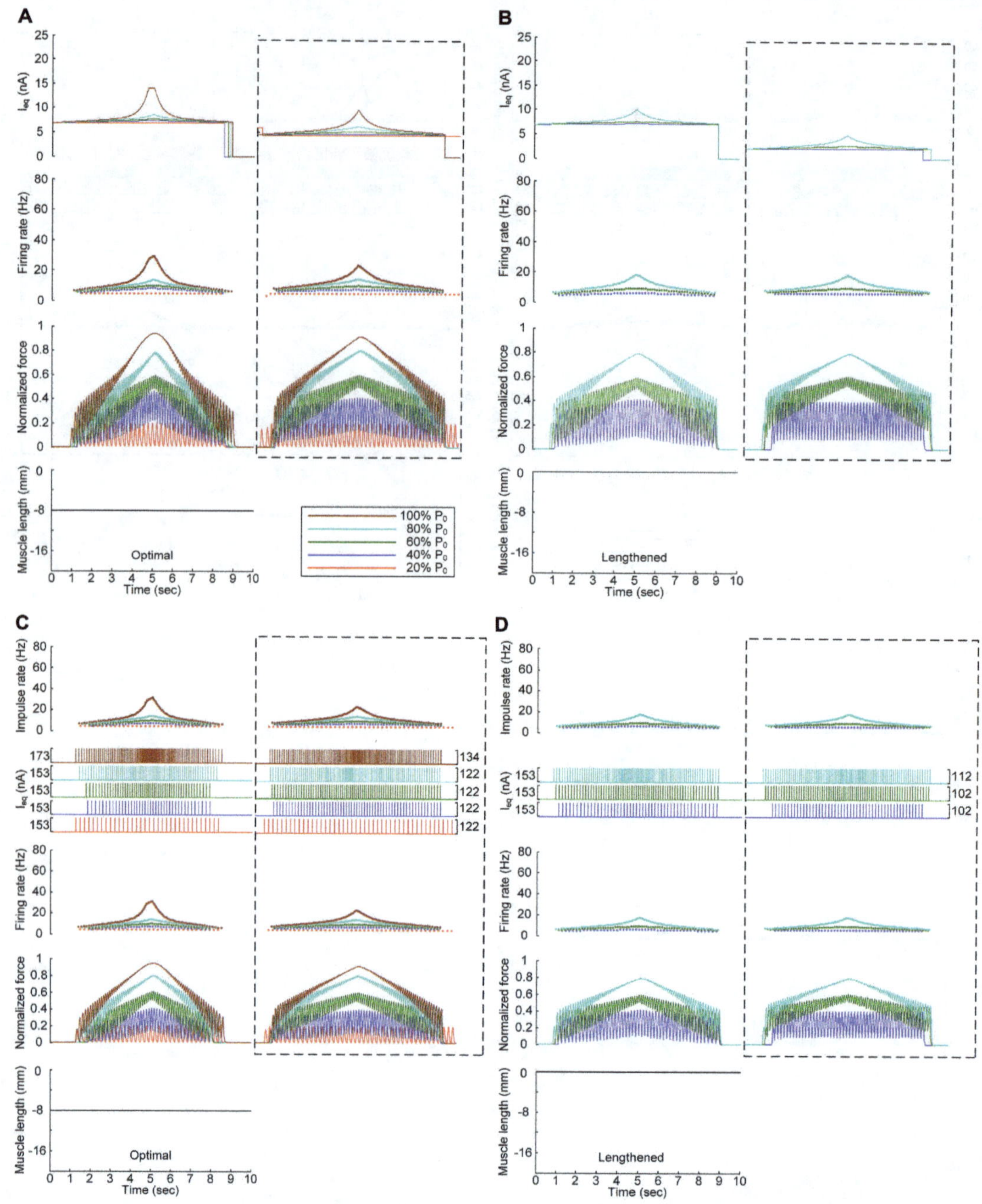

FIGURE 7 | Influence of muscle spindle feedback on the stimulation waveforms. **(A,B)** Intensities of continuous current stimulation (I_{eq}) applied to the somatic compartment (*top*), instantaneous firing rate (*upper middle*) in the motoneuron, and normalized muscle force (*lower middle*) produced by the muscle unit at the two muscle lengths (*bottom*): physiologically optimal and maximum muscle lengths. **(C,D)** Frequency and amplitude (two *top panels*) of impulse current stimulation (I_{eq}) applied to the somatic compartment, instantaneous firing rate (*upper middle*) in the motoneuron, and normalized muscle force (*lower middle*) generated by the muscle unit at the two muscle lengths (*bottom*): physiologically optimal and maximum muscle lengths. The level of force production produced by the motor unit is denoted as a percentage of the maximal isometric force (P_0) at the optimal muscle length and indicated with different colors. The dashed-line rectangles indicate the simulation results with the motoneuron PIC channels, as shown in **Figures 3**, **4** for the purpose of comparison.

and the current intensity limitation and stimulation waveform disruption observed under continuous stimulation conditions.

Figure 6 shows the stimulation waveforms under discrete stimulation conditions without PIC channels over the motoneuron dendrites. Overall, the stimulation waveforms were comparable to those in the case with PIC channels over the motoneuron dendrites. The stimulation rate first exponentially increased and then decreased during linear force development and relaxation within the full range (i.e., from 20 to 100% of P_0). However, the amplitude of the current impulses increased

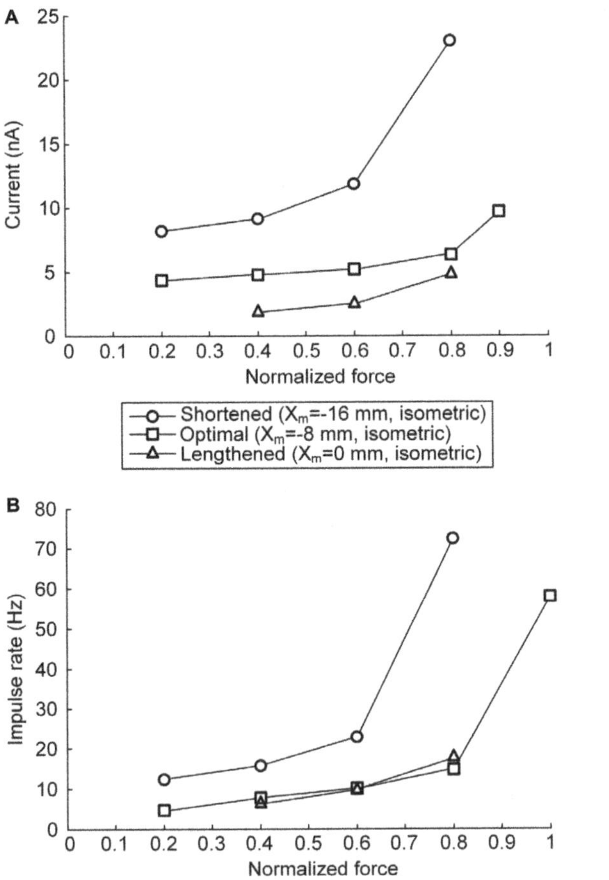

FIGURE 8 | Relationship between current stimulation and force genesis at the various muscle lengths. **(A)** Peak current amplitude eliciting the peak force during triangular force production under continuous stimulation conditions. **(B)** Peak impulse frequency eliciting the peak force during triangular force production under discrete stimulation conditions. The peak force is normalized based on the maximal force isometrically produced at the optimal muscle length. The three symbols (circles, squares, and triangles) indicate the physiological minimal (X_m = −16 mm), optimal (X_m = −8 mm), and maximal (X_m = 0 mm) muscle lengths, respectively.

to compensate for the absence of an intrinsic PIC current in the motoneuron. The amplitude increment increased with increasing force level at all muscle lengths (please refer to the dashed-line boxes in **Figure 6** representing the PIC activation case). It should be noted that under discrete current stimulation, the model motor unit produced 20% of P_0 (**Supplementary File 5**), in addition to the maximal force at the optimal muscle length in the absence of PIC channels over the motoneuron dendrites.

These results reinforce the robustness of discrete stimulation under short-width current pulses for muscle force control purposes regardless of the presence of PICs over the motoneuron dendrites.

Influence of the Muscle Afferent Inputs on the Stimulation Waveforms

We also assessed the influence of muscle afferent feedback on the stimulation waveforms for force speed and magnitude control purposes. **Figure 7** shows the stimulation waveforms estimated with and without muscle afferent inputs over the motoneuron model, as shown in **Figures 3, 4**, respectively. Under both continuous and discrete stimulation conditions, the current stimulation amplitude increased to compensate for the lack of muscle afferent inputs to the motoneuron at the optimal and lengthened muscle lengths. In addition, the peak current intensity under continuous current stimulation conditions was relatively high to prevent the full activation of the PIC channels over the motoneuron in the ascending force production phase. This result could be explained by the absence of muscle afferent-mediated facilitation of PIC activation over the motoneuron dendrites (**Figure 2A**). However, the model motor unit without muscle afferent feedback did not fully reach the maximal force level at the optimal muscle length under continuous motoneuron current stimulation conditions (**Figure 7A**). Importantly, in the case of discrete current stimulation, the stimulus rate increased until the maximal force level was reached without the full activation of motoneuron PIC channels (**Supplementary File 6**).

The comparison analysis results indicate that muscle afferent feedback may exacerbate the limitation of the current intensity to prevent full PIC activation during continuous stimulation, and this limitation may also be avoided under discrete stimulation conditions with short-width current pulses.

DISCUSSION

We estimated the waveforms under extracellular microstimulation near the initial segment and cell body of a spinal motoneuron that control the speed and level of force production by the motor unit during isometric contraction at the various muscle lengths. In terms of both the continuous and discrete stimulation types, the non-linearity of the stimulation waveform systematically increased with increasing force speed and level and with decreasing muscle length. Furthermore, the presence of neuromodulatory inputs from the brainstem and afferent feedback originating from the muscle spindle reduced the current stimulation intensity for linear force production. These results may provide a template for the design of stimulation waveforms under varying force profile, muscle length, and neuromodulation conditions.

Continuous Versus Discrete Stimulation Protocols

The non-linearity of the stimulation waveform was assessed by evaluating the difference between the areas under the linear and stimulation curves, i.e., between the lowest and highest points of the stimulation curve (Emancipator and Kroll, 1993). In the present study, the variation in the non-linearity of the stimulation waveform was approximated as the variation in the highest point of the stimulation curve because the lowest point of the stimulation curve remained similar at all produced force levels during isometric contraction at a specific muscle length. Under both the continuous and discrete stimulation protocols, the non-linearity of the current stimulation waveform substantially increased during linear force generation, particularly higher than

60% of the maximal isometric force (i.e., P_0) at shorter-than-optimal muscle lengths (**Figure 8**). In addition, the current amplitude increased in the absence of motoneuron PIC channels (please refer to **Figures 5, 6**) and muscle afferent inputs (**Figure 7**), indicating the influence of neuromodulation from the brainstem and sensory feedback originating from the muscle on the current stimulation pattern.

The non-linear current stimulation waveforms at the soma of the motoneuron were captured with an exponential function within a broad range of speeds and force production levels at muscle lengths larger than the optimal length (**Table 1**). In terms of the shortened muscles, however, the stimulation waveforms were considerably distorted to prevent the saturation of motoneuron PICs to achieve linear force relaxation in the descending stimulation phase under continuous stimulation conditions (see **Figure 3A**). Furthermore, the model motor unit did not fully reach the maximum force at the optimal muscle length without full PIC activation over the motoneuron dendrites in the ascending phase under continuous stimulation (**Figure 8A**). In contrast, the model motor unit reached all force levels within the full physiological range of the muscle length under discrete stimulation conditions (**Figure 8B**). This result indicates that at a high level of force generation, continuous current stimulation may sufficiently depolarize the membrane potential of the motoneuron dendrites to fully activate the dendritic PIC channels. However, the activation kinetics of dendritic PIC channels have been reported to be slow (i.e., ~60 ms) (Carlin et al., 2000). Furthermore, attenuation of the alternating electrical signals tends to be much more severe than that of the direct electrical signals when propagating to the distal dendritic areas in the motoneuron (Kim and Jones, 2012). Thus, discrete current stimulation with a small pulse width (i.e., 0.5 ms) may effectively control the firing output of the motoneuron, thus avoiding the full activation of PIC channels over the motoneuron dendrites.

To this end, under the various conditions of brainstem neuromodulation and muscle length, the discrete stimulation protocol is more suitable than the continuous stimulation protocol for the precise modulation of the muscle force at the motor unit level.

Comparison to Previous Studies

The motor unit model considered in the present study accurately replicated the non-linear input–output relationship of the motoneuron and muscle unit, as separately investigated in previous experimental studies. The motoneuron model captured the acceleration in firing rate above the recruitment threshold in the ascending phase and the persistence of firing below the recruitment threshold in the descending phase during triangular current injection at the soma in the presence of monoamines (Lee and Heckman, 1998a, 1999). The muscle unit model also reproduced the sigmoidal force production in response to a linear increase and decrease in the stimulation frequency, as experimentally reported in previous studies (Rack and Westbury, 1969; Mrowczynski et al., 2006). The muscle length dependence of the non-linear behavior of the motoneuron and muscle fibers is consistent with the results obtained in a previous computational study involving an anatomically realistic model of the spinal motoneuron (Kim, 2017). Thus, the model motor unit constructed in the PyMUS software environment in this study may provide an efficient computational platform for the estimation of the stimulation waveforms required for force control at the motor unit level under a wide range of physiological conditions, including neuromodulation from the brainstem and sensory feedback originating from the muscle spindle.

To our knowledge, the waveform under intraspinal microstimulation has not yet been systematically investigated for muscle force control under various force profile and muscle length conditions. Seminal work has demonstrated, based on both extracellular and intracellular microelectrodes, that spinal motoneurons may be directly activated at the lowest threshold with a stimulating electrode near the initial segment (Gustafsson and Jankowska, 1976). Recently, a field model of the spinal cord coupled with realistic motoneuron models has been analyzed, suggesting that local cells may be selectively activated without activation of bypassing nerve fibers through asymmetric modulation of the duration and amplitude of the cathodic and anodic phases of the biphasic stimulus current pulse (McIntyre and Grill, 2002). This form of the stimulus current pulse may be applied to the discrete stimulation waveforms estimated in this study to improve the selectivity of the target motoneuron. In addition, the previous study has revealed that the stimulus amplitude must be increased to elicit firing in a one-to-one manner at high stimulation frequencies (McIntyre and Grill, 2002). This phenomenon was also observed in the current study with increasing force level (**Figure 4**). Furthermore, the motoneuronal output during extracellular microstimulation near the cell body has been evaluated with respect to several factors, including the dendritic active conductance and synaptic contact. The previous analysis has suggested that dendritic active conductance and synaptic contact activation may reduce the current threshold for firing initiation with little effect on the motoneuronal output (McIntyre and Grill, 2002). These results are consistent with those obtained in the present study. The amplitude of the current pulses was lowered with PIC activation over the motoneuron dendrites (**Figure 6**). The influence of synaptic activation was evaluated by increasing the excitatory synaptic conductance over the somatic compartment of the reduced motoneuron. This increase in the excitatory synaptic conductance reduced the amplitude of the current impulses with little difference observed between the stimulation waveforms (not shown).

The present study was conducted in regard to the direct activation of a spinal motoneuron *via* a microelectrode placed near the initial segment and cell body (Gustafsson and Jankowska, 1976). In contrast, indirect transsynaptic activation of the motoneuron has been verified to mostly occur when the microelectrode is located in dendritic regions likely including PIC channels (Gustafsson and Jankowska, 1976). The aforementioned dendritic location of the excitatory synaptic contacts may greatly facilitate the saturation of dendritic PIC channels, resulting in non-responsiveness of the dendrites to synaptic activation at a low force production level (Heckman et al., 2008). Thus, the effective type and waveform required for extracellular microstimulation might differ in the case of transsynaptic activation of the motoneuron and should be further investigated considering the addition of an additional excitatory synaptic conductance to the dendritic compartment of the reduced motoneuron model constructed in this study.

With the above considerations, the present study extends previous investigations by proposing the effective type (i.e., discrete) and waveform (i.e., exponential) of current stimulation for spinal motoneurons that may lead to the precise control of force production at the motor unit level.

Potential Contributions to Spinal Cord Modulation

Spinal cord stimulation has been applied to effectively restore complex motor functions through the modulation of neuronal networks in the spinal cord (Harkema et al., 2011; Megia Garcia et al., 2020). Intraspinal microstimulation with a multielectrode array may represent an efficient technique to stimulate and modulate the motor output of targeted motor units for the precise control of muscle forces and voluntary movements. From this perspective, this study may provide a basis to design the type and waveform of current stimulation for the precise control of voluntary muscle contractions. The predictions obtained in this study may be testable with recently developed experimental techniques. The force output of a single motor unit in response to current stimulation intracellularly injected at the soma of a spinal motoneuron has been characterized *via in vivo* mouse preparation (Manuel and Heckman, 2011). In addition, the multielectrode array interface developed for spinal cord stimulation (Meacham et al., 2011) and nerve cuff and flexible split ring electrode developed for selective stimulation of the motor nerve (Deurloo et al., 2003; Lee et al., 2017) could also be employed to test the stimulation waveforms required for force control predicted at the motor unit level in the present study. It should be noted that further analysis is needed for the indirect control of spinal motoneurons through current stimulation *via* the skin on the back (Gogeascoechea et al., 2020) or the epidural portion (Ahmed, 2016) of the spinal cord, which typically involves a variety of interneurons and afferents.

Modeling Considerations

The fundamental limitations of the reduced modeling approach of spinal motoneurons and muscle fibers have been fully addressed in previous studies (Kim et al., 2014, 2015). To estimate the stimulation pattern more physiologically, several issues should be resolved by improving the current motor unit model in future studies. First, the influence of the dendritic structure and PIC distribution on the motoneuron output should be reflected in the prediction of the stimulation pattern under pathological conditions (Elbasiouny et al., 2010). Second, the active membrane mechanisms over the dendrites of spinal motoneurons should be considered in detail, including calcium-activated potassium currents (Li and Bennett, 2007) and hyperpolarization-activated cation channels (Manuel et al., 2007). Third, the present study was conducted particularly considering slow fatigue-resistible motor units. To evaluate other types of motor units, such as fast fatigable motor units, the stimulation waveforms estimated in this study should be adjusted considering the discrepancy in electrical and mechanical properties, particularly in regard to the somatic input resistance, system time constant, rheobase current, afterhyperpolarization potential, and PIC dynamics in spinal motoneurons (Lee and Heckman, 1999; Heckman and Enoka, 2012), twitch rate and amplitude, progressive force reduction phenomenon (i.e., the sag observed over short contraction time <2 s and fatigue over a long contraction time >2 min), and length- and velocity-tension properties of muscle fibers (Brown et al., 1999; Burke, 2011). Fourth, the present study did not consider the shape of the current pulse (Anderson et al., 2019). Thus, the waveforms predicted in the current study might vary according to the shape of the current pulse. Finally, further investigation is required in terms of the stimulation waveforms to control the force production with the whole muscle, considering the organization of spinal motoneurons exhibiting different anatomical and electrical properties (Zengel et al., 1985; Capogrosso et al., 2013). In addition, the influence of spinal interneurons and peripheral afferents should be considered, particularly in the case of skin or epidural stimulation of the spinal cord (Harkema et al., 2011; Takei and Seki, 2013; Gogeascoechea et al., 2020).

Concluding Remarks

In principle, the waveform obtained with a microelectrode near the motoneuron cell body to realize isometric force control of the motor unit strongly depends on the stimulation type, neuromodulatory input, and muscle length. Compared to continuous current stimulation, discrete current stimulation more suitably prevents the non-linearities induced by the full activation of PIC-generating channels over the motoneuron dendrites, including muscle spindle feedback. Thus, motor unit function modulation may be more effectively achieved by stimulating spinal motoneurons with short-width current pulses. The model-based approach and waveform equations developed in the present study may provide a basis for the design of stimulation patterns applicable to spinal motoneurons to better understand neuromuscular physiology and neuromodulation of movement disorders *via* a neural interface.

AUTHOR CONTRIBUTIONS

HK conceived and designed the study and wrote the manuscript. YJ and HK performed the simulations and analyzed the data. Both authors contributed to the article and approved the submitted version.

ACKNOWLEDGMENTS

The authors thank Minjung Kim for her help with updating the PyMUS software for this study.

SUPPLEMENTARY MATERIAL

Supplementary File 1 | Equations and descriptions of the model motor unit.

Supplementary File 2 | Computer codes of the models and simulations.

Supplementary File 3 | Dataset of the current stimulation levels applied to the motoneuron for force production of the muscle unit at the various speeds and levels, as shown in **Figures 3–7**.

Supplementary File 4 | Production of 100% of the maximal force by the model motor unit, as shown in **Figure 4**, at the optimal muscle length under discrete current stimulation.

Supplementary File 5 | Production of 20% of the maximal force by the model motor unit, as shown in **Figure 6**, at the optimal muscle length under discrete current stimulation conditions.

Supplementary File 6 | Production of 100% of the maximal force by the model motor unit, as shown in **Figure 7**, at the optimal muscle length under discrete current stimulation conditions.

REFERENCES

Ahmed, Z. (2016). Modulation of gamma and alpha spinal motor neurons activity by trans-spinal direct current stimulation: effects on reflexive actions and locomotor activity. *Physiol. Rep.* 4:e12696. doi: 10.14814/phy2.12696

Anderson, D. J., Kipke, D. R., Nagel, S. J., Lempka, S. F., Machado, A. G., Holland, M. T., et al. (2019). Intradural spinal cord stimulation: performance modeling of a new modality. *Front. Neurosci.* 13:253. doi: 10.3389/fnins.2019.00253

Booth, V., Rinzel, J., and Kiehn, O. (1997). Compartmental model of vertebrate motoneurons for Ca2+-dependent spiking and plateau potentials under pharmacological treatment. *J. Neurophysiol.* 78, 3371–3385. doi: 10.1152/jn.1997.78.6.3371

Brown, I. E., Cheng, E. J., and Loeb, G. E. (1999). Measured and modeled properties of mammalian skeletal muscle. II. The effects of stimulus frequency on force-length and force-velocity relationships. *J. Muscle Res. Cell Motil.* 20, 627–643.

Burke, R. E. (2011). *Motor Units: Anatomy, Physiology, and Functional Organization. Comprehensive Physiology.* Hoboken, NJ: John Wiley & Sons, Inc.

Capogrosso, M., Wenger, N., Raspopovic, S., Musienko, P., Beauparlant, J., Bassi Luciani, L., et al. (2013). A computational model for epidural electrical stimulation of spinal sensorimotor circuits. *J. Neurosci.* 33, 19326–19340. doi: 10.1523/jneurosci.1688-13.2013

Carlin, K. P., Jones, K. E., Jiang, Z., Jordan, L. M., and Brownstone, R. M. (2000). Dendritic L-type calcium currents in mouse spinal motoneurons: implications for bistability. *Eur. J. Neurosci.* 12, 1635–1646. doi: 10.1046/j.1460-9568.2000.00055.x

Deurloo, K. E., Holsheimer, J., and Bergveld, P. (2003). Fascicular selectivity in transverse stimulation with a nerve cuff electrode: a theoretical approach. *Neuromodulation* 6, 258–269. doi: 10.1046/j.1525-1403.2003.03034.x

Elbasiouny, S. M., Amendola, J., Durand, J., and Heckman, C. J. (2010). Evidence from computer simulations for alterations in the membrane biophysical properties and dendritic processing of synaptic inputs in mutant superoxide dismutase-1 motoneurons. *J. Neurosci.* 30, 5544–5558. doi: 10.1523/jneurosci.0434-10.2010

Emancipator, K., and Kroll, M. H. (1993). A quantitative measure of nonlinearity. *Clin. Chem.* 39, 766–772. doi: 10.1093/clinchem/39.5.766

Gogeascoechea, A., Kuck, A., van Asseldonk, E., Negro, F., Buitenweg, J. R., Yavuz, U. S., et al. (2020). Interfacing with alpha motor neurons in spinal cord injury patients receiving trans-spinal electrical stimulation. *Front. Neurol.* 11:493. doi: 10.3389/fneur.2020.00493

Goslow, G. E. Jr., Reinking, R. M., and Stuart, D. G. (1973). The cat step cycle: hind limb joint angles and muscle lengths during unrestrained locomotion. *J. Morphol.* 141, 1–41. doi: 10.1002/jmor.1051410102

Gustafsson, B., and Jankowska, E. (1976). Direct and indirect activation of nerve cells by electrical pulses applied extracellularly. *J. Physiol.* 258, 33–61. doi: 10.1113/jphysiol.1976.sp011405

Harkema, S., Gerasimenko, Y., Hodes, J., Burdick, J., Angeli, C., Chen, Y., et al. (2011). Effect of epidural stimulation of the lumbosacral spinal cord on voluntary movement, standing, and assisted stepping after motor complete paraplegia: a case study. *Lancet* 377, 1938–1947. doi: 10.1016/s0140-6736(11)60547-3

Heckman, C. J., and Enoka, R. M. (2012). Motor unit. *Compr. Physiol.* 2, 2629–2682.

Heckman, C. J., Hyngstrom, A. S., and Johnson, M. D. (2008). Active properties of motoneurone dendrites: diffuse descending neuromodulation, focused local inhibition. *J. Physiol.* 586, 1225–1231. doi: 10.1113/jphysiol.2007.145078

Heckman, C. J., Lee, R. H., and Brownstone, R. M. (2003). Hyperexcitable dendrites in motoneurons and their neuromodulatory control during motor behavior. *Trends Neurosci.* 26, 688–695. doi: 10.1016/j.tins.2003.10.002

Heckmann, C. J., Gorassini, M. A., and Bennett, D. J. (2005). Persistent inward currents in motoneuron dendrites: implications for motor output. *Muscle Nerve* 31, 135–156. doi: 10.1002/mus.20261

Hochman, S., and McCrea, D. A. (1994). Effects of chronic spinalization on ankle extensor motoneurons. II. Motoneuron electrical properties. *J. Neurophysiol.* 71, 1468–1479. doi: 10.1152/jn.1994.71.4.1468

Holsheimer, J. (1998). Concepts and methods in neuromodulation and functional electrical stimulation: an introduction. *Neuromodulation* 1, 57–61. doi: 10.1111/j.1525-1403.1998.tb00018.x

Hornby, T. G., McDonagh, J. C., Reinking, R. M., and Stuart, D. G. (2002). Motoneurons: a preferred firing range across vertebrate species? *Muscle Nerve* 25, 632–648. doi: 10.1002/mus.10105

Hounsgaard, J., Hultborn, H., Jespersen, B., and Kiehn, O. (1984). Intrinsic membrane properties causing a bistable behaviour of alpha-motoneurones. *Exp. Brain Res.* 55, 391–394.

Hounsgaard, J., Hultborn, H., Jespersen, B., and Kiehn, O. (1988). Bistability of alpha-motoneurones in the decerebrate cat and in the acute spinal cat after intravenous 5-hydroxytryptophan. *J. Physiol.* 405, 345–367. doi: 10.1113/jphysiol.1988.sp017336

Kim, H. (2017). Muscle length-dependent contribution of motoneuron Cav1.3 channels to force production in model slow motor unit. *J. Appl. Physiol.* 123, 88–105. doi: 10.1152/japplphysiol.00491.2016

Kim, H., and Jones, K. E. (2012). The retrograde frequency response of passive dendritic trees constrains the nonlinear firing behaviour of a reduced neuron model. *PLoS One* 7:e43654. doi: 10.1371/journal.pone.0043654

Kim, H., Jones, K. E., and Heckman, C. J. (2014). Asymmetry in signal propagation between the soma and dendrites plays a key role in determining dendritic excitability in motoneurons. *PLoS One* 9:e95454. doi: 10.1371/journal.pone.0095454

Kim, H., and Kim, M. (2018). PyMUS: python-based simulation software for virtual experiments on motor unit system. *Front. Neuroinform.* 12:15. doi: 10.3389/fninf.2018.00015

Kim, H., Sandercock, T. G., and Heckman, C. J. (2015). An action potential-driven model of soleus muscle activation dynamics for locomotor-like movements. *J. Neural. Eng.* 12:046025. doi: 10.1088/1741-2560/12/4/046025

Lee, R. H., and Heckman, C. J. (1998b). Bistability in spinal motoneurons in vivo: systematic variations in rhythmic firing patterns. *J. Neurophysiol.* 80, 572–582. doi: 10.1152/jn.1998.80.2.572

Lee, R. H., and Heckman, C. J. (1998a). Bistability in spinal motoneurons in vivo: systematic variations in persistent inward currents. *J. Neurophysiol.* 80, 583–593. doi: 10.1152/jn.1998.80.2.583

Lee, R. H., and Heckman, C. J. (1999). Paradoxical effect of QX-314 on persistent inward currents and bistable behavior in spinal motoneurons in vivo. *J. Neurophysiol.* 82, 2518–2527. doi: 10.1152/jn.1999.82.5.2518

Lee, R. H., Kuo, J. J., Jiang, M. C., and Heckman, C. J. (2003). Influence of active dendritic currents on input-output processing in spinal motoneurons in vivo. *J. Neurophysiol.* 89, 27–39. doi: 10.1152/jn.00137.2002

Lee, S., Sheshadri, S., Xiang, Z. L., Delgado-Martinez, I., Xue, N., Sun, T., et al. (2017). Selective stimulation and neural recording on peripheral nerves using flexible split ring electrodes. *Sens. Actuators B Chem.* 242, 1165–1170. doi: 10.1016/j.snb.2016.09.127

Li, X., and Bennett, D. J. (2007). Apamin-sensitive calcium-activated potassium currents (SK) are activated by persistent calcium currents in rat motoneurons. *J. Neurophysiol.* 97, 3314–3330. doi: 10.1152/jn.01068.2006

Manuel, M., and Heckman, C. J. (2011). Adult mouse motor units develop almost all of their force in the subprimary range: a new all-or-none strategy for force recruitment? *J. Neurosci.* 31, 15188–15194.

Manuel, M., Meunier, C., Donnet, M., and Zytnicki, D. (2007). Resonant or not, two amplification modes of proprioceptive inputs by persistent inward currents in spinal motoneurons. *J. Neurosci.* 27, 12977–12988. doi: 10.1523/jneurosci.3299-07.2007

McIntyre, C. C., and Grill, W. M. (2000). Selective microstimulation of central nervous system neurons. *Ann. Biomed. Eng.* 28, 219–233. doi: 10.1114/1.262

McIntyre, C. C., and Grill, W. M. (2002). Extracellular stimulation of central neurons: influence of stimulus waveform and frequency on neuronal output. *J. Neurophysiol.* 88, 1592–1604. doi: 10.1152/jn.2002.88.4.1592

Meacham, K. W., Guo, L., Deweerth, S. P., and Hochman, S. (2011). Selective stimulation of the spinal cord surface using a stretchable microelectrode array. *Front. Neuroeng.* 4:5. doi: 10.3389/fneng.2011.00005

Megia Garcia, A., Serrano-Munoz, D., Taylor, J., Avendano-Coy, J., and Gomez-Soriano, J. (2020). Transcutaneous spinal cord stimulation and motor rehabilitation in spinal cord injury: a systematic review. *Neurorehabil. Neural Repair* 34, 3–12.

Mrowczynski, W., Celichowski, J., and Krutki, P. (2006). Interspecies differences in the force-frequency relationship of the medial gastrocnemius motor units. *J. Physiol. Pharmacol.* 57, 491–501.

Mushahwar, V. K., and Horch, K. W. (1998). Selective activation and graded recruitment of functional muscle groups through spinal cord stimulation. *Ann. N. Y. Acad. Sci.* 860, 531–535. doi: 10.1111/j.1749-6632.1998.tb09096.x

Perreault, E. J., Heckman, C. J., and Sandercock, T. G. (2003). Hill muscle model errors during movement are greatest within the physiologically relevant range of motor unit firing rates. *J. Biomech.* 36, 211–218. doi: 10.1016/s0021-9290(02)00332-9

Rack, P. M., and Westbury, D. R. (1969). The effects of length and stimulus rate on tension in the isometric cat soleus muscle. *J. Physiol.* 204, 443–460. doi: 10.1113/jphysiol.1969.sp008923

Radivojevic, M., Jackel, D., Altermatt, M., Muller, J., Viswam, V., Hierlemann, A., et al. (2016). Electrical identification and selective microstimulation of neuronal compartments based on features of extracellular action potentials. *Sci. Rep.* 6:31332.

Sandercock, T. G., and Heckman, C. J. (1997). Force from cat soleus muscle during imposed locomotor-like movements: experimental data versus Hill-type model predictions. *J. Neurophysiol.* 77, 1538–1552. doi: 10.1152/jn.1997.77.3.1538

Scott, S. H., Brown, I. E., and Loeb, G. E. (1996). Mechanics of feline soleus: I. Effect of fascicle length and velocity on force output. *J. Muscle Res. Cell Motil.* 17, 207–219. doi: 10.1007/bf00124243

Segev, I., Fleshman, J. W. Jr., and Burke, R. E. (1990). Computer simulation of group Ia EPSPs using morphologically realistic models of cat alpha-motoneurons. *J. Neurophysiol.* 64, 648–660. doi: 10.1152/jn.1990.64.2.648

Shames, D. M., Baker, A. J., Weiner, M. W., and Camacho, S. A. (1996). Ca(2+)-force relationship of frog skeletal muscle: a dynamic model for parameter estimation. *Am. J. Physiol.* 271(6 Pt 1), C2062–C2071.

Spruston, N., Jaffe, D. B., and Johnston, D. (1994). Dendritic attenuation of synaptic potentials and currents: the role of passive membrane properties. *Trends Neurosci.* 17, 161–166. doi: 10.1016/0166-2236(94)90094-9

Sunshine, M. D., Cho, F. S., Lockwood, D. R., Fechko, A. S., Kasten, M. R., and Moritz, C. T. (2013). Cervical intraspinal microstimulation evokes robust forelimb movements before and after injury. *J. Neural Eng.* 10:036001. doi: 10.1088/1741-2560/10/3/036001

Sunshine, M. D., Ganji, C. N., Reier, P. J., Fuller, D. D., and Moritz, C. T. (2018). Intraspinal microstimulation for respiratory muscle activation. *Exp. Neurol.* 302, 93–103. doi: 10.1016/j.expneurol.2017.12.014

Takei, T., and Seki, K. (2013). Spinal premotor interneurons mediate dynamic and static motor commands for precision grip in monkeys. *J. Neurosci.* 33, 8850–8860. doi: 10.1523/jneurosci.4032-12.2013

Wagner, F. B., Mignardot, J. B., Le Goff-Mignardot, C. G., Demesmaeker, R., Komi, S., Capogrosso, M., et al. (2018). Targeted neurotechnology restores walking in humans with spinal cord injury. *Nature* 563, 65–71.

Wang, Q., Millard, D. C., Zheng, H. J., and Stanley, G. B. (2012). Voltage-sensitive dye imaging reveals improved topographic activation of cortex in response to manipulation of thalamic microstimulation parameters. *J. Neural Eng.* 9:026008. doi: 10.1088/1741-2560/9/2/026008

Warman, E. N., Grill, W. M., and Durand, D. (1992). Modeling the effects of electric fields on nerve fibers: determination of excitation thresholds. *IEEE Trans. Biomed. Eng.* 39, 1244–1254. doi: 10.1109/10.184700

Westerblad, H., and Allen, D. G. (1994). The role of sarcoplasmic reticulum in relaxation of mouse muscle; effects of 2,5-di(tert-butyl)-1,4-benzohydroquinone. *J. Physiol.* 474, 291–301. doi: 10.1113/jphysiol.1994.sp020022

Winters, T. M., Takahashi, M., Lieber, R. L., and Ward, S. R. (2011). Whole muscle length-tension relationships are accurately modeled as scaled sarcomeres in rabbit hindlimb muscles. *J. Biomech.* 44, 109–115. doi: 10.1016/j.jbiomech.2010.08.033

Zengel, J. E., Reid, S. A., Sypert, G. W., and Munson, J. B. (1985). Membrane electrical properties and prediction of motor-unit type of medial gastrocnemius motoneurons in the cat. *J. Neurophysiol.* 53, 1323–1344. doi: 10.1152/jn.1985.53.5.1323

Permissions

All chapters in this book were first published by Frontiers; hereby published with permission under the Creative Commons Attribution License or equivalent. Every chapter published in this book has been scrutinized by our experts. Their significance has been extensively debated. The topics covered herein carry significant findings which will fuel the growth of the discipline. They may even be implemented as practical applications or may be referred to as a beginning point for another development.

The contributors of this book come from diverse backgrounds, making this book a truly international effort. This book will bring forth new frontiers with its revolutionizing research information and detailed analysis of the nascent developments around the world.

We would like to thank all the contributing authors for lending their expertise to make the book truly unique. They have played a crucial role in the development of this book. Without their invaluable contributions this book wouldn't have been possible. They have made vital efforts to compile up to date information on the varied aspects of this subject to make this book a valuable addition to the collection of many professionals and students.

This book was conceptualized with the vision of imparting up-to-date information and advanced data in this field. To ensure the same, a matchless editorial board was set up. Every individual on the board went through rigorous rounds of assessment to prove their worth. After which they invested a large part of their time researching and compiling the most relevant data for our readers.

The editorial board has been involved in producing this book since its inception. They have spent rigorous hours researching and exploring the diverse topics which have resulted in the successful publishing of this book. They have passed on their knowledge of decades through this book. To expedite this challenging task, the publisher supported the team at every step. A small team of assistant editors was also appointed to further simplify the editing procedure and attain best results for the readers.

Apart from the editorial board, the designing team has also invested a significant amount of their time in understanding the subject and creating the most relevant covers. They scrutinized every image to scout for the most suitable representation of the subject and create an appropriate cover for the book.

The publishing team has been an ardent support to the editorial, designing and production team. Their endless efforts to recruit the best for this project, has resulted in the accomplishment of this book. They are a veteran in the field of academics and their pool of knowledge is as vast as their experience in printing. Their expertise and guidance has proved useful at every step. Their uncompromising quality standards have made this book an exceptional effort. Their encouragement from time to time has been an inspiration for everyone.

The publisher and the editorial board hope that this book will prove to be a valuable piece of knowledge for researchers, students, practitioners and scholars across the globe.

List of Contributors

Xia Wang, Ruijuan Guan, Xiaomei Zhao and Danian Zhu
Department of Physiology and Pathophysiology, School of Basic Medical Sciences, Fudan University, Shanghai, China

Nana Song
Division of Nephrology, Zhongshan Hospital, Fudan University, Shanghai, China

Linlin Shen
Department of Physiology and Pathophysiology, School of Basic Medical Sciences, Fudan University, Shanghai, China
Shanghai Key Laboratory of Medical Imaging Computing and Computer-Assisted Intervention, Fudan University, Shanghai, China

Ioan Opris, Dawn M. G. Johnson, Francisco J. Sanchez, Luz M. Villamil, Songtao Xie, Cecelia R. Lee-Hauser, Stephano Chang and Brian R. Noga
The Miami Project to Cure Paralysis, Department of Neurological Surgery, University of Miami Miller School of Medicine, Miami, FL, United States

Xiaohong Dai and Larry M. Jordan
Department of Physiology, Spinal Cord Research Centre, University of Manitoba, Winnipeg, MB, Canada

Tian-jian Luo, Jitu Lv, Fei Chao and Changle Zhou
Fujian Provincal Key Lab of Brain-Inspired Computing, Department of Cognitive Science, School of Informatics, Xiamen University, Xiamen, China

Chang-Wei Wei, Ting Luo, Shan-Shan Zou and An-Shi Wu
Department of Anesthesiology, Beijing Chao-Yang Hospital, Capital Medical University, Beijing, China

Ashim Maharjan
Department of Anatomy, School of Biomedical Sciences, University of Otago, Dunedin, New Zealand

Mei Peng
Department of Food Science, University of Otago, Dunedin, New Zealand

Yusuf O. Cakmak
Department of Anatomy, School of Biomedical Sciences, University of Otago, Dunedin, New Zealand
Brain Health Research Centre, Division of Sciences, University of Otago, Dunedin, New Zealand
Medical Technologies Centre of Research Excellence, Auckland, New Zealand

Sheng Li and Gerard E. Francisco
Department of Physical Medicine and Rehabilitation, University of Texas Health Science Center, Houston, TX, United States
TIRR Memorial Hermann Research Center, TIRR Memorial Hermann, Houston, TX, United States

Ping Zhou
Department of Physical Medicine and Rehabilitation, University of Texas Health Science Center, Houston, TX, United States
TIRR Memorial Hermann Research Center, TIRR Memorial Hermann, Houston, TX, United States
Guangdong Work Injury Rehabilitation Center, Guangzhou, China

Jacob G. McPherson
Department of Biomedical Engineering, Florida International University, Miami, FL, United States
Department of Physical Therapy and Human Movement Sciences, Northwestern University Feinberg School of Medicine, Chicago, IL, United States

Laura M. McPherson
Department of Biomedical Engineering, Florida International University, Miami, FL, United States
Department of Physical Therapy and Human Movement Sciences, Northwestern University Feinberg School of Medicine, Chicago, IL, United States
Department of Physical Therapy, Florida International University, Miami, FL, United States

Christopher K. Thompson
Department of Physical Therapy, Temple University, Philadelphia, PA, United States
Department of Physiology, Northwestern University Feinberg School of Medicine, Chicago, IL, United States

Michael D. Ellis
Department of Physical Therapy and Human Movement Sciences, Northwestern University Feinberg School of Medicine, Chicago, IL, United States

Charles J. Heckman
Department of Physical Therapy and Human Movement Sciences, Northwestern University Feinberg School of Medicine, Chicago, IL, United States
Department of Physiology, Northwestern University Feinberg School of Medicine, Chicago, IL, United States

Julius P. A. Dewald
Department of Physical Therapy and Human Movement Sciences, Northwestern University Feinberg School of Medicine, Chicago, IL, United States
Department of Biomedical Engineering, Northwestern University, Evanston, IL, United States

Samantha Meneely, Mai-Lynne Dinkins, Miki Kassai and Stefan Clemens
Department of Physiology, Brody School of Medicine, East Carolina University, Greenville, NC, United States

Shangru Lyu and Yuning Liu
Department of Neurology, College of Medicine, University of Florida, Gainesville, FL, United States

Chien-Te Lin
Department of Physiology, Brody School of Medicine, East Carolina University, Greenville, NC, United States
East Carolina Diabetes and Obesity Institute, Brody School of Medicine, East Carolina University, Greenville, NC, United States

Kori Brewer
Department of Emergency Medicine, Brody School of Medicine, East Carolina University, Greenville, NC, United States

Yuqing Li
Department of Neurology, College of Medicine, University of Florida, Gainesville, FL, United States
Wuxi Medical School, Jiangnan University, Wuxi, China

Liang Li, Qingguang Qin, Yutian Yu, Xiang Cui, Peijing Rong and Bing Zhu
Institute of Acupuncture and Moxibustion, China Academy of Chinese Medical Sciences, Beijing, China

Lingling Yu
Department of Neurology, Tongji Hospital, Tongji Medical College, Huazhong University of Science and Technology, Wuhan, China
Institute of Acupuncture and Moxibustion, China Academy of Chinese Medical Sciences, Beijing, China

Haifang Li, Rong Yao, Xiaoluan Xia, Guimei Yin, Hongxia Deng and Pengfei Yang
College of Information and Computer, Taiyuan University of Technology, Taiyuan, China

Harumi Hotta, Harue Suzuki, Kaori Iimura and Nobuhiro Watanabe
Department of Autonomic Neuroscience, Tokyo Metropolitan Institute of Gerontology, Tokyo, Japan

Liping Jiang, Xuan Zhou, Hongyu Yang, Yanlei Xin, Jijiang Wang and Jin Wang
Department of Physiology and Pathophysiology, School of Basic Medical Sciences, Fudan University, Shanghai, China

Shulan Ma
Training Center of Medical Experiments, School of Basic Medical Sciences, Fudan University, Shanghai, China

German G. Miroshnichenko, Saara M. Rissanen and Pasi A. Karjalainen
Biosignal Analysis and Medical Imaging Group, Department of Applied Physics, Faculty of Science and Forestry, University of Eastern Finland, Kuopio, Finland

Alexander Yu Meigal
Laboratory for Novel Methods in Physiology, Institute of High-Tech Biomedical Solutions, Petrozavodsk State University, Petrozavodsk, Russia

Irina V. Saenko
Laboratory of Gravitational Physiology of Sensorimotor System, Department of Sensorimotor Physiology and Countermeasure, Institute of BioMedical Problems, Russian Academy of Sciences, Moscow, Russia

Liudmila I. Gerasimova-Meigal
Department of Human and Animal Physiology, Physiopathology, Histology, Petrozavodsk State University, Petrozavodsk, Russia

Liudmila A. Chernikova
Department of Neurorehabilitation and Physiotherapy, Research Center of Neurology, Russian Academy of Medical Sciences, Moscow, Russia

Natalia S. Subbotina
Department of Neurology, Psychiatry, and Microbiology, Petrozavodsk State University, Petrozavodsk, Russia

Robert M. Brownstone and Jeremy W. Chopek
Sobell Department of Motor Neuroscience and Movement Disorders, Institute of Neurology, University College London, London, United Kingdom

Kathrin Koblinger, Céline Jean-Xavier, Sandeep Sharma, Leanne Young, Shane E. A. Eaton and Charlie Hong Ting Kwok
Hotchkiss Brain Institute, University of Calgary, Calgary, AB, Canada
Department of Comparative Biology and Experimental Medicine, University of Calgary, Calgary, AB, Canada

Tamás Füzesi and Jaideep Singh Bains
Hotchkiss Brain Institute, University of Calgary, Calgary, AB, Canada Department of Physiology and Pharmacology, University of Calgary, Calgary, AB, Canada

Patrick J. Whelan
Hotchkiss Brain Institute, University of Calgary, Calgary, AB, Canada
Department of Comparative Biology and Experimental Medicine, University of Calgary, Calgary, AB, Canada
Department of Physiology and Pharmacology, University of Calgary, Calgary, AB, Canada

Simon N. Jacob and Hendrikje Nienborg
Department of Neurosurgery, Klinikum Rechts der Isar, Technical University of Munich, Munich, Germany
Werner Reichardt Centre for Integrative Neuroscience, University of Tübingen, Tübingen, Germany

Hojeong Kim
Division of Biotechnology, DGIST, Daegu, South Korea

Youngchang Ju
Department of Brain and Cognitive Sciences, DGIST, Daegu, South Korea

Index

A

Acid-sensing Ion Channels, 1-2, 9-10

Action Observation, 36-37, 48-50

Alzheimer's Disease, 51, 55, 57-60, 134-135, 173

Amiloride, 1-2

Analgesia, 101, 113-114, 117, 119-121, 198

Analysis Of Variance, 62, 67, 139, 151, 189

Artificial Cerebrospinal Fluid, 1, 6, 148, 188

B

Bupivacaine, 1-2, 6

C

Cerebellum, 70-71, 78, 160, 166, 176, 185

Cerebrospinal Fluid, 1-2, 6, 148, 188

Chemoreception, 1-2, 4-5, 9-10, 29

Choline Acetyltransferase, 11, 13, 19, 22, 33, 177, 213

Colorectal Distension, 113-114

Correlation Dimension, 159, 165-168

Cuneiform, 11-12, 14, 26, 33-35, 180

D

Diencephalon, 176, 186-187, 196-197

Dopamine Transporter, 191, 200, 213

Dopaminergic Cells, 58, 187, 208

Dry Immersion, 159-162, 164-173

E

Electroacupuncture, 63, 72-75, 113-114, 116, 120-121, 158

Electroencephalography, 36-37, 123

Electrostimulation, 62-63, 69-71, 74

F

Fictive Locomotion, 11, 13, 16, 18, 20, 22-25, 29, 33-34, 108, 179, 184, 196

Fluorescence In Situ Hybridization, 148, 150

G

Gene Expression, 32, 51-53, 57-60, 149, 151, 158

Glutamatergic Neurons, 26-27, 30, 32, 148-149, 152-157, 176, 180

H

Homeostasis, 2, 4, 55, 58, 60, 100, 110

Human Mirror Neuron System, 36, 49

Huntington's Disease, 51, 56-59

Hypertension, 148-149, 151-152, 155-158, 161

I

Immunofluorescence, 3, 5

Intermediolateral Column, 148-150

L

Labeled Magnitude Scale, 62-63, 65, 67, 69, 73

Lateral Paragigantocellular Nucleus, 1, 3, 176-177

Locus Coeruleus, 2, 31-33, 71-72, 74, 183, 204, 212-216

M

Mauthner Cells, 177-178, 181

Mean Arterial Blood Pressure, 29, 148, 155

Mechanoreceptors, 137, 141, 143, 145-147

Median Nerve Stimulation, 62, 64, 67, 74

Mesencephalic Locomotor Region, 11-12, 26, 31-35, 78, 176, 179, 183-186, 196

Microcircuits, 12, 176, 181-182

Microgravity, 159-162, 171-172, 174-175

Microinjection, 1-4, 6-9, 148-150, 152-156, 185

Microstimulation, 37, 179, 184, 218-219, 221, 231-233, 235

Monoamines, 28, 91-93, 95-97, 187, 191, 196, 198, 201, 212-213, 215, 219, 232

Morphine, 99-102, 104, 106, 109-110, 112

Motoneurons, 9, 21, 26, 33, 35, 83-85, 92-99, 111, 168, 176-180, 182-185, 187, 198, 218-220, 226, 232-235

Motor Imagery, 36-37, 49-50, 79, 135

Muscle Hypertonicity, 160, 166

Muscle Tone, 35, 79, 97-98, 159-161, 166, 172, 174-175, 178, 180, 184-185

Mutual Information, 159, 165-167, 169, 171, 173-174

N

Near-infrared Spectroscopy, 62-65, 67, 69, 73

Neurodegenerative Diseases, 51-52, 55-60, 123

Neuronal Excitability, 1-2, 7, 53, 198, 211

O

Odor Identification Test, 65, 67

Open Reading Frame, 51-52

Orbitofrontal Cortex, 62-63, 65, 75, 208

P

Parkinson's Disease, 12, 34, 48, 50-51, 55, 57-61, 123, 159-161, 164, 172-175, 182

Pedunculopontine Nucleus, 11, 32-34, 176, 180

Phrenic Nerve Discharge, 1-3, 6

R

Raphe Nucleus, 71, 199, 202-203
Reactive Oxygen Species, 148-149, 154, 157-158
Recurrence Quantification Analysis, 161, 165
Restless Legs Syndrome, 99-100, 110-112, 187, 198-199
Reticular Formation, 11-12, 14, 24, 26-29, 32-35, 78, 120, 176-177, 181, 183-186, 196
Reticulospinal Neurons, 31-32, 34-35, 176-185
Rostral Ventrolateral Medulla, 12, 24, 148-149, 153, 157-158
Ruthenium Red, 1-2, 7

S

Sample Entropy, 159, 165-166, 168, 172, 174
Senile Plaques, 55
Sleep Atonia, 176, 180-181
Somatosensory Cortex, 69, 145, 202-206, 209, 211-214
Spinal Cord Injury, 12, 93, 96, 182, 199, 219, 234-235
Stretch Reflex, 79, 82, 84-85, 92, 95-98, 160, 166
Subnucleus Reticularis Dorsalis, 113, 120
Substantia Nigra, 27, 187, 190-191, 208, 215
Support Vector Machine, 41, 126
Surface Electromyogram, 159, 162, 164-172, 174
Synaptic Plasticity, 53-54, 57, 59
Synchronization, 48-49, 122-131, 133-136, 161, 167-168, 171, 173-174
Systolic Blood Pressure, 139, 148-149, 151-152

T

Tonic Vibration Reflexes, 84-85, 89, 96
Tyrosine Hydroxylase, 33, 186, 199-200, 208, 214, 216

V

Vascular Parkinsonism, 159, 161, 164, 172
Ventral Tegmental Area, 11-12, 17, 74, 187, 190-191, 208
Ventrolateral Medulla, 1-2, 4, 10-12, 24, 148-150, 153, 157-158
Vestibular Nuclei, 11, 18, 29, 32
Visceral Pain, 113, 117, 119-120

W

Western Blot Analyses, 99-100
Working Memory, 122-123, 127-128, 135-136, 216

www.ingramcontent.com/pod-product-compliance
Lightning Source LLC
LaVergne TN
LVHW082142200926
848484LV00008B/2097